Fundamentals
of
CHIROPRACTIC

Fundamentals

of

CHIROPRACTIC

Edited by

DANIEL REDWOOD, DC
Private Practice
Virginia Beach, Virginia

CARL S. CLEVELAND III, DC
President, Cleveland Chiropractic College
Kansas City, Missouri and Los Angeles, California

Editorial advisor

MARC MICOZZI, MD, PHD
Director of the Policy Institute for Integrative Medicine
Thomas Jefferson University Hospital

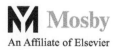
Mosby
An Affiliate of Elsevier

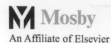

An Affiliate of Elsevier

11830 Westline Industrial Drive
St. Louis, Missouri 63146

ISBN-13: 978-0-323-01812-8
ISBN-10: 0-323-01812-2

Publishing Director: Linda Duncan
Managing Editor: Christie Hart
Publishing Services Manager: Linda McKinley
Senior Project Manager: Julie Eddy
Editorial Assistant: Jennifer Clark
Designer: Amy Buxton
Cover Designer: Studio Montage

CONTRIBUTORS

Joel Alcantara, BsC, DC
Research director, International Chiropractic
  Pediatric Association
Media, Pennsylvania
Private practice
San Jose, California

Claudia A. Anrig, DC
Private practice
Fresno, California
Postgraduate faculty, Life Chiropractic
  College West
Hayward, California
Postgraduate faculty, Life Chiropractic College
Marietta, Georgia
Postgraduate faculty, Cleveland Chiropractic
  College
Kansas City, Missouri
Los Angeles, California
Postgraduate faculty, Parker Chiropractic College
Dallas, Texas
Postgraduate faculty, Northwestern Health
  Sciences University
Bloomington, Minnesota

Geoffrey Bove, DC, PhD
Assistant professor, Beth Israel Deaconess
  Medical Center and Harvard Medical School,
  Department of Anesthesia and Critical Care
Boston, Massachusetts

Carol Claus, MA, DC, FICPA
Chair, Chiropractic Sciences Department,
  Cleveland Chiropractic College
Los Angeles, California

Ashley Cleveland, MA, DC
Associate dean and associate professor,
  Cleveland Chiropractic College
Kansas City, Missouri

Carl S. Cleveland III, DC
President, Cleveland Chiropractic College
Kansas City, Missouri
Los Angeles, California

Gerard W. Clum, DC
President, Life Chiropractic College West
Hayward, California

Robert Cooperstein, MA, DC
Director of technique and research, Palmer
  College of Chiropractic West
San Jose, California

Patrick Coughlin, PhD
Professor, Department of Anatomy
Coordinator, Distance and Distributed Learning
  Systems
Philadelphia College of Osteopathic Medicine
Philadelphia, Pennsylvania

Alan Dumoff, JD, MSW
Attorney-at-law, private practice
President, LifeTree Consulting
Rockville, Maryland

Leonard John Faye, DC, FCCSS (Canada)
  Honorary affiliated
Postgraduate faculty, Cleveland Chiropractic
  College, Kansas City, Missouri and Los
  Angeles, California
Private practice,
Los Angeles, California

David P. Gilkey, DC, PhD, DACBO,
DACBOH, FICC
Assistant professor and director of
undergraduate education, The Department
  of Environmental and Radiological Health
  Sciences
Colorado State University
Fort Collins, Colorado

Gary Guebert, DC, DABCR
Associate professor of radiology, Logan College
  of Chiropractic
Maryland Heights, Missouri

Warren Hammer, DC, MS, DABCO
Postgraduate faculty, National University
of Health Sciences
Postgraduate faculty, Northwestern Health
Sciences University
Postgraduate faculty, Cleveland Chiropractic
College, Kansas City, Missouri and Los
Angeles, California
Private Practice
Norwalk, Connecticut

Jennifer Jamison, MBBCh, PhD, EdD
Professor of diagnostic sciences, Department of
Complementary Medicine, RMIT University,
Melbourne, Australia

Lisa Zaynab Killinger, DC
Assistant professor of research and diagnosis,
Palmer College of Chiropractic
Davenport, Iowa

William J. Lauretti, DC
Private practice
Bethesda, Maryland

Craig Liebenson, DC
Private practice
Postgraduate faculty, Southern California
University of Health Sciences
Postgraduate faculty, Murdoch University
Postgraduate faculty, Anglo-European College
of Chiropractic
Los Angeles, California

Charles S. Masarsky, DC
Private practice
Vienna, Virginia
Co-director, Neurological Fitness
Postgraduate faculty, Cleveland Chiropractic
College
Kansas City, Missouri and Los Angeles,
California

Jerome F. McAndrews, DC
Board of directors, NCMIC Insurance Company
National spokesperson, American Chiropractic
Association
Past president, Palmer College of Chiropractic
Claremore, Oklahoma

William Meeker, DC, MPH
Vice president for research, Palmer
Chiropractic University Foundation
Director, Palmer Center for Chiropractic
Research
National Advisory Council, National
Institutes of Health, National Center
for Complementary and Alternative Medicine
Davenport, Iowa

Joseph Morley, DC, PhD, PG Cert (Oxford)
Youngstown, Ohio

Marino Passero, DC
Senior vice president, NCMIC Insurance
Company
New Canaan, Connecticut

Stephen M. Perle, MS, DC
Associate professor of clinical sciences, College
of Chiropractic
Adjunct professor of mechanical engineering,
School of Engineering, University of
Bridgeport
Bridgeport, Connecticut

Reed Phillips, DC, PhD
President, Southern California University of
Health Sciences
Whittier, California

Gregory Plaugher, DC
Director of research, Life Chiropractic College
West
Director of research, Gonstead Clinical Studies
Society
Hayward, Calfornia

Daniel Redwood, DC
Private practice
Virginia Beach, Virginia

Anthony L. Rosner, PhD, LL.D. (Honorary)
Director of research and education,
Foundation for Chiropractic Education
and Research
Brookline, Massachusetts

John G. Scaringe, DC, DACBSP
Dean of Clinical Education, Chief of Staff,
    Southern California University of Health
    Sciences
Whittier, California

Clayton Skaggs, DC
Research associate, Logan College of
    Chiropractic
Adjunct faculty, Washington University School
    of Medicine
Private practice
St. Louis, Missouri

Louis Sportelli, DC
President, NCMIC Insurance Company
Former chairman of the board,
American Chiropractic Association
Palmerton, Pennsylvania

Rand Swenson, DC, MD, PhD
Associate professor of medicine, neurology and
    anatomy, Dartmouth Medical School
Hanover, New Hampshire

Marion Todres-Masarsky, DC
Private practice
Co-director, Neurological Fitness
Vienna, Virginia

Howard Vernon DC, FCCS, PhD (candidate)
Director, Center for Studies of the Cervical
    Spine, Canadian Memorial Chiropractic
    College
Toronto, Ontario, Canada

Glenda C. Wiese, MA
Special collections librarian and archivist,
    David D. Palmer Health Sciences Library,
    Palmer College of Chiropractic
Davenport, Iowa

John C. Willis, MA, DC
Editor, *Chiropractic History, The Archives and
    Journal of the Association for the History of
    Chiropractic*
Private practice
Richlands, Virginia

Terry Yochum, DC, DACBR, FICC, Fellow,
    ACCR
Director, Rocky Mountain Chiropractic
    Radiological Center
Denver, Colorado
Adjunct professor of radiology, Southern
    California University of Health Sciences
Los Angeles, California
Instructor, skeletal radiology, University of
    Colorado School of Medicine
Denver, Colorado

ABOUT THE AUTHORS

DANIEL REDWOOD

Daniel Redwood serves on the editorial board of the *Journal of the American Chiropractic Association* and is associate editor of *The Journal of Alternative and Complementary Medicine*. He has lectured on chiropractic at the National Institutes of Health and at the Medical College of Virginia. He has been widely published in both professional and lay publications. Churchill Livingstone published his text, *Contemporary Chiropractic,* in 1997.

A 1979 graduate of Palmer College of Chiropractic, where he was student council president, Dr. Redwood is a former vice president and legislative committee chair for the chiropractic state association in the District of Columbia. He has a private practice in Virginia Beach, Virginia.

CARL S. CLEVELAND III

Carl S. Cleveland III is president of the Cleveland Chiropractic College with campuses in Kansas City and Los Angeles. He has served as president of both the Association of Chiropractic Colleges (ACC) and the Council on Chiropractic Education. Dr. Cleveland has been the National Spokesperson for the Alliance for Chiropractic Progress of the American Chiropractic Association (ACA), International Chiropractors Association (ICA), and ACC, and has served as chair of the Philosophy Council of the California Chiropractic Association. He presently chairs the Unity Committee of the National Chiropractic Leadership Forum and is a board member of the Association for the History of Chiropractic, the Chiropractic Centennial Foundation, and the New Zealand College of Chiropractic. Dr. Cleveland has taught in the classroom for over 3 decades and is internationally known as a chiropractic lecturer, author, and educator. He is a fourth-generation doctor of chiropractic.

FOREWORD

Fundamentals of Chiropractic is a high-quality textbook that we strongly recommend to chiropractors, chiropractic students, and educators, as well as members of other health care professions. It fills a need in chiropractic education for a comprehensive, entry-level textbook designed to introduce readers to the key principles and practices of the profession. We have great respect for this text—its conception, its contributors, and its editors.

Dr. Daniel Redwood is a skilled organizer, author, and editor with outstanding dedication to his chosen profession. Through recent contributions to a variety of scholarly and general readership publications, he has emerged as one of the foremost writers on chiropractic and integrative health care, effectively translating and interpreting chiropractic to members of other health care professions and to the general public. Among chiropractors in full-time private practice, he is arguably the most prolific writer in the profession.

Dr. Carl Cleveland III is a fourth-generation chiropractor and a third-generation chiropractic college president, serving in this role for the Cleveland Chiropractic College with campuses in Kansas City and Los Angeles. In a profession with a broad diversity of opinion, Dr. Cleveland has always served as a unifying force and is highly respected across the chiropractic spectrum. Aside from his leadership at Cleveland College, his tireless efforts on behalf of the profession have included extensive work for national and state chiropractic associations, countless speaking engagements, and the authorship of numerous journal articles and book chapters. He has served as president of both the Association of Chiropractic Colleges and the Council on Chiropractic Education and has taught in the classroom for over 3 decades, playing a central role in the remarkable educational advances of the past generation.

The combined breadth of skills and experience represented by Drs. Redwood and Cleveland has resulted in an exceptional textbook that intro-

duces the reader to the fundamentals of the science, philosophy, and art of chiropractic. Terms are carefully defined in the text and in the extensive glossary. Concepts are explained, enabling first- and second-year students to grasp them readily. Facts on anatomy and physiology, palpation and technique, patient care, research, safety, legal and ethical issues, and much more are presented in a logical progression that is extremely user-friendly for both faculty and students. *Fundamentals of Chiropractic* will become a standard entry-level text for the chiropractic profession.

Chiropractic started a century ago as an alternative to the medical mainstream with a focus on the relationship of the spine and nervous system to overall function and health. The chiropractic profession is now in the process of becoming mainstream in the early twenty-first century, as the social movement behind popular medicine recognizes health care alternatives in a renewed and positive light. Many of the chapters in this text illustrate the basic and clinical science research that is fundamental to understanding the effectiveness of chiropractic procedures. Such research has been a primary driving force behind the recent enhanced interprofessional cooperation between doctors of chiropractic and medical physicians.

It is no coincidence that chiropractic's most impressive strides toward acceptance and integration have occurred between 1970 and the present—the era of the profession's great leap forward in the quality of its education and research. Starting around 1970, leaders in the profession embarked on an intensive project of educational and professional advancement. Numerous achievements are the result: the expansion of chiropractic licensure that includes all of North America and many other nations; the governmental recognition of the Council on Chiropractic Education; the development of chiropractic programs in universities in several nations; the inclusion of chiropractic in Medicare; the first conference on spinal manipulation offered by the National Institutes of Health; and the acknowledgment of spinal manipulation by the Agency for Health Care Policy and Research as one of the most effective procedures in the management low back pain.

Landmark events since the mid-1990s have included the initiation of an annual national Research Agenda Conference, the Chiropractic Demonstration Grants Program at the U.S. Health Resources and Services Administration, the first research funding of chiropractic institutions by the National Institutes of Health's National Center for Complementary and Alternative Medicine, inclusion of chiropractic in U.S. Department of Defense and Veterans Administration health care, and the demonstration project under which chiropractic students are eligible for student loan reimbursement through the National Health Services Corps program for graduates committing to practice in underserved areas of the United States. The remarkable achievements of this era continue today.

As it is for all professions, ever-increasing quality of its educational institutions is crucial to the further development of chiropractic. Both in the colleges and in the profession at large, a heightened understanding and appreciation of the scientific process and endorsement of evidence-based practice must be encouraged, with doctors at all stages of their careers committed to changing and updating their practices when newly emerging evidence clearly calls for such changes. Aside from its value as a teaching tool in chiropractic colleges worldwide, one of the most important uses of *Fundamentals of Chiropractic* will be as a source of informed guidance—a software update as it were—for practicing chiropractors.

A new health care paradigm is on the horizon that can include the core concepts of chiropractic—the link between structure and function, the effectiveness of manual adjustment/manipulation, and the crucial mediating role of the nervous system. This new perspective may allow consideration of various nonallopathic methods as part of a more inclusive and expansive model of health care that accommodates rather than subsumes these alternatives. Chiropractic is on the cusp of this significant transition in the new millennium.

For example, the high cost of medical liability insurance has reached a crisis point in many places. Low back pain is the most common cause of disability in American workers. Those practitioners performing surgery on the spine carry liability insurance that, in some cases, costs hundreds of thousands of dollars per year, requiring hundreds of such procedures to be performed annually simply to offset the cost of this insurance. Public policy discussion has focused on how we pay for health care rather than how it is practiced. The high costs and risks of health care, however, reside not only in providing new drugs, technologies, and procedures through scientific innovation, but also in the management of the known and accepted side effects of these powerful protocols.

Although health care technology has advanced, renewed interest in methods once known as alternative or complementary has led to increasing research, establishing their safety and effectiveness. Along these lines, it is useful to arrange various practices according to their degree of invasiveness, because this characteristic is strongly associated with both risks and costs. From least invasive to most invasive, these practices would be meditation, talk therapies, hands-on healing, massage, adjustment/manipulation, insertion, ingestion, injection, and surgery (see Appendix II).

To illustrate how the level of invasiveness applies in the real world, consider the aforementioned case of back surgery where inherent risks have led to the unacceptably high cost of insurance. It is possible that inappropriate procedures may be performed simply to enable the practitioner to offer the service, or such procedures may be ultimately priced out of the market. By comparison, proven alternatives for the treatment of back pain are available at lower cost with lower risk. For example, spinal adjustment/manipulation provided by chiropractors and certain other professionals is effective at reducing pain and restoring function in many people with low back pain. In addition, liability insurance for chiropractors in the United States averages only $1500 annually. Procedures that work effectively at lower risk and with lower cost are not complementary or alternative; rather, they are simply good health care that make good public policy.

William Meeker, DC, MPH
Vice President of Research at
Palmer College of Chiropractic
Principal Investigator at the Consortial
Center for Chiropractic Research

Marc Micozzi, MD, PhD
Director of the Policy Institute
for Integrative Medicine
Thomas Jefferson University Hospital
Editor, *Medical Guides to Complementary*
& Alternative Medicine
Editor of the quarterly review journal,
Seminars in Integrative Medicine

PREFACE

Fundamentals of Chiropractic meets a long-standing need in chiropractic education for a wide-ranging, introductory textbook constructed in a format fully accessible to first- and second-year students; one that presents the fundamental paradigm of chiropractic with its history, its principles and practices, and its science and research; and one with an overview of the most significant contemporary issues in the profession.

Fundamentals of Chiropractic is designed to serve as an effective core textbook that introduces the beginning chiropractic student or interested health science practitioner to the central elements of chiropractic practice and its emerging role as part of the mainstream health delivery system. Faculty will find multiple applications for *Fundamentals of Chiropractic* as a required text for class instruction in the introductory chiropractic principles and practices, an effective resource for national and state examination review, and a valuable compendium for introducing other health care practitioners to the concepts of chiropractic.

In this era of accelerating change, grounding a book in its historical context is essential. The opening section of *Fundamentals of Chiropractic*, "History, Philosophy, and Sociology," has three chapters that trace the origins and development of chiropractic. In "Forerunners of the Chiropractic Adjustment," John Willis, editor of the journal *Chiropractic History*, surveys and examines forms of manual manipulation before Daniel David Palmer's discovery of chiropractic. This chapter is followed by "The Chiropractic Paradigm," a unique collaboration by Ashley Cleveland, associate dean of instruction for Cleveland Chiropractic College, Kansas City campus, the profession's first fifth-generation chiropractor, and two chiropractic college presidents, Reed Phillips of Southern California University of Health Sciences and Gerard Clum of Life Chiropractic College West. These authors, representing diverse perspectives, have jointly crafted an introduction to the science, art, and philosophy of chiropractic that will be of value to all who wish to understand chiropractic. In the third chapter in this section, "Major Themes in Chiropractic History," Glenda Wiese, special collections librarian and archivist at the David D. Palmer Health Sciences Library and co-author of *Chiropractic: An Illustrated History,* describes the profession's landmark historical events and the individuals and groups that helped shape them.

The "Anatomy, Biomechanics, and Physiology" section is made up of six chapters that provide students with the means to begin the daunting task of understanding the basic functions of the human body, with special emphasis on chiropractic applications. Although a general text such as this cannot replace the great classics such as *Gray's Anatomy* or *Guyton's Physiology,* it does provide a focused and well-contextualized introduction for entry-level students, a concentrated review for national board examinations in these fundamental subjects, and a useful "back to basics" resource for the practicing doctor of chiropractic. The "Spinal Anatomy" and "Spinal Neurology" chapters written by Patrick Coughlin, professor of anatomy at the Philadelphia College of Osteopathic Medicine, offer a clear, well-organized presentation of this core chiropractic material with helpful explanations of its clinical relevance. Space did not allow us to include detailed information on spine-related musculature and fascial anatomy. For these topics, we refer readers to the many available standard texts.

Joseph Morley's chapter "Basic Biomechanics" expands on the foundations presented in the anatomy and neurology chapters, introducing the basic terms and concepts of this central element of the chiropractor's specialty. Carl Cleveland's chapter, "Vertebral Subluxation" follows and describes the development of this essential chiropractic construct through the profession's history, up to and including contemporary models of the vertebral subluxation complex. Cleveland's "Neurobiologic Relations and Chiropractic Applications" offers a wide-ranging presentation of the chiropractic theories and research that are opening new vistas of understanding and possibilities for interdisciplinary study at the dawn of the twenty-first century. The final chapter in this section, Geoffrey Bove and Rand Swenson's "Nociceptors, Pain, and Chiropractic," provides a detailed introduction to the neurophysiology of pain, with particular emphasis on the International Association for the Study of Pain definitions and nociceptive and neuroinflammatory processes. Dr. Bove is assistant professor in anesthesia and critical care at Harvard Medical School, and Dr. Swenson is associate professor of anatomy and medicine (neurology) at Dartmouth Medical School.

Two chapters make up the "Spinal Analysis and Diagnostic Procedures" section. In "Palpation: The Art of Manual Assessment," John Scaringe, dean of clinical education and chief of staff at the Southern California University of Health Sciences, and Leonard John Faye, who serves on the postgraduate faculty at Cleveland Chiropractic College, describe the manual examination procedures central to chiropractic practice. Particular emphasis is given to the role of palpation in evaluating the mechanics of spinal and extraspinal joints. In "Introduction to Diagnostic Imaging," chiropractic radiologists Gary Guebert, assistant professor of radiology at Logan College of Chiropractic, and Terry Yochum, director of the Rocky Mountain Chiropractic Radiological Center, and instructor in skeletal radiology at University of Colorado School of Medicine, survey the uses of the various imaging techniques commonly in use today. We believe it is important to note that the chiropractor's diagnostic process involves more than palpation and diagnostic imaging. Orthopedic and neurologic testing and laboratory procedures are essential components of chiropractic training and practice. For discussions on these topics, we refer the reader to the many available standard texts.

"Chiropractic Care" is the largest section in *Fundamentals of Chiropractic* with 10 chapters whose primary goal is to offer the reader a solid introduction to the key areas of focus in the typical chiropractic practice. John Scaringe, serving as co-author with innovative technique author and instructor Robert Cooperstein, director of

technique and research at Palmer College of Chiropractic West, begin this section with a discussion on the cornerstones of chiropractic the manual adjustment and related hands-on procedures. "Manual Soft Tissue Procedures" follows, in which Warren Hammer, who serves on the postgraduate faculties of the National University of Health Sciences, Northwestern Health Sciences University, and Cleveland Chiropractic College, provides both the rationale for soft tissue work and a well-guided tour through many of the most widely used contemporary methods. Next, in "Reactivation and Rehabilitation," Craig Liebenson, who serves on the Murdoch University, Anglo-European College of Chiropractic, and Southern California University of Health Sciences postgraduate faculties, and Clayton Skaggs, an adjunct faculty member at the Washington University School of Medicine and Southern California University of Health Sciences, describe contemporary methods of rehabilitation through which patients become active participants in their own recovery.

The care of children and older adults has been part of chiropractic practice since the profession's inception. The "Pediatrics" chapter by Joel Alcantara, Gregory Plaugher, and Claudia Anrig describes the biomechanical features unique to the pediatric spine. This chapter provides the rationale and foundation for their discussion of pediatric adjusting. Alcantara is research director of the International Chiropractic Pediatric Association, Plaugher serves as director of Research at Life Chiropractic College West, and Anrig is on the postgraduate faculties of the following chiropractic colleges: Life, Life West, Cleveland, Parker, and Northwestern. This chapter is followed by "Caring for the Aging Patient" by Lisa Zaynab Killinger, assistant professor of diagnosis at Palmer College of Chiropractic, which addresses the special needs of older patients. Her chapter emphasizes the appropriate choice of case management methods and counseling on age-related changes. Killinger and Carol Claus, associate professor and chair of the Los Angeles campus of the Chiropractic Sciences department at the Cleveland Chiropractic College, collaborated on "Adjusting the Aging Patient," which describes the ways chiropractors can adapt adjustive techniques to accommodate the degenerative and osteoporotic changes that are more common with increased age, in the interest of enhanced patient comfort and safety.

"Occupational Health," by David Gilkey, a past president of the American Chiropractic Association's Council on Occupational Health, and currently assistant professor and director of undergraduate education, The Department of Environmental and Radiological Health Sciences, Colorado State University, offers a thorough discussion of occupational health. This chapter demonstrates that the traditional chiropractic emphasis on the treatment of work-related injuries has been expanded to include prevention, ergonomic analysis, and interdisciplinary case management. In "Sports Chiropractic," Stephen Perle, associate professor of clinical sciences at the University of Bridgeport—College of Chiropractic, discusses the important roles chiropractors play in helping athletes to perform safely and to recover from injuries. In "Wellness: A Lifestyle," Jennifer Jamison, professor of diagnostic sciences at RMIT University in Australia and author of *Maintaining Health in Primary Care,* explains the crucial roles of diet, exercise, and stress management in chiropractic practice. Louis Sportelli, president of the National Chiropractic Mutual Insurance Company, former chairperson of the board of the American Chiropractic Association, and author of *Introduction to Chiropractic,* demonstrates in "A Patient's Introduction to Chiropractic" that explaining chiropractic principles and practices to patients and potential patients is a crucial skill for students to master. This chapter offers the reader a basic outline for introducing the patient to chiropractic's role in health care and to the importance of proper spinal health.

Because research is a linchpin of professional growth and development, we have devoted four extensive chapters to this topic, providing up-to-date summaries of the relevant literature, along with interpretations of its significance. For the entry-level student, a solid, step-by-step introduction to the terminology and to the purposes and types of research is an absolute necessity.

"Research Essentials" by Daniel Redwood and William Meeker, vice president for Research of the Palmer Chiropractic University and director of research at the Palmer Center for Chiropractic Research, offers this introduction. "Musculoskeletal Disorders Research" by Anthony Rosner, director of research and education for the Foundation for Chiropractic Education and Research, demonstrates the dramatic progress in chiropractic research over the past generation. Howard Vernon's chapter on headaches follows, which thoroughly discusses research on headaches, as well as providing a valuable introduction to differential diagnosis and case management options. Chiropractic research on visceral conditions is currently at an earlier stage of development than research on musculoskeletal disorders, but as Charles Masarsky and Marion Todres-Masarsky, postgraduate faculty members at Cleveland Chiropractic College and authors of *Somatovisceral Aspects of Chiropractic: An Evidence-Based Approach*, discuss in "Somatovisceral Research," a promising basis exists for what may prove a fertile area for chiropractic research in the coming years.

The closing section, "Contemporary Issues in Chiropractic Practice," is intended to stimulate thought and discussion. William Lauretti's "The Comparative Safety of Chiropractic," is a solidly documented summary of critical safety issues by one of the profession's leading authorities on this subject, with special emphasis on cerebrovascular accidents. Lauretti's key original contribution is his comparison between chiropractic neck adjustments and the most common medical treatment for neck pain—the use of nonsteroidal antiinflammatory drugs. Lauretti powerfully demonstrates the relative safety of chiropractic while offering cautionary instruction on how to minimize the likelihood of negative reactions to chiropractic care. Attorney Alan Dumoff's "Chiropractic and the Law" discusses the essentials of legal matters, including licensure, scope of practice, insurance reimbursement, and malpractice, as well as the landmark case of *Wilk v. AMA*. J.F. McAndrews, a past president of Palmer College who has also held leadership positions for both the American Chiropractic Association and the International Chiropractors Association, has been one of the chiropractic profession's leading spokespersons for decades. In "Appropriate Care, Ethics, and Practice Guidelines," McAndrews contends that although the profession has made great strides toward maturity, substantial improvement is still required in two pivotal areas: (1) respect for reasonable, objectively based practice guidelines and (2) the development of a profession-wide ethic of financial fairness. "Managed Care" by Marino Passero of NCMIC Insurance Company and Daniel Redwood addresses issues central to delivery of care and reimbursement for services.

Daniel Redwood's closing chapter, "Pathways for an Evolving Profession," begins with the question, "How can chiropractors and chiropractic students help the profession evolve so that it more fully reflects our noblest aspirations?" Redwood offers 10 touchstones to guide the process, including distinguishing clearly among the proven, the probable, and the speculative; promoting a healing partnership with patients; recognizing that the doctor must strive to model the healthy lifestyle choices he or she recommends; cultivating an attitude of tolerance and openmindedness; minimizing patient dependency; and serving those who cannot afford our services.

Each chapter begins with a list of key terms to help readers focus on its essential points. All key terms are defined in the glossary at the back of the book. At the close of each chapter review and concept questions are provided.

We are aware that readers outside the United States will have to contend with parts of a few chapters (particularly those relating to legal matters and managed care) in which the focus is on issues specific to chiropractic in the United States. However, the vast majority of the text should be directly relevant to students and practitioners from all nations.

Daniel Redwood, DC
Carl S. Cleveland III, DC

ACKNOWLEDGMENTS

I wish to thank my parents, Norman and Jewel, for sharing my passion for chiropractic and other health-affirming endeavors; my wife, Beth, for her loving encouragement, thoughtfulness, and companionship on our journey through life; my children, Reuben and Jessica, for following their dreams as I have tried to follow mine; Marc Micozzi, for years of friendship and collaboration and his pioneering role in bridging the gap between alternative and mainstream health care; William Meeker, for his patience, good humor, and dedication to chiropractic research; Dana Lawrence, for his level-headed editorial judgment and prompt and remarkably helpful responses to my questions; and the late Jing-Nuan Wu, for always encouraging me to look more deeply and to focus on what matters most. Thanks as well to Ron Hendrickson, Mac McClelland, J.F. McAndrews, Joseph Keating, Christopher Kent, and Claire Cassidy.

—DR

I dedicate my role in the development of this text to the three generations of chiropractic family members who have stood before me. I acknowledge my great grandmother, Sylva L. Ashworth, DC, a 1910 Palmer graduate, who became the first woman to practice chiropractic in the state of Nebraska. She was a woman of influence during the emergence of a new profession in an era when being a woman in any profession stirred controversy. I acknowledge my grandparents, C.S. Cleveland Sr., DC, and Ruth R. Ashworth-Cleveland, DC, Palmer graduates of 1917 and founders of Cleveland Chiropractic College. Their struggle and sacrifice led to the establishment of licensure of doctors of chiropractic—now in all 50 states. Finally, I acknowledge my parents, Carl S. Cleveland Jr., DC, and Mildred G. Cleveland, DC, for their commitment to instill in me and so many others the science, philosophy, and art of chiropractic. They were pioneers. They lit a torch and have passed the torch to future generations. We must sustain the flame.

—CSC

Drs. Redwood and Cleveland both wish to thank all the chapter authors for their expertise and hard work and to gratefully acknowledge Kellie White, Christie Hart, and Julie Eddy, of Mosby and its parent company Elsevier, for their enthusiastic support of this textbook.

CONTENTS

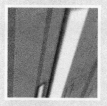

PART **ONE**

HISTORY, PHILOSOPHY, AND SOCIOLOGY

Forerunners of the Chiropractic Adjustment

John Willis, DC

Key Terms

ADJUSTMENT	HIPPOCRATES	MAGNETIC HEALING
ANDREW TAYLOR PALMER	HUMORS	MANIPULATION
AYURVEDIC MEDICINE	LAYING ON OF HANDS	MASSAGE
BONESETTING	LESION	NEI JING
BROAD OSTEOPATHS	LESION OSTEOPATHS	OSTEOPATHY
D.D. PALMER	LUMBAGO	

Although its origins are lost deep in history, the practice of **manipulation** is close to being universal,[1] because "to **massage** and manipulate an aching muscle and limb"[2] is a natural tendency. Only a small step separates adding pressure from rubbing an aching joint, especially when a popping noise and some degree of relief is often the reward. The first episodes of spinal manipulation certainly occurred well before the first known recordings of its use. What had been performed and orally passed on for unknown years was eventually written down.

Sociologist Walter I. Wardwell, a pre-eminent observer of chiropractic, warns about the problems of language when studying the forerunners of the chiropractic adjustment.[3] Although **D.D. Palmer** and chiropractors termed chiropractic manipulation the **adjustment** and gave it a relatively precise meaning, manipulation itself is a generic term. At various times, manipulation may refer to the reduction of a fracture, massage, mobilization, and other related activities. Unlike the chiropractic adjustment, manipulation is not limited to the spine. Ancient and modern documents frequently fail to specify the type of manipulation to which they refer.

Wardwell provides an excellent categorization system for the study of prechiropractic spinal manipulation:

The pre-Palmer literature on spinal manipulation can be put in several categories. First would be manipulative practices of ancient civilizations—Chinese, Japanese, Indian, Egyptian, Greek, Roman, and others. Second would be the often similar practices of primitive peoples. Third would be the bonesetters and similar folk practitioners in Western societies, some of whom practiced well into the present century. Fourth, mention will be made of the orthodox medical literature on "spinal irritation" which appeared in the nineteenth century. Finally there is osteopathy, which began pre-Palmer and is unquestionably similar to chiropractic though not identical in theory or technique. As is well known, both Palmers took great pains to differentiate chiropractic from it.[3]

MANIPULATIVE PRACTICES OF ANCIENT CIVILIZATIONS

Joint manipulation seems to have always been a part of Chinese medicine.[4] From the beginning it was linked to massage; only rather recently was joint manipulation separated as a distinct discipline. As in other geographic areas, its use was based on the results of empirical findings. It was perpetuated from generation to generation through the heritage and teachings of its disciples; consequently, early records of its use are fragmentary.

The first book pertaining to manipulation was briefly mentioned in the **Nei Jing** *(The Yellow Emperor's Classic of Medicine)* about three centuries BC; unfortunately, the book was lost. Early practitioners of the manipulative arts performed massage, reduced dislocations and fractures, and manipulated joints for traumatic injuries, such as those seen in war. However, from a chiropractic perspective, it is interesting that from the outset, Chinese manipulative arts were used to treat some internal disorders. The first known description of manipulation is recorded in the writings of Pien Chiao in about the fifth century BC. In his writings, he recommended manipulation for fatigue, rheumatism, nervous disorders, insomnia, **lumbago**, and for some forms of paralysis. As with most forms of the healing arts, manipulation had its periods of exaltation, as during the Tang dynasty, and periods during which it was held in low esteem. Especially during periods of high use, it was used not only curatively but also as an aid in preventing disease. However, most of its use may have been soft tissue work or massage.

The Mongol conquest strongly influenced Chinese manipulation. The wandering, warlike Mongols developed skills necessitated by their active way of life, including the ubiquitous horseback riding involved in their far-ranging wars. However, as with any forerunner, techniques used by the ancient (and even relatively recent) Chinese practitioners would seem cumbersome or even harsh to the current chiropractor. For example, one technique for torticollis used one hand to steady the head while the other held the chin, thereby extending the neck in a gross maneuver[4] (Fig. 1-1).

D.D. Palmer was aware of Chinese medicine. He recorded an incident involving a Chinese "houseboy" suffering from cholera. He stated that the Chinese healer "was prodding him [the houseboy] under the tongue with a long needle,"[5] and he also recorded having seen a physiologic chart used in Chinese medicine. Nevertheless, no definitive evidence suggests that the Chinese influenced Palmer's adjusting.

Other Eastern medical traditions, including those of India, also contained forms of spinal manipulation. However, manipulation of joints

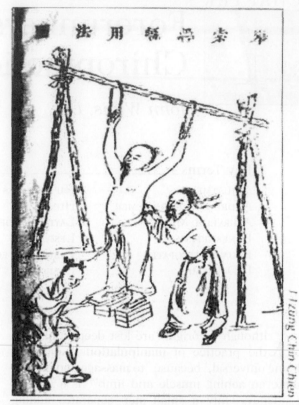

Fig. **1-1** Lumbar manipulation during the use of gravity traction as practiced in ancient China. *(From The Golden Mirror of Medicine.)*

was usually performed by bath attendants, because it was considered a part of hygiene, not a medical procedure.[6] In fairness, it should be noted that preventive measures such as hygiene, diet, and proper living are of great importance in **Ayurvedic** (Indian) **medicine**, not simply peripheral items as observed during periods of recent history.

Although most modern chiropractors, osteopathic practitioners, and medical manipulators are proud to trace their lineage to **Hippocrates** (fifth century), the techniques he used bear little resemblance to modern methods. A minority opinion advanced by K.A. Ligeros, MD, PhD, claims that Hippocrates and Greek physicians of Hippocrates' day actually performed manipulation of the spine in a manner similar to that performed by chiropractors today.[6] Ligeros appears to extrapolate the facts of Hippocrates' knowledge of the spine and nervous system, as well as his recorded use of manipulation, to a point in which similarities to modern chiropractic manipulation seem inevitable. Ligeros states that the methods rediscovered and known as chiropractic were also known and practiced by Aesculapius and his followers 420 years before the Christian era. A famous votive relief depicting Aesculapius manipulating a person's upper thoracic spine serves as part of Ligeros' proof.[7] However, little further evidence supports the view of a proto-chiropractic discipline during that era. Most historians might agree with Elizabeth Lomax who states, "Only further scholarly research could establish whether the Greeks merely attempted to reposition vertebrae

displaced through trauma, the conventional interpretation, or indeed frequently manipulated spines as therapy for a wide variety of dysfunctions."[8] It is still interesting to note that D.D. Palmer referred to Aesculapius and his teachings as a foundation for what he termed chiropractic[5] (Fig. 1-2).

The Persian physician and philosopher Avicenna (AD 980-1037), known as Ibn Sina, also used and wrote of manipulation. His work was, for all practical purposes, a rewrite of Galen's that, in turn, was descended from that of Hippocrates.[9]

Pierre Gaucher-Peslherbe wrote, "Well into the seventeenth century and regardless of whether they were Greek, Roman, Byzantine, Cretan,

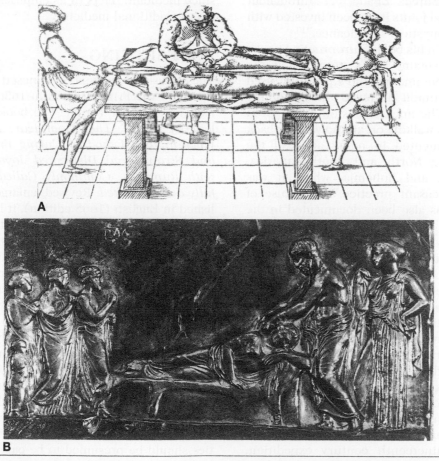

Fig. 1-2 **A,** Typical spinal manipulation from classical Greek period into the seventeenth century. **B,** Votive relief depicting Aesculapius manipulating an individual's upper thoracic spine. (*A courtesy Biblioteca Universitaria, Aarchiginnas, Bologna, Italy. B courtesy Palmer College of Chiropractic, Library Special Collections.*)

Arabic, Spanish, Turkish, Italian, French, or German, all published authors resorted to the same method. The patient was bandaged and lay on a board; traction was applied toward the head and feet while pressure was exerted onto a selected spinal area."[6] The pressure or thrust was delivered by using the practitioner's hands, feet, or even buttocks by simply sitting on the patient's spine. Occasionally, a piece of wood might have also been used as a lever.

Forms of manipulation practiced among primitive peoples were similar to these practiced in ancient civilizations, but they were often accompanied by more extensive religious ritual or magic. The interconnection of religion and healing was always present. In reference to manipulation, Gaucher-Peslherbe quotes the noted anthropologist, Mircea Eliade, ". . . throughout history bones and joints have been invested with a symbolic and mystical significance."[10]

Chester Wilk in his book *Chiropractic Speaks Out* recounts Captain Cook's story of how the techniques of "pummeling and squeezing" used by Tahitian women relieved his crippling rheumatism.[11] The ancient custom of children and small adults walking on an individual's back has been documented in many areas of the world, including North and South America, Polynesia, Asia, and Bohemia, where it was known as a "peasant practice."[12] The use of manipulation has also been documented in the Americas.

From the records of the early Spanish Friars of the sixteenth century, chiropractor and anthropologist C.W. Weiant relates that Aztecs distinguished between what they called a "true doctor" and a "false doctor" or witch doctor. One of the qualifications for true doctors was their knowledge of how the joints worked properly.[13]

North American Indians predating the Jamestown settlement (1607) used forms of manipulation as a part of daily life. Stories of their appreciation of spinal manipulation have become so commonplace that they have crept into popular literature. In a novel on Lewis and Clark's early nineteenth century expedition, James Alexander Thom relates how Clark kept the Nez Perce busy for most of a day "adjusting" their spines, anachronistically using Palmer's

word for spinal manipulation, which would not come into common usage until after another century had passed.[14]

In South America, Ronald L. Firestone cites evidence of extensive use of manipulation in pre-Columbian culture (Firestone R, e-mail communication to author, 11/19/01). "One of the best indicators of such would be the prevalence of this method in the current practices of the Quechua and Aymara traditional practitioners." Firestone shows great respect for these practitioners, known as Callahullas or Yatiri (Fig. 1-3). Describing the work of these practitioners from an innovative perspective, he suggests, "I actually think that we in chiropractic should begin referring to those who practice, or have practiced, in this manner as traditional chiropractors since medicine refers to its empirical practitioners as traditional medicine."

BONESETTING

The earliest known text on **bonesetting** was published by the Friar Moulton in 1656 and republished by Robert Turner. The book, despite its lengthy title, *The Compleat Bone-Setter, Wherein the Method of Curing Broken Bones and Strains and Dislocated Joynts, together with Ruptures, Commonly Called Bellyes, is fully demonstrated.* Revised, enlarged, and published in English (1665 edition), it had only two pages that described manipulative techniques.[15] Although *The Compleat Bone-Setter* was written during a period in which physicians still used manipulation, the book merely commended its use but did not teach it. Most of the teaching was left to one-on-one contact.

Lomax states that manipulation was ubiquitous, and its utility was not seriously questioned until the eighteenth century.[8] She attributes spinal manipulation's falling out of favor with medical physicians to the tuberculosis caries of the spine, which were frequently diagnosed during this period. Eminent physicians, such as Sir Percival Pott, believed all spinal deformities should be presumed to be caused by caries and therefore should not be manipulated. They considered it malpractice to do so, stating clearly that the preferred treatment for spinal

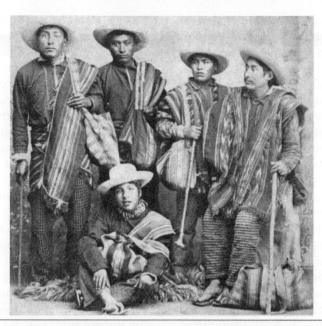

Fig. 1-3 The Callahullas, or Yatiri, of South America. *(Courtesy Ronald Firestone, D.C.)*

deformities should be rest and induced local ulceration.

Not all historians agree with Lomax as to the reason manipulation fell from grace; they only agree that it did. Johan Schultes, who died in 1645, was the last published author to teach spinal manipulation as a part of regular medicine.[15] Although the discontinuation of manipulation by medical physicians took place over a period of more than 100 years, no evidence of its use after the end of the seventeenth century can be found. Johannes Fossgreen suggests another cause may have been fear of contagious contact.[15] This argument is supported by evidence from physicians in the seventeenth and eighteenth centuries, distancing themselves from their patients in the wake of such contagious diseases as the highly virulent form of syphilis brought back to Europe from the Americas by the adventurers who had themselves introduced smallpox to the American Indians.

In his seminal 1993 work, *Chiropractic: Early Concepts in Their Historical Setting,* Pierre Gaucher-Peslherbe discusses a more complicated and subtle scenario.[6] To oversimplify Gaucher's work, culture changed. In medicine, the soft tissue and particularly the muscle became the center of attention, and vertebral dislocations and subluxations were discarded from medical attention. As a result, massage became a recommended treatment, and manipulation or reduction was condemned because of the supposed progress in therapy. These changes fit the cultural image of the time. Medicine was becoming professionalized. Anything traditional, such as bonesetting, was associated with lay practitioners and thus rejected.

A remarkably effective process had begun following the surgeons' condemnation of those practices they did not wish to see continued; incidentally, more to mark their newly acquired professional status by setting themselves apart, than because of any real objection to the practices themselves, which they now dismissed on the grounds that they were unprofessional.[16]

The bonesetter or layperson's speech was criticized. Greater importance was placed on how an individual communicated (flowery imagery often became more important than what it represented). It followed that the plain speech of laypeople was of little value because it lacked eloquence and was therefore unprofessional. Because manipulation was performed by nonprofessionals who could not speak as professionals spoke, it followed that manipulation could not and should not be a part of the profession of medicine.

Anderson and Gaucher-Peslherbe are in agreement that pompous arguments concerning theory are diversionary and explain little of why physicians abandoned manipulation and then castigated the bonesetters who filled the void they had left.[16] Essentially, bonesetters based their practices on pragmatism. What was deemed to work was used. Attempts to explain the reasons procedures worked were often inadequate and, by standards of that society, considered unprofessional. Largely because of this failure to articulate theories in a manner acceptable to the medical profession, bonesetter procedures were rejected. One is reminded of C.S. Lewis' discussion of scientists' depiction of the atom. He describes how the scientists' belief of a mathematical formula is given in such a manner that the layperson can create a mental picture. The mental picture is meant to be helpful; however, if it ceases to be helpful, it should be dropped, not confused with what it symbolizes.[17] Apparently, the flowery language of individuals such as Pouteau, with its love of imagery and metaphor, was carried so far that critical sense was sometimes lost.[16] This was the language that the lay manipulators could not duplicate.

When medical physicians abandoned manipulation in the seventeenth century, it became identified with the humble oral traditions of the uneducated ordinary people.[15] As members of the ruling class, traditional physicians had no desire to emulate the common folk, even when manipulation showed success. The physicians and other members of the ruling class ". . . dedicated themselves to their whole body of custom as symbolic of discreteness from other classes of society. They took pride in being different, and by definition of different, superior."[18] Excellent examples of this phenomenon can be found in the stories of many bonesetters of medieval France. When their successes became well-known, they were often summoned to serve the French Court. Once ensconced inside the society of the day, these bonesetters had opportunities to advance academic studies and solidify bonesetting into a profession. Instead, they moved quickly to separate themselves from their common past and dedicated themselves to becoming part of the elite. In so doing, they abandoned bonesetting, and many became " 'hereditary [passed from parent to child by virtue of birth] physicians' whose families flourished in France until the seventeenth century and who touched for dog bites and other mishaps."[6]

A number of well-known bonesetters practiced in Great Britain and the United States. They seemed to arise in their communities when the need arose. Although most performed other jobs for their livelihood (as did many early chiropractors), some were full-time practitioners. Among the more famous was Sir Herbert Barker (d.1950), a British bonesetter knighted for helping humanity[19] (Fig. 1-4). Although the son of a solicitor, Barker learned bonesetting through a tutorship under his cousin. He reportedly refined and developed his techniques to a higher

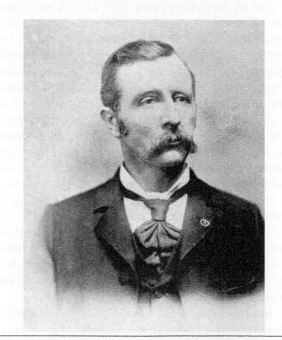

Fig. 1-4 The British bonesetter Sir Herbert Barker. (*Courtesy David D. Palmer Health Sciences Library, Palmer College of Chiropractic, Davenport, Iowa.*)

standard, eventually coining the term "manipulative surgery" as an accurate description of his work. He often invited physicians to witness his work, but few accepted his offers. After a malpractice case that Barker suspected was "trumped-up" by physicians, the bonesetter's reputation and practice grew, although he lost the case. As an old man, he was invited by the British Orthopaedic Association to demonstrate his techniques. Although Barker believed the demonstration capped his career with a crowning victory, it had little or no effect on the medical profession during the years that followed (Fig. 1-5).

The history of bonesetting as observed in Barker's case is important to the history of forerunners of the chiropractic adjustment, not only from the aspect of manipulative technique but also (and possibly more significantly) in the manner in which it "demonstrates the obvious depth of feeling by organized medicine against health practitioners outside the medical establishment on grounds which are, in principle, understandable."[20] The Barker episode was used by the 1979 New Zealand government commission's report on chiropractic to help explain the attitude of New Zealand's organized medicine toward chiropractic. The commission believed that many clear parallels existed between Barker's episode and

chiropractic, including the lack of formal medical qualifications and Barker's inability to explain his methods. The commission went on to point out that the latter problem should not be considered as only an elitist way of separating the professional from the nonprofessional. Accepting Barker's unexplained method, even had he been a qualified medical practitioner, would have placed the medical profession in a difficult position were it to be faced with "the claims of anyone else who might say that he had discovered a miracle cure by using a technique that could not adequately be explained: The typical equipment of the quack."[20] In other words, there was no doubt that prejudice existed, but there was also no doubt that bonesetters, as many other healers before and after them, must be able to explain themselves.

However, the stigma of bonesetting's association with the humble and uneducated could not be overcome even when physicians such as Dr. Edward Harrison used its techniques. Although well educated and articulate, he could not overcome the emotional resistance of the medical profession. His reputation among them was at best tenuous. One anonymous colleague would not go so far as to call Harrison a charlatan but would say that what he was doing was certainly well adapted to charlatanism.[8]

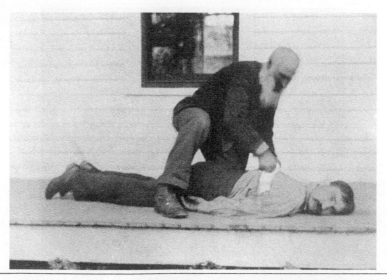

Fig. 1-5 A bonesetter practicing near Cedar Rapids, Iowa, at the turn of the twentieth century. *(From Smith OG, Langworthy SM, Paxson MC:* Modernized chiropractic, *Cedar Rapids, Iowa, 1906, American School of Chiropractic.)*

Some of the more famous names among American bonesetters are Reese, Sweet, Tiesten, and Orton. As bonesetting with its lack of formal education and credentialing began to fade, entire families adopted the professions. The Sweets became orthopedists, whereas the Tiestens and Ortons became chiropractors.[21-23]

An often-overlooked antecedent of the chiropractic adjustment is **magnetic healing**, the form of healing that D.D. Palmer practiced for 9 years before founding the chiropractic profession (Fig. 1-6). **Andrew Taylor Still**, the founder of osteopathy, also was a magnetic healer in and around 1875 (Fig. 1-7). The hands-on technique of magnetic healing often involved vigorous rubbing and probably manipulation of various kinds.[3] Wardwell was intrigued when learning that often the practitioners of magnetism, faith healing, and mental healing did more than simply the **laying on of hands**. Gevitz describes how Andrew Jackson Davis, a leading nineteenth century exponent of spiritualism, and Warren Felt Evans emphasized "vigorous rubbing along the spinal column."[24]

Homola adds:

The Mormon leader, Joseph Smith, Jr., practiced faith healing employing the use of bonesetting. One of his elders advertised to "set bones through faith in Christ" stating that "while commanding the bones, they came together, making a noise like the crushing of an old basket." Only the joints of the spine can be made to give out with such sounds as the "crushing of an old basket."

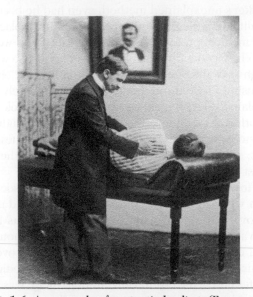

Fig. 1-6 An example of magnetic healing. *(From Weltmer SA: Revised illustrated mail course of instruction in magnetic healing, 1901, self-published.)*

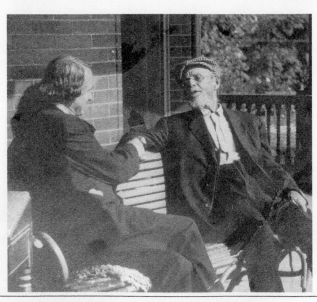

Fig. 1-7 Andrew Taylor Still with his friend Elbert Hubbard, an author who was also a friend of B.J. Palmer. *(Courtesy Still Osteopathic Museum and National Center for Osteopathic History.)*

Obviously, the laying on of hands in this faith-healing procedure was performed with considerable force.[2]

Gevitz states that Still was able to synthesize many of the major aspects of magnetic healing and bonesetting into "one unified doctrine," and the same could be said of Palmer. Far from attempting to hide his background in magnetic healing, Palmer wrote that "quite a portion of that which now constitutes Chiropractic I had collected during the previous nine years" (the years spent practicing magnetic healing).[5] Again, as noted earlier, a natural tendency to rub an aching joint exists, and from there, it takes only a small step to add the necessary pressure to the joint to move it. Both Still and Palmer took that step.

OSTEOPATHY

Finally, the last of chiropractic's antecedents, **osteopathy**, is reached in this discussion. Osteopathy's position as a forerunner of chiropractic, based on its common use of manipulation, may be a contentious one for the **osteopath** and, at least at times, an unappreciated one. When this author wrote to a renowned Virginia osteopath, he was firmly told that the osteopaths were complete physicians and that he, for one, performed no manipulation at all. When Still first announced his philosophy a mere 21 years before D.D. Palmer's founding of chiropractic, he did not mention manipulation. It was not until 1879 that Still began using manipulation and structural diagnosis in the manner associated with classical osteopathy.[25] However, even in his time, Still was a complete physician. Siehl explains the founding:

Remember, Dr. Still founded osteopathy to improve upon the present practice of medicine, surgery, and obstetrics. He did not say "no drugs." He merely stated that the drugs then in vogue were harmful and largely useless. He did not say "no surgery." In fact, the ASO (American School of Osteopathy) Hospital had a surgery suite and relatives of Dr. Still were the early chief surgeons in the ASO Hospital. Kirksville became quite a surgical center as well as a center for osteopathic manipulative treatment at the turn of the century. Dr. Still did not say to avoid diagnostic procedures other than palpatory diagnosis. He empha-

sized physical diagnosis. He emphasized that other methods were necessary.[25]

That Still's osteopathy, like Palmer's chiropractic, was not confined to low back pain, stiff necks, and typical musculoskeletal complaints is as much a cause for celebration of their similarities as is the fact that both use manipulation. Neither man intended to simply add the modality of manipulation to the accepted system. Both meant to establish a new and superior system that dealt with the entire person. It was not a wryneck or the proverbial "hitch-in-your-get-along" that motivated Still; it was the dysentery and spinal meningitis that ravaged his family. Neither Still nor Palmer considered his system as merely manual medicine.

Chiropractic and osteopathy have always emphasized their differences. The reasons for this emphasis are varied, ranging from political to personal to economic. Both were evangelistic in their desire to spread the good news of the new professions. An early osteopath from North Carolina quoted a Moravian tenet, wishing it to be adopted by osteopaths: "Go as a missionary yourself, or take the fruits of your own labor and support someone else in the field of missionary endeavor."[26]

When Still "flung to the breeze the banner of osteopathy" in 1889, it was an act against the primitive state of medicine as he saw it, as well as the hubris of the physicians themselves.[27] The same could be said of Palmer.

Whether Palmer took from Still or Still from Palmer or both from each other, the debate has been taken on by many including Brantingham, Gaucher-Peslherbe, and others but to the full satisfaction of few.[28] Both the founders and their professions had always significant differences, as well as similarities. Although different terminology was used, both professions initially emphasized the body's inherent ability to maintain health and the use of manipulation as a primary technique. Osteopathy's focus was on "the rule of the artery" and the use of nonspecific manipulation to enhance the flow of blood. Gaucher-Peslherbe makes the argument of osteopathy's ties with the ancient Greek doctrine of body **humors**, the predominant medical philosophy into the nineteenth century. (In medieval physiology, a humor one of the four elemental fluids of the body—blood, phlegm, black bile and yellow bile—and the fluids' relative proportions determined an individual's physical and mental makeup.) Chiropractic, on the other hand, gave emphasis to the specific spinal adjustment, which meant to release energy that traveled through the nervous system, a break from the humoral doctrine. However, caution must be used in these debates because neither profession sprang forth from their respective shells in full-blown maturity. Both professions underwent considerable legal trauma, which helped define them. The early inclusion of drugs and surgery into osteopathy also made the debates about the differences between the professions more obvious. Indeed, Palmer's first theory of manipulation was as much concerned with circulation as it was with the nervous system.

Debates between the **lesion osteopaths**, those most closely adhering to manipulation and Still's early tenets, and the **broad osteopaths**, those aligned more strongly with drugs and surgery, have also declined with time. The osteopathic **lesion,** later called *somatic dysfunction,* is a disturbance of musculoskeletal structure and/or function, which may include accompanying disturbances of other biological mechanisms. Early legal battles that were used to show osteopathy's distinctness from medicine, thereby establishing it as a separate healing art, later turned to battles that were used to show it equal and similar to medicine.

Ironically, a 1982 study in Ohio surveying osteopathic practitioners found that they viewed osteopathic manipulative treatments as the least important of the five main concepts stressed by osteopathy: (1) holistic medicine, (2) doctor-patient relations, (3) emphasis on general practice, (4) the body's ability to heal itself, and (5) manipulation. Yet, from the patient's perspective, the study showed the more that individuals favored osteopathic manipulative therapy (OMT), the greater their tendency to rate osteopaths as well qualified, at least as well qualified as medical physicians.[29] The same study showed that most osteopaths surveyed believed that patients receive less OMT in osteopathic hospitals than they need. This comes at a time

when there are no longer any chiropractic hospitals, and the number of osteopathic hospitals (there are approximately 140 in the United States) appears to be waning. However, as Westview Hospital in Indiana is discovering, the reason for this reduction may not be that osteopathic hospitals are too different; rather, it may be because they do not provide enough difference to acquire special status.[30] Without special status, they are similar to most small hospitals, which cannot absorb the discounts demanded by aggressive third party payers and therefore find survival difficult.

CONCLUSION

The forerunners of the chiropractic adjustment have been many and varied. Most in Western culture have managed musculoskeletal problems such as fractures, sprains, and strains. This is probably true of most cultures. If Ligeros is correct, some ancient Greeks may have practiced as proto-chiropractors. The evidence is strong that the Chinese also saw merit for manipulative treatment of nonmusculoskeletal illnesses, but it appears that this area was not much more than an aside to the mainstream of manipulation. The Middle Ages in Europe were preoccupied with the straightness of the spine as a sign of virtue and knightly stature, and the treatments provided, both regular and otherwise, were primarily aimed toward orthopedic problems. Practices of primitive peoples, though more steeped in religious aspects, still aimed predominately at helping structure, dislocations, and related ailments, such as Captain Cook's rheumatism. Only osteopathy (or magnetic healing, if it can be considered a manipulative healing art) has a philosophy of care, which, like chiropractic, definitively goes beyond the musculoskeletal system to the management of visceral problems. Both osteopathy and chiropractic aimed at being independent health care systems, not merely adjuncts to regular medicine. In addition, both, after achieving positions of relative esteem, continue to find themselves still battered by old prejudices and the ubiquitous struggle for the health-care dollar. Yet, with the revival of public demand for spinal manipulation, osteopaths are enjoying a renaissance in the heritage and application of Dr. Still's favorite modality, a heritage chiropractic has never abandoned.

Review *Questions*

1. What manual methods may be included under the generic term manipulation?
2. What are some of the health conditions for which joint manipulation was used in ancient China?
3. Who were the "bonesetters," and how were they trained?
4. What were the relations between British bonesetters and medical physicians in the seventeenth and eighteenth centuries?
5. To what does historian Elizabeth Lomax attribute manipulation's falling out of favor in the eighteenth century?
6. Why did bonesetting fail to move toward full professional status after bonesetters were invited to serve the French Court?
7. To what extent did social class (commoners versus professionals) influence the acceptance or rejection of joint manipulation in Europe?
8. Some of the best-established families of American bonesetters joined which two professions when bonesetting declined?
9. In what ways was magnetic healing similar to chiropractic? In what ways did the two differ?
10. What were the similarities between early osteopathy and chiropractic? What were the differences?

Concept *Questions*

1. A.T. Still, the founder of osteopathy, was originally a medical physician, whereas D.D. Palmer, the founder of chiropractic, was originally a magnetic healer. In what ways does the evolution of the professions they founded reflect the different backgrounds of the founders?
2. Do you agree or disagree with Ronald Firestone's suggestion that ancient or indigenous practitioners of spinal manipulation should be referred to as "traditional chiropractors." Why?

REFERENCES

1. Dintenfass J: *Chiropractic: a modern way to health,* New York, 1995, Pyramid Books.
2. Homola S: *Bonesetting, chiropractic and cultism,* Panama City, Fla, 1963, Critique Books.
3. Wardwell WI: Before the Palmers: an overview of chiropractic antecedents, *Chiropr Hist* 7(2):27, 1987.
4. Shu Yan Ng: A brief review of manipulation in Chinese history, *Eur J Chiropr* 34(1-2):24, 1986.
5. Palmer DD: *The science, art, and philosophy of chiropractic,* Portland, Ore, 1910, Portland Printing House.
6. Gaucher-Peslherbe PL: Antecedents to chiropractic: a cultural approach from ancient myths to modern mythologies. In Petersen D, Wiese G, editors: *Chiropractic: an illustrated history,* St Louis, 1995, Mosby.
7. The ancient art of manipulation depicted in 5th century votive tablet, *Chiropr Hist* 7(2):26, 1987.
8. Lomax E: Manipulative therapy: an historical approach. In Burger AA, Tohis JS, editors: *Approaches to the validation of manipulation therapy,* Springfield, Ill, 1977, Charles C Thomas.
9. Victory KS: Spinal manipulation in the 11th century Middle East, *Chiropr Hist* 13(1):12, 1970.
10. Gaucher-Peslherbe PL: *Chiropractic: early concepts in their historical setting,* Lombard, Ill, 1993, National College of Chiropractic.
11. Wilk CA: *Chiropractic speaks out: a reply to medical propaganda, bigotry and ignorance,* Park Ridge, Ill, 1973, Wilk Publishing.
12. Zarbuch MV: A profession for "bohemian chiropractic": Oakley Smith and the evolution of naprapathy, *Chiropr Hist* 7:77, 1986.
13. Thom JA: *Sign-talker: the adventure of George Drouillard on the Lewis and Clark expedition,* New York, 2000, Ballentine Books.
14. Weiant CW: *Medicine and chiropractic,* Lombard, Ill, 1975, National College of Chiropractic.
15. Anderson RT: On doctors and bonesetters in the 16th and 17th centuries, *Chiropr Hist* 3(1):12, 1983.
16. Anderson RT: Bonesetting: a medical bone of contention, *J Am Chiropr Assoc* 15:5, 1981.
17. Lewis CS: *Mere Christianity,* New York, 1975, Simon & Schuster.
18. Anderson RT: *Traditional Europe: a study of anthropology and history,* Belmont, Calif, 1971, Wadsworth Publishing.
19. Taylor HH: Sir Herbert Baker: bone-setter and early advocate of "bloodless surgery," *J Am Chiropr Assoc* 32(7):27, 1995.
20. *Chiropractic in New Zealand: report of the commission of inquiry,* Wellington, New Zealand, 1979, PD Hasselberg, Government Printer.
21. Janse J: *Principles and practices of chiropractic,* Lombard, Ill, 1976, National College of Chiropractic.
22. Orton E: A touching story, *the Canastota (South Dakota) clipper,* 1985.

23. Master RO Sr: A history of the chiropractic adjustment, *Dig Chiropr Econ* 3(a):24, 1998.
24. Gevitz N: *The DO's osteopathic medicine in America,* Baltimore, 1982, Johns Hopkins University.
25. Siehl D: The osteopathic differences: is it only manipulation? *J Am Osteopath Assoc* 101(10):630, 2001.
26. Meachum WB: Destiny of the osteopathic profession, *J Am Osteopath Assoc* 101(10):621, 2001.
27. Klafhorn WK, Dodson JL: *Osteopathic medicine: a photographic history,* Greenwich, Conn, 1995, Greenwich Press.
28. Brantingham JW: Still and Palmer: the impact of the first osteopath and the first chiropractor, *Chiropr Hist* 6:12, 1986.
29. Culbertson HM, Stompel GH III: *A study of the public relations posture of osteopathic medicine in Ohio,* Columbus, Ohio, 1982, Ohio Osteopathic Association.
30. Swiatek J: Beyond osteopathy—hospital looks for health-care niche, *The Indianapolis Star,* Sunday, 30 September 2001, sec. E1.

CHAPTER
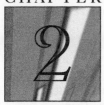

The Chiropractic Paradigm

Ashley Cleveland, MA, DC, Reed Phillips, DC, PhD, Gerard Clum, DC

Key Terms

ACUPUNCTURE	DANIEL DAVID PALMER	OSTEOPATHY
ADJUSTMENT	DIAGNOSIS	PHYSIOTHERAPY
ALLOPATHIC	HOMEOPATHY	SAMUEL HAHNEMANN
AMERICAN CHIROPRACTIC	HYDROTHERAPY	SCOPE OF PRACTICE
ASSOCIATION	INNATE INTELLIGENCE	SOMATIC DYSFUNCTION
ANDREW TAYLOR STILL	INTERNATIONAL	STRAIGHT
ANTON MESMER	CHIROPRACTORS	SUBLUXATION
ASSOCIATION OF	ASSOCIATION	THOMSONIANISM
CHIROPRACTIC COLLEGES	INTERVENTIONS	TONE
PARADIGM	J.F. ALAN HOWARD	TREATMENT
B.J. PALMER	LESION	VITALISM
BIOPSYCHOSOCIAL	MAGNETIC HEALING	WORLD CHIROPRACTIC
CANADIAN CHIROPRACTIC	MANIPULATION	ALLIANCE
ASSOCIATION	MASSAGE	WORLD FEDERATION OF
CONGRESS OF CHIROPRACTIC	MIXER	CHIROPRACTIC
STATE ASSOCIATIONS	ONE CAUSE–ONE CURE	

The chiropractic profession traces its roots to the American Midwest at end of the nineteenth century. **Daniel David Palmer,** a man in many ways characteristic of his times, wove together the threads of his era's metaphysical and scientific thought to create a philosophy, science, and art of healing that has now entered its second century. Palmer's varied health-related interests ranged from what was known in his day as *magnetism* and ***magnetic healing*** to his signature contribution—identifying a fundamental relationship between functional skeletal abnormality and the potential for adverse effects on the nervous system.

Attention to the human skeleton did not begin with Palmer. As described in Chapter 1, "Forerunners of the Chiropractic Adjustment," throughout history countless people have been acknowledged for their talent in caring for various components of the skeletal system. Such

manually applied skills, in one form or another, have been found in all cultures on all continents.

What was it that made Palmer's contribution sufficiently noteworthy to form the basis of a profession that, a century later, spans the globe? Similar to his contemporary, **Andrew Taylor Still,** the founder of **osteopathy,** Palmer did not view the spine, or even the full skeleton, as an isolated body part to be tended solely at the site where symptoms arose. Rather, each person articulated a paradigm of human health in which the spine played a central role. A.T. Still related the integrity of the spine and skeleton to the proper functioning of the circulatory system and theorized a broad impact on health and well being as a consequence of alterations of that relationship. Palmer, on the other hand, emphasized the relationship between the skeleton (especially the spine) and the nervous system and theorized a system-wide interdependence, in which a person's state of health depends on proper integration between skeletal structures and the function of the nervous system.

Perhaps Palmer's greatest contribution was not the delivery of a spinal adjustment but rather his concentrated focus on the effects of spinal dynamics on nerve function, as well as the development of a body of knowledge and clinical skills to address the clinical manifestations of these effects. Palmer was not the first to discover that the human body is capable of self-regulation and healing, nor was he the first healer to use manual techniques. Palmer was, however, the originator of an approach to healing that incorporated specific manual techniques into a paradigm that accorded supremacy to the role of the nervous system (rather than the circulatory system) in physiologic regulation and healing.

HEALTH CARE AND PHILOSOPHIC LANDSCAPE IN D.D. PALMER'S ERA

To understand how Palmer arrived at his unique synthesis, it is essential to understand the state of late nineteenth century health care in the United States. **Allopathic** doctors of the time did not yet enjoy the status they now possess and did not have to meet the same rigorous educational and licensing standards as today. Much of medical practice emphasized using so-called *heroic* therapies, such as leeching, cupping, and bleeding. Because the public often perceived these methods as worse than the ailments they sought to cure, Americans were hungry for alternative approaches to their health problems.[1]

Several more *natural* healing systems, less invasive than allopathic medicine, gained popularity during the nineteenth century. Among these systems were[2]:

1. **Homeopathy,** founded by the German physician **Samuel Hahnemann,** which used as its medicines highly diluted quantities of various substances, primarily from plant and mineral sources
2. **Thomsonianism,** a system of healing founded by the American herbalist Samuel Thomson, in which overexposure to cold was considered a central cause of disease

3. **Hydrotherapy,** which emphasized the internal and external therapeutic uses of water
4. Nature Cure, which used a vegetarian diet, along with light and air
5. Hygienic System, which amalgamated the hydrotherapy and Nature Cure movements
6. Osteopathy, founded by Andrew Taylor Still, which used manual therapy for correcting osseous lesions (referred to as the *osteopathic lesion*) proposed to exert a negative effect on circulation and thereby on overall health

These approaches to healing shared a preference for conservative, minimally invasive **interventions** that were believed to allow the body to heal itself. (See Appendix II regarding the relative invasiveness of various health interventions.)

Health care practitioners in this era ranged from those trained in formal university settings to villagers who apprenticed under local doctors and at some point were themselves recognized as doctors. Health education and practice-related legislation were minimal. Many systems of health and healing were freely espoused throughout the United States, each proclaiming its own superiority and the failings of its competitors. Numerous health fads gained adherents and then lost them, only to be supplanted by newer approaches.

Gevitz, a historian of osteopathy, outlined a life cycle for these developments, noting that "movements such as osteopathy, homeopathy, and eclecticism, generally have a natural life cycle. They are conceived by a crisis in medical care; their youth is marked by a broadening of their ideas; and their decline occurs whenever whatever distinctive notions they have as to patient management are allowed to wither. At this point, no longer having a compelling reason for existence, they die."[3] To survive for many generations, a healing art must provide a unique and valuable service, as allopathic medicine, dentistry, chiropractic, and other professions have done. Similarly, its practitioners must not lose sight of its basic purpose: to restore patients when ill and to aid them in their daily quest for health.

PALMER'S MAGNETIC HEALING AND METAPHYSICAL INTERESTS

Palmer's interests extended beyond the purely physical aspects of health and healing as he explored the energetics of the body, as well as paranormal phenomena. During the nineteenth century, the American religious landscape included various forms of spiritualist and metaphysical speculation, and Palmer's curiosity was piqued by these influences. **Anton Mesmer's** concept of *animal magnetism* was used by many individual practitioners such as Palmer and adapted by Mary Baker Eddy for use in her Christian Science, although Benjamin Franklin had dealt the concept a nearly fatal blow in a famous experiment in the royal court of France early in the nineteenth century. In this early example of a blinded clinical trial, Franklin demonstrated that healing effects occurred when patients believed they were being *mesmerized,* although no healing effects were noted if patients were ignorant of Mesmer's *magnetic passes.*[4]

Mesmer used magnetic healing methods to treat a wide range of disorders, including hysterical blindness, paralysis, headaches, and joint pains. Magnetic healing primarily involved "laying on of hands" to transmit healing energy and may also have included vigorous rubbing, **manipulation,** or both. (See Chapter 1 for greater detail.) In his work with magnetic healing, D.D. Palmer believed that he was able to attain a higher degree of specificity than other magnetics.[5]

During this same era, spiritualism, the belief that consciousness survives beyond death and that it is possible to contact the spirits of those who have died, also gained in popularity. Mediums purporting to facilitate this contact traveled the country, and séances were held in the parlors of many well-respected members of society. D.D. Palmer was part of the metaphysical movement of his day, attending spiritualist meetings then common in the Midwest. Other major philosophic influences in that era were the transcendentalist philosophers Henry David Thoreau and Ralph Waldo Emerson, whose love of nature and fierce independence of thought and action resonated with the individualistic spirit of many Americans and provided a supportive milieu for the pioneers of new healing methods.[6]

D.D. PALMER'S CORE CHIROPRACTIC CONCEPTS

Though the individual components of Palmer's chiropractic philosophy did not originate with him, he was able to blend recognized spiritual and metaphysical concepts together with the then-current scientific principles to create a unique ethos for the chiropractic healing art. The relationship between the structure and function of the body formed the essence of chiropractic's approach to health care. Chiropractors sought to influence the body's capacity to heal itself through the nervous system by applying specific forces to the spine. According to Palmer, function of the nervous system can be altered by a subtle change in position of a vertebral segment. Once function of the nervous system was altered, the entire organism can become predisposed to incoordination (dis-ease) and, ultimately, disease.

Stated in a current conceptual framework, "a structural problem within the spine contributes to diminished neurologic ability to cope with the environment, and the ability of the body to heal itself is decreased. Palmer believed the cause of most disease is displaced vertebrae; the disease is an effect of that displacement."[7]

Although few contemporary chiropractors would now endorse a **one cause–one cure** explanation of human health and illness (with subluxation being the cause and adjustment being the cure), the interdependence of structure of the spine and function of the nervous system remains a cornerstone of the philosophy and practice of chiropractic today.

D.D. Palmer conceived of nerve function in the context of vibration and **tone,** common explanations for his time. Disease, he claimed, resulted from fluctuations in nerve tone, "nerves too tense or too slack."[8] Palmer asserted that either "too much or not enough energy is disease."[8] and that disease, rather than being something external that invades the body, is instead the result of internal imbalances involving hyperfunction or hypofunction of organs and systems. From this perspective, the resistance of the host is more significant than the power of the pathogen. Chiropractors are not now, nor were they in Palmer's time, the only health care practitioners to place primary emphasis on strengthening the internal resistive forces of the body. The uniqueness of chiropractic lies in its assertion that the spine provides a key to affecting the nervous system, the controlling and coordinating system of the body. Thus according to Palmer, the mechanical process of spinal adjustment was employed for vitalistic purposes.

Vitalism is an explanatory model that suggests the body requires something greater than physical and chemical processes to function. In its more extreme forms, this something greater is given theologic significance.[9] Chiropractors have generally looked at the physiologic processes of the body as expressive of *intelligence,* or a *wisdom of the body.* Some early chiropractors philosophized about the source of that intelligence; however, many chiropractors have been content to acknowledge that the functions of the body are not wholly explicable by mere physical and chemical laws and that the nervous system seems to function largely to express the body's integrative capability.

Palmer noted that the physical structure of the body is challenged through the activities of daily living and theorized that these challenges, or stressors, take three primary forms, the three Ts—trauma, toxins, and thoughts. Current discussions of the philosophy of chiropractic continue to include these three challenges (often expressed as physical, chemical, and emotional) and their adverse influence on tone or function of the nervous system, as well as in the causation of subluxation and illness.

REINTERPRETING PALMER'S ORIGINAL CONCEPTS

Palmer may have crystallized an idea and defined a philosophic context within which to employ it, but he was unable to constrain others, including his son, from modifying and reinterpreting chiropractic and its clinical application.

Similar to many sons, Bartlett Joshua, or B.J., followed in the footsteps of his father; and similar to many sons, he did not see eye to eye with his father. A nearly legendary level of disagreement, rivalry, and antagonism arose between the two. These disagreements did not end at the family dinner table but reverberated throughout the chiropractic profession.

D.D. envisioned chiropractic as a way to treat the full skeleton and also saw it integrated with matters of thought, trauma, and toxicity. D.D. theorized that the three Ts lead to skeletal manifestations, which continue to compromise the body's capacity for well being. B.J. focused much more specifically on the mechanics of the spine, with correction of vertebral malposition and attendant neural compromise, together known as **subluxation,** assuming a primary role in helping sick people get well.

Although many chiropractors, then and now, have maintained that spinal or vertebral subluxations have more profound effects on health than subluxations of the extremities, **B.J. Palmer** went further. He simply stopped correcting subluxations beyond the spine, as a matter of both practice and philosophy, declaring such nonspinal subluxations to be of little significance to the chiropractor. Eventually, B.J. asserted that the only area of the spine capable of true subluxation was the upper cervical spine, the occipito-atlanto-axial region. For decades, between the early to mid-1930s and mid-1950s, the Palmer School's technique department taught only upper cervical methods (H.M. Himes, unpublished notes, 1956).

The split between the Palmers was one among many in the early years of the profession. In the first decade of the twentieth century, many competing schools of chiropractic were founded, such as the National School of Chiropractic (later National College of Chiropractic and now National University of Health Sciences), founded in 1906 by Palmer graduate **J.F. Alan Howard.** Many of these new schools were not simply new institutions, but also new schools of thought based on alternate interpretations of the most appropriate and efficient application of the ideas first expressed by D.D. Palmer a few years earlier.

AREAS OF CONTROVERSY

From this environment of creativity and controversy emerged various factions and viewpoints within the chiropractic community that still exist today. The key elements of division center on the following:

- Procedures that should appropriately be included and applied in the scope of chiropractic practice
- Range of effects of chiropractic care for the patient
- Clinical value of subluxation correction
- Appropriate terminology with which to describe chiropractic methods and their effects
- Questions that are related to isolation from or integration with other health care practitioners and professions, especially allopathic practitioners

SCOPE AND APPLICATION OF CHIROPRACTIC SERVICES

Differences of opinion as to the range of services that doctors of chiropractic should provide led early in the profession's history to the development of the labels *straight* and *mixer*. Most **straight** chiropractors focused almost exclusively on the vertebral subluxation and its manual adjustment. In contrast, many **mixer** practitioners used additional clinical approaches as adjuncts to adjusting the spine. Depending on state law and individual preference, such adjunctive therapies have included, but are not limited to, **physiotherapy**, dietary counseling and nutritional supplementation, **acupuncture**, midwifery, herbology, and **massage.**

An examination of their approaches to diagnosis provides further distinction between straight and mixer chiropractors. Before discussing these distinctions, it is important to note that all North American doctors of chiropractic, regardless of philosophic allegiances, are qualified as portal-of-entry providers and have the responsibility to determine whether a patient will likely benefit from chiropractic care and whether a patient should be referred for other care for a nonchiropractic health condition. In some cases, co-management with another practitioner is the appropriate choice.

Grouping chiropractors into straight and mixer categories is an oversimplification. Chiropractors' attitudes regarding diagnosis and methods of intervention vary substantially even within the straight and mixer categories. The following examples illustrate some of these combinations. The order of these examples is not intended to indicate the authors' preferences:

1. Chiropractors who primarily perform a musculoskeletal diagnostic workup and use adjustment as their sole intervention
2. Those who primarily perform a musculoskeletal diagnostic workup and use adjustments along with exercise, dietary recommendations, rehabilitation, other adjunctive procedures, or any combination
3. Those who perform no diagnosis beyond the analysis of spinal subluxations and use adjustments as their sole intervention
4. Those who perform a broad diagnostic workup, including the musculoskeletal and other systems, and practice as musculoskeletal specialists, using adjustments and various adjunctive procedures primarily for treating musculoskeletal disorders
5. Those who perform a broad diagnostic workup, including the musculoskeletal and other systems, and practice as complementary care generalists, using adjustments and adjunctive procedures with a strong emphasis on nutritional therapy, including supplements for treating disease
6. Those who limit their practice to diagnosis, specifically diagnostic imaging (chiropractic radiologists), and who serve as consulting specialists

A common denominator in examples 1 through 5 is the use of spinal adjustments to improve and maintain musculoskeletal function and to support the body's homeostatic mechanisms through the adjustment's effects on the nervous system, thus helping the body heal itself.

VALUE OF THE ADJUSTMENT, RANGE OF ITS CLINICAL EFFECTS

Many people who were trained in the early Palmer tradition viewed chiropractic care as a panacea or near-panacea for all ills of the human body. Correcting the vertebral subluxation was understood to be all that patients needed, and once this was accomplished, little else remained to consider or to do, other than to ensure that no new subluxations developed. Other practitioners viewed the adjustment as one among many natural approaches to bring aid and comfort to patients.

Currently, doctors of chiropractic, as well as some outside the profession, continue to debate the full clinical value of the chiropractic adjustment/manipulation and correcting subluxation or joint dysfunction. To pose the central question: Is the chiropractic adjustment the key to all the ills of humankind, or is its influence limited to musculoskeletal complaints? Although the vast majority of chiropractors hold positions in the broad middle ground between these extremes, the question of how to resolve conflicts among scientific evidence, anecdotal observation, belief, and tradition remains unanswered. At this time, despite advances in chiropractic research, many issues cannot be resolved based on firm evidence. Nevertheless, the way the profession ultimately addresses the inevitable conflicts between newly emerging evidence and traditional beliefs will undoubtedly shape its future.

LANGUAGE FOR DESCRIBING CHIROPRACTIC

Words have power, and the words used to describe the principles and practices of chiropractic continue to stir controversy. To some chiropractors, the issue is purely semantic; to others, it is a matter of principle in which the choice of terminology is a strong indicator of one's stance on major issues confronting the profession.

Should the chiropractor's primary manual intervention be called *adjustment* or *manipulation?* Is chiropractic care a form of **treatment** or does this term indicate something strictly allopathic? Similarly, is the chiropractic adjustment/manipulation a *therapy,* with *therapeutic effects,* or is it better termed an *intervention* or a *procedure?* Is the entity addressed by adjustment/manipulation a *subluxation, segmental dysfunction,* or *somatic joint dysfunction?* Is the practitioner of chiropractic to be known as a *chiropractor* or *chiropractic physician?* Doctors of chiropractic have argued over these and related matters for almost the entire history of the profession. This text cannot resolve such questions, but it can frame the issues in a nonadversarial context so that entry-level students and other readers can understand both points of view.

Notably, many uniquely chiropractic terms were first introduced so as to avoid criminal conviction for the illegal practice of medicine. On the advice of attorney Tom Morris in the 1907 *Morikubo v. Wisconsin* case,[10] the chiropractor argued that chiropractors analyze rather than diagnose, adjust rather than treat, that chiropractic is not therapeutic, and that chiropractors do not treat disease but instead adjust to remove subluxation, the cause of disease. Thus according to this reasoning, if medicine is defined as the diagnosis and treatment of disease, chiropractors were not guilty of practicing medicine.

To a great extent, controversy regarding choice of language in chiropractic springs from a concern on the part of straight chiropractors that adopting the language that the medical and osteopathic professions use (i.e., *manipulation, treatment* or *therapy*, and **lesion** or **somatic dysfunction** rather than *adjustment, intervention,* and *subluxation*) represents an unacceptable compromise for the sake of acceptance within the mainstream health care system. A parallel concern on the part of mixer chiropractors is that failing to adopt the terminology in widespread use throughout the health professions will contribute to the continued marginalization of chiropractic.

INTERPROFESSIONAL RELATIONS

Historically, relations between doctors of chiropractic and medical physicians have often been difficult, although this has begun to diminish in recent years. Having been disparaged by most medical physicians and attacked by political medicine since the profession's inception, many chiropractors have been understandably cautious in seeking alliances with medical physicians or integration into the mainstream medical delivery system. Although some chiropractors have always wanted to ally and integrate with the medical profession, others have staunchly opposed such moves. Ironically, the decision to integrate did not belong to the chiropractors; thus chiropractors remained outside of mainstream health care. This is finally changing.

As a profession matures, its relations with other professions must mature as well. Healthy interprofessional relations must be based on mutual respect and understanding. A key question for chiropractic's future is: How can chiropractic be integrated into the mainstream health care delivery system so that chiropractic services are readily available to all who can benefit from them? Moreover, of equal significance: How can such integration be achieved without diluting the unique identity of chiropractic to the point at which it is unrecognizable?

Probably, no single answer to these questions exists. The future shape of the profession will likely be worked out, step by step, in numerous pilot projects in a wide range of settings—in private chiropractic and medical practices in which interprofessional referral *in both directions* becomes the norm; in interdisciplinary (including joint chiropractic-medical) practices in which practitioners work out the best ways to cooperate for the benefit of their patients; and in larger-scale enterprises such as the health care systems serving veterans and the active duty military, in which chiropractic inclusion is now in its early stages. In each of these situations, it is important not to mistake uncertain beginnings for failures. Inevitably, as new relationships are developed and tested, both successes and difficulties will occur. Creating positive, sustainable interprofessional relations depends on a willingness by all involved parties to build on their successes and learn from their mistakes.

CONTEMPORARY EXPRESSIONS OF THE CHIROPRACTIC PARADIGM

Example One: Traditional Paradigm

Traditionally, the core chiropractic paradigm has included the following:

1. The body is a self-regulating and self-healing organism.
2. The nervous system is the master system that regulates and controls all other organs and tissues and relates the individual to his or her environment.
3. Spinal biomechanical dysfunction in the form of vertebral subluxation complex may adversely affect the nervous system's ability to regulate function.
4. The central focus of the doctor of chiropractic is to optimize patient health by correcting, managing, or minimizing vertebral subluxation through the chiropractic spinal adjustment.

These four points constitute the foundation of traditional chiropractic. Moreover, they convey this essence without metaphysical terminology. Chiropractors comfortable with the term *innate intelligence* will recognize this concept in the first component. Similarly, those chiropractors who prefer to think of self-regulation and healing in terms of homeostasis and normal physiologic function are accommodated. Notably, the relationship between structure and function as mediated by the nervous system is given prominence here. This principle is the essence, the distinctive feature, of chiropractic thought and practice.

Example Two: Biopsychosocial Paradigm

Other recent expressions of chiropractic's essence build on these core concepts, explicitly incorporating a contemporary *biopsychosocial* model of health. One such description[11] expresses the chiropractic paradigm as follows:

1. Health is the natural state of individuals, and any departure from this state represents a failure of the individual to

adapt to the internal and external environment or is the result of adverse adaptation. The innate tendency of the body is to restore and maintain health by (compensating) homeostatic mechanisms, reparative processes, and adaptive responses to genetic and acquired limitations.

2. Health is an expression of biologic, psychologic, social, and spiritual factors, and disease and illness is multicausal. This view is a holistic philosophy of health.

3. Optimal health is unique for any individual. Health involves enabling individuals to fulfill their biologic, human, and social potentials realistically. This viewpoint also implies individual responsibility for health. The chiropractor is simply the facilitator and, through cooperation with the patient, patient education, and adherence, they together achieve health for the patient. Health also implies a belief in healthy living (good nutrition, constructive exercise, stress management, and good posture).

4. The structure and functioning of the neuromusculoskeletal system is central to maintaining good health and combating disease. The functioning of the musculoskeletal system is integrated with neurologic function and is expressed by the various regulatory systems of the body.

Although they express the chiropractic paradigm in different terms, these two models have much in common and no overt areas of disagreement. The second model includes all the basic chiropractic premises of the first, with additional emphasis on the social and spiritual dimensions of health, the cooperative nature of the chiropractor-patient relationship, and the value of health-promoting self-care activities such as diet and exercise. As Ian Coulter, a professor at schools of dentistry and chiropractic who has written extensively on chiropractic and its role in the health care system, aptly notes in his book, *Chiropractic: A Philosophy for Alternative Health Care,*[9] when it comes to chiropractic intraprofessional philosophic disagreements, "to an outside observer, the differences in

terms of philosophy are less than the similarities," adding that "[t]hose external to the profession have had great difficulty in understanding the nature and importance of these philosophical issues."

Example Three: Association of Chiropractic Colleges Paradigm[12]

The preeminent contemporary expression of the chiropractic paradigm was written in 1996 by the presidents of all North American chiropractic colleges under the auspices of the **Association of Chiropractic Colleges** (ACC). These institutions, many of which were founded by early chiropractic leaders, represent the full spectrum of mainstream chiropractic thought. In a landmark of professional unity, every North American chiropractic college president agreed to a common paradigm (Fig. 2-1) that defines the purpose, principle, and practice of chiropractic. In the years following development of this ACC consensus document, other chiropractic organizations (including the **American Chiropractic Association, International Chiropractors Association, Canadian Chiropractic Association, World Federation of Chiropractic, Congress of Chiropractic State Associations,** and **World Chiropractic Alliance**) have endorsed it as a description of the paradigm under which chiropractors from all points on the spectrum practice (see Appendix III).

ASSOCIATION OF CHIROPRACTIC COLLEGES CONSENSUS DEFINITIONS

On chiropractic:

Chiropractic is a health-care discipline which emphasizes the inherent recuperative powers of the body to heal itself without the use of drugs or surgery.

The practice of chiropractic focuses on the relationship between structure (primarily of the spine) and function (as coordinated by the nervous system) and how that relationship affects the preservation and restoration of health.

Doctors of Chiropractic recognize the value and responsibility of working in cooperation with other health care practitioners when in the best interest of the patient.

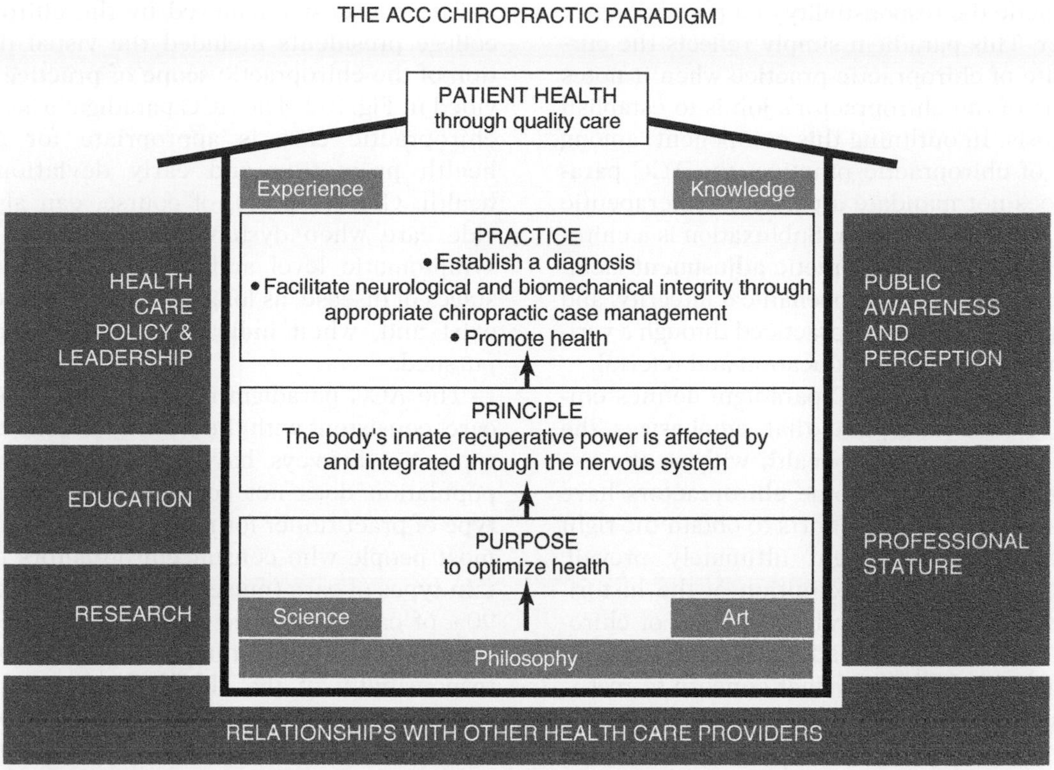

THE ACC CHIROPRACTIC PARADIGM

PATIENT HEALTH
through quality care

Experience | Knowledge

PRACTICE
- Establish a diagnosis
- Facilitate neurological and biomechanical integrity through appropriate chiropractic case management
- Promote health

PRINCIPLE
The body's innate recuperative power is affected by and integrated through the nervous system

PURPOSE
to optimize health

Science | Art

Philosophy

HEALTH CARE POLICY & LEADERSHIP

EDUCATION

RESEARCH

PUBLIC AWARENESS AND PERCEPTION

PROFESSIONAL STATURE

RELATIONSHIPS WITH OTHER HEALTH CARE PROVIDERS

Fig. 2-1 The ACC Chiropractic Paradigm, 1996. (*Association of Chiropractic Colleges, with permission.*)

The ACC continues to foster a unique, distinct chiropractic profession that serves as a health care discipline for all. The ACC advocates a profession that generates, develops, and utilizes the highest level of evidence possible in the provision of effective, prudent and cost-conscious patient evaluation and care.

On subluxation:

A subluxation is a complex of functional, structural, and/or pathological articular changes that compromise neural integrity and may influence organ system function and general health.

A subluxation is evaluated, diagnosed and managed through the use of chiropractic procedures based on the best available rational and empirical evidence.

The preservation and restoration of health is enhanced through the correction of the subluxation.

Examining several components of this paradigm in greater depth is instructive. First, the ACC paradigm emphasizes that the fundamental purpose of chiropractic is "to optimize health" and that "the body's innate recuperative power is

affected by and integrated through the nervous system." Across all differences in style, the substance of chiropractic rests on this foundation—that the body is self-regulating and self-healing and that the nervous system is the primary receptor, integrator, effector, and coordinator.

The practice of chiropractic is described to include appropriate diagnosis, facilitating neurologic and biomechanical integrity through chiropractic methods and promoting health. The attention given to the diagnostic responsibility of the doctor of chiropractic in this paradigm is noteworthy. Throughout the course of chiropractic history, chiropractors have debated the appropriateness of not only the term *diagnosis,* but also of the process that it entails. Some chiropractors have maintained that diagnosis is purely the purview of the allopathic practitioner and that because chiropractors do not focus on treating disease, an emphasis on the diagnosis of disease is contradictory. Current accreditation and licensing standards give to all doctors of chiropractic the responsibility of a portal of entry provider. This paradigm simply reflects the current state of chiropractic practice when it notes that part of the chiropractor's job is to establish a diagnosis. In outlining this component, among others, of chiropractic practice, the ACC paradigm does not mandate a particular therapeutic or management approach. Subluxation is a chiropractic diagnosis. Chiropractic **adjustment** facilitates neurologic and biomechanical integrity, and health promotion can be practiced through a variety of means, including education and referral.

Significantly, the ACC paradigm defines chiropractic as a discipline that emphasizes the body's ability to restore health without the use of drugs and surgery. Some chiropractors have expressed concern that efforts to obtain the right to prescribe drugs might ultimately prevail, resulting in a major redefinition of the historically conservative, natural orientation of chiropractic thought. The broad support for the ACC paradigm should help lay that concern to rest.

Addressing discord within the profession surrounding the meaningfulness of the term *subluxation,* the ACC paradigm stands behind continued use of this term, describing it as capable of compromising neural integrity and potentially influencing organ system function and general health.

The consensus achieved by the chiropractic college presidents included the visual description of the chiropractic **scope of practice** is provided in Fig. 2-2. The ACC paradigm asserts that chiropractic care is appropriate for general health promotion and early deviation from health. Chiropractors, of course, can also provide care when dysfunction progresses to the symptomatic level and even at the advanced stages of disease, as long as no contraindications exist and, when indicated, co-management is pursued.

The ACC paradigm encourages collaborative care, consistent with the way Americans use chiropractic. Surveys have documented that the population does not generally select only one type of practitioner for their health care. In fact, most people who consult chiropractors for certain types of care (musculoskeletal conditions in 90% of cases) also see a medical physician for other needs.[13] Implicit in the ACC diagram is the responsibility of the chiropractor to recognize when co-management and referral are appropriate. If the patient has a vertebral subluxation, the doctor of chiropractic is the most appropriate practitioner to manage that condition; however, the patient may have a concomitant problem that requires concurrent care by another health care

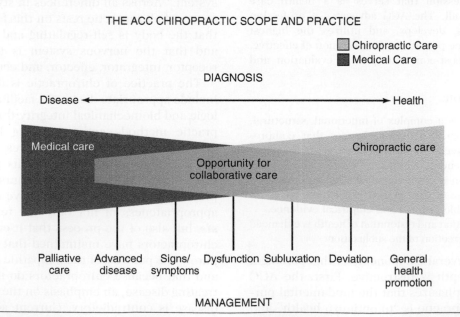

THE ACC CHIROPRACTIC SCOPE AND PRACTICE

☐ Chiropractic Care
■ Medical Care

DIAGNOSIS

Disease ←――――――――――――――――――――→ Health

Medical care   Chiropractic care

Opportunity for
collaborative care

Palliative   Advanced   Signs/   Dysfunction   Subluxation   Deviation   General
care   disease   symptoms   health
                                                                          promotion

MANAGEMENT

Fig. 2-2 ACC Chiropractic Scope and Practice. (*Association of Chiropractic Colleges, with permission.*)

practitioner. In some cases (e.g., an apparent malignancy on x-ray films), referring the patient out for immediate medical care before initiating chiropractic care is necessary.

Chiropractors have long used the Biologic Spectrum[14] or Health Continuum (Fig. 2-3) to educate patients about the processes of good health and the significance of preventive self-care activities.

These visual tools in combination with the ACC Scope and Practice diagram help demonstrate that health is not a state but rather a process. Further, they emphasize that disease is generally the result of long-standing alterations in the body's regulatory functions (pathophysiology) that may produce no symptoms and are thus undetected. In many cases, health care does not begin until symptoms are present. However, by the time symptoms are exhibited, the patient has often truly been "sick" for a very long time (Fig. 2-4).

Chiropractors, along with other nonallopathic practitioners, emphasize the value of care at the presymptomatic stage, when the patient is experiencing stress to the body-mind system. Intervention at this point seeks to prevent presymptomatic abnormalities from developing into disease. At this stage, the chiropractor acts largely as a health coach, advising the patient about conservative self-care strategies such as diet, exercise, and stress-management techniques. Similarly, the chiropractor checks the patient's spine for subluxations and provides adjustments to address spinal biomechanics to foster optimal functioning of the nervous system and thus to maintain health.

As the patient's condition progresses toward the right of the spectrum, the chiropractor or other doctor will be required to play a greater role in care. Self-care is still important; however, intervention to reduce symptoms and prevent progression is the focus. In some cases, this intervention may need to come from practitioners of various other disciplines and specialties.

ROLE OF PHILOSOPHY IN CHIROPRACTIC

The philosophy of chiropractic is alive and well in the profession. Growing numbers of chiropractic educators, practitioners, and researchers are

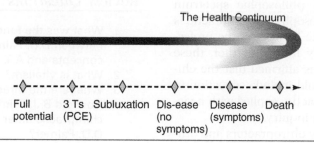

Fig. 2-3 Health continuum. Three Ts—Trauma, Thoughts, and Toxicity. *PCE*, Physical, chemical, emotional.

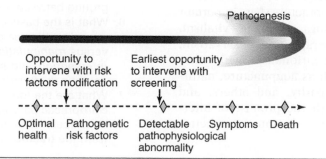

Fig. 2-4 Pathogenesis.[15]

engaging in spirited philosophic inquiry and discourse in professional publications and presentations. At a World Federation of Chiropractic (WFC) conference in November 2000, educators from chiropractic colleges around the world met to consider the role of philosophy in chiropractic education. That conference produced a series of consensus statements, including the following[16]:

1. A shared approach to health and healing, based upon a shared philosophy of chiropractic, is important for the identity and future of the chiropractic profession.
2. Chiropractic is a unique discipline, but it exists as part of a broader entity—the health care system. Accordingly, the discussion of philosophy as a discipline and the philosophy of health care, as well as specifically the philosophy of chiropractic, should be important components in every chiropractic curriculum.
3. The philosophy of chiropractic should be taught and developed in a manner that is intellectually defensible in the discipline of philosophy.

Significantly, chiropractic educators and representatives of chiropractic professional associations from all points on the philosophic spectrum agreed that a shared philosophy of chiropractic is important not only for the identity of the profession, but also for its very future. Further, these educators and associations affirmed that the chiropractic curriculum should include education in the philosophy of chiropractic, applied with a vigorous spirit of intellectual inquiry.

Recent publications by chiropractors and others have suggested that a robust philosophy of chiropractic does not require abandoning traditional chiropractic principles. These authors[9,17] have suggested that chiropractors share important philosophic underpinnings, including vitalism, holism, naturalism, therapeutic conservatism, humanism, and critical rationalism, with other healing disciplines, such as acupuncture, naturopathy, classical osteopathy, and others, and therefore they hold forth the promise of interdisciplinary cooperation in the interest of better serving patients.

DEALING WITH DUALISM

Chiropractic thought grew out of a seeming dualism of matter and intelligence that piqued D.D. Palmer's curiosity. Perhaps it should come as no surprise, then, that the profession that Palmer founded still struggles with this dualism, with thinkers and practitioners striving to understand science and philosophy, matter and intelligence, and structure and function. Seeing things in terms of either-or rather than both-and appears to be a general human tendency, and chiropractic is no stranger to this tendency. Various historic figures aligned themselves more closely with either vitalism or science. However, inferring that those who embraced the vitalistic philosophy were unable to understand science or were uninterested in its findings would be a mistake. Similarly mistaken is the notion that those chiropractors who strongly supported scientific exploration are not "principled" chiropractors. A need exists for both science and philosophy in the profession; there is room for both not only in the profession as a whole, but also within individual chiropractors.

Review *Questions*

1. What was the fundamental distinction between D.D. Palmer's chiropractic concepts and A.T. Still's osteopathy?
2. What is vitalism?
3. What are the three Ts?
4. How did B.J. Palmer's approach to chiropractic differ from that of D.D. Palmer?
5. What are some of the differences between the straight and mixer approaches to chiropractic? What are the areas of common ground between these approaches?
6. What is the basis of the controversy regarding the use of the terms *adjustment* versus *manipulation, treatment* versus *intervention,* and *subluxation* versus *somatic dysfunction?*
7. What are the four points in the traditional chiropractic paradigm?
8. How does the biopsychosocial model differ from the traditional model?

9. What are the main points of the ACC paradigm? What is unique about the development of this model?
10. What are the ACC definitions for *chiropractic* and *subluxation?*

Concept *Questions*

1. Is vitalism a necessary component of chiropractic? In what ways is the concept of vitalism consistent or inconsistent with contemporary health science?
2. What is philosophy? What is the philosophy of chiropractic? What is the appropriate role of philosophy in contemporary chiropractic?

REFERENCES

1. Moore JS: *Chiropractic in America: the history of a medical alternative,* Baltimore, 1993, Johns Hopkins University Press.
2. Pizzorno JE: Naturopathic medicine. In Micozzi MS, editor: *Fundamentals of complementary and alternative medicine,* New York, 1996, Churchill Livingstone.
3. Gevitz N: *The DOs: osteopathic medicine in America,* Baltimore, 1982, Johns Hopkins University Press.
4. Kaptchuk TJ: History of vitalism. In Micozzi MS, editor: *Fundamentals of complementary and alternative medicine,* ed 2, New York, 2001, Churchill Livingstone.
5. Gielow V: *Old dad chiro: a biography of D.D. Palmer, founder of chiropractic,* Davenport, Iowa, 1981, Bawden Bros.
6. Miller A: Transcendentalism's inspiration to chiropractic philosophy and practice, *Today's Chiropractic* 29:2, 2000.
7. Waagen G, Strang V: Origin and development of traditional chiropractic philosophy. In Haldeman S, editor: *Principles and practice of chiropractic,* ed 2, San Mateo, Calif, 1992, Appleton & Lange.
8. Palmer DD: *The chiropractor's adjustor,* Portland, Ore, 1910, Portland Printing House.
9. Coulter ID: *Chiropractic: a philosophy for alternative health care,* Oxford, 1999, Butterworth-Heinemann.
10. Rehm WS: Legally defensible: chiropractic in the courtroom, 1907 and after, *Chiropr Hist* 6:50, 1986.
11. Phillips RB et al: A contemporary philosophy of chiropractic for the Los Angeles College of Chiropractic, *J Chiropr Human* 4:20, 1994.
12. Association of Chiropractic Colleges, Minutes, Chicago, July 1, 1996.
13. Eisenberg DM et al: Perceptions about complementary therapies relative to conventional therapies among adults who use both: results from a national survey, *Ann Int Med* 135:344, 2001.
14. Strang V: *Essential principles of chiropractic,* Davenport, Iowa, 1984, Palmer College of Chiropractic.
15. Woolf SH, Jonas S, Lawrence RS, editors: *Health promotion and disease prevention in clinical practice,* Baltimore, 1996, Williams & Wilkins.
16. Chapman-Smith D, editor: New international consensus on philosophy, *Chiropractic Report* 15:1, 2001.
17. Gatterman M: A patient-centered paradigm: a model for chiropractic education and research, *J Altern Complement Med* 1:371, 1995.

9. What are the main points of the ACC paradigm? What is unique about the development of this model?

10. What are the ACC conditions for chiropractic and subluxation?

Concept Questions

1. Is vitalism a necessary component of chiropractic? In what ways is the concept of vitalism consistent or inconsistent with contemporary health sciences?

2. What is philosophy? What is the philosophy of chiropractic? What is the appropriate role of philosophy in contemporary chiropractic?

REFERENCES

1. Moore JS. Chiropractic in America: the Story of a medical alternative. Baltimore: 1993, Johns Hopkins University Press.

2. Wardwell WI. Chiropractic history and evolution of a new profession. New York: 1996, Mosby.

3. Gevitz N. The DOs: osteopathic medicine in America (2nd ed). 1982, Johns Hopkins University Press.

4. Keating JC. History of vitalism. In Morter MT, editor. Dynamic chiropractic: a comprehensive text reference. New York: 2001, Churchill Livingstone.

CHAPTER 3

Major Themes in Chiropractic History

Glenda Wiese, MA

Key Terms

AMERICAN CHIROPRACTIC
ASSOCIATION
ASSOCIATION OF
CHIROPRACTIC COLLEGES
BASIC SCIENCE LAWS
COMMITTEE ON QUACKERY
COUNCIL ON CHIROPRACTIC
EDUCATION
INTERNATIONAL
CHIROPRACTORS
ASSOCIATION

MANAGED CARE
ORGANIZATION
MEDICAID
MEDICARE
NATIONAL BOARD
OF CHIROPRACTIC
EXAMINERS
NATIONAL CHIROPRACTIC
ASSOCIATION
NATIONAL INSTITUTES OF
HEALTH

NEUROCALOMETER
PHYSIOLOGICAL
THERAPEUTICS
SUBLUXATION
UNIVERSAL CHIROPRACTORS
ASSOCIATION
WILK V. AMERICAN MEDICAL
ASSOCIATION
WORLD FEDERATION OF
CHIROPRACTIC

Within 5 years, chiropractic celebrated its centennial, chiropractic education celebrated 100 years, and a third millennium was ushered in. These times are appropriate to stop and consider the major themes in chiropractic history. The major themes of chiropractic are identified in this chapter and, when possible, are chronologically discussed. Although selection of any list of major events in chiropractic is, of course, a subjective process, this text relies heavily on the works of Walter Wardwell, Russell Gibbons, William Rehm, Herbert Vear, Vern Gielow, Pierre Louis Gaucher-Peslherbe, and Joseph Keating, Jr. in developing the selections and expounding on the themes that are discussed. The author of this text is indebted to these scholars of chiropractic history.

DANIEL DAVID PALMER AND THE FORMULATION OF THE CHIROPRACTIC THEORY

The occasion of the first chiropractic adjustment is, of course, the first major event in chiropractic.

Daniel David (D.D.) Palmer, Canadian by birth, performed the first adjustment on an African-American man, Harvey Lillard, on September 18, 1895, in Davenport, Iowa (Fig. 3-1). Palmer, who was 50 years old at the time, tells the story:

He had been so deaf for seventeen years that he could not hear the racket of a wagon or the ticking of a watch. I made inquiry as to the cause of his deafness, and was told that when he was exerting himself in a cramped, stooping position, he felt something give way in his back and immediately became deaf. An examination showed a vertebra racked from its normal position. I reasoned that if the vertebra was replaced, the man's hearing could be restored. I racked it into position by using the spinous process as a lever, and soon the man could hear as before. There was nothing "accidental" about this as it was accomplished with an objective in view, and the result expected was obtained.[1]

Palmer had been studying and practicing magnetic healing* since 1886, and his evolution

---

*Magnetic healing was a form of energy healing involving the laying on of hands. It may also have included vigorous rubbing and manipulation of various kinds.

from magnetic healing to chiropractic was gradual. He was well read in the fields of anatomy, physiology, neurology, and pathology[2] and used his extensive knowledge to develop a theory to explain his clinical successes. When Palmer applied his newly developed technique to other patients, he observed that other disorders responded to the thrusts he used to reposition vertebrae. One of his patients had a heart condition that had failed to respond to the usual medical care. Palmer examined the patient's spine and found a displaced fourth dorsal vertebra that he theorized was pressing against the nerves that segmentally innervate the heart. After he adjusted this segment of the spine, the patient experienced relief. Of this second attempt, Palmer said, "Then I began to reason, if two diseases, so dissimilar as deafness and heart trouble, came from impingement, a pressure on the nerves, were not other diseases due to a similar cause?"[3]

D.D. Palmer accepted his first student in 1897, and soon students were graduating from his Palmer School and Infirmary (later renamed Palmer School of Chiropractic [PSC]) to both practice and teach chiropractic. In 1903, D.D. Palmer and his son Bartlett Joshua (B.J.) formed an equal partnership, which was to continue until 1906. In that year, D.D. Palmer was tried and found guilty in Scott County, Iowa, of prac-

ticing medicine without a license, after which he sold his share of the PSC to his son and moved west, where he opened schools in Oklahoma, Oregon, and California.

After leaving Davenport, D.D. Palmer assembled a collection of his writings in his 1000-page magnum opus, *The Chiropractor's Adjuster: A Textbook of the Science, Art, and Philosophy of Chiropractic for Students and Practitioners* (1910). Undoubtedly, D.D. Palmer's formulation of the theory of chiropractic and its elucidation through his writings are the seminal and most important event in the history of chiropractic.

B.J. PALMER AND THE DEVELOPMENT OF CHIROPRACTIC

B.J. Palmer was the second major influence on the development of chiropractic (Fig. 3-2). Always careful to describe his father as the

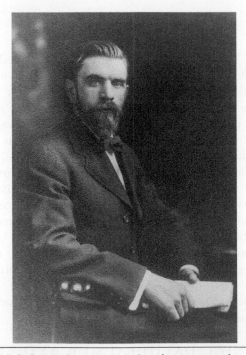

Fig. 3-2 B.J. Palmer, D.D. Palmer's son, president of the Palmer School of Chiropractic (PSC) from 1906 until his death in 1961 and a leading force in the development of chiropractic. (*Courtesy Library Special Collections, Palmer College of Chiropractic, Davenport, Iowa.*)

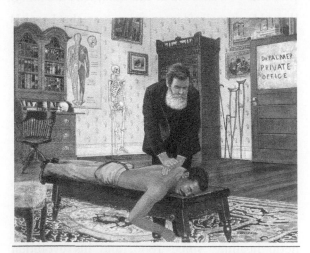

Fig. 3-1 Artist John Dyeuss' rendering of the first adjustment, performed by D.D. Palmer on Harvey Lillard, September 1895. (*Courtesy Chiropractic Centennial Foundation, Davenport, Iowa.*)

"founder" of chiropractic, B.J. Palmer considered himself the "developer" of chiropractic, and proceeded to do so in style. On purchasing his father's half of PSC, B.J. began developing it into one of the largest health practitioner schools in the country, with the school's population growing from 400 in 1911 to 3000 by 1923.[4] Both Gibbons[5] and Wardwell[6] attribute the survival of the fledgling chiropractic profession to B.J. Palmer's flamboyant marketing and his dogged insistence that chiropractic remain "pure and unadulterated." According to Wardwell, "Without B.J. chiropractic might not have survived. A colorful multimedia salesman for chiropractic, he used lectures, pamphlets, 27 books, and his own radio station to spread the word about chiropractic to students, patients, and the public."[7] B.J. was a charismatic and energetic speaker who traveled around the country, boosting chiropractic and testifying on behalf of chiropractors before courts and state legislatures. Although B.J. was a controversial figure, his pronouncements against raising educational standards (he declared that they were "veneer and polish..., which [would] weaken the profession and cause a large reduction in the number of chiropractors,") were used in the courtroom against chiropractic; however, not a man or woman who knew him questioned his undying loyalty to chiropractic.

DEFENSE OF CHIROPRACTIC IN COURT

A third major event or series of events in the history of chiropractic was the struggle to defend chiropractors in court against the charge of practicing medicine without a license. Although D.D. Palmer was not the first to be accused of practicing medicine or osteopathy without a license (he was tried and found guilty of the offense in 1906), the trial of Shegataro Morikubo (PSC graduate, 1903) in La Crosse, Wisconsin, in 1907 was a watershed event that helped determine the strategy that chiropractors would adopt to defend themselves against future charges of unlicensed medical practice.

The jury acquitted Morikubo. The defense attorney, Tom Morris, convinced the jury that

chiropractic was not osteopathy or medicine; rather, it was a new form of treatment. B.J. Palmer retained Tom Morris as counsel for the **Universal Chiropractors Association** (UCA), and they proceeded to use the argument that chiropractic was a separate and distinct science from medicine. The central purpose of the UCA, with B.J. Palmer serving as its secretary for 20 years, was to raise funds to pay bail and fines for arrested chiropractors who adhered to the "straight" chiropractic philosophy. In addition, its purpose was to defend chiropractors in court and to lobby for state licensure of chiropractors, separate and distinct from medical practice acts. By 1927 the UCA had defended chiropractors in 3300 court cases.[8]

OTHER PIONEERS

Although B.J. Palmer casts a giant shadow on the landscape of chiropractic history, several other influential pioneers deserve mention.

Solon Langworthy, the founder of the first school to provide serious competition to D.D. Palmer's PSC, was very influential in early chiropractic history (Fig. 3-3). With Oakley Smith and Minora Paxson, Solon Langworthy published the first textbook on chiropractic in 1906, *A Textbook of Modernized Chiropractic*. He also published an early journal, *The Backbone*, which D.D. and B.J. used as a model for their journal, *The Chiropractor*. Langworthy also organized the first chiropractic association in 1905, the **American Chiropractic Association** (ACA) (not related to the current ACA). Although Langworthy's school, journal, and association did not last long, his impact was far reaching on the early profession.

Willard Carver had been a friend and sometimes legal counsel for D.D. Palmer, but he graduated from the Charles Ray Parker School of Chiropractic in Ottumwa, Iowa, in 1906, rather than from PSC. Carver referred to himself as the "constructor" of chiropractic, as opposed to B.J. Palmer being called the "developer," and he referred to his college in Oklahoma City as the "Science Head," in contrast to B.J. Palmer's "Fountainhead." Carver went on to preside over four separate institutions in Oklahoma City,

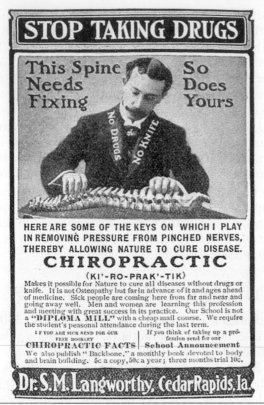

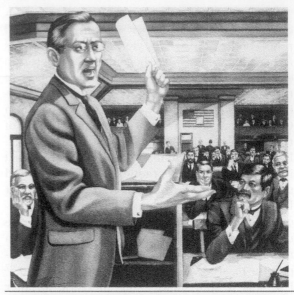

Fig. 3-4 Willard Carver fighting for chiropractic legislation in Oklahoma. *(Painted by Robert Lawson. Courtesy Chiropractic Centennial Foundation, Davenport, Iowa.)*

Fig. 3-3 Solon Langworthy, president of the American School of Chiropractic in Cedar Rapids, Iowa, co-author of the first chiropractic textbook, editor of the early journal *The Backbone*, and the first serious competitor to the PSC. (*Courtesy Library Special Collections, Palmer College of Chiropractic, Davenport, Iowa.*)

Washington, D.C., New York, and Denver, which eventually merged with other schools. When the new Oklahoma legislature convened in 1907, Carver introduced the first bill to legalize chiropractic in that state (Fig. 3-4). It did not pass. For years, his training as a lawyer would be used when called on to testify for chiropractic in legislative hearings. Carver authored 18 books and exerted a great influence on the new profession.

John Howard, a 1905 graduate of the PSC, resigned from the PSC faculty in 1906 and started a competing school in the same building in which D.D. Palmer first practiced and formulated his theory of chiropractic. Howard moved his National School of Chiropractic (NSC) to Chicago in 1908, where it was able to take advan-

tage of its proximity to Cook County Hospital to offer observation of surgeries. By 1912 the school was offering **physiological therapeutics** and had several medical physicians on its faculty. In 1914, Howard sold the NSC to one of its faculty, William Schultz, M.D. Under Schultz's leadership, NSC became the major broad scope chiropractic influence. It was eclectic in its approach, and it offered physiologic therapeutics, naturopathy, and various other adjunctive procedures, in strong contrast to B.J. Palmer's straight, hands-only approach to chiropractic.

Tullius Ratledge, another early chiropractic educator, heavily influenced the development of the profession in California. He moved his school from Kansas to California in 1911 and continued as President of the Ratledge College of Chiropractic until he sold it in 1951 to Carl Cleveland, Sr. Ratledge served 75 days in jail in California in 1916 rather than pay his fine. In one year alone, 450 chiropractors were jailed in California for practicing medicine without a license.[9] Ratledge was active in the 1922 California referendum, which won licensure for chiropractors. California Governor

Friend Richardson pardoned all chiropractors in jail at the time of the referendum's passage, declaring they had been unjustly accused.

Sylva Ashworth, the last pioneer in this attenuated list, graduated from the PSC in 1910 and became active in Nebraska state politics, serving on the first chiropractic board of examiners for that state. Her daughter, Ruth, and son-in-law, Carl Cleveland (1917 PSC graduates), started the Central College of Chiropractic in Kansas City in 1922, renaming it the Cleveland Chiropractic College in 1924. In 1951, Carl Cleveland took leadership of the Ratledge College of Chiropractic, renaming it the Cleveland Chiropractic College of Los Angeles in 1955. Sylva's great-great grand-daughter, Ashley, became the world's first fifth-generation chiropractor, and she currently serves as an administrator and faculty member at Cleveland Chiropractic College–Kansas City (Fig. 3-5, A-G).

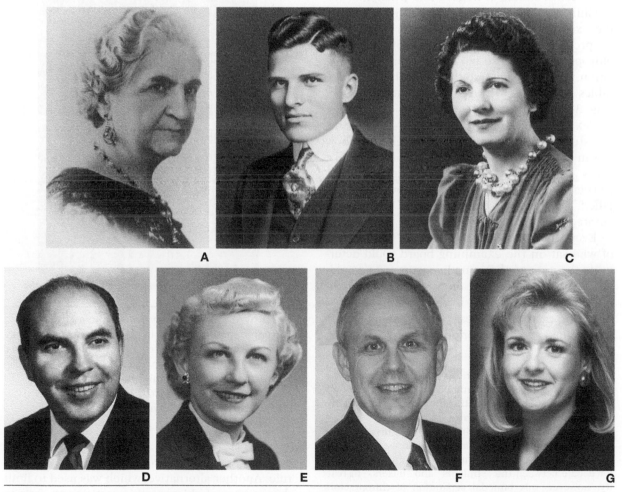

Fig. 3-5 The first five-generation chiropractic family. **A,** Sylva L. Ashworth, PSC 1910; **B,** Carl S. Cleveland, Sr., PSC 1917; **C,** Ruth R. (Ashworth) Cleveland, PSC 1917; **D,** Carl S. Cleveland, Jr., CCC 1942; **E,** Mildred G. Cleveland, DC, CCC 1954. **F,** Carl S. Cleveland, III, CCC 1975. **G,** Ashley E. Cleveland, CCC 1995. *(Courtesy Cleveland Chiropractic College, Kansas City, Mo.)*

STRUGGLE FOR LICENSING LEGISLATION

The fifth major event—actually, a series of events—that chronicle chiropractic's struggle for state licensure, was an effort that would require diligence for over 60 years. Politics, both that of organized medicine against chiropractic and that of "mixer" and "straight" chiropractors against each other,* extended the process in the United States from before 1913 when the first state, Kansas, licensed chiropractors, until 1974, when legislation for chiropractic was passed in Louisiana.[10] The years between are filled with hundreds of stories of tragedy and triumph.

Chiropractors in California provided a striking example of success after years of struggle. As previously noted, more than 450 California chiropractors went to jail rather than pay a fine. Often, they would set up their portable adjusting tables and proceed to treat their patients in jail (Fig. 3-6, A).

Texan Charles Lemley (1892-1970) was arrested 66 times. A parade was held for fellow Texan Paul Meyers, complete with patients and a brass band, when he was released from jail. Herbert Reaver held the record for the "most jailed," having paid eight fines and been incarcerated four times in Ohio (Fig. 3-6, B).

Even when licensing was granted, the question of who sat on the examining board could determine the ease of obtaining licensure for a would-be practitioner. States dominated by straight chiropractors tended to have boards dominated by chiropractors, whereas states dominated by mixers had medically oriented boards in many

---

*"Mixers" have been historically referred to as chiropractors who use ancillary methods to treat their patients in addition to the chiropractic adjustment. These methods may include electrotherapy, hydrotherapy, acupuncture, acupressure, and vitamin therapy. The disagreement over whether these ancillary procedures are within the purview of the chiropractor has formed the basis for debate between the "straights" and "mixers." In reality, however, this bimodal separation of chiropractors has never existed. In a statistical sense, there is a "normal" distribution, with most chiropractors falling somewhere in the middle (see Chapter 2 for further discussion).

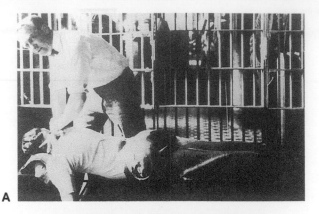

A

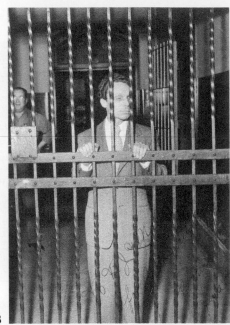

B

Fig. 3-6 A, Fred Courtney, one of the many chiropractors prosecuted in California for practicing medicine without a license, is shown adjusting from his jail cell in Los Angeles, circa 1921. B, Herbert Reaver, the most jailed chiropractor. (A *from Fountainhead News 19(26), 1921.* B *courtesy Library Special Collections, Palmer College of Chiropractic, Davenport, Iowa.)*

cases, although there are many exceptions to this rule. Another alternative, which was used to limit the number of chiropractic practitioners, was to examine all practitioners—medical, osteopathic, and chiropractic—by the same "basic-science board."

INTRODUCTION OF THE NEUROCALOMETER

In August 1924 in a speech entitled, "The Hour Has Struck," B.J. Palmer introduced the **neurocalometer** to the profession. It was a hand-held, heat-sensing instrument, which he insisted was necessary for the chiropractor to detect subluxations. It could be leased for a fee that would include lessons in how to use it and periodic checks and repairs. Many B.J. supporters believed the cost of leasing the instrument was exorbitant and that B.J.'s insistence on its use downplayed the efficacy of palpation in detecting subluxations. The neurocalometer controversy, the sixth event in the history of chiropractic selected in this text, coincided with B.J. Palmer's dramatic transition from using full-spine adjusting techniques to using the upper cervical-only Hole-in-One (HIO) technique, and it marked the beginning of the decline of B.J. Palmer's influence in the field. Although he would continue to exert a powerful influence on the profession, he would no longer be its undisputed leader.

DEVELOPMENT OF TWO STRONG NATIONAL ASSOCIATIONS

The development of two strong national associations was the seventh influence to shape chiropractic. Partially as a result of the erosion of support for B.J. Palmer and partially as a result of tougher **basic science laws*** and a renewed medical assault, by 1929, PSC's enrollment had dropped by 90%.[11] By 1930 the importance and influence of the UCA declined, with a 50% drop

---

*Basic science laws established examinations that certified candidates from all major healing arts in the basic sciences of anatomy, pathology, physiology, chemistry, and public health. These laws were enacted with the purpose of excluding chiropractors and other practitioners with supposedly inadequate training. The basic science laws elevated educational standards in those professions in which students had difficulty passing the examinations. By 1969, chiropractic education had improved to the point that four state basic science boards recognized the chiropractic board examinations as being equivalent. By 1980, all states had repealed their basic science laws.

in membership. B.J. Palmer resigned as secretary-treasurer, and the UCA merged with the original ACA to form the fledgling **National Chiropractic Association** (NCA). B.J. Palmer continued to exert his influence through the Chiropractic Health Bureau, renamed the **International Chiropractors Association** (ICA) in 1941. A campaign to merge the two national associations in 1963 resulted in a new ACA, with a resulting smaller membership in the ICA.

In 1987 a renewed effort to merge the two national associations led to their first joint convention in Las Vegas, Nevada. Promerger forces led by ICA president Michael Pedigo and vice-president Virgil Strang secured a majority vote of ICA members in favor of the merger, but they failed to achieve the constitutionally required two-thirds vote. Antimerger forces were led by Sid Williams, who became president of a smaller ICA after some in the promerger camp (including Pedigo and J.F. McAndrews) left to join ACA. Pedigo later became the first and only chiropractor to have served as president of both ICA and ACA; McAndrews, a former ICA executive director and former president of Palmer College, became ACA's Vice-President for Professional Affairs. The two organizations continue to remain separate, and the straight-mixer, narrowscope-broadscope split that began over 100 years ago continues to this day.

CAMPAIGN BY THE AMERICAN MEDICAL ASSOCIATION TO "CONTAIN AND ELIMINATE" CHIROPRACTIC

The eighth event, the American Medical Association's (AMA's) campaign to eliminate chiropractic, first started in the 1920s and accelerated in 1963 when the AMA founded its **Committee on Quackery** (originally called the Committee on Chiropractic). When chiropractic sought inclusion in **Medicare**, the Secretary of Health, Education, and Welfare's report recommended that chiropractic not be included, because it was "not based upon the body of basic knowledge . . . that has been widely accepted by the scientific community," and that "the scope and quality of chiropractic education do not prepare the practitioner to make an adequate diagnosis and provide appropriate treatment."[12] It was later revealed in internal AMA documents in the landmark **Wilk v. AMA** et al. antitrust case that the AMA heavily influenced the results of Secretary Cohen's report and that these results had been determined in advance.

Next, the AMA launched an aggressive campaign against chiropractic in popular journals such as *Reader's Digest, Consumer Reports,* and *Good Housekeeping*. In response to the vitriolic campaign against chiropractors, the ICA and ACA worked together to publish *Chiropractic's White Paper on Health, Education, and Welfare Secretary's Report* (1969), contesting the data and its conclusions. Since then, the ICA and ACA have held a joint legislative conference in Washington, D.C. (1983) and have frequently joined forces to respond to legislative threats.

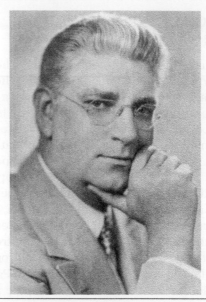

Fig. 3-7 John Nugent, PSC 1922, spearheaded early reforms in chiropractic education. *(From The National Chiropractic Journal, November 1941.)*

COUNCIL ON CHIROPRACTIC EDUCATION (ACCREDITATION)

The ninth event to influence chiropractic history was the recognition of a national chiropractic accrediting agency. Early chiropractic education lacked consistent standards; significant variations in the duration and quality of educational curricula existed. John Nugent, often referred to as the "Abraham Flexner" of chiropractic, was appointed chair of the NCA's committee on educational standards in 1935 (Fig. 3-7). For the next 30 years he cajoled and threatened the heads of the chiropractic schools, mostly for-profit educational enterprises, to adopt stricter, more stringent standards. He believed that chiropractic education must be raised to a level that the academic community and the federal and professional accrediting agencies would recognize. The numbers tell the story. In 1930, 42 chiropractic institutions existed, most with courses of 18 months or less. When Nugent retired in 1963. 15 chiropractic educational institutions were operating in the United States with all but 3 having made the transition to professionally owned, not-for-profit educational institutions with independent boards of directors.[13]

The NCA Committee on Educational Standards became the **Council on Chiropractic Education** (CCE) in 1947. In 1953 the CCE made the 4-year curriculum standard, and by 1968 it had adopted the 2-year preprofessional requirement. In 1974 the U.S. Office of Education recognized the CCE as the official accrediting agency for all chiropractic colleges.

Currently, 16 U.S. and 2 Canadian chiropractic colleges are operating in North America; all are nonprofit and require a minimum of 3 years prechiropractic collegiate studies, and they all offer a 4- to 5-academic-year chiropractic program. With the advent of Bachelor programs in biology and Master programs in anatomy, nutrition, and sports chiropractic, most colleges have achieved regional accreditation, as well as CCE recognition.

As the sole educational accrediting agency for chiropractic colleges, CCE was the first entity to bridge the gap among the various factions in chiropractic education effectively, bringing all of the key stakeholders to the same table. This fact is as important as CCE's role in standardizing chiropractic education and elevating its standards.

CHIROPRACTIC COVERAGE BY MEDICARE AND OTHER INSURANCE PLANS

The inclusion of chiropractic in insurance plans is the tenth key event in chiropractic history. According to Wardwell,[14] chiropractors competed on a level playing field, economically speaking, until third parties began paying for health care. As Medicare, **Medicaid**, and employee group health insurance plans paid for more health care services in the United States after World War II, chiropractors faced a crisis. Patients would only pay chiropractors out-of-pocket, forgoing their insurance, if they were wealthy, dedicated, or desperate. Chiropractors used political action to pass "insurance equality laws." Despite the AMA's strongest opposition, Congress voted to include chiropractors under Medicare in 1972. Currently, more than one half of all federal, state, and private health plans include chiropractic coverage, although there are often restrictions on the number of patient visits or the modalities used.

THE NATIONAL INSTITUTE FOR NEUROLOGICAL AND COMMUNICATIVE DISEASES AND STROKE CONFERENCE

The eleventh event was a conference held in 1975 at the Bethesda, Maryland, campus of **National Institutes of Health** (NIH), sponsored by the U.S. Congress as an "independent, unbiased study of the fundamentals of the chiropractic profession." Medical physicians, osteopaths, and chiropractors assembled to discuss spinal manipulative therapy. In the resulting document, *The Research Status of Spinal Manipulative Therapy*, edited by osteopathic physician Murray Goldstein, most of the participants concluded that spinal manipulation:

Provides relief from pain, particularly back pain, and sometimes cures, and may be dangerous, particularly if used by non-physicians; [there was] a difference of opinion focusing on the issues of indications, contraindications, and the precise scientific basis for the results obtained.[15]

In the years following the National Institute for Neurological and Communicative Diseases and Stroke (NINCDS) Conference, other interdisciplinary conferences on the spine took place; in 1982 the American Back Society was founded to promote interdisciplinary conferences of chiropractors, osteopaths, physical therapists, and medical physicians. The 1990s witnessed the beginning of significant interdisciplinary research and substantial NIH grants to chiropractic colleges to study chiropractic scientific principles and the clinical benefits of chiropractic care.

WILK ANTITRUST SUIT

In 1976, Chester Wilk and four other chiropractors, Patricia Arthur, James Bryden, Steven Lumsden, and Michael Pedigo, launched the twelfth event—an antitrust suit against the AMA and 10 other medical organizations (Fig. 3-8).

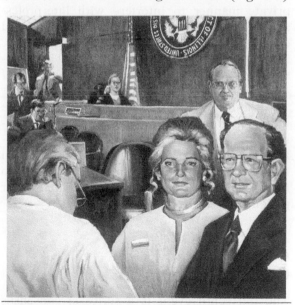

Fig. 3-8 Artist Kirk Miller's rendering of the Wilk and colleagues courtroom victory. In October 1976, five chiropractors filed suit against the American Medical Association (AMA) and 10 other health care associations to stop the boycott against chiropractic. Depicted in the foreground (*left to right*) are Michael Pedigo, Patricia Arthur, and Chester Wilk. In the background is attorney for the plaintiffs, George McAndrews. Seated behind the bench is Judge Susan Getzendanner. (*Courtesy Chiropractic Centennial Foundation.*)

They charged that the AMA and others had engaged in a conspiracy to monopolize health care and restrain competition by making voluntary professional associations between doctors of medicine and doctors of chiropractic unethical. Further, they contended that the AMA had been working with medical physician–dominated insurance companies to strangle the chiropractic profession economically. After two 8-week court trials and two appeals to the United States Court of Appeals for the Seventh Circuit (and one petition to the United States Supreme Court by the defendant medical societies, which was denied), United States District Judge Susan Getzendanner found the AMA guilty in late 1987 of an illegal effort to destroy the profession of chiropractic through boycott. She entered an injunction, national in scope (which is still in force today), prohibiting the AMA and all who act in concert with the AMA from acting in any private manner to interfere with interprofessional relations between medical physicians and doctors of chiropractic and their institutions. She also required the AMA to publish her decision in *The Journal of the American Medical Association*.

Although interprofessional relations have improved in the last 15 years, the economic reality is that medical physicians and their organizations continue to use their influence on insurance companies, hospitals, and media to influence doctors of chiropractic and their patients adversely.

ASSOCIATION OF CHIROPRACTIC COLLEGES PARADIGM

The thirteenth event is a series of consensus statements. In July 1996 the **Association of Chiropractic Colleges** (ACC), represented by the presidents of all seventeen CCE accredited schools, presented a series of consensus statements,[16] which sought "to clarify professional common ground" and to define chiropractic's role within the health care system. For the first time in 100 years of chiropractic education, all U.S. chiropractic college presidents reached a unanimous consensus on definitions fundamental to

chiropractic. The ACC position on chiropractic follows:

- Chiropractic is a health care discipline that emphasizes the inherent recuperative power of the body to heal itself without the use of drugs or surgery.
- The practice of chiropractic focuses on the relationship between structure (primarily the spine) and function (as coordinated by the nervous system) and how that relationship affects the preservation and restoration of health. In addition, doctors of chiropractic recognize the value and responsibility of working in cooperation with other health care practitioners when it is in the best interest of the patient to do so.
- The ACC continues to foster a unique, distinct chiropractic profession that serves as a health care discipline for all. The ACC advocates a profession that generates, develops, and uses the highest level of evidence possible in the provision of effective, prudent, and cost-conscious patient evaluation and care.[17]

The ACC's position on **subluxation** is:

- Chiropractic is concerned with the preservation and restoration of health and focuses particular attention on subluxation.
- Subluxation is a complex of functional or structural (or both) and/or pathologic articular changes that compromise neural integrity and may influence organ system function and general health.
- A subluxation is evaluated, diagnosed, and managed through the use of chiropractic procedures based on the best available rational and empirical evidence.[18]

See Chapter 2 for further discussion of the ACC paradigm.

In November 2000 the **World Federation of Chiropractic** (WFC), in association with the ACC and the **National Board of Chiropractic Examiners**, met in Fort Lauderdale, Florida, to discuss philosophy in chiropractic education. From that meeting came the following consensus statements:

- A shared approach to health and healing, based upon a shared philosophy of chiropractic, is important for the identity and future of the chiropractic profession.

- Chiropractic is a unique discipline, but it exists as part of a broader entity—the health care system. Accordingly, the discussion of philosophy as a discipline and the philosophy of health care, as well as the philosophy of chiropractic specifically, should be important components in every chiropractic curriculum.
- The philosophy of chiropractic should be taught and developed in a manner that is intellectually defensible in the discipline of philosophy.[19]

CHIROPRACTIC IN THE MILITARY

In January 2002, President Bush signed the Department of Veterans Affairs Health Care Programs Enhancement Act of 2001. The bill included a mandate to establish a permanent chiropractic benefit within the Department of Veterans Affairs (DVA) health care system. The passage of this bill represented a victory in a struggle that began in 1944 when Representative J.H. Tolan of California first introduced similar legislation. The bill was sponsored by House Veterans Committee Chairman Christopher Smith (R-New Jersey) and personally championed in the Senate by Majority Leader Tom Daschle (D-South Dakota).

This legislation authorized the hiring of chiropractors in the DVA health system; it set a broad scope of chiropractic practice and allowed the chiropractic profession to participate in the implementation of the new benefits through an advisory committee partially composed of chiropractors.

Key provisions of the DVA law include (1) immediate phase-in of the program, (2) designation of at least one DVA medical center in each geographic service area of the Veterans Health Administration to provide chiropractic services, and (3) a scope of chiropractic services that provides a variety of chiropractic care with services for neuromusculoskeletal conditions, including the subluxation complex.

For years, the chiropractic profession had also lobbied, with little success, the Department of Defense (DoD) to open its health care facilities to chiropractors. In 1995 the DoD agreed to a 5-year Chiropractic Health Care Demonstration Program with test sites at 13 different military installations. The Oversight Advisory Committee evaluating this project reported that 81.5% of the chiropractic patients described the improvement in their condition as "excellent," and that incorporating chiropractic could save the military $28 million in lost work days as a result of back pain and other musculoskeletal conditions. In response to the overwhelmingly positive results of the demonstration project, President Clinton signed P.L. 106-398 into law in October 2000, mandating that chiropractic care be made available to all active-duty personnel.

These two events, the passage of the DVA and Veterans Affairs bills, coming as they did within 15 months of each other, are the fourteenth major event in the history of chiropractic. Another area of the military in which the chiropractic profession continues to seek recognition is the awarding of commissions similar to those received by podiatrists, optometrists, and psychologists.

CHIROPRACTORS IN HOSPITAL AND INTEGRATED SETTINGS

Early in the history of chiropractic, some chiropractors could admit patients to hospitals and treat them there. With the AMA's antichiropractic campaign in the 1960s and its insistence on a strict adherence to the Code of Medical Ethics (which prohibited association with a chiropractor), hospitals were unable to admit chiropractors on their staffs if they wished to gain or keep accreditation. After the chiropractic victory in the antitrust suit, hospitals began to open their doors slowly to chiropractors, which represents the fifteenth major event in chiropractic history. The first hospital to accept chiropractors on its staff was Lindell Hospital in St. Louis in 1984.[20] By 1990, at least 60 hospitals and ambulatory surgical centers had chiropractors on staff[21]; by 1997, that number had grown to approximately 200.[22] Although the number of hospitals granting privileges to chiropractors continues to grow, they remain a minority.

Another consequence of the AMA's removal of the ban on medical physicians cooperating with chiropractors has been the increase in the formation of multidisciplinary clinics and practices. Most opportunities for chiropractors to practice in integrated settings involve family practice or pain management groups. Other opportunities lie with acupuncturists, naturopaths, massage therapists, psychologists, and other complementary practitioners. The complexities of starting such a practice are many, but the potential for improved patient care is great. "If managed by caring, competent, and compassionate people, the multidisciplinary practice holds forth the possibility of a more integrated, patient-centered model."[23]

RESEARCH RESULTING IN RECOGNITION BY THE UNITED STATES, GREAT BRITAIN, AND CANADA

During the 1990s, several research reports were favorable toward chiropractic. These reports represent the sixteenth major event in chiropractic history. The RAND study (1992)[23] found that spinal manipulation benefits some patients with acute low back pain, and it is appropriate for many patients with acute low back pain and for some patients with subacute low back pain. In a study published in the *British Medical Journal*, Meade and colleagues (1995) found a "29% greater improvement in patients with back pain treated with chiropractic compared to those treated with hospital outpatient management."[24] In Canada, two studies commissioned by the provincial government of Ontario, authored by health economist Pran Manga in 1993[25] and 1998,[26] recommended that the government increase coverage of chiropractic, expand chiropractic privileges, and facilitate more cooperation between chiropractic and medical professionals. In 1994 the U.S. Agency for Health Care Policy and Research released its *Clinical Guideline Number 14: Acute Low Back Problems in Adults*,[27] which concluded that

spinal manipulation is one of the most effective and safest treatments for low back pain.

IMPACT OF MANAGED CARE

Because **managed care organizations** (MCOs) currently play a dominant role in the American health care marketplace, their policies toward chiropractic are critical to the future of chiropractic and represent the seventeenth event influencing chiropractic. MCOs have been slow to accept chiropractic, and when they accept chiropractic services, the range of covered services is often narrowly defined. In addition, MCOs seldom grant chiropractors status as primary care providers, which means that in some cases, referral from a medical physician is required to receive reimbursement. A key struggle for chiropractic in the new century will be its full participation in managed care plans. Although 41 states mandate insurance reimbursements for chiropractic services,[28] most managed care providers claimed that state-mandated insurance coverage was not an important factor in determining chiropractic coverage. All six of the new MCOs in 2000 who responded to a survey listed market demand and consumer interest as primary motivators for offering coverage for complementary and alternative services. Of the six MCOs responding to the survey, all but one included some degree of chiropractic care. (For a more detailed discussion on managed care, see Chapter 29.)

CONCLUSION

The Palmers and the other pioneers that followed were of a different time, yet their concepts have weathered an entire century. Chiropractic has responded to forces similar to those that challenged nineteenth century medical sectarians—and it has survived. The political climate, educational reforms, and legislative trends, as well as the rise of a strong medical community and the increased research in chiropractic efficacy, are factors that are enormously influential in the marketplace of health care. Chiropractic has survived and flourished in a century that witnessed the demise or assimilation of several other healing disciplines. Understanding our history, Santayana suggests, may help us avoid the mistakes or pitfalls of the past.

Review *Questions*

1. How did D.D. Palmer found chiropractic?
2. What was the neurocalometer? Why was it controversial when introduced?
3. What was the first national chiropractic association? Who organized it?
4. What were the first and last states in the United States to license chiropractors? In what years were these licenses granted?
5. Historically, what issues divided straight and mixer chiropractors?
6. In the Morikubo case, what was the basis for the chiropractor's defense against charges of practicing medicine without a license?
7. Which chiropractor was arrested 66 times on charges of practicing medicine without a license?
8. When did the U.S. Office of Education recognize the CCE as the official accrediting agency for all chiropractic colleges?
9. What was the final verdict in the Wilk v. AMA case?
10. What is the current status of chiropractic in military and veterans health care in the United States?

Concept *Questions*

1. What are the advantages (if any) and disadvantages (if any) of having two major national chiropractic associations rather than one?
2. What unifying beliefs and objectives are common to all groups in the chiropractic profession? How might these be used to support the advancement of chiropractic?
3. What might be some of the major events in chiropractic in the next 50 years?

REFERENCES

1. Palmer DD: *The science, art and philosophy of chiropractic*, Portland, Ore, 1910, Portland Printing House.
2. Gaucher PL, Donahue J, Wiese GC: Daniel David Palmer's medical library: the founder was "into the literature," *Chiropr Hist* 15(2):63, 1995.
3. Palmer DD: *The science, art and philosophy of chiropractic*, Portland, Ore, 1910, Portland Printing House.
4. Wiese GC, Peterson DR: An overview of chiropractic educational institutions, 1896 to the present, *J Chiropr Ed* 4(4):104, 1991.
5. Gibbons RW: The rise of the chiropractic educational establishment: 1897-1980. In Dzaman FL, editor: *Who's who in chiropractic*, Littleton, Colo, 1980, Who's Who in Chiropractic International Publishing.
6. Wardwell WI: *Chiropractic: history and evolution of a new profession*, St Louis, 1992, Mosby.
7. Wardwell WI: Sixteen major events in chiropractic history, *Chiropr Hist* 16(1):66, 1996.
8. Turner C: *The rise of chiropractic*, Los Angeles, 1931, Powell Publishing.
9. Reed L: *The healing cults*, Chicago, 1932, University of Chicago Press.
10. Wardwell WI: *Chiropractic: history and evolution of a new profession*, St Louis, 1992, Mosby.
11. Wiese GC, Peterson DR: An overview of chiropractic educational institutions, 1896 to the present, *J Chiropr Ed* 4(4):104, 1991.
12. Cohen WJ: *Independent practitioners under Medicare: a report to Congress*, Washington, DC, 1968, US Department of Health, Education, and Welfare.
13. Gibbons RW: Chiropractic history: turbulence and triumph—the survival of a profession. In Dzaman FL, editor: *Who's who in chiropractic international 1976-78*, Littleton, Colo, 1978, Who's Who in Chiropractic International Publishing.
14. Wardwell WI: *Chiropractic: history and evolution of a new profession*, St Louis, 1992, Mosby.
15. Goldstein M: *The research status of spinal manipulative therapy.* A Workshop held at the NIH, Feb. 2-4, 1975, Bethesda, Md. DHEW pub. No. (NIH 76-998), NINCDS.
16. Cleveland CS III: Vertebral subluxation. In Redwood D, editor: *Contemporary chiropractic*, New York, 1997, Churchill Livingstone.
17. Association of Chiropractic Colleges: *The chiropractic paradigm: ACC position on chiropractic.* Retrieved February 4, 2002, http://www.chirocolleges.com.
18. Association of Chiropractic Colleges: *The chiropractic paradigm: the subluxation.* Retrieved February 4, 2002, http://www.chirocolleges.com.
19. World Federation of Chiropractic: *Proceeding from a conference on philosophy in chiropractic education*, Fort Lauderdale, Fla, 2000, WFC.
20. King J: Hospital privileges: yesterday's dream, today's reality, *ICA Review* 40(2):41, 1984.
21. Wardwell WI: *Chiropractic: history and evolution of a new profession*, St Louis, 1992, Mosby.
22. Francis RS, Buriak J, Ladenheim CJ: Chiropractic in hospitals and integrated settings. In Redwood D, editor: *Contemporary chiropractic*, New York, 1997, Churchill Livingstone.

23. Shekelle PG et al: Spinal manipulation for low-back pain, *Ann Intern Med* 117(7):590, 1992.
24. Meade TW et al: Randomized comparison of chiropractic and hospital outpatient management for low back pain; results from extended follow up, *BMJ* 311(5 August):349, 1995.
25. Manga P et al: *The effectiveness and cost-effectiveness of chiropractic management of low-back pain*, Ottawa, Ontario, 1993, the author.
26. Manga P, Angus D: *Enhanced chiropractic coverage under OHIP as a means of reducing health care costs, attaining better health outcomes and achieving equitable access to health services*. [online].

Ontario Chiropractic Association. Available from Internet: http://www.chiropractic.on.ca/execsummary.html.
27. Bigos SJ et al: *Acute low back problems in adults: clinical practice guideline No. 14*. Rockville, Md, 1994, Agency for Health Care Policy and Research, Public Health Service, U.S. Department of Health and Human Services.
28. Pelletier KR, Astin JA: Integration and reimbursement of complementary and alternative medicine by managed care and insurance providers: 2000 update and cohort analysis, *Altern Ther Health Med* 8(1):38, 42, 2002.

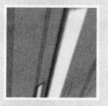

PART **TWO**

ANATOMY, BIOMECHANICS, AND PHYSIOLOGY

CHAPTER 4

Spinal Anatomy

Patrick Coughlin, PhD

Key Terms

AFFERENT
ALAR LIGAMENTS
ANASTOMOSES
ANNULUS FIBROSUS
ANTERIOR LONGITUDINAL
   LIGAMENT
ANTIGENIC
APICAL LIGAMENT
APOPHYSEAL JOINTS
ARACHNOID MATER
ARTICULAR PROCESSES
ASSOCIATION NEURONS
ATLAS
AXIS
CAUDA EQUINA
COLLATERAL CIRCULATION
CONDYLES
CONUS MEDULLARIS
CORONAL
DENTICULATE LIGAMENT
DERMATOME
DISK HERNIATION
DORSAL HORN
DORSAL ROOT GANGLION
DURA MATER
ECTODERM
EFFERENT
ENDODERM
EPINEURIUM
EQUILIBRIAL TRIAD
EXTENSION
FACET JOINTS
FALSE PELVIS
FALX CEREBELLI
FALX CEREBRI
FASCIA
FASCICULI
FILUM TERMINALE
FLEXION

FORAMEN MAGNUM
FORAMEN TRANSVERSARIUM
FUNCTIONAL SPINAL UNIT
GLIA
GOLGI TENDON ORGANS
GRAY MATTER
HERNIATE
HUNCHBACK
ILIOLUMBAR LIGAMENTS
INFARCTION
INION
INSERTION
INTERCRISTAL LINE
INTERNEURONS
INTERSPINOUS LIGAMENTS
INTERTRANSVERSE
   LIGAMENTS
INTERVERTEBRAL DISK
INTERVERTEBRAL FORAMEN
ISCHEMIA
KYPHOSIS
LAMINAE
LATERAL FLEXION
LIGAMENTS
LIGAMENTUM FLAVUM
LIGAMENTUM NUCHAE
LINEA TERMINALIS
LORDOSIS
LYMPHATIC
MAMMILLARY PROCESS
MENINGES
MESODERM
MUSCLE SPINDLES
MYOTOMES
NEURAL ARCH
NEURAL CRESTS
NEUROVASCULAR BUNDLE
NUCLEUS PULPOSUS
ORIGIN

PEDICLES
PELVIC GIRDLE
PIA MATER
PIAL ARTERIAL PLEXUS
POSTERIOR LONGITUDINAL
   LIGAMENT
PROPRIOCEPTIVE
RAMI
SACROSPINOUS LIGAMENT
SACROTUBEROUS LIGAMENT
SAGITTAL
SCHMORL'S NODES
SCLEROTOME
SINUVERTEBRAL NERVES
SOFT TISSUE
SOMITES
SPINAL ARTERIES
SPINOUS PROCESSES
SUBARACHNOID SPACE
SUPRASPINOUS LIGAMENT
SWAYBACK
SYNOVIAL
TENDONS
TENSEGRITY
TENTORIUM CEREBELLI
TRACTS
TRANSVERSE PROCESSES
TROPISM
TRUE PELVIS
VALSALVA MANEUVERS
VENOUS PLEXUSES
VENTRAL HORN
VERTEBRAL FORAMEN
VESTIBULAR SYSTEM
VISCERA
WHITE MATTER
WOLFF'S LAW
ZYGAPOPHYSEAL JOINTS

45

In the study of the anatomy of the axial skeleton and its related **soft tissues,** several foundational concepts must be understood. First is that of bilateral symmetry. In theory (although this is almost never the case), the left side of the body should be an identical mirror image of the right side. Although this symmetry is ideally true of the musculoskeletal system, it is not true of the visceral organs.

The ability to adapt to changing conditions is another trait of living organisms. In humans, this ability takes the form of maintaining balance while negotiating changing or uneven terrain (or sometimes even while standing or sitting still) or while responding to various external stimuli (e.g., antigens, emotional stresses, the occasional life-threatening event).

Postural adaptations are accomplished through a system that can be referred to as the **equilibrial triad.** This system is composed of three elements: (1) the **proprioceptive** system, found throughout the body in the **Golgi tendon organs** (GTOs), the **muscle spindles,** and the nerves that innervate these receptors; (2) the **vestibular system,** found in the inner ear, which signals the nervous system regarding the position of the head; and (3) the visual system.

Adaptations to **antigenic** challenges are primarily mediated thorough the immune system. However, as more evidence accumulates, the immune system is clearly interrelated with and is heavily influenced by both the endocrine and nervous systems.

Responses to other forms of stress are processed through the *autonomic nervous system,* which is discussed in some detail later in this chapter. Understanding this system, how it innervates the **viscera,** and its interplay with the *somatic nervous system* (that which innervates the muscles, joints, **fascia,** and skin) is absolutely crucial to the informed practice of the adjustive/manipulative arts.

Familiarity with the principles of **tensegrity** will provide a more thorough understanding of the operation of the musculoskeletal system and the proper maintenance of posture and balance. Tensegrity is a concept originated by the artist Kenneth Snelson and the architect Buckminster Fuller, which posits a balance of compressional and tensional forces through a body that exists in a gravitational field. Simplistically speaking, the bones and disks of the vertebral column are built to withstand compressional forces, and the muscles and **ligaments** are the tensional elements of the axial skeleton. In addition, the tensional elements are *preloaded* (i.e., muscle tone and connective tissue tension are *at rest*), which adds to the stability of the system. When compression and tension are in balance, an upright posture can be maintained with a minimum of work. Within this framework, the words **origin** and **insertion** will not be used to describe the attachments of the muscles. These common terms have been used over the years based on certain assumptions of the kinetics of the body. Specifically, the word *origin* has been used to describe a more proximal or stable attachment, and *insertion* is ascribed to the distal or mobile attachment of a muscle. However, especially relative to the muscles that influence the spine, an important point to realize is that either muscle attachment can produce movement, sometimes simultaneously, and thus it is believed that these two terms are too limiting.

The embryologic development of the human organism establishes a time line for the early period of life. A basic knowledge of this early history allows for a more thorough understanding of the ultimate arrangement of the human body, as well as the existence of anatomic variations and, in some cases, birth defects.

Wolff's law is a concept with which all students of anatomy should be familiar. Wolff's law simply states that when stress is placed on a bone, it undergoes a tissue reaction whereby its form may change to fit its function. An important point to remember is that bone is living tissue, and as such, it will react to stress and its local environment. An example of this phenomenon is the difference in size and shape of the vertebrae of a large, physically active man, compared with a small, inactive woman. The vertebra of the man would bear more weight and be subjected to greater stresses. Therefore the vertebral body would be larger, and the processes would be longer and perhaps broader and thicker, given that the muscles attached to these parts of the vertebra would be pulling harder to perform more work. This concept, although not specifically stated, can also be extended to soft tissues, such as ligaments, **tendons,** and other connective tissues, which also respond to the forces placed on them.

The various rhythms and oscillations of the body are also important for the clinician to appreciate. Most notable are cardiorespiratory rhythms and the (hopefully unimpeded) movement of the diaphragms of the body. These rhythms can be exploited in manual procedures to the advantage of both the clinician and the patient.

VERTEBRAL COLUMN AS A WHOLE

Anatomically, the human body is arranged lengthwise as a series of building blocks or segments. This arrangement can be observed most directly by looking at the individual vertebrae that make up the spinal column, which extends from the base of the skull to the "tail bone," or the coccyx. Just above the coccyx is the sacrum, which is a single bone resulting from the fusion of five vertebrae. This fusion is significant because the sacrum articulates with the pelvic bones that, in turn, articulate with the femurs. This relationship produces an arch, which has the sacrum as its keystone.

The spine, or vertebral column, is usually composed of 33 individual vertebrae. Proceeding from superior to inferior, these vertebrae are 7 cervical, 12 thoracic, 5 lumbar, 5 fused vertebrae forming the sacrum, and 4 rudimentary vertebrae, usually fused, forming the coccyx (Fig. 4-1).

Each region of the spine is curved in the **sagittal** (front to back) plane of the body. The cervical and lumbar regions are curved with a posterior concavity, referred to as **lordosis,** or a lordotic curvature. The thoracic and sacral regions possess an anteriorly concave curvature, referred to as **kyphosis,** or a kyphotic curvature. Both of these curvatures exist within a normal range. However, curvatures outside the normal range will be seen. For example, excessive thoracic **kyphosis** (hyperkyphosis) is commonly referred to as **hunchback** (especially when combined with scoliosis, as described later), and

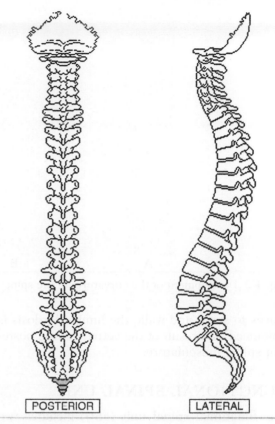

| POSTERIOR | | LATERAL |

Fig. 4-1 Posterior and lateral views of the spine.

excessive lumbar lordosis is commonly referred to as **swayback.**

Under ideal conditions, the spine is vertical in the *frontal* (side-to-side) plane of the body. Lateral curvatures are referred to as scoliosis and can exist separately or in combination with hyperkyphosis (hunchback) or hyperlordotic curves.

The curvatures of the spine are sometimes referred to as primary and secondary. Early in embryonic development, the spine is C-shaped (Fig. 4-2), that is, a single kyphotic curve (primary). As time passes, the spine gradually straightens, until at birth, two secondary lordotic curves begin to appear in the cervical and lumbar regions (secondary). As the infant learns to raise and hold his or her head erect with the supporting muscles of the neck, the cervical lordotic curve is enlarged. Later, as the infant

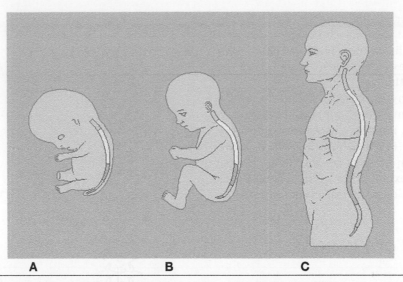

Fig. 4-2 Development of the curvatures of the spine; **A,** fetus; **B,** infant; **C,** adult.

learns to stand and walk, the lumbar lordosis is enhanced as a result of the activity of the posterior spinal musculature.

FUNCTIONAL SPINAL UNIT

The **functional spinal unit** (FSU) includes two adjacent vertebrae and the joints that link them, as well as the skeletal muscles that move the joints. The FSU is closely related to the body segment (see the Embryonic Segmental Development section in this chapter), which also includes the spinal nerves, blood and **lymphatic** vessels, and fascia. Other bones, muscles, and associated fascia (e.g., ribs, intercostal muscles in the thoracic region), as well as visceral structures within the body cavities that receive innervation from the autonomic portion of the spinal nerves, should also be considered elements of individual segments.

VERTEBRAL CHARACTERISTICS

Although the vertebrae vary considerably in size and shape from region to region and within specific regions, certain characteristics are common to all (Fig. 4-3). Each structure has an anterior body and a posterior vertebral arch, or **neural arch.** The arch consists of four elements: the pedicles, the transverse processes, the laminae,

and the spinous processes. The **pedicles,** which are short and stout, attach to the vertebral body posterolaterally. The pedicles form part of the boundaries of the intervertebral foramina through which pass the spinal nerves and other structures (see later discussion). The **transverse processes,** which extend laterally from the ends of the pedicles, are of varying length. The **laminae,** which are generally broad and flat, project posteromedially from the transverse processes or pedicles. The **spinous processes,** which extend posteriorly from the midline junction of the laminae, are of varying length, shape, and angulation and can, in many cases, be easily palpated.

The posterior aspect of the vertebral body and vertebral arch forms the **vertebral foramen.** The collective group of vertebral foramina creates the vertebral or spinal canal, which contains the spinal cord and related structures.

Projecting in both superior and inferior directions from the laminae are the superior and inferior **articular processes,** which form part of the **synovial** joints with the vertebrae above and below. The angle of the joint plane is of great significance because it will direct the motion of the FSU.

The vertebrae develop from the embryonic **sclerotome** (see later discussion), which contains several specific elements that are common

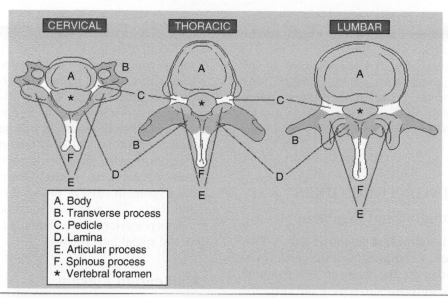

Fig. 4-3 The parts of the vertebrae.

A. Body
B. Transverse process
C. Pedicle
D. Lamina
E. Articular process
F. Spinous process
* Vertebral foramen

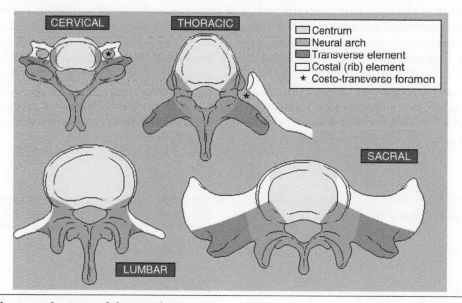

Centrum
Neural arch
Transverse element
Costal (rib) element
* Costo-transverse foramen

Fig. 4-4 Developmental origins of the vertebrae.

to all vertebrae. The vertebral body corresponds to the centrum (or central element, Fig. 4-4). The pedicles, base of the transverse processes, laminae, and spinous processes correspond to the neural arch element. The transverse elements form the transverse processes. In addition, costal elements may be found, which in the thoracic region become the ribs but which also persist in other regions and will be described later. The costal element is often overlooked, especially in the cervical and lumbar regions. The costal element makes up the anterior portion, including the anterior tubercle of the cervical vertebra, and forms the majority of the transverse processes of the lumbar vertebra, as well as the anterior portion of the ala of the sacrum. The costotransverse foramen exists solely in the cervical and thoracic regions. The significance of the costotransverse foramen in the cervical vertebrae is the formation of the foramen transversarium for the passage (and presumably for the protection) of the vertebral artery. Failure of midline fusion of the posterior arch results in spina bifida, a potentially serious condition.

SUPPORTING STRUCTURES

Anterior Longitudinal Ligament

The **anterior longitudinal ligament** (Fig. 4-5) is broad and thick. Extending from the basilar portion of the atlas to the sacrum, the ligament attaches to the anterior surfaces of the vertebral bodies and intervertebral disks. Superiorly, the anterior longitudinal ligament extends from the anterior arch of the atlas to the occiput as the anterior atlanto-occipital membrane and inferiorly as the anterior sacrococcygeal ligament. The anterior longitudinal ligament limits anterior protrusion of the intervertebral disks and hyperextension of the spine. This ligament is prone to damage in whiplash-type injuries in which the spine is hyperextended as a result of rapid acceleration (or a blow from behind).

Posterior Longitudinal Ligament

This ligament is found on the posterior surfaces of the vertebral bodies and intervertebral disks. Within the vertebral canal, the **posterior longitudinal ligament** (Fig. 4-6) is much narrower than the anterior longitudinal ligament. Extending from the axis to the sacrum, this ligament is continuous superiorly with the tectorial membrane and inferiorly with the deep dorsal sacrococcygeal ligament. Lateral extensions of the posterior longitudinal ligament exist at the level of the intervertebral disks. The posterior longitudinal ligament prevents posterior protrusion of the intervertebral disk and spinal hyperflexion.

Ligamentum Flavum

These ligaments (Fig. 4-7) are found extending from the articular process to the spinous process and connect adjacent vertebral laminae and attach to the anterior surface of the lamina above and the posterior surface of the lamina below. The word *flavum* (L. for yellow) is used to describe these ligaments because of their yellow coloration resulting from the predominance of elastic tissue. These ligaments are the most important of the posterior ligaments in limiting **flexion** of the spine.

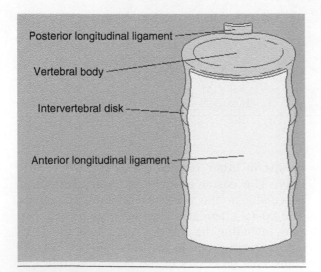

Fig. **4-5** The anterior longitudinal ligament.

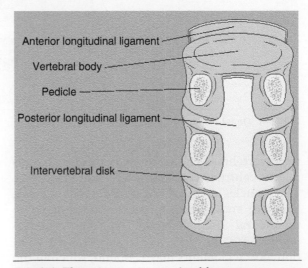

Fig. **4-6** The posterior longitudinal ligament.

Intervertebral Disk

The anterior fibrous joints (symphyses) between the vertebral bodies are formed by the **intervertebral disks** (Fig. 4-8). The disks are found between the vertebral bodies from the C2-C3 to the lumbosacral junction. A small, rudimentary disk also exists between the sacrum and coccyx and possibly between caudal coccygeal segments. The intervertebral disk consists of two basic components: a central, gelatinous **nucleus pulposus** (a remnant of the embryonic notochord) and a peripheral, fibrocartilaginous **annulus fibrosus.**

The **annulus fibrosus** is arranged in concentric rings. The collagen fibers in each ring run obliquely from one vertebra to the next, and in each succeeding ring, the fibers run in the opposite direction; that is, one set of fibers runs clockwise, the next counterclockwise, and so forth. This arrangement limits the amount of torsion allowed on the disk and the amount of rotation of

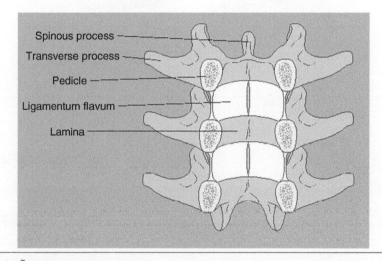

Spinous process

Transverse process

Pedicle

Ligamentum flavum

Lamina

Fig. 4-7 The ligamenta flava.

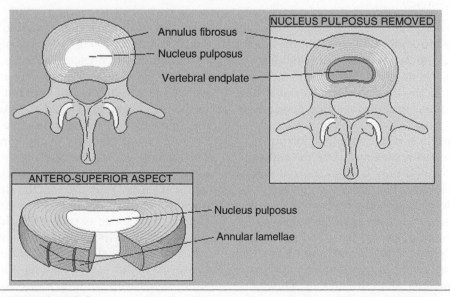

Annulus fibrosus

Nucleus pulposus

Vertebral endplate

NUCLEUS PULPOSUS REMOVED

ANTERO-SUPERIOR ASPECT

Nucleus pulposus

Annular lamellae

Fig. 4-8 The intervertebral disk.

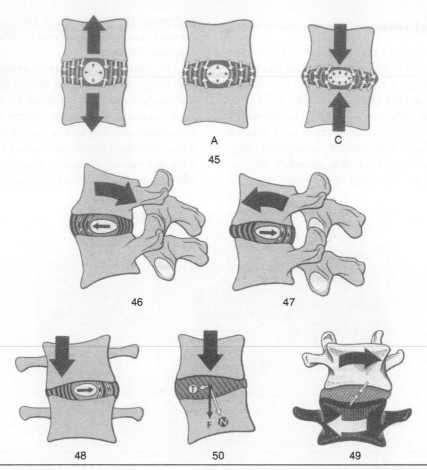

Fig. 4-9 Deformation of the intervertebral disk. *(From Kapandji IA:* Physiology of the joints, New York, *1990, Churchill Livingstone.)*

the vertebrae relative to one another. In addition, the fibers are under tension, creating a preloading effect, which increases the stability of the joint when it is not under stress, and increasing the ability of the disk to adapt to the stress placed on it, similar to the cables in a suspension bridge.

The outer portion of the annulus fibrosus has a blood supply and is innervated by the **sinuvertebral nerves,** which may be the cause of much idiopathic back pain. The inner portion has neither innervation nor blood supply and is nourished by diffusion, as is the nucleus pulposus.

The nucleus pulposus is composed mainly of water, which is bound to a gelatinous matrix by high concentrations of hyaluronic acid. As mentioned, the nucleus is nourished by diffusion, primarily from the periphery of the disk. Dynamic

weight bearing has a demonstrable effect on the shape of the disk (Fig. 4-9). During movements of the spine, the nucleus, because of its relative incompressibility, acts as a swivel or pivot around which one vertebra in the FSU can move relative to the other vertebra (Fig. 4-10). Additionally, as the spine moves, the shape of the disk changes because of the elasticity of the annulus fibrosus. This change causes the nucleus to move in various directions, depending on the action of the moment. The pressure of the incompressible nucleus, in turn, causes the annulus to bulge slightly. The bulge is typically held in check by the integrity of its own fibers, as well as by the anterior and posterior longitudinal ligaments. However, under severe loading, these fibers can rupture, creating an injury referred to as a *herniated nucleus pulposus* (HNP) or "slipped"

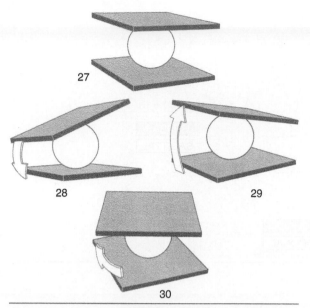

Fig. 4-10 Intervertebral disk acting as a swivel in vertebral motion. *(From Kapandji IA:* Physiology of the joints, *New York, 1990, Churchill Livingstone.)*

disk. During the aging process, the water content of the annulus gradually decreases, and collagen cross-linking increases, which causes the annulus to become less elastic and more brittle. Consequently, the probability of incurring an HNP during certain lifting maneuvers is increased yet can be prevented by proper posture during this activity ("Lift with the legs, not the back."). The arrangement of the anterior and posterior longitudinal ligaments holding the annulus in check predisposes herniation in a posterolateral direction, which unfortunately is in the direction of the **intervertebral foramen.** Often, *nerve impingement and severe pain accompany disk herniation.* Occasionally, the nucleus can **herniate** in a superior or inferior direction, creating a defect in the vertebral bodies, known as **Schmorl's nodes,** which can be visualized radiographically.

Other Ligaments

The additional *intervertebral ligaments* are described as being part of the fibrous intervertebral joints but can also be thought of as check ligaments. These additional ligaments are found between the transverse processes **(intertransverse ligaments)** and spinous processes **(interspinous ligaments).** A long, thick ligament is also found extending between and over the tips of the spinous processes, the **supraspinous ligament,** which extends from the axis to the sacrum. In the cervical region, this ligament forms an attachment point for the ligamentum nuchae. The interspinous and supraspinous ligaments in the cervical region are quite strong and, in deceleration-hyperflexion injuries, can actually avulse the spinous process of the vertebra.

Zygapophyseal Joints

The **zygapophyseal joints** (also called **apophyseal joints** or **facet joints**) occur between the superior and inferior articular processes of the vertebrae. Zygapophyseal joints are synovial joints with a thin, loose, somewhat elastic fibrous capsule and are of the gliding type. The joint facets are covered with hyaline cartilage and are oriented at oblique angles, which are region specific (Fig. 4-11). These joints significantly affect the movements of the vertebrae. Owing to their oblique orientation, motions in the transverse plane (rotation) and frontal plane **(lateral flexion** or sidebending) are said to be coupled. Although a very small amount of pure rotation or lateral flexion is allowed because of the intervening joint space, the facets engage quickly, and the direction of motion changes to conform to the facet plane. Although the plane of the facets is region specific, a gradual change in orientation takes place so that abrupt changes do not occur (e.g., between the cervical and thoracic regions). However, vertebrae do exist that exhibit characteristics of one region in the superior articular processes and of the caudal region with the inferior articular processes. Such vertebrae are described as transitional (Fig. 4-12).

BLOOD SUPPLY AND INNERVATION OF THE VERTEBRAE AND JOINTS

The blood supply to the spine and related tissues differs from region to region. In the cervical region, the vertebral artery and its branches

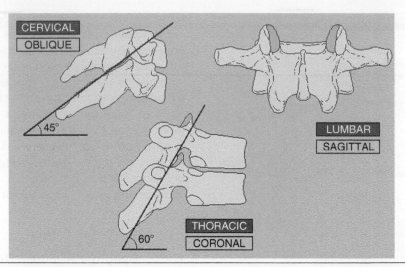

Fig. 4-11 Orientation of the zygapophyseal joints.

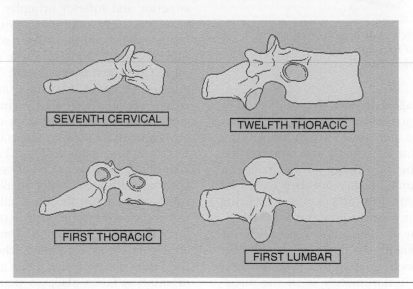

Fig. 4-12 Transitional vertebrae.

provide the primary blood supply to the vertebrae. In the thoracic and lumbar regions, typical segmental arteries supply the vertebrae. In the sacral region, the blood supply is derived from the lateral sacral branches of the internal iliac arteries (Fig. 4-13).

Segmental Artery

The typical *segmental artery* is similar in distribution to that of the spinal nerve (Fig. 4-14). Many of the segmental arteries are branches of

the aorta. The descending aorta lies slightly to the left of the midline; therefore the right segmental branch must cross the midline (i.e., the vertebral body) to reach the right side of the body. As the artery crosses the vertebral body, it sends off small branches to supply it, the anterior longitudinal ligament, and the anterolateral portion of the intervertebral disk.

The primary segmental artery sends its first (major) branch back toward the midline structures and is thus sometimes referred to as the *recurrent* or *spinal artery*. The spinal artery has

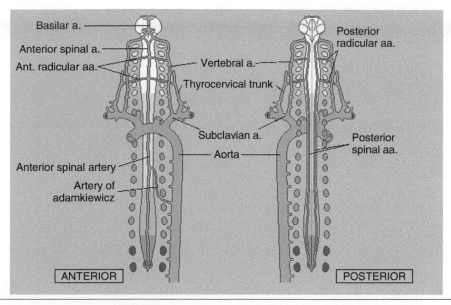

Fig. 4-13 Arterial supply of the axial skeleton.

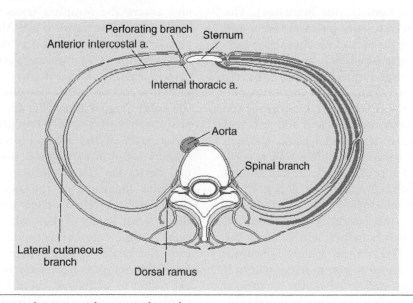

Fig. 4-14 The segmental artery and its main branches.

several important branches (Fig. 4-15). Radicular branches course along the spinal nerve and supply its proximal portion, including the dorsal root ganglion. The radicular arteries terminate in **anastomoses** with the anterior and posterior spinal arteries (of the spinal cord). Branches from both sides anastomose as the anterior spinal artery, an important collateralization for the spinal cord. The spinal arteries continue into the vertebral canal and send off dural and vertebral branches, which supply the meninges, the vertebral body and posterior arch, the ligaments within the vertebral canal, and the posterior portion of the intervertebral disk.

The next branch point of the segmental artery follows the pattern of a spinal nerve, that is, the

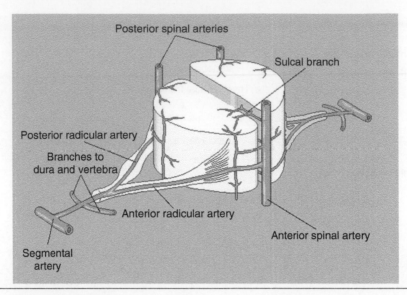

Fig. **4-15** Branches of the spinal artery.

dorsal and ventral **rami** (L. for branches). The dorsal ramus penetrates the paraxial fascia and muscles, supplying them, and reaches the superficial fascia, where it supplies it and the overlying skin. The ventral ramus proceeds laterally and enters what is referred to as the neurovascular plane, between (in the thoracic region) the innermost intercostal muscle and the internal intercostal muscle. In this fascial plane, the segmental nerve and its corresponding vein accompany the artery. At approximately the midaxillary line, a lateral branch is given off, which penetrates the muscles and comes to lie in the superficial fascia. At this point, the lateral branch sends off anterior and posterior branches, which supply the fascia and skin. The ventral ramus continues anteriorly to just lateral to the midline, where it penetrates the body wall to reach the superficial fascia (the anterior cutaneous branches) and skin. In the thoracic region, the anterior intercostal artery anastomoses with the internal thoracic artery. A vein of the same name accompanies each branch of the artery.

Vertebral Artery

The *vertebral artery* branches directly from the subclavian artery (Fig. 4-16). The vertebral artery runs deep to the anterior scalene muscle and enters the foramen transversarium of the sixth cervical vertebra (C6). Although an intervertebral foramen is found at the seventh cervical vertebra (C7) for the vertebral vein, the vertebral artery does not enter it. The artery follows this course until it traverses the foramen of the atlas (Fig. 4-17). The artery then courses posteriorly and medially in a groove on the posterior arch of the atlas, pierces the posterior atlanto-occipital membrane, and enters the cranial cavity via the posterolateral aspect of the **foramen magnum** of the occiput. From this point, each vertebral artery courses forward to the anterior aspect of the brainstem, and the two vessels come together at the level of the pons to form the basilar artery. A high degree of elasticity of this artery is necessary in the upper cervical region to withstand the torque generated by normal range of motion of the atlanto-axial joint (90 degrees). Because the artery is held stable in the foramina intertransversarii of both the **atlas** and **axis**, significant stretching of this artery occurs during normal rotational excursion of the head. Range-of-motion testing and impulse-oriented manual techniques in this area can put this artery at risk, especially in older patients with atherosclerosis. Patients may also exhibit rotational dysfunctions resulting from developing or congenital insufficiency of this artery.

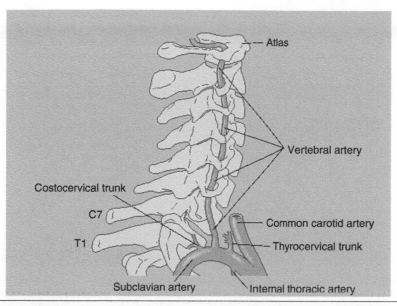

Fig. 4-16 The vertebral artery.

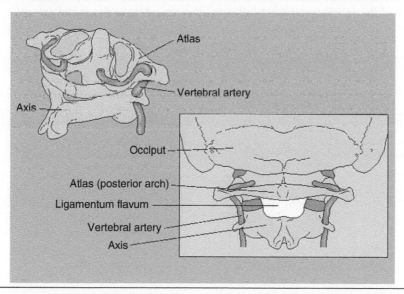

Fig. 4-17 The vertebral artery, upper section. Two views of this critical part of the pathway of the vertebral artery are shown here. In the superior view, the posterior turn that the artery takes can be seen when it passes through the foramen transversarium of the atlas, as well as the medial turn as it crosses the posterior arch of the atlas (in the groove) to reach the foramen magnum of the occiput. The reader should be aware of the elastic nature of this artery and realize that its structural integrity can be severely compromised by atherosclerosis.

VENOUS DRAINAGE OF THE SPINE

Rather than a single arterial supply of various structures, the venous return of the spine is a series of plexuses, which ultimately drain into the caval system (Fig. 4-18). Within the spinal canal, two *epidural plexuses* may be found, one anterior and the other posterior. These veins drain the spinal cord and meninges, as well as

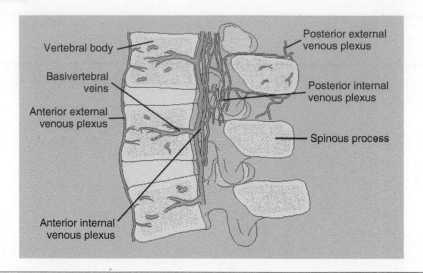

Fig. 4-18 The spinal venous plexus. This cutaway section of the lumbar vertebrae shows the venous plexuses and their communications with one another. The reader should note the basivertebral veins draining the vertebral body and the communications of the internal venous plexuses and the external venous plexuses, as well as the existence of the spinal (intervertebral) vein, corresponding to the spinal artery.

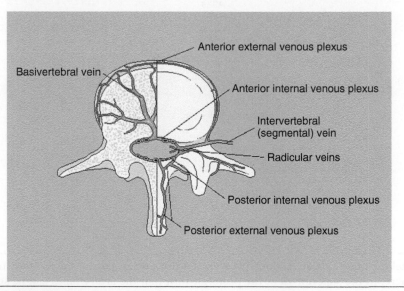

Fig. 4-19 Venous drainage of the lumbar vertebra.

the vertebrae via the basivertebral veins. The plexuses will communicate with the spinal veins through the intervertebral foramina and with the anterior and posterior external venous plexuses adjacent to the vertebral bodies and spinous processes, respectively (Fig. 4-19). These plexuses, in turn, communicate with other veins in their respective regions, including the pelvic cavity. Of clinical significance is the fact that these veins contain no valves, thus blood may flow in either direction within them. This characteristic becomes problematic in men with malignancies of the prostate in which metastatic cells can travel through these veins to the vertebral column and seed there, or they can travel all the way to the brain.

INNERVATION OF THE SPINE AND RELATED STRUCTURES

Recurrent branches of the primary dorsal rami of the spinal nerves innervate the vertebrae, joints, dura, and intervertebral disks. These recurrent nerves are also referred to as *sinuvertebral nerves,* which are distributed with the spinal arteries external to the vertebrae and reenter the spinal canal through intervertebral foramina. The sinuvertebral nerves contain nociceptive (pain) fibers, as well as proprioceptive fibers, which innervate the zygapophyseal joints. Autonomic fibers are also present, which innervate the vessels in the area. Because of the intersegmental nature of the vertebrae, sinuvertebral nerves from the nerve above and below will innervate each vertebra and its associated zygapophyseal joints.

REGIONAL SPECIALIZATIONS
Occiput, Atlas, Axis

The *occiput* is one of the bones that make up the base of the skull (Fig. 4-20). This structure artic-

ulates with the two temporal and parietal bones through uneven, fibrous joints known as sutures. The exterior surface of the occiput has two lines, the superior and inferior nuchal lines, for muscle attachments, and a palpable, midline external occipital protuberance **(inion).** The inion serves as an attachment site for the ligamentum nuchae. The foramen magnum, located at the base of the occiput, serves as the bony landmark, indicating the transition point of the central nervous system from brainstem to spinal cord. The occiput has two convex articular processes, the occipital **condyles,** which articulate with the atlas. In addition, the occiput contains the hypoglossal canals through which the twelfth cranial nerves (hypoglossal) pass on their way from the brainstem to the muscles of the tongue.

The interior surface of the occiput displays features related to the structures that attach to it, pass through it, or articulate with it (Fig. 4-21). Anteriorly, the occiput has a postlike, basilar terminal, which articulates with the body of the sphenoid bone. In addition, a small tubercle forms part of the jugular foramen, the origin of the internal jugular vein. On the interior surface, several ridges and grooves are visible. The ridges are the attachment sites of the dura as it reflects off the occiput to contribute to the

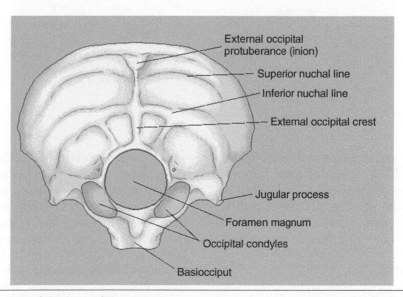

Fig. 4-20 External view of the base of the occiput.

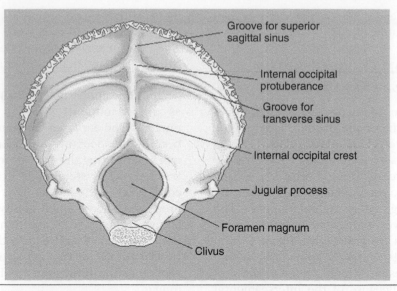

Fig. **4-21** Internal surfaces of the occiput.

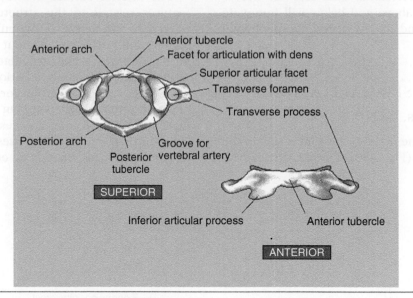

Fig. **4-22** The atlas.

formation of the dural venous sinuses, which drain most of the blood from the brain. Grooves in the occiput represent spaces where the arteries that supply the meningeal tissue course. Centrally located is the foramen magnum, which serves as the egress point of the brainstem from the cranial cavity as it establishes continuity with the spinal cord.

The *atlas* (C1), as its name implies, holds up the globe of the skull, through its articulation with the occiput (Fig. 4-22). The atlas is an atypical cervical vertebra in that part of its body is lost by migration and fusion to the axis during development, the remainder being known as the anterior arch, which has a facet for articulation with the dens of the axis. In addition, the spinous process is modified and is known as the posterior arch. The superior articular processes of the atlas are concave and almost horizontal in orientation. This configuration allows for signifi-

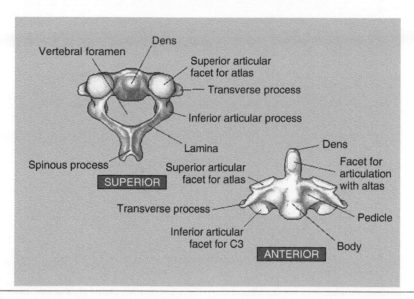

Fig. 4-23 The axis.

cant flexion-extension of the occipito-atlantal joint, as in nodding the head. The "cupping" of the facets allows only small amounts of sidebending or rotation, these motions being accomplished by the combined actions at the other intercervical joints. However, the convex-concave relationship of the occipital condyles with the superior articular processes of the atlas creates a modified ball-and-socket joint in which movements in all three planes of space are possible. Bilateral grooves in the laminae adjacent to the superior articular processes form a support structure for the vertebral arteries as they travel from the foramina intertransversaria of the atlas to the foramen magnum of the occiput.

The *axis* is an atypical cervical vertebra for several reasons (Fig. 4-23). The vertebral body differs significantly from other cervical vertebrae in that it contains a superior **extension,** known as the dens (L. for tooth). The dens actually represents the embryonic vertebral body of the atlas, which undergoes dissociation from the atlas and absorption into the body of the axis during development. This process results in a large degree of rotation between the atlas and axis (approximately 90 degrees under normal circumstances). The dens also has a facet for articulation with the anterior arch of the atlas. The superior articular processes are positioned more anteriorly in relation to the transverse processes, actually associating with the pedicle, as opposed to the inferior articular processes, which are more typically associated with the lamina. The angle of the superior facet is more horizontally (axially) arranged than the more coronally (or paracoronally) arranged inferior facet. The spinous process is bifid but is considerably longer posteriorly than both the posterior arch of the atlas and the spinous process of the third cervical vertebra. Consequently, this is the first cervical spinous process that can be palpated. The relationship of the foramen intertransversarium is important. The foramen is directly inferior to the superior articular facet. In the anatomic position, this foramen is also inferior to the foramen transversarium of the atlas. However, the degree of rotation available at this joint, can endanger the vertebral artery, especially in the presence of pathologic conditions such as atherosclerosis and vertebrobasilar insufficiency.

When grouped together, the occiput, atlas, and axis display complex yet interesting relationships, which follow the function of the joints that connect them (Fig. 4-24). The superior and inferior articular facets of the atlas are angled in opposite directions. That is, the superior articular facets wedge inward (medially), and the inferior

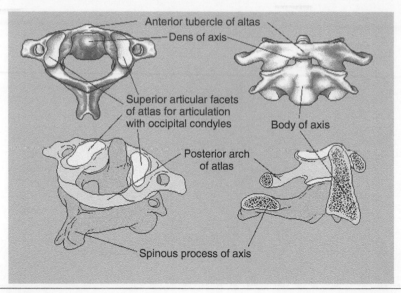

Fig. 4-24 C1-C2 relationships.

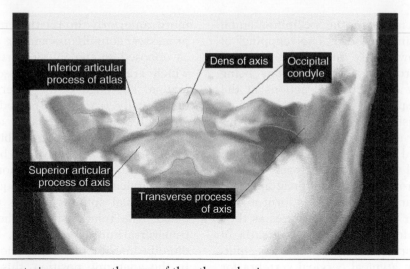

Fig. 4-25 Anterior-posterior open mouth x-ray of the atlas and axis.

articular facets wedge outward (laterally) (Fig. 4-25). When a severe blow to the top of the head is incurred, the atlas can fracture, and given this arrangement, each lateral mass will be forced laterally, which can be seen on x-ray examination (Fig. 4-26).

The planes of the facets directly affect the type of motion allowed in this joint. The atlas and axis articulate so that approximately 90 degrees total or 45 degrees in each direction is allowed to rotate of the head. The center of the

dens acts as the axis of rotation of the joint. An important point to remember is that the dens begins during development as the body of the atlas but subsequently separates from it to fuse with the body of the axis. The facet (zygapophyseal) joints, which are between these two bones, are almost in a transverse (horizontal) plane, again to allow free rotation. As mentioned previously, the course of the vertebral artery as it passes between these two bones is important. Because of the degree of movement allowed here,

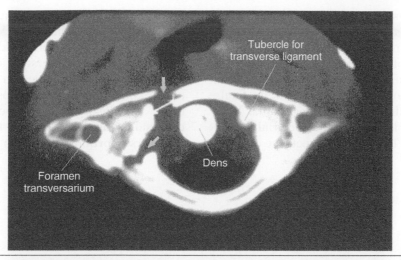

Fig. 4-26 Jefferson fracture of the atlas.

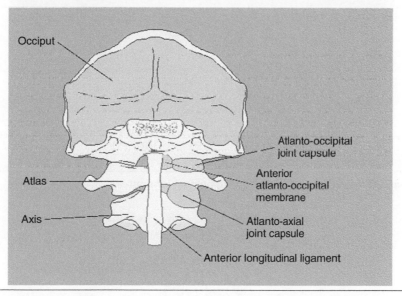

Fig. 4-27 Supporting structures of the occipito-atlanto-axial complex (anterior view).

the artery has developed a significant amount of slack (as well as elastic fibers in its wall), which takes the form of a kink at this location.

Occipito-Atlanto-Axial Ligaments

The occipito-atlanto-axial (OAA) region contains supporting soft tissues that are unique to this area. Anteriorly, three groupings of ligamentous structures exist, two of which are typical of the vertebral column (Fig. 4-27). The joint capsules of the occipito-atlantal (OA) joint and the atlanto-axial (AA) joint make up one group, and the anterior longitudinal ligament make up the second group. Additional atypical supporting elements are also present: the anterior atlanto-occipital membrane and a medial extension of the atlanto-axial joint capsule. The laxity and elasticity of these ligaments allow the anatomic range of motion at these joints. However, the supporting role of these joints is of extreme importance because dislocations in this area can be life threatening.

The AA joint is complex because of its primary function of allowing significant rotation in the transverse plane. The ligaments, which serve to hold the dens of the axis close to the anterior arch of the atlas, are of the greatest significance, because dislocation in this area can be fatal. A deep layer of the posterior longitudinal ligament is present, known as the tectorial membrane (Fig. 4-28). The layer connects the occiput to the axis by spanning the distance between the dens and foramen magnum. Deep to the tectorial membrane are several additional ligaments (Fig. 4-29). The transverse ligament of the dens extends from two tubercles on the anterior arch of the atlas tubercles and slips posterior to the dens. This ligament has superior and inferior extensions **(fasciculi)**, which together with the transverse portion are known as the cruciform

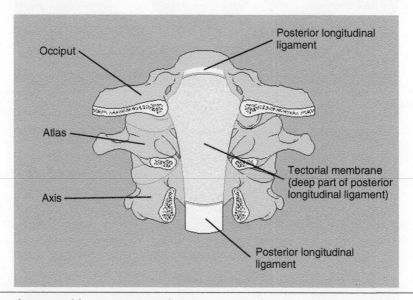

Fig. 4-28 Occipito-atlanto-axial laminectomy and supporting structures.

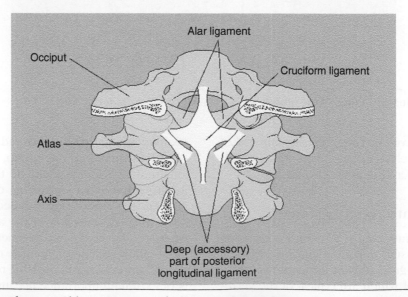

Fig. 4-29 Occipito-atlanto-axial laminectomy and supporting structures.

(L. for similar to a cross) ligament. In addition, the **alar ligaments** extend upward and outward from the apex of the dens toward the occiput. The **apical ligament** of the dens extends from the tip of the dens and attaches to the occiput. The median AA joint has two components consisting of an anterior synovial cavity and a posterior bursal sac (Fig. 4-30). The alar ligaments separate the joint into two separate compartments. The *transverse ligament of the dens* supports the posterior compartment posteriorly. This ligament holds the dens snugly against the posterior arch and prevents posterior displacement, which can seriously jeopardize the spinal cord. The existence of these two synovial cavities is of great importance because of the lubricating properties of the synovial fluid. The amount of friction that would result if these bones were approximated without lubrication would be substantial, especially considering the number of times the head is turned in a single day. In median section, the continuity of the posterior atlanto-occipital membrane with the **ligamentum flavum** can be visualized (Fig. 4-31).

Cervical

Typical cervical vertebrae are specialized in several ways (Fig. 4-32). The bodies are smaller than the vertebrae below, which bear more weight. The vertebrae also have anterolateral lips, the uncinate processes. Associated with the uncinate processes are additional synovial joints known as the *uncovertebral joints* (of Luschka), which are unique to the cervical vertebrae. The space between the vertebral bodies, occupied by the intervertebral disks, is larger in the cervical region than the space in the thoracic region because of the relative height (or thickness) of the disks. This difference is one factor that predisposes these disks to herniation. The transverse process contains a **foramen transversarium,** the conduit for the vertebral artery. The anterior portion of the transverse process, containing the anterior tubercle (an attachment site for the anterior intertransversarii muscle group), represents the costal element of the cervical vertebrae. The tip of the transverse process, termed the posterior tubercle, represents part of the true transverse process and is an attachment site for the posterior intertransversarii muscle group. The articular processes are thickened to form what are commonly referred to as *articular pillars.* The designation *pillars* stems from the fact that the interarticular (zygapophyseal or facet) joints in this region are arranged in the transverse plane, thus the articular processes sit atop one another, similar to blocks of a column

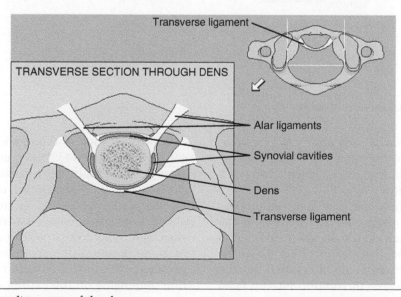

Fig. 4-30 Supporting ligaments of the dens.

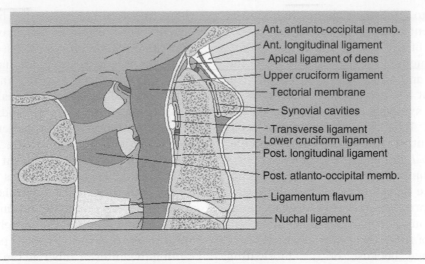

Fig. 4-31 Supporting structures of the occipito-atlanto-axial complex.

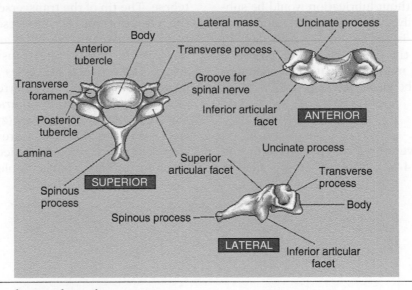

Fig. 4-32 The typical cervical vertebra.

(Fig. 4-33). The trend as one proceeds in an inferior direction is for the angles of the facet joints to change from a transverse orientation to a **coronal** orientation.

Cervical vertebrae have a spinous process that is bifid, accounting for the pairing of the interspinales muscle group in this region. The arrangement of the articular facets of the cervical vertebra represents an adaptation to the need for a high degree of rotation for the head and neck (for visual scanning: approximately 7 to 8 degrees each, totaling about 45 degrees to each side) (Fig. 4-34). However, the angle of the facet joints is such that rotation is coupled with sidebending (lateral flexion) to the same side. Conversely, sidebending in this region is also allowed, which is coupled with rotation to the same side. The degree of flexion allowed in each of these joints will permit herniation of the nucleus pulposus in a posterior and lateral direction, impinging on the exiting nerve. Herniation does not usually occur directly posteriorly

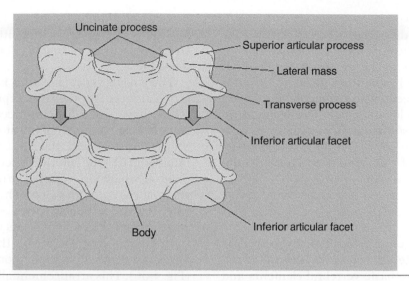

Fig. 4-33 Relationships of the cervical articular joints.

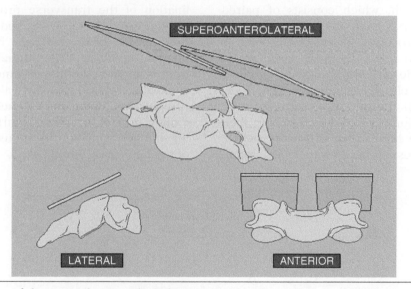

Fig. 4-34 The plane of the cervical zygapophyseal joints.

because of the presence of the posterior longitudinal ligament. The intervertebral foramen is located just between the articular process and the vertebral body. The cervical nerve, exiting the foramen, passes just posterior to the vertebral artery (which is traveling through the foramen transversarium) and is "guided" to the periphery by a groove in the transverse process. The uncovertebral joint is just anterior to the

intervertebral foramen. Degenerative disease of this joint can also cause nerve impingement.

The supporting ligaments and joint capsules of the cervical vertebrae and their respective intervertebral joints are flexible enough to allow the range of motion necessary for appropriate functional movement of the head. However, these supports will also limit motion such that dislocation does not occur, or any action that might be damaging to the spinal cord (via shear, torque), which would be disastrous. (See Chapter 6 for descriptions of shear, torque, and other biomechanical concepts.) The posterior longitudinal ligament and the ligamentum flavum both limit flexion of the neck. The ligamenta flava also limit rotation to a lesser degree. The **ligamentum nuchae,** which also functions as a major muscle attachment in the cervical region, virtually surrounds the tips of the spinous processes in the sagittal plane.

Thoracic

The thoracic vertebra is traditionally known as the "typical" vertebra, primarily because of the presence of all the basic vertebral elements and the lack of special features (Fig. 4-35). The thoracic vertebra is composed of an anterior body and posterior arch, which consists of paired pedicles, transverse processes, laminae, and a single spinous process. The spinous process is angled downward in the thoracic vertebrae. In the upper thoracic vertebra, the spinous process is only slightly declined, resembling that of a cervical vertebra. In the mid-thoracic region, the angle of declination reaches a peak, which then decreases as the lumbar region is approached. The spinous process of the lower thoracics resembles that of a lumbar vertebra. This process again illustrates the gradual transition in vertebral structure, which adds considerable stability to the spine.

The singular specialization is the presence of articular facets for the ribs. Typical thoracic vertebrae have two rib *demi-facets.* The superior facet is located at the point at which the vertebra articulates with the rib, which shares its number (T6). The inferior facet is located at the point at which the vertebra articulates with the rib from the segment below. The first and twelfth ribs, though, articulate with a single thoracic vertebra and thus only possess a single rib facet.

In the mid-thoracic region the zygapophyseal joints are coronally (or paracoronally) arranged (Fig. 4-36). This arrangement allows a significant amount of flexion (forward bending). Extension would also be allowed if not for the angle of declination of the transverse process. Significant rotation would also be allowed, were it not for the presence of the rib cage. From superior to inferior, the plane of the thoracic facets changes from a horizontal-oblique plane (similar to the cervical vertebrae) to a vertical-oblique or paracoronal plane in the mid-thoracic region, then to a more sagittal (or parasagittal) plane, completing another transition to the usual arrangement of the lumbar vertebral facets.

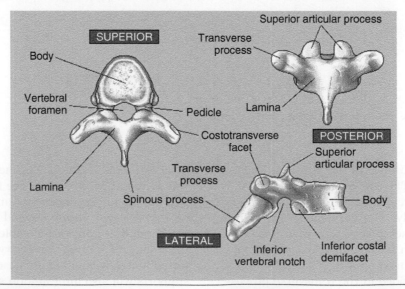

Fig. **4-35** The thoracic vertebra.

The anterior longitudinal ligament in the thoracic region is typically broad and limits extension (along with the oblique angle of the spinous processes). The interspinous ligaments, supraspinous ligaments, and the posterior longitudinal ligament conversely limit flexion. The ligamenta flava, which also limit flexion, form the posterior borders of the intervertebral foramina. The intervertebral disks are relatively thin compared with those in the cervical and lumbar regions

(Fig. 4-37). This differential in thickness accounts for the relative rarity of **disk herniation** in this region.

Lumbar

The lumbar vertebra has a body that reflects the amount of weight it bears (Fig. 4-38). The pedicles and laminae are thick and broad, and they surround a spinal canal, which is generally oval

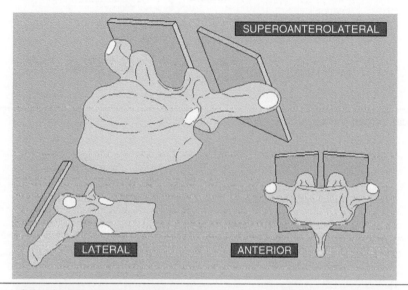

Fig. 4-36 The plane of the thoracic zygapophyseal joints.

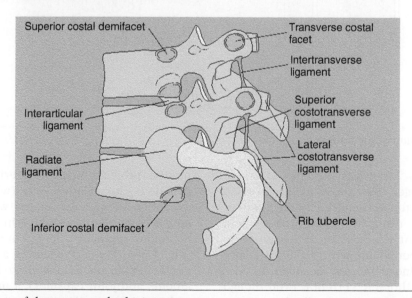

Fig. 4-37 Ligaments of the costovertebral joints.

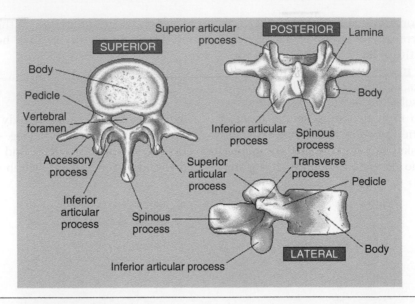

Fig. 4-38 The typical lumbar vertebra.

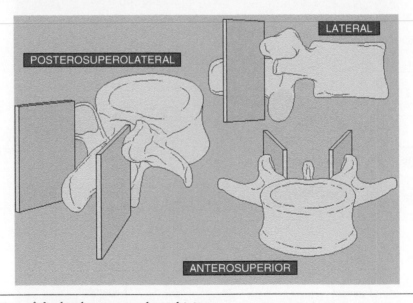

Fig. 4-39 Orientation of the lumbar zygapophyseal joints.

or heart shaped. The transverse processes are considerably longer than those in the thoracic region. This difference is caused by the fact that developmentally the transverse process is a costal element. At the base of each transverse process is a tubercle known as the accessory process. The spinous process is much broader than that of the thoracic vertebra. Even though it is considerably shorter overall, the spinous process projects further posteriorly and can be palpated with relative ease (with the possible exception of L5). Associated with the laminae are the articular processes, which in the lumbar region are typically oriented in the sagittal plane (Fig. 4-39). This arrangement allows for considerable flexion and extension (to be limited by ligaments and joint capsules), a moderate amount of lateral flexion, but little rotation (about 1.5

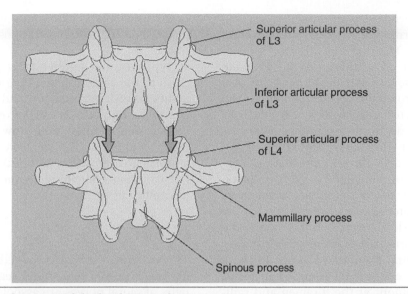

Fig. 4-40 The articular joints of the lumbar vertebrae.

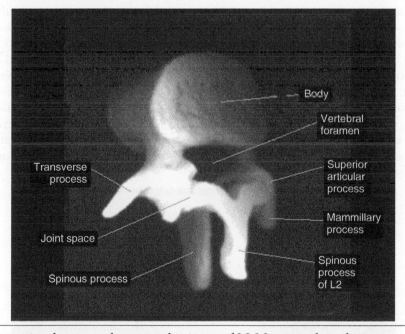

Fig. 4-41 Three-dimensional computed tomographic image of L2-L3 zygapophyseal joints.

degrees to each side per segment). The superior and inferior articular processes are arranged so that the upper lumbar vertebra fits inside of the one below it, similar to a telescope (Figs. 4-40 and 4-41). The superior articular process of the lower vertebra flares out to allow the inferior articular process of the upper vertebra to slip down inside it. The superior process has a ridge

lateral to it known as the **mammillary process,** which serves as an attachment site for the multifidus muscle. The oblique orientation of the facet joints also guides rotation (along the longitudinal axis) so that when rotation takes place, lateral flexion (sidebending) is coupled to it.

The lordotic curve in the lumbar region and the height differential of the anterior and posterior borders of the vertebral bodies cause a varying amount of deformation of the intervertebral disks (Fig. 4-42). The disks in this area are significantly thicker than those in the thoracic region, allowing for greater cushioning but also increasing the probability of herniation. In the normal lordotic curve, the forces of gravity and weight bearing tend to push the nucleus pulposus in an anterior direction, accounting for the slight bulge in the disk. As aging progresses, however, the height of individual disks decreases, which decreases the longitudinal dimension (height) of the intervertebral foramina, thereby increasing the risk of nerve impingement. The ligamenta flava form part of the posterior border of the intervertebral foramina. Injuries to these ligaments, which cause local edema, can result in nerve impingement at the foramen and radiating pain (radiculopathy). In the case of the nerves below L1, this pain can radiate down the lower limb. In the case of a disk bulge or herniation into the lumbar spinal canal, more than one nerve root can be impinged because of the presence of the **cauda equina** (the collection of spinal roots that occupy the vertebral canal below the inferior end of the spinal cord), resulting in additional symptoms. Clinicians should check all local **dermatomes** and **myotomes** (strength testing and reflexes) to determine the exact location and extent of any pathologic condition, bearing in mind the possibility of multiple bulges.

Typically, the lumbar facet joint is oriented close to the sagittal plane (see Fig. 4-39), which allows considerable flexion and extension, some lateral flexion, but very little rotation. The lower lumbar facets may turn toward the coronal plane, similar to the thoracics. This situation allows a greater degree of rotation at these levels but can also contribute to the development of instability in the area.

Sacrum

The *sacrum* is a wedge-shaped bone representing the fusion of five spinal segments (thus five pairs of sacral nerves are associated with it). The *base* of the sacrum faces superiorly, articulating with L5, and the *apex* points inferiorly, providing an articulation with the coccyx (Figs. 4-43 and 4-44). Two *alae* (L. for wings) can be seen to extend laterally from the sacral base to articulate with the ilia at the sacroiliac joints. Four anterior and posterior foramina are present, which transmit the primary ventral and dorsal divisions of the sacral nerves. The fifth sacral nerve does not usually exit via a foramen but slips under the notch just medial to the inferior lateral angle.

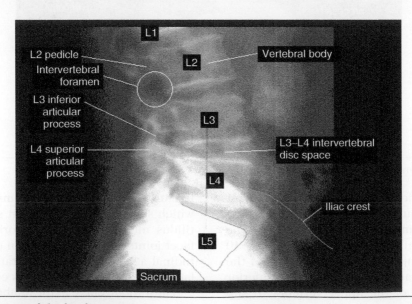

Fig. 4-42 Lateral view of the lumbar spine.

Several articular surfaces are present: the two auricular surfaces for articulation with the iliac bones of the pelvis, the superior articular processes for articulation with the inferior articular processes of L5, and the articular surfaces for joining the sacrum to the coccyx. The facets of the superior processes can be aligned in the sagittal plane, similar to the typical lumbar facet alignment, or more toward the coronal plane, representing a departure from the lumbar orientation and contributing somewhat to rotational instability in the area. Asymmetry in these joints (facet **tropism**) can result in the predisposition to significant musculoskeletal problems, resulting principally from the amount of force brought to bear in this area.

Rather than the smooth surface of the anterior sacrum, three longitudinal bony protuberances may be found on its posterior aspect. The median sacral crest displays the remnants of

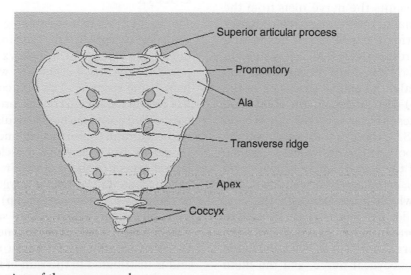

Fig. 4-43 Anterior view of the sacrum and coccyx.

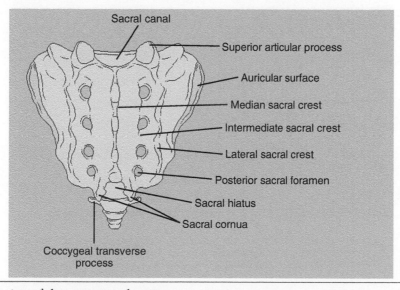

Fig. 4-44 Posterior view of the sacrum and coccyx.

the spinous processes of the original unfused sacral segments and serves as an attachment site for the erector spinae and multifidus muscles. The intermediate sacral crest, which lies just lateral to the posterior sacral foramina, represents fused articular processes, also serving as a muscular attachment site. The lateral sacral crest lies just medial to the auricular surface and is the site of attachment of the posterior sacroiliac ligaments and joint capsule.

Medial to the articular processes is the sacral canal, which transmits the nerve roots from the lumbar spinal canal to the anterior and posterior sacral foramina (for the passage of the ventral and dorsal rami, respectively). Also contained in the triangular sacral canal are the **meninges** and the **filum terminale,** the caudal extension of the pia mater (Fig. 4-45). Although the *dural sac* usually terminates at the level of the second sacral vertebra (S2), the dural sleeves continue with the nerve roots to the individual foramina. The distal end of the sacral canal opens to form the sacral hiatus, with two protuberances, the sacral *cornua* (which articulate with the coccyx), on either side. This opening can be used in certain clinical situations to gain access to the dural sac or subarachnoid space. The last sacral nerve (S5), the coccygeal nerve, and the filum

terminale exit the sacral hiatus. The S5 leaves the hiatus, with its ventral ramus proceeding in an anterior direction just adjacent to the inferior lateral angle of the sacrum. The dorsal ramus of the coccygeal nerve (mixed with fibers of S5) provides cutaneous sensory innervation of the area around the coccyx. The filum terminale attaches to the dorsal aspect of the coccyx to give longitudinal support to the spinal cord.

Coccyx

The *coccyx,* though resembling the tail of a rattlesnake, is actually the remains of the vestigial tail of the human. The coccyx is usually composed of four fused segments, with the first perhaps being separate. The first coccygeal segment has remnants of the articular processes and pedicles, called cornua, which articulate with the apex of the sacrum; it also has rudimentary transverse processes. The coccygeus muscle attaches to the lateral aspect of the coccyx. From the tip of the sacrum extend the pubococcygeus muscle (part of the levator ani muscle group) and the anococcygeal ligament, which help to support the pelvic diaphragm. A single coccygeal nerve is associated the coccyx, which has only a sensory function and is distributed to the skin of the natal cleft.

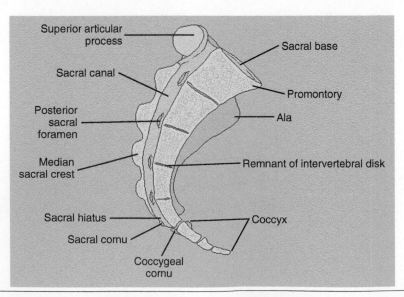

Fig. 4-45 Median section of the sacrum and coccyx.

Pelvic Bone (Innominate Bone, Hip Bone)

The pelvic bone represents the fusion of the *ilium*, *ischium*, and *pubis* (Fig. 4-46). The point of fusion, close to the center of the *acetabular fossa*, is the point at which the head of the femur resides to make up the hip joint. Fusion generally takes place between the ages of 20 and 25 years. Following this terminology, the various features of each bone are named thus (e.g., iliac crest, ischial tuberosity). Above the acetabulum is thickening of the ilium known as the iliopectineal or iliopubic eminence. This eminence increases the weight-bearing capacity of the pelvis.

Many of the protuberances of the pelvic bones can be palpated on the body surface, providing a valuable diagnostic tool for the trained professional (Figs. 4-47 and 4-48). The *iliac crest, posterior superior iliac spine* (PSIS, as indicated by the dimpling on the skin), *anterior superior iliac spine* (ASIS), *ischial tuberosity*, and *pubic tubercle* are all normally palpable on the patient. The *ischial spine* (site of attachment of the sacrospinous ligament) and anterior inferior iliac spine (AIIS) are generally not palpable. Posteriorly, between the PSIS and ischial tuberosity, is the *sciatic notch*, which has important relations with the *sciatic nerve* and *piriformis* muscle and forms the anterior border of the *greater sciatic foramen*. The outer surface of the ilium is the point of the attachment of the gluteal musculature hence the term *gluteal surface*. Below the gluteal surface of the ilium is the socketlike acetabulum, the site of articulation with the femur. The acetabulum presents an incomplete outer rim and an inner fossa. In the fossa is a cartilage-covered lunate surface, which is the actual site of femoral articulation (and weight bearing).

The arc of the coxal bone from the PSIS to the ischial spine forms a notch. This notch is known as the *greater sciatic* or *ischiadic notch* and is very significant in that both the piriformis muscle and the sciatic (also called ischiadic) nerve pass by to reach the lower limb from the pelvic cavity. In the lateral view, the relations of the *iliosacral articulation* are more apparent. The reader should note that a line drawn from the ASIS to the anterior margin of the pubic bone is vertical. In addition, the angle formed by a line drawn from the top of the pubic bone to the sacral promontory is approximately 60 degrees from the horizontal.

The pubic bone presents superior and inferior rami that fuse with the ilium and ischium, respectively. The fusion results in a deficient area in the bone, the *obturator foramen*. In life, this

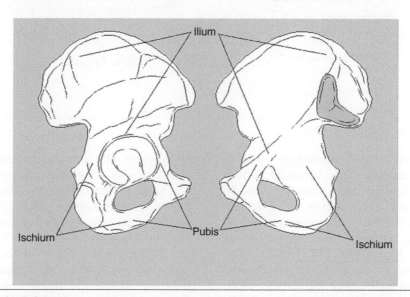

Fig. 4-46 Parts of the pelvis.

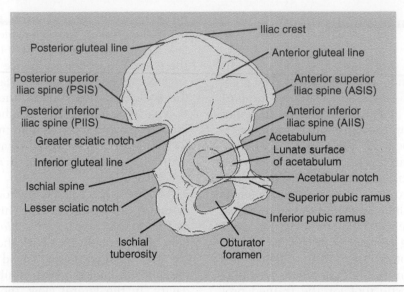

Fig. 4-47 Lateral view of the pelvic bone.

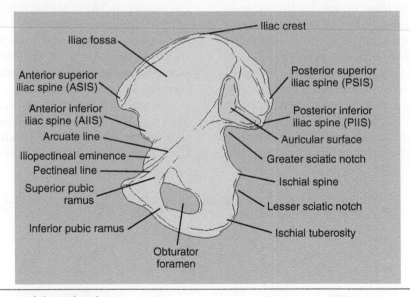

Fig. 4-48 Medial view of the pelvic bone.

foramen is covered by the connective tissue of the obturator membrane. The obturator artery and nerve pass through this membrane and it, along with the pubic rami, serves as an attachment site for the obturator internus and externus muscles. The ischial spinae and tuberosity are the two major landmarks of the ischium. The ischial spine is the attachment site for the coccygeus muscle, as well as for the sacrospinous ligament. The *ischial tuberosity*, which is the

attachment site for the hamstring muscles, is also the bone on which a person sits.

The inner surface of the iliac portion of the pelvic bone possesses the concave iliac fossa, providing an attachment site for the iliacus muscle (the fossa also forms part of the **false pelvis,** which houses a portion of the abdominal viscera) (see Fig. 4-48). The auricular surface is the point at which the ilium articulates with the sacrum. Projecting forward from the auricular

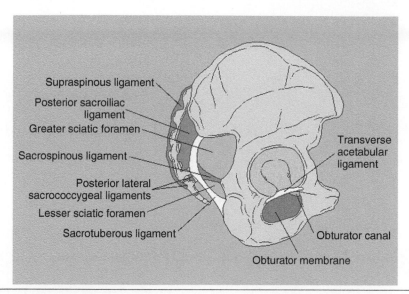

Fig. 4-49 Lateral view of the pelvic girdle.

surface and continuous with the pectineal line is the arcuate line, which forms the posterior component of the **linea terminalis** (the pelvic brim, or dividing line between the **true pelvis** and the false pelvis). The anterior portion of the pubic bone articulates with the pubic bone from the opposite side via the fibrocartilaginous *pubic symphysis*. The two inferior pubic rami form an angle, which varies from men to women. In women, the angle is considerably more obtuse, which, in effect, increases the distance between the ischial tuberosities for easier passage of a baby through the birth canal.

Two important ligaments extend from the sacrum to the pelvic bone (Fig. 4-49). The sacrotuberous and sacrospinous ligaments form two separate foramina of the pelvis. The **sacrotuberous ligament** extends from the inferolateral aspect of the sacrum to the ischial tuberosity (the part of the pelvis on which a person sits). The **sacrospinous ligament** extends from the sacrum, just anterior to the **sacrotuberous ligament,** to the spine of the ischium. In their relationship to the sciatic notch of the pelvis and to each other, the two ligaments form the *greater sciatic foramen*, whereas the sacrotuberous ligament in association with the sacrospinous ligament forms the *lesser sciatic foramen*. A significant number of structures pass through these

foramina from the pelvic cavity to the lower limb and perineum. In addition, a set of **iliolumbar ligaments** may be found, which add support to the lumbar spine by spanning the distance between the transverse processes of L4 and L5 and the iliac crest.

Pelvic Girdle and Sacroiliac Joint

The articulation of the two coxal bones, the sacrum, and coccyx is what is referred to as the **pelvic girdle** (Fig. 4-50). The angles of the acetabula are angled downward and slightly forward, which is important for proper weight bearing by the lower limb.

The pelvic girdle forms a closed biomechanical system for weight bearing. The center of mass of the body is located within the pelvic cavity, approximately at the level of second sacral vertebra (S2). The two femurs, as they articulate with the pelvis, form two buttresses that support the pelvic girdle. The sacrum actually forms the keystone of an arch, which is made up of the head and neck of each femur, the acetabulum, ilium, and sacrum. When considering the weight of the torso, upper limbs, and the head being borne from above, as well as the articulation between the lumbar spine and pelvic girdle, it is easy to rationalize the existence of strong supporting

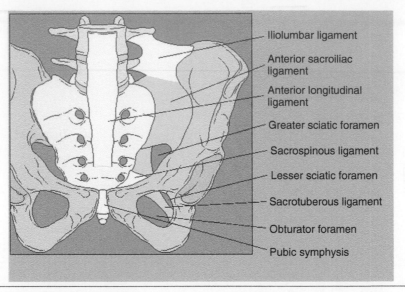

Iliolumbar ligament

Anterior sacroiliac ligament

Anterior longitudinal ligament

Greater sciatic foramen

Sacrospinous ligament

Lesser sciatic foramen

Sacrotuberous ligament

Obturator foramen

Pubic symphysis

Fig. **4-50** Anterior view of the pelvic girdle.

structures to assist in this task. It is also easy to understand the preponderance of low back pain given the amount of force that must be tolerated by these structures over time.

A line drawn across the top of the iliac crests is referred to as the **intercristal line,** which usually passes through the inferior end of L4 (or in many cases through the L4-L5 disk). If a structural variant places the intercristal line abnormally low, the result is abnormally long (and possibly unstable) iliolumbar ligaments, predisposing the individual to lumbar sprain and strain.

The *sacroiliac joint* is somewhat complex. The sacroiliac joint is a synovial joint that, over time, develops a varying amount of fibrocartilaginous attachments, referred to as interosseous ligaments. The unusual arrangement of the articular surface of the sacroiliac joint is described by various authors as "L" shaped, "hockey stick" shaped, or "golf club" shaped (see Fig. 4-49). Because the sacroiliac joint is subjected to tremendous force during weight bearing, very strong ligaments must support it. In addition to the interosseous ligaments, two sets anterior and posterior sacroiliac ligaments may be found (Fig. 4-51; see also Fig. 4-50) The *anterior sacroiliac ligaments* are an extension of the joint capsule and are thickest at the level of the third sacral vertebra (S3). The *posterior sacroiliac ligaments* extend from the

spinous processes of the sacrum laterally to the PSIS and beyond and inferiorly to the sacrotuberous ligament.

CONTENTS OF THE VERTEBRAL CANAL
Meninges

The *meninges* are connective tissue coverings arranged in three distinct layers that cover and protect the spinal cord from excessive movement and damage (Fig. 4-52). These layers consist of the dura mater (L. for tough mother), arachnoid (L. for weblike) mater, and pia (L. for loving mother) mater. Between the arachnoid and pia is a space, the **subarachnoid space,** which contains the cerebrospinal fluid (Fig. 4-53). The cerebrospinal fluid, which bathes the brain and spinal cord, both protects and nourishes these vital structures.

The most external layer of the meninges, the **dura mater,** is a thick, tough connective tissue layer (Fig. 4-54). The dura mater is continuous from the cranial cavity to the sacrum (S2) and is composed of two distinct layers: the periosteal dura (attached to the internal surfaces of the skull and spinal canal) and the meningeal dura. These two layers split at strategic locations. In

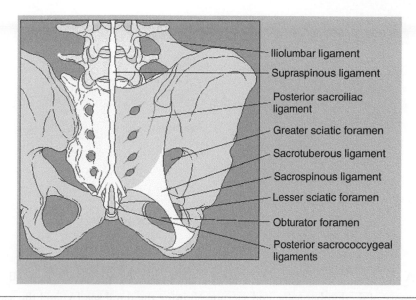

Fig. 4-51 Posterior view of the pelvic girdle.

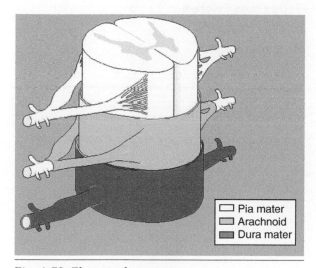

Fig. 4-52 The spinal meninges.

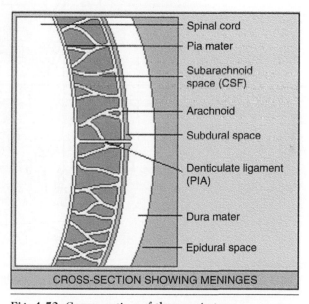

CROSS-SECTION SHOWING MENINGES

Fig. 4-53 Cross-section of the meninges.

the cranial cavity, both layers become lined with endothelium, creating the dural venous sinuses, which drain the large portion of blood from the brain and also serve as a major reabsorption point for the cerebrospinal fluid. The meningeal dura also reflects from the inner surface of the cranial cavity to form the **falx cerebri** and **falx cerebelli** that separate the cerebral and cerebellar hemispheres and the **tentorium cerebelli,** which separates the cerebrum from the cerebellum.

The dura is firmly attached to the internal surface of the skull and to the vertebral foramina of the atlas and axis. The layer then separates from the vertebral surface, creating an epidural space, which contains the blood vessels that supply the vertebrae and contents of the vertebral canal. This space continues to the level of vertebra S2, at which point the dura then firmly

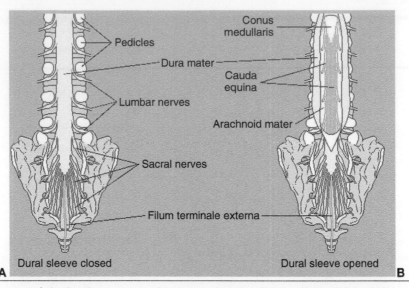

Fig. 4-54 Laminectomy of the lumbar spine and sacrum, showing the dural sac (**A**) and the sac opened (**B**).

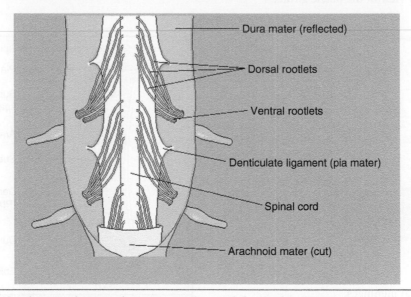

Fig. 4-55 Opened dural space showing the nerve rootlets and denticulate ligament.

reattaches to the interior of the sacral canal. The dura covers the individual nerve roots and nerves as they exit the spinal canal, fusing to the pedicles at the intervertebral foramina.

The **arachnoid mater** is a more delicate, avascular membrane, which is attached to the inner surface of the dura. Thin, weblike projections extend from the arachnoid to the pia, which are responsible for its name. The arachnoid extends along the nerve roots, as does the subarachnoid space, and both terminate approximately at the intervertebral foramen.

The **pia mater** is a single-cell connective tissue layer that adheres directly to the surface of the neural tissue, including the individual cranial and spinal nerve rootlets. The pia has two specializations (Fig. 4-55; see also Fig. 4-54): the *filum terminale*, which extends from the end of the spinal cord to the sacrum and coccyx, thereby tethering it longitudinally, and the denticulate ligament, which supports the cord later-ally. The **denticulate ligament** is a series of pial projections, located primarily in the thoracic region, which project from the lateral surface of the spinal cord, penetrate the arachnoid, and anchor to the dura.

In the lumbosacral region, the dural sac extends to the level of S2, beyond which the individual dural sleeves pass out toward the sacral foramina (see Fig. 4-55). When the dural sac is opened, the end of the spinal cord is seen at L2. Inferior to this level is the cauda equina, consisting of the dorsal and ventral roots of the remaining lumbar and sacral nerves. Also present in this area is an inferior extension of the pia mater, known as the filum terminale. This connective tissue element extends from the tip of the spinal cord **(conus medullaris),** through the sacral hiatus, to attach to the external-posterior aspect of the apex of the sacrum and coccyx. This tissue anchors the spinal cord longitudinally and prevents excessive movement within the canal.

Spinal Cord and Spinal Nerves

Passing through the intervertebral foramina between the vertebrae and proceeding from the spinal cord to the periphery are 31 pairs of spinal nerves (one for each side, with the excep-tion of the coccygeal nerve, which is fused at the midline). Each of these spinal nerves contains sensory and motor nerve fibers that are distributed to the periphery. In many cases, the nerves are accompanied by arteries, which supply blood to the same region supplied by the spinal nerve (Fig. 4-56). In addition, the **neurovascular bundle** contains veins and lymphatic vessels, which serve to drain away waste products from the same territory. Each segment may appear to function as a separate entity, but this is not the case. Because of significant overlap both inside and outside the central nervous system, in a sense each segment is aware of activity that transpires in the segments adjacent to it.

Individual nerve rootlets course inferiorly and are surrounded by the dura and arachnoid as they coalesce to form the spinal nerve (see Fig. 4-56). The sleeves of dura follow the nerves to the intervertebral foramina and also surround a swelling, which represents the location of the **dorsal root ganglion,** the point at which the cell bodies of sensory **(afferent)** neurons reside. This fascial layer is continuous with the connective tissue covering of the peripheral nerve, also known on the histologic level as the **epineurium.** The individual nerve roots are suspended in the cerebrospinal fluid present in the subarachnoid space, thus affording additional protection from trauma.

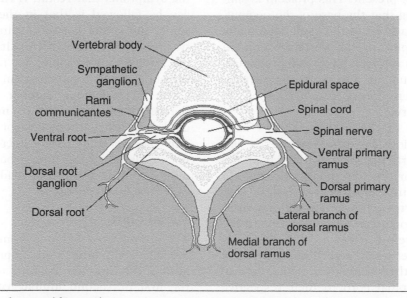

Fig. 4-56 The spinal nerve (thoracic).

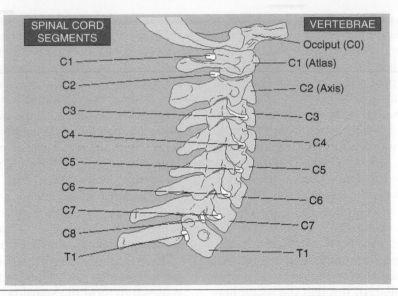

Fig. 4-57 The cervical nerves.

The points of exit of the spinal nerves in the cervical region are deserving of special note (Fig. 4-57). Convention describes the C1 nerve as exiting between the occiput and atlas (i.e., superior to C1 vertebra), C2 between the atlas and axis (superior to C2 vertebra), C3 nerve between C2 and C3 vertebrae, and so on until nerve C8, which exits inferior to vertebra C7. Thus eight cervical nerves may be found, and only seven cervical vertebrae are present. This problem is simplified by realizing that the base of the occiput, in spite of being a bone of the skull, is actually embryologically part of the vertebral column and is sometimes referred to by authors as C0. In the thoracic, lumbar, and sacral regions, the total number of vertebrae corresponds exactly to the number of nerves.

The exit path of the nerves changes from superior to inferior. The first two nerves exit posterior to the articular pillars, whereas all the rest exit anterior to the pillars. Nerves C3 through C7 exit in a more typical fashion (for cervical nerves), traveling in a small groove in the transverse process and just posterior to the course of the vertebral artery.

As the spinal nerves proceed from the cervical region caudally, the declination of the path of the roots from spinal cord to their respective intervertebral foramina significantly increases

(Fig. 4-58). This increase is caused by the differential growth rate and size of the spinal cord relative to the vertebral column. This difference results in the tip of the spinal cord (conus medullaris) residing approximately at the L2 vertebral level. Knowing the location of the vertebral segment relative to the spinal cord segment is important when dealing with vertebral injuries that affect the spinal cord and predicting the symptoms that result. A rule of thumb that can be followed is that in the upper thoracic spine, the spinal nerves decline approximately two vertebral levels before exiting the canal. In the lower thoracic spine, the nerves pass three vertebral levels before exiting the foramina. Given that the upper lumbar spine represents the beginning of the **conus medullaris** of the cord, injuries to these vertebrae usually affect only the sacral spinal cord segments (which is not to minimize the injury, because these segments control bowel and bladder function, as well as sexual responses).

Spinal Cord

The *spinal cord* extends from the end of the medulla of the brain stem, approximately at the level of the foramen magnum of the occiput, to the first or second lumbar vertebrae. At this point, the spinal cord tapers to a point, known as

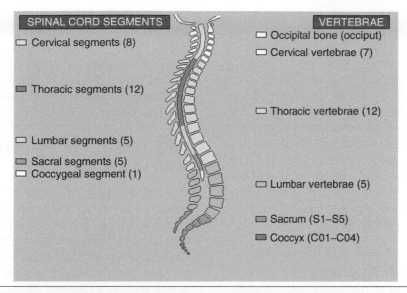

Fig. 4-58 Relationships between the spinal cord segments and vertebral segments.

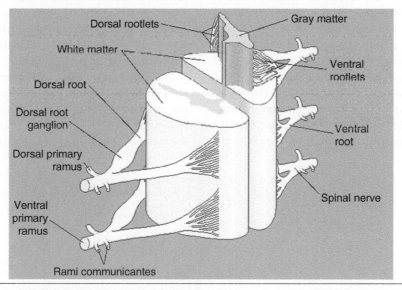

Fig. 4-59 The spinal cord and spinal nerve roots and branches.

the conus medullaris. The cord is made up of neurons and supporting cells known as **glia,** of which there are several types. In cross section (Fig. 4-59), the spinal cord has **gray matter** and **white matter.** The designations *gray* and *white* are the result of the appearance of the tissue before fixation, histologic staining, or both. The white matter, which surrounds the gray, is made up primarily of myelinated neuronal processes,

which are running longitudinally along the cord. Collections of functionally related fibers are organized into **tracts,** which have similar origins and destinations inside or outside the central nervous system.

The gray matter consists of neuronal cell bodies and supporting tissue, along with a substantial number of small blood vessels and capillaries. The gray matter typically has a shape that is described as being as a butterfly. **Dorsal** and **ventral horns** (or columns if viewed three-dimensionally) are present. The dorsal part of the gray matter is populated by neurons, which are principally involved in sensory functions, and the ventral wing contains neurons whose primary function is motor. Interspersed throughout the gray matter all along the cord are **association neurons** or **interneurons,** which interconnect sensory neurons to each other, and to motor neurons. In the thoracic region, a lateral extension of the gray matter exists, known as the intermediolateral cell column, which is the site of preganglionic sympathetic nerve cell bodies.

Spinal Nerves

Afferent and **efferent** fibers enter and leave the cord respectively as rootlets that then coalesce peripherally into dorsal (afferent) and ventral (efferent) roots. These roots then merge to form the spinal nerve, which exits the spinal canal at the intervertebral foramen (see Fig. 4-56). After leaving the spinal canal, the spinal nerve begins to break up into branches (rami), which proceed to their respective targets of innervation. An analogy can be made to a tree that has its roots in the spinal canal, its trunk at the intervertebral foramen, and its branches out in the periphery. The dorsal roots contain a swelling, which represents the dorsal root ganglion, the location of cell bodies of the afferent nerve fibers. These cells are derived from the neural crests. The connection between the segmental nerve and the sympathetic chain (via gray and white rami communicantes) occurs immediately outside the spinal canal (Fig. 4-60).

BLOOD SUPPLY OF THE SPINAL CORD

The blood supply of the spinal cord is derived primarily from anterior and posterior **spinal arteries,** which are branches of the vertebral arteries within the cranial cavity (see Fig. 4-15). These arteries run the length of the spinal cord and are supplemented at intervals by anastomoses with branches of the segmental arteries. Below the arch of the aorta, the *segmental arteries* are branches of the descending aorta. Above the aortic arch, the segmental arteries are branches either of the ascending vertebral arteries or of the ascending cervical branch of the thyrocervical trunk.

The importance of **collateral circulation** in this area cannot be overstated. However, two areas present an increased risk as a result of lower perfusion pressure. These areas are the transition zones between the cervical and tho-

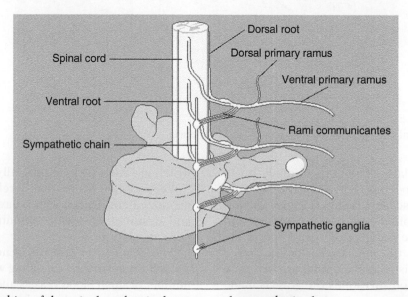

Fig. 4-60 Relationships of the spinal cord, spinal nerves, and sympathetic chain.

racic cord segments and between the thoracic and lumbar cord. Occlusions in these "watershed" areas can lead to significant ischemic lesions of the spinal cord. In the mid-thoracic region, an artery is generally somewhat larger in caliber than other arteries in the region. This type of artery is known as the *artery of Adamkiewicz* (see Fig. 4-13).

The segmental arteries send spinal branches into the intervertebral foramen. Radicular branches stem from these arteries, which follow the spinal nerves back toward the spinal cord. As these nerves break up into the dorsal and ventral roots, the radiculars send off anterior and posterior branches, which follow the roots to the cord. These arteries, in turn, give off smaller arteries that directly supply the tissues of the central nervous system. This arterial system is referred to as the **pial arterial plexus.** These small arteries course on the surface of the cord, sending penetrating branches into the deeper layers. The vessels of the ventrolateral plexus represent an anastomosis of the posterior and anterior spinal arteries; the posterior plexus is anastomosis of the two posterior spinal arteries. The *sulcal artery*, which runs deep within the anterior sulcus of the spinal cord, supplies through its penetrating branches the central area of the spinal cord. Although some overlap of distribution occurs, this by no means implies full collateralization. Occlusion of any of these arteries results in tissue **ischemia** or **infarction,** leading to major neurologic deficits.

The venous drainage of the spinal cord and vertebrae is extensive (see Fig. 4-18). Extending the length of the spine are four continuous plexuses of veins, designated internal and external, anterior and posterior. The reader should note that the internal **venous plexuses** lie in the epidural space, embedded in the epidural fat. The veins draining the neural tissue are similar in course to the arteries, with the exception that only one main posterior spinal vein exists. These veins contain no valves, thus blood may flow in either direction. In addition, the veins form a significant route for the spread of infection, as well as for the metastasis of tumors. As noted earlier, in men, prostate tumor cells can use this route to seed into the individual vertebrae and all the way to the brain. The valveless nature of these veins

also provides a conduit for the release of venous pressure during **Valsalva maneuvers** (forcible exhalation effort against a closed glottis), sneezing, and coughing. Unfortunately, paroxysmal increases in intravenous pressure can occasionally cause disk herniation.

EMBRYONIC SEGMENTAL DEVELOPMENT

During the third and fourth weeks of development, the embryo consists of three layers of tissue: the dorsal **ectoderm,** the ventral **endoderm,** and an intermediate tissue layer, the **mesoderm.** Subsequently, the trilaminar germ disk undergoes folding along a longitudinal axis, resulting in the development of the *neural tube* (Fig. 4-61). While neural tube fusion is taking place, a small number of cells at the apical region of the neural folds separates from the neural tube and come to lie just lateral to it. These cells, collectively known as the **neural crests,** will give rise to a wide variety of tissues in the embryo. The mesoderm just lateral to the neural tube (paraxial mesoderm) forms a segmented series of tissue blocks known as **somites,** which extend from the occipital region of the head to the tail of the embryo. While this is happening, neural derivatives of the neural crests and neural tube are growing into the somites, which ultimately provide sensory and motor innervation to these structures and their derivatives. As such, these somites will also migrate into any location in the embryo, following the migration patterns of the structures to be innervated. This same phenomenon also occurs with the blood supply to these structures, although the ultimate arrangement of arteries is considerably more variable than that of nerves.

The somites undergo further differentiation into a *sclerotome*, which resides in a ventromedial location, and a *dermomyotome*, which lies dorsolateral (Fig. 4-62). The dermomyotome then splits into a superficial dermatome and a deeper myotome. The dermatome and myotome begin then to migrate in a lateral and ventral direction, conforming to the pattern established earlier by the lateral folding of the embryo. The cells of the sclerotome do not, however, undergo extensive migration. As a result of differential

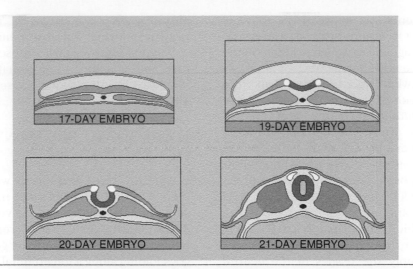

Fig. 4-61 Neural tube formation and development of the somite.

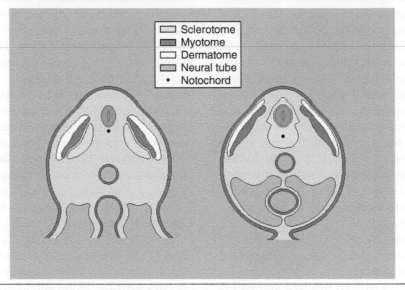

Fig. 4-62 Development of the somite: dermatome, myotome, and sclerotome.

growth, their position shifts, gradually moving around the neural tube and *notochord* to fuse with their counterparts from the opposite side. This tissue ultimately forms the vertebrae and intervertebral disks. At this point, the peripheral process of the segmental dorsal root (cell bodies derived from the neural crest) has grown into the somite, and as it splits into its respective parts (dermatome, myotome, sclerotome), these nerve processes also split and follow the tissues to wherever they migrate in the embryo.

The central process of the segmental dorsal root grows into the developing spinal cord and makes connections with the appropriate neurons within the appropriate segment of the developing central nervous system. The cell bodies continue to reside adjacent to the vertebrae and will become the neuronal cell bodies of the dorsal root ganglion.

By the fourth week of development, the sclerotomes corresponding to the somites are separated by loosely arranged intersegmental mesenchyme

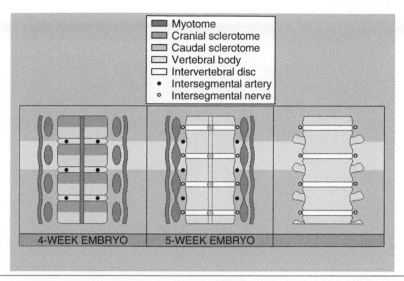

Fig. 4-63 Development of the vertebrae and intervertebral disks.

(Fig. 4-63). As time passes, the cells at caudal end of each sclerotome proliferate and condense, fusing with the cephalic end of the sclerotome below. This portion of the sclerotome forms the vertebral body, which, because of this fusion, is intersegmental. Meanwhile, the sclerotomal tissue between the cephalic and caudal ends fails to proliferate, thereby leaving an area of less dense tissue between the vertebral bodies above and below. This tissue contributes to the formation of the annulus fibrosus of the intervertebral disk. The remaining notochordal tissue persists as the nucleus pulposus. This tissue is the only remnant of the notochord in the newborn and adult, the remainder being obliterated by the formation of the vertebral bodies. At this stage, because of the intersegmental nature of the vertebrae, the myotomes are in a position corresponding to the intervertebral disks. The peripheral process of the corresponding segmental nerve has already grown into the myotome (as well as the dermatome and sclerotome) to innervate it. Given the nomenclature of the vertebra, each nerve is said to exit the spinal canal below (or above as in the cases of C1 through C7) its corresponding numbered vertebra. As the myotome migrates to its final destination in the embryo, the nerve that innervates it will follow.

As the myotome begins to migrate in a ventrolateral direction, it splits into two parts: a dorsal epimere and a ventral hypomere (Fig. 4-64). As the myotome splits, so does the nerve that innervates it, forming a dorsal ramus (epimeric) and a ventral ramus (hypomeric). The *epimere* ultimately becomes the intrinsic muscles of the back (erector spinae, transversospinal group), which are innervated by dorsal rami. The *hypomere* eventually develops into the extrinsic muscles of the back (as well as contributing to the development of the muscles of the limb), which are innervated by ventral rami of the spinal nerves. The reader should also note that the hypomere splits additionally into three layers and that the innervating nerve comes to lie between the deepest and next deepest layers. This fascial plane becomes known as the neurovascular plane. The three layers of the body wall are consistent throughout the trunk, forming part of the thoracic and abdominal walls. In the adult, these muscles have been given different names (e.g., intercostal muscles viz. abdominal obliques), relative to their locations, but their derivation is the same, the principal difference being the presence of a fully developed rib cage in the thoracic region.

The organization of myotomes in the embryo roughly resembles that of the dermatomes. This relationship diverges somewhat as muscles migrate to their ultimate destinations, especially in the limbs. Certain myotomes at either end of

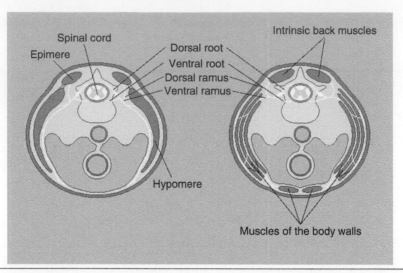

Fig. **4-64** Development of the myotomes-spinal nerves.

the embryo are reabsorbed (e.g., most of the occipital and coccygeal myotomes). Insofar as segmentation and innervation are considered, the relationship established earlier in development between the dermatome, myotome, and sclerotome is maintained. Understanding of segmentation is clinically important in differential diagnosis between peripheral nerve and nerve root lesions, as well as in recognizing reflex patterns, segmental dysfunctions, and the relationship between superficial structures and underlying viscera.

Changes occur in the relationship between the vertebral column and the spinal cord during development as a result of differential growth (see Fig. 4-59). At approximately 3 months in utero, the spinal cord reaches to the end of the vertebral column. As the fetus increases in length, growth of the spinal gradually slows, effectively resulting in a cephalad movement of the end of the cord and the creation of the lumbar cistern, cauda equina, and filum terminale. At birth, the cord resides approximately at the level of the third lumbar vertebra. Continued growth in the newborn changes the relationship further until the cord attains its final position between vertebrae L1 and L2. Notably, in spite of this differential growth and movement, the spinal cord is still tethered longitudinally by the filum terminale. Being aware of variation in this positioning is important, especially if lumbar puncture to obtain cerebrospinal fluid is indicated. Fluid must

be obtained without endangering the cord, necessitating the lumbar approach. Lumbar puncture performed below L2 or lower will generally avoid risk.

Review *Questions*

1. What are the three elements of the equilibrial triad through which postural adaptation is accomplished?
2. Explain the concept of tensegrity as it applies to the musculoskeletal system.
3. What are the components of the FSU?
4. What are the primary functions of the anterior and posterior longitudinal ligaments?
5. What is involved in disk herniation?
6. In what ways are the atlas and axis vertebrae atypical?
7. Which ligaments are unique to the upper cervical area?
8. Why is facet tropism a complicating factor in case management?
9. Describe the structure and function of the meninges.
10. What are the primary functions of the dorsal and ventral horns of the spinal cord?

Concept *Questions*

1. How do the intrinsic muscles of the back maintain the spine as a tensegrity structure?

2. What motions are allowed or restricted by the zygapophyseal joints in each region of the spine, and how does this relate to coupled motion?

3. How does the proprioceptive system of the vertebral column function to maintain erect posture within the conceptual framework of compensation?

SUGGESTED READINGS

Coughlin P, editor: *Principles and practice of manual therapeutics*, New York, 2002, Churchill-Livingstone.

Kapandji IA: *The physiology of the joints, volume three: the trunk and vertebral column*, ed 2, Edinburgh, 1974, Churchill-Livingstone.

Larsen WJ: *Anatomy: development, function, clinical correlations*, Philadelphia, 2002, WB Saunders.

Sadler TW: *Langman's medical embryology*, ed 8, Baltimore, 2000, Williams and Wilkins.

White AA, Panjabi MM: *Clinical biomechanics of the spine*, ed 2, Philadelphia, 1990, Lippincott.

Williams PL, editor: *Gray's anatomy*, ed 38, New York, 1996, Churchill-Livingstone.

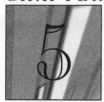

Spinal Neurology

Patrick Coughlin, PhD

Key Terms

ACETYLCHOLINE	GAMMA MOTOR NEURONS	REFLEXES
ACTION POTENTIAL	GANGLION	RETICULAR FORMATION
ADRENERGIC	GUARDING	SENSITIZATION
AFFERENT INHIBITION	HYPERALGESIA	SENSORY
A FIBERS	INTEROCEPTORS	SENSORY FIELD
ALLODYNIA	MECHANORECEPTORS	SOMA
ALLOSTATIC RESPONSE	MOTOR	SOMATOSOMATIC REFLEX
ALPHA MOTOR NEURONS	MYELINATED	SOMATOVISCERAL REFLEX
ANAPHYLAXIS	NEURAXIS	SPLINTING
AUTONOMIC NERVOUS SYSTEM	NEUROTRANSMITTERS	STIMULUS-INDUCED ANALGESIA
AXON	NEUROTRANSMITTER SPILLOVER	SUBSTANCE P
CENTRAL NERVOUS SYSTEM	OLIGODENDROCYTES	SUPERIOR CERVICAL GANGLION
C FIBERS	PARASYMPATHETIC	SYMPATHETIC
CHOLINERGIC	PARAVERTEBRAL SYMPATHETIC CHAIN	SYMPATHETIC GANGLION
COLLATERALIZE	PERIAQUEDUCTAL GRAY	THERMORECEPTORS
CONVERGENCE	PERINEURIUM	TONIC RECEPTORS
DENDRITE	PERIPHERAL NERVOUS SYSTEM	VASA NERVORUM
DIVERGENCE	PHASIC RECEPTORS	VISCERA
DORSAL ROOT GANGLION	POSTGANGLIONIC NEURON	VISCERO-SOMATIC REFLEX
ENDOGENOUS OPIATES	PREGANGLIONIC NEURON	VISCERO-VISCERAL REFLEX
ENDONEURIUM	PROPRIOCEPTORS	WITHDRAWAL REFLEX
EPINEURIUM	RAMI COMMUNICANTES	
EXTEROCEPTORS		
FACILITATION		

A thorough understanding of the spinal nerve and its implications in diagnosis and case management necessitates a review of its development in the embryo, as discussed in Chapter 4. In this light, the basic architecture of the nerve and its components (i.e., the tree analogy) becomes clear. This chapter offers a more functional approach, with emphasis on *information processing* in the peripheral nervous system and its relationship to certain activities in the central nervous system. The information presented here is by no means comprehensive, but it serves as a springboard for further study (see Suggested Reading).

Neurons convey information in the form of impulses or action potentials, which typically travel in a specific direction. The **peripheral nervous system** (PNS), which consists of the spinal nerve roots, spinal nerves, and peripheral nerves, is responsible for bringing information about the external and internal environments to the **central nervous system** (CNS), which consists of the brain and spinal cord. This type of input information is referred to as **sensory** or *afferent*.

The PNS also transmits responses to sensory stimuli, bringing **motor** or *efferent* output information from the CNS to target tissues in the periphery.

BASIC STRUCTURE OF THE NEURON

The neuron is made up of three basic parts. The **soma,** or *cell body,* is the point at which the cell nucleus resides along with other cellular organelles (Fig. 5-1). Extending from the soma are two types of processes. The **dendrite,** which receives signaling information from the local environment, contains, or is associated with, receptors that are designed to sense specific stimuli or react to specific chemical transmitters. Neurons may have hundreds or even thousands of dendrites, depending on the size and complexity of their receptive fields. The second type of cellular process is the **axon,** along which a signal travels as an **action potential.** Action potentials are typically generated in an axon via the summation of signals received from the dendrites, which can be either stimulatory or inhibitory. When the action potential reaches the end of the axon, it causes the release of one or more **neurotransmitters,** which signal either other neurons or specific target tissues. Axons can branch extensively, allowing a single neuron to communicate with and send signals to many other neurons. This phenomenon is known as **divergence** and is significant when the spread of information is desirable for the organism (Fig. 5-2). In this case, the signal is said to be *amplified.* Conversely, when signals from multiple neuronal sources terminate on a single neuron, **convergence** is said to exist (Fig. 5-3). When convergence exists, some signals may be excitatory; others may be inhibitory. As with all neu-

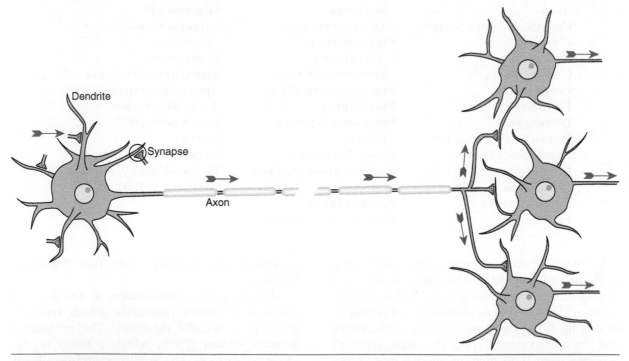

Fig. 5-1 Schematic view of a typical neuron, indicating synaptic inputs to its dendrites (although other sites are possible) and information flow down its axon, reaching synaptic endings on other neurons. Information flow is unidirectional because of molecular specializations of various parts of neurons. The segments covering the axon represent the myelin sheath that coats many axons, and the gap in the axon represents a missing extent that might be as long as 1 meter in length. *(From Nolte J: The human brain: an introduction to its functional anatomy, ed 5, St Louis, 2002, Mosby.)*

rons, the summation of signals may (or may not) reach the threshold for the stimulated neuron to generate an action potential.

FACTORS INFLUENCING CONDUCTION VELOCITY

Neurons of the PNS are associated with *Schwann cells (myelin)*. These cells are responsible for supporting and insulating axons, allowing for more efficient propagation of action potentials. Neurons are said to be **myelinated** or *unmyelinated*, depending on the number of times a Schwann cell wraps around a given axon (often referred to as a fiber) (Fig. 5-4).

Action potentials are propagated along axons with varying speeds. The speed of an action potential depends primarily on two factors: the diameter of the axon and the degree of myelination. Larger diameter and heavily myelinated axons **(A fibers)** convey impulses considerably faster than smaller diameter unmyelinated axons **(C fibers)**. The difference in propagation speeds becomes important when discussing the transmission of pain (see later discussion).

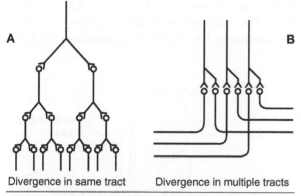

Fig. 5-2 Divergence in neuronal pathways; **A,** divergence within a pathway to cause amplification of the signal; **B,** divergence into multiple tracts to transmit the signal to separate areas. *(From Guyton AC: Hall J: Textbook of medical physiology, ed 10, Philadelphia, 2001, WB Saunders.)*

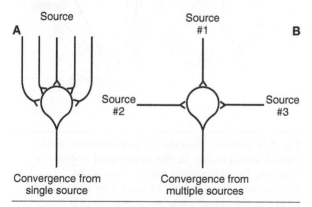

Fig. 5-3 Convergence of multiple input fibers onto a single neuron; **A,** multiple input fibers from a single source; **B,** input fibers from multiple sources. *(From Guyton AC: Hall J: Textbook of medical physiology, ed 10, Philadelphia, 2001, WB Saunders.)*

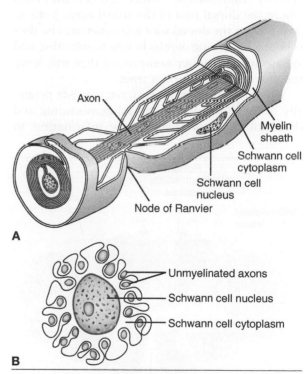

Fig. 5-4 Function of the Schwann cell to insulate nerve fibers; **A,** the wrapping of a Schwann cell membrane around a large axon to form the myelin sheath of the myelinated nerve fiber. *(Modified from Leeson TS, Leeson R: Histology, Philadelphia: 1979, WB Saunders.)* **B,** Partial wrapping of the membrane and cytoplasm of a Schwann cell around multiple unmyelinated nerve fibers (shown in cross section). *(From Guyton AC: Hall J: Textbook of medical physiology, ed 10, Philadelphia, 2001, WB Saunders.)*

BASIC STRUCTURE OF THE SPINAL CORD

A cross section of the spinal cord reveals two basic components: gray matter and white matter (Fig. 5-5). The *gray matter* is a butterfly-shaped column of nerve cell bodies, axons, and dendrites. Because of the metabolic needs of the neuronal cell bodies, a robust blood supply is contained in the gray matter, providing its characteristic appearance. The *butterfly* is subdivided into a pair of dorsal (or posterior) horns, or columns (when seen three dimensionally), and a pair of ventral (or anterior) horns, or columns. The dorsal horns are responsible for processing sensory information, which enters the cord where the dorsal root of the spinal nerve joins it. Axons from the dorsal root will penetrate the dorsal horn to varying depths before terminating and synapsing with other neurons, or they will leave the gray matter to form a tract.

The *white matter,* in contrast, consists primarily of myelinated axons forming ascending and descending tracts that convey information to other areas of the CNS. Specialized cells called **oligodendrocytes** are responsible for myelination in the CNS. The white matter is subdivided into columns or funiculi, whose names are derived from their relationship with the gray matter: anterior, posterior, and lateral. The fatty myelin sheaths are responsible for the coloration of the white matter.

SENSORY NEURONS

The sensory neurons contained in the spinal nerves are of the pseudounipolar variety (Fig. 5-6). The cell bodies of these sensory neurons are located in the **dorsal root ganglion** (DRG).

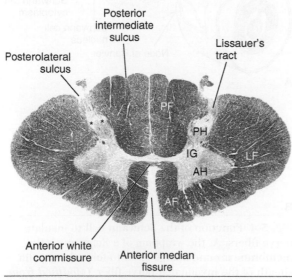

Fig. **5-5** General cross sectional anatomy of the spinal cord, represented in this case by the eighth cervical segment. *PF,* Posterior funiculus; *AF,* anterior funiculus; *LF,* lateral funiculus; *PH,* posterior horn; *AH,* anterior horn; *IG,* intermediate gray. *(From Nolte J: The human brain: an introduction to its functional anatomy, ed 5, St Louis, 2002, Mosby.)*

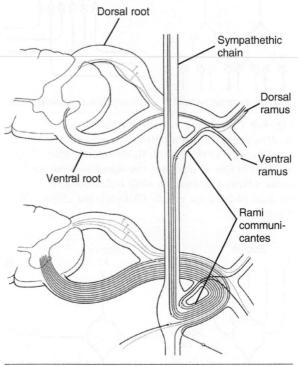

Fig. **5-6** Scheme showing the constitution of a typical spinal nerve. In the *upper part* of the diagram, the spinal cord nerve roots show the somatic components. In the *lower part* of the diagram, the spinal roots show the visceral components, somatic efferent and preganglionic sympathetic fibers, somatic afferent and visceral afferent fibers, and postganglionic sympathetic fibers. *(From Williams PL, editor: Gray's anatomy, ed 38, London, 1995, Churchill-Livingstone.)*

Each DRG neuron contains a peripheral process, which extends to the periphery along the path taken by the spinal nerve and its branches, and a central process, which extends into the CNS as the dorsal root of the spinal nerve. Even though the peripheral process of the DRG neuron is technically a *dendrite,* it is more often called an axon because an action potential travels along it toward the spinal cord. There are many classes of DRG neurons, but the most common neurons that transmit pain are the A fibers (fast-conducting) and C fibers (slow-conducting).

These nerves convey a wide range of sensations. Each specific sensation is referred to as a *modality.* Some examples are light touch, proprioceptive sensations (giving a sense of position to the body), and pain. These and other modalities are discussed later in this chapter. Specific receptors exist for each modality (Fig. 5-7). Sensory receptors are divided into three basic types: **exteroceptors,** which carry information that originates outside or on the surface of the body, **interoceptors,** which convey information originating from inside the body, and **proprioceptors,** which provide information on body position and movement. Subclasses of the exteroceptors include:

- Mechanoreceptive (touch, hearing)
- Thermoreceptive (temperature)
- Nociceptive (pain)
- Chemoreceptive (smell, taste)
- Electromagnetic (vision)

GANGLION

A *ganglion* is a collection of functionally related nerve cell bodies outside the central nervous system. Nerves whose cell bodies reside in ganglia can be sensory (somatic or visceral), or motor (visceral). All ganglion cells are derived from the embryonic neural crest.

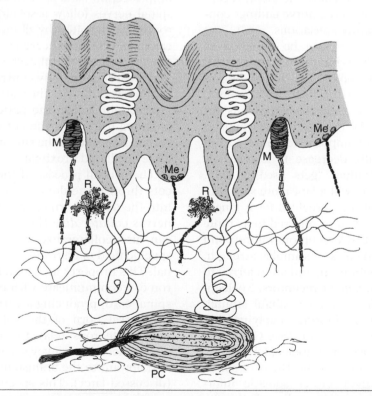

Fig. 5-7 Some of the sensory endings found in glabrous (smooth and bare) skin. *M,* Meissner corpuscle; *Me,* Merkel cell; *PC,* Pacinian corpuscle; *R,* Ruffini ending. *(From Nolte J: The human brain: an introduction to its functional anatomy, ed 5, St Louis, 2002, Mosby.)*

Subclasses of the interoceptors include:

- Mechanoreceptive (stretch, pressure)
- Chemoreceptive (pO_2, pCO_2, blood levels of glucose, fatty acids, amino acids)
- Nociceptive (pain)

The proprioceptors, which respond to mechanical stimuli, such as the state of contraction of a muscle (muscle spindles) or the tension on a tendon or joint (Golgi tendon organs), are also classified as **mechanoreceptors.**

Sensory receptors generate an action potential by changing the neuronal cell membrane in some way. This action can take the form of physical deformation (mechanoreceptors) or interaction of chemicals with the membrane. Both types of stimuli cause the opening of ion channels in the cell membrane. In addition, changes in temperature **(thermoreceptors)** or electromagnetic radiation (visual) can alter membrane permeability. The receptors of spinal nerves can also be classified as encapsulated or free nerve endings. Encapsulated receptors include the touch receptors and proprioceptors. Free nerve endings convey pain and temperature sensations.

Most sensory receptors can be classified as slowly adapting (SA) or rapidly adapting (RA). In either case, the receptors are responding to some type of change in the local environment. Adaptation of receptors occurs when a constant stimulus is applied. As the stimulus is applied over time, the rate of impulse response to the stimulus will gradually decrease to a very low level (i.e., The individual "gets used to it."). Therefore SA receptors will adapt more slowly to a stimulus, and it will be perceived for a longer period. SA receptors are also referred to as **tonic receptors.** In contrast, RA receptors will respond more efficiently to changes in stimulus strength, such as occurs with vibration, and are referred to as **phasic,** *rate,* or *movement* **receptors.** Nociceptors, or receptors that perceive painful stimuli, are referred to as *nonadapting,* implying that there is no getting used to pain. (See Chapter 9 for an extensive discussion of nociceptors.)

The neurons contained in the DRGs of spinal nerves generally convey either somatic information from the body surface, walls of body cavities, and extremities or visceral information from the internal organs and contents of body cavities.

The special senses (smell, vision, hearing, and taste) are conveyed by the cranial nerves. An important point to remember is that each neuron has a specific receptor or set of receptors on its peripheral end that are consistent with the type of information that the neuron conveys (i.e., neurons are modality specific). Also worthy of note is that some DRG neurons are quite long. For example, a single neuron carrying pain information from the foot might be 3 to 4 feet or longer, depending on the height of the individual.

The peripheral distribution of the sensory neuron conforms to its distribution in the embryo and fetus (see Chapter 4). In addition, these neurons can branch or **collateralize** quite extensively on their peripheral ends. This branching can result in an extensive **sensory field** for a single neuron. Thus the sensory component (along with the motor component) of the spinal nerve is distributed to the dermatome (for touch, temperature, and pain), the myotome, and the sclerotome (for proprioception and pain). The dermatomes of the spinal nerves follow a specific pattern, which is routinely exploited by clinicians (Fig. 5-8). For example, if a spinal nerve is damaged, the patient may experience numbness or tingling along the nerve's dermatome. By contrast, if a spinal nerve is impinged by another structure such as an intervertebral disk, the patient may experience radiating pain along the entire length of the dermatome, in spite of the site of impingement being quite small and proximal.

The central process of the DRG neuron projects through the dorsal root of the spinal nerve into the dorsal horn of the spinal cord. As these nerves *collateralize* (branch) peripherally, they can also collateralize centrally, resulting in a specific field of distribution for the incoming signal. This property means that a single DRG neuron can communicate with many neurons in the spinal cord, producing a variety of effects. From the dorsal horn of the spinal cord, modality-specific neurons relay to or directly enter the nerve tracts that convey specific types of information upward to the brainstem and cerebral cortex (discussed later). This specificity in conveying a specific type of information from the periphery to a specific tract and subsequently to a specific area of the CNS is known as a *labeled line.*

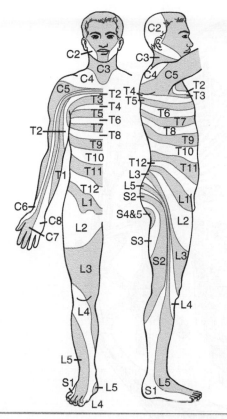

Fig. 5-8 Dermatomes. *(Modified from Grinker RR, Sahs AL: Neurology, Springfield, Ill, 1996, Charles C Thomas; cited in Guyton AC: Hall J: Textbook of medical physiology, ed 10, Philadelphia, 2001, WB Saunders.)*

Somatic Motor Neurons

Somatic motor neurons come in two varieties: alpha and gamma (Aα and Aγ) motor neurons. **Alpha motor neurons** are responsible for innervating and activating skeletal muscle fibers through the myoneural junction. These neurons fall into the category of large diameter, fast-conducting nerve fibers. **Acetylcholine** is secreted into the myoneural junction, which, in turn, stimulates the muscle to contract. **Gamma motor neurons** are responsible for innervating muscle spindles, which establish a set point for muscle tone (Fig. 5-9). These neurons are somewhat smaller in diameter than alpha motor neurons and thus conduct impulses at a somewhat slower velocity. Motor neurons, similar to sensory neurons, can have exceedingly long axons, projecting from the spinal cord all the way to the target muscle.

STRUCTURE OF THE SPINAL NERVE

The spinal nerve derives its nomenclature from the early anatomists whose descriptions compared it with a tree, with roots, a trunk, and branches (Fig. 5-10). Because of its position in the body, the nerve is said to have a dorsal (or posterior) root, a ventral (or anterior) root, each of which penetrates the spinal cord (as roots penetrating the ground). The roots unite to form the spinal nerve (the tree trunk). Shortly there-

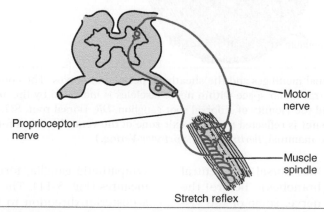

Fig. 5-9 Neuronal circuit of the stretch reflex. *(From Guyton AC: Hall J: Textbook of medical physiology, ed 10, Philadelphia, 2001, WB Saunders.)*

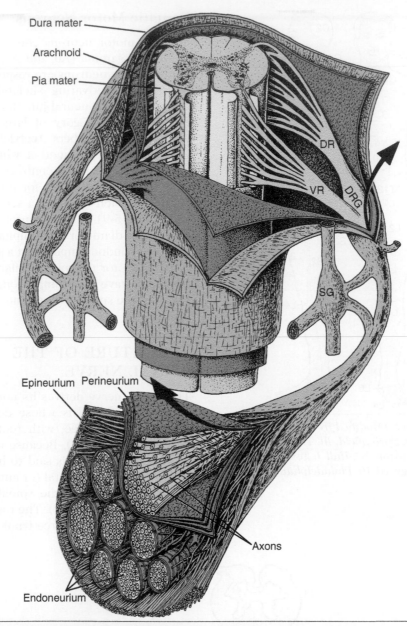

Fig. 5-10 Continuity of spinal meninges and the sheaths of peripheral nerves. The continuity between spinal subarachnoid space and extracellular space within nerve fascicles is indicated by the arrow emerging from both the cut end of the nerve and the vicinity of a dorsal root ganglion. *DR,* Dorsal root; *SG,* sympathetic ganglion; *VR,* ventral root. The pia mater is reflected from the exit zone of the ventral rootlets for clarity. *(From Krstic RV: General histology of the mammal, Berlin, 1985, Springer-Verlag.)*

after, the nerve divides into dorsal and ventral primary rami (L. for branches). Before the branching of the spinal nerve, some of the visceral afferents and efferents branch from the nerve to connect with the paravertebral chain of sympathetic ganglia, forming the **rami communicantes** (Fig. 5-11). The dorsal rami proceed in a posterior direction to innervate the skin and intrinsic muscles of the back. The ventral rami continue in a ventrolateral direction and give off

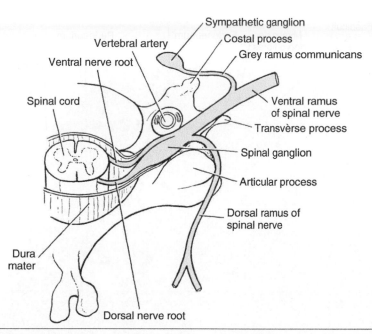

Fig. 5-11 Scheme showing the relations of a cervical nerve and its ganglion to a cervical vertebra. *(From Williams PL, editor: Gray's anatomy, ed 38, London, 1995, Churchill-Livingstone.)*

a varying number of additional branches to innervate the skin and muscles of the trunk and limbs.

The organization of the spinal nerve may seem confusing at first, but with some reasoning (and repetition), the concept should become intuitive. If the spinal cord is compared with a computer, then it can be viewed as an information processor. Sensory information can be considered input data (similar to that obtained from a mouse or keyboard). Motor information, in turn, can be considered output (similar to an image on a monitor or sound from a speaker). As the structures that carry information (in this case the nerve roots) approach the processor (the spinal cord), they separate and enter the part of the computer that is responsible for processing the type of information being conveyed. Because the dorsal horn of the cord is responsible for processing sensory information, the dorsal root conveys sensory information to it. Similarly, the ventral root transports motor (efferent or output) information from the ventral horn of the spinal cord, which processes motor information, to the target organ (in this case the skeletal muscle).

Once the roots of the spinal nerve join, the information they carry becomes mixed (sensory plus motor). When the spinal nerve begins to branch distally (i.e., the rami), both sensory and motor information are carried to the target area. Thus in the case of the dorsal ramus, sensory information is being gathered from the skin of the back, and the motor component is providing innervation (stimulation) to the intrinsic muscles of the back (e.g., the erector spinae).

CONNECTIVE TISSUE COMPONENTS

The conduit of a spinal nerve and its branches is made up of connective tissue, which together with myelin sheaths supports and protects the impulse-conducting axons. Three distinct divisions of this connective tissue have been described:

- **Epineurium**, which surrounds an entire nerve and its major branches
- **Perineurium**, which surrounds smaller bundles of nerve fibers
- **Endoneurium**, which surrounds individual nerve fibers (Fig. 5-12)

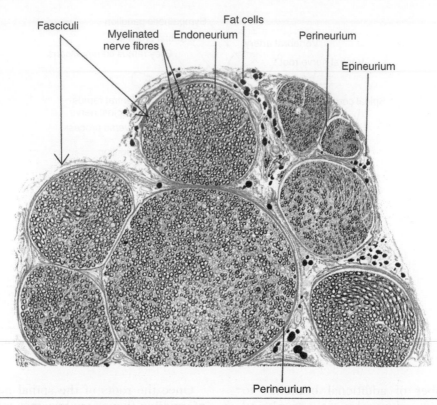

Fasciculi
Myelinated
nerve fibres
Endoneurium
Fat cells
Perineurium
Epineurium
Perineurium

Fig. **5-12** Cross-section of a peripheral nerve. *(From Williams PL, editor:* Gray's anatomy, *ed 38, London, 1995, Churchill-Livingstone.)*

This connective tissue becomes apparent as the spinal nerves exit the intervertebral foramina. If the relative diameter of the nerve roots inside the vertebral canal is compared with the diameter of the nerves in the periphery, it becomes clear that a significant amount of connective tissue has been added to the nerve for its protection and support. For example, the nerve roots that comprise the sciatic nerve might collectively approximate the diameter of a small pencil, yet the sciatic nerve is typically the diameter of the human thumb!

In addition to the connective tissue cells and matrix elements, the tissue of the nerve has a vascular component. Small arteries (**vasa nervorum**) supply the nerves and small local veins, and lymphatics drain them.

AUTONOMIC NERVOUS SYSTEM

The **autonomic nervous system** (ANS) controls or influences many of the involuntary (visceral) functions of the body. The ANS differs from the somatic part of the peripheral nervous system in the types of sensory information it conducts, the way the information is processed in the CNS, and the degree to which it reaches consciousness (usually not). In addition, the ANS differs from the somatic system in the way motor information is conveyed. Rather than having a single neuron sending a signal all the way from the CNS to a target muscle, the ANS relays this information to its target tissues via a two-neuron hookup (Fig. 5-13). The first neuron in the series is referred to as the *presynaptic* or **preganglionic neuron,** the second being named the *postsynaptic* or **postganglionic neuron.** As can be inferred by these names, the two neurons in the series communicate with each other via a synapse, which takes place within an intervening **sympathetic ganglion.** Sympathetic ganglia are located in the **paravertebral sympathetic chain,** which extends from the upper cervical spine to the coccyx, and in preaortic (preverte-

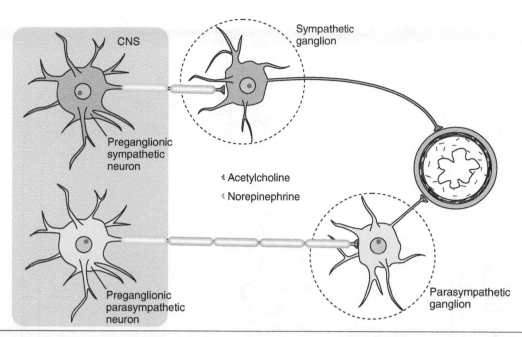

Fig. 5-13 Scheme of the two-neuron hookup between the central nervous system and the target organ. *(From Nolte J: The human brain: an introduction to its functional anatomy, ed 5, St Louis, 2002, Mosby.)*

bral) ganglia, located on the anterior surface of the abdominal aorta.

The ANS is responsible for innervating four types of tissues in the body:

- Smooth muscle (found in all blood vessels except capillaries, the gut tube, the bronchial tree, the bladder, and in many other strategic locations)
- Cardiac muscle (the heart)
- Glandular epithelium (organized into discrete structures, such as salivary and sweat glands, exocrine glands of the pancreas, and as sheets of tissue lining the body cavities)
- Lymphoid tissue (e.g., the spleen, lymph nodes, thymus, tonsils)

The ANS has two divisions or subsystems, which are antagonistic to one another and, under normal circumstances, exist in homeostatic balance with one another (the yin-yang principle). These subsystems are referred to as the **sympathetic** and **parasympathetic** divisions. Synonyms for these divisions, which are perhaps more descriptive, are the *thoracolumbar* and *craniosacral* divisions or systems (Fig. 5-14). The rationale for these terms is simple: they describe the loca-

tions in the CNS of the cell bodies of the presynaptic motor neurons of each division. Thus the cell bodies of the presynaptic neurons of the sympathetic division are located in the thoracic and lumbar segments of the spinal cord, usually from T1 to L2, whereas those of the parasympathetic division are located within the brainstem (those associated with cranial nerves 3 [oculomotor], 7 [facial], 9 [glossopharyngeal], and 10 [vagus]), and sacral segments of the spinal cord (S2 to S4). From a functional standpoint, the sympathetic division of the ANS is designed to stimulate the body to react to a threat, the *fight or flight* response, and its motor portion is distributed to the entire body. Conversely, the parasympathetic division is designed for metabolic functions, the *rest and digest* system, and its distribution is restricted to organs within body cavities, and in the head with structures primarily associated with the visceral tube. These two divisions are also sometimes referred to as **adrenergic** and **cholinergic,** respectively, because the principal neurotransmitter of the postsynaptic sympathetic neurons is epinephrine (adrenaline) and that of the postsynaptic parasympathetics is acetylcholine.

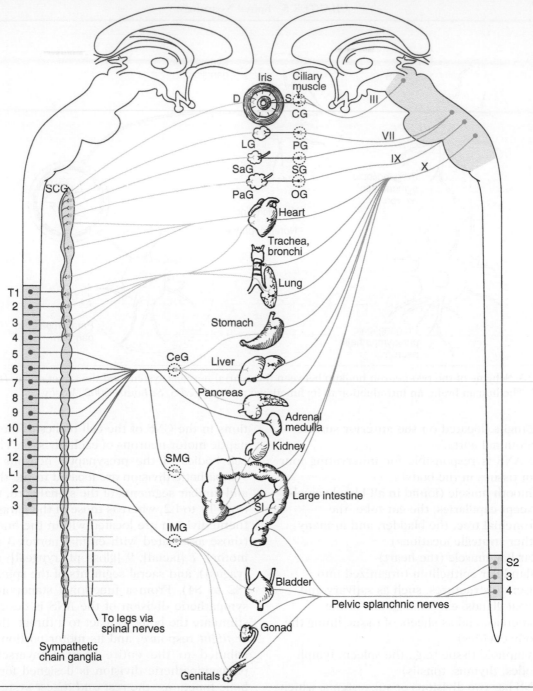

Fig. 5-14 Origin and distribution of sympathetic (*left*) and parasympathetic (*right*) efferents. Postganglionic neurons that live in sympathetic chain ganglia and project to the body wall and upper extremity are omitted from the diagram to avoid excessive complexity. Their axons travel in spinal nerves in a way analogous to that indicated for the lower-extremity supply. Although the cranial nerves have distinct and separate parasympathetic contents, substantial overlap exists in the contents of ventral roots S2 to S4. *CG,* Ciliary ganglion; *CeG,* celiac ganglion; *D,* pupillary dilator; *IMG,* inferior mesenteric ganglion; *LG,* lacrimal gland; *OG,* otic ganglion; *PaG,* parotid gland; *PG,* pterygopalatine ganglion; *S,* pupillary sphincter; *SaG,* submandibular and sublingual salivary glands; *SCG,* superior cervical ganglion; *SG,* submandibular ganglion; *SMG,* superior mesenteric ganglion. *(Modified from Mettler FA: Neuroanatomy, ed 2, St Louis, 1948, Mosby; cited in Nolte J: The human brain: an introduction to its functional anatomy, ed 5, St Louis, 2002, Mosby.)*

Probably the most important function of the ANS is to regulate blood flow to different areas of the body, supplying the most blood to the organs and tissues that need it most in any given situation (e.g., shunting blood away from gut organs and into skeletal muscle during the fight-or-flight response).

DISTRIBUTION OF SYMPATHETIC MOTOR NEURONS

Because the sympathetic efferents originate located only in the thoracolumbar spinal cord and yet are ultimately found throughout the body, four peripheral distribution strategies are employed. These pathways can be categorized as follows.

Schéma 1: Intrasegmental (T1 through L2)

In this pathway, the presynaptic neuron exits the cord in the ventral root, joins the spinal nerve, and passes through the intervertebral foramen. The neuron then leaves the spinal nerve and enters the sympathetic chain **ganglion** through the white ramus communicans (so named because the preganglionic neurons are myelinated), where it terminates in a synapse with the postsynaptic neuron. The postsynaptic neuron sends its axon back to the (same) spinal nerve through the gray ramus communicans (so named because the axons are unmyelinated) to be distributed to the target tissues within that segment.

Schéma 2: Intersegmental

At this point, the preganglionic neuron exits the cord through the ventral ramus, joins the spinal nerve, and leaves the nerve to enter the sympathetic chain through the white ramus communicans. Rather than terminating in a synapse, however, the axon continues through the ganglion and ascends or descends through the chain to another segment. This pathway allows for distribution of the preganglionic sympathetic neurons not only within the T1 through L2 cord segments, but also up to the head and neck (through the cervical extension of the chain)

and to the chain ganglia below L2. Once the preganglionic neuron terminates in a chain ganglion and synapses, the postganglionic axon reenters the spinal nerve through the gray ramus communicans. This process is how sympathetics are distributed to the upper and lower extremities. Because the spinal nerves are not distributed to the head (other than the posterior scalp), the sympathetics use another pathway to reach these targets. At this point, the preganglionic axons terminate in the **superior cervical ganglion** (the most superior limit of the sympathetic chain) (Fig. 5-15). Once the signal is transmitted through the synapse, the postsynaptic axons project to a plexus contained within the walls of the carotid arteries (internal and external), which supply the head. Not only do these nerves innervate these arteries, but they also follow them to other target tissues in the head.

Schéma 3: To the Organs of the Thoracic Cavity (T1 through T4)

In this pathway, preganglionic axons (from segments T1 through T4) reach the sympathetic chain as described earlier and terminate in the chain ganglia. Postsynaptic fibers then project from the chain directly to the organs of the thoracic cavity as the *cardiac nerves,* which travel through the *cardiopulmonary plexus* (which includes parasympathetic contribution from the vagus nerve) located on the aorta and base of the heart and the roots of the lungs.

Schéma 4: To the Organs of the Abdomen, Pelvis, and Perineum (T5 through L2)

At this point, the presynaptic axons pass from the spinal cord to the sympathetic chain as previously described. Once in the chain, however, this population of axons does not terminate, but rather bypasses the chain without synapse. These axons then coalesce with other segmental groups to form the splanchnic nerves, which are divided into four sets. The greater splanchnic nerves receive contributions from segments T5 through T9 (which ultimately innervate the organs of the foregut), the lesser splanchnic

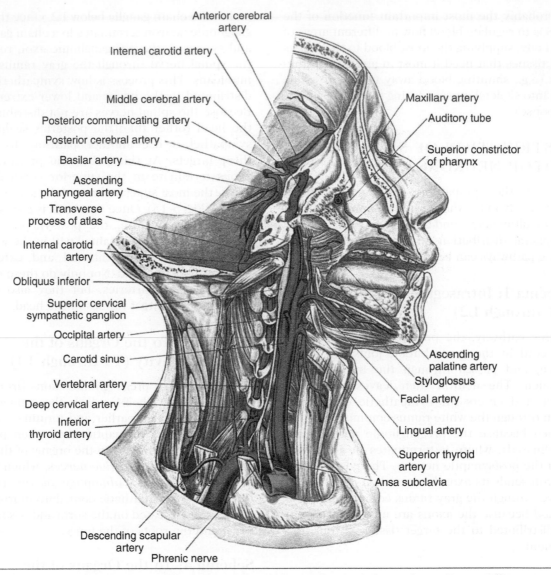

Fig. 5-15 Dissection showing the major arteries of the neck and the sympathetic chain. *(From Williams PL, editor:* Gray's anatomy, *ed 38, London, 1995, Churchill-Livingstone.)*

nerves receive contributions from T10 and T11 (which innervate the organs of the midgut and the gonads), the least splanchnic nerves from T12 (which innervates the kidneys), and the lumbar splanchnics from L1 and L2 (which innervate the organs of the hindgut, pelvis, and perineum). All but the lumbar splanchnics cross the diaphragm to the abdominal cavity, at which point they synapse with postganglionic sympathetic neurons whose cell bodies are located in the various preaortic ganglia. The postganglionics then follow the branches of the aorta to the target organs and tissues in the abdomen, pelvis, and perineum. In the case of the pelvic and perineal structures, the nerves travel in a large group of neurons called the *hypogastric plexus.*

An important point to remember is that significant divergence occurs in the sympathetic ganglia. That is, a single presynaptic sympathetic neuron may collateralize and stimulate multiple postsynaptic neurons. This action is one way that the arousal response is amplified to guarantee an adequate response from the body. Of course, occasionally, this response is inappropriately strong or prolonged, resulting in dysfunction.

DISTRIBUTION OF PARASYMPATHETIC MOTOR NEURONS

As mentioned previously, the parasympathetic division of the ANS is also known as the *craniosacral* division, because the presynaptic neuronal cell bodies are located in the brain stem and sacral spinal cord. As the axons of these nerves exit the **neuraxis** (from the brain, spinal cord, or both), they are associated with four of the cranial nerves (CNs 3, 7, 9, and 10), as well as with sacral nerves 2, 3, and 4 (S2 through S4). The presynaptic parasympathetic neurons associated with cranial nerves 3 (oculomotor), 7 (facial), and 9

ADRENAL MEDULIA

The adrenal medulla consists of secretory cells that are actually neurons, specifically postsynaptic sympathetics. The function of these neurons is to secrete epinephrine (and norepinephrine) directly into the bloodstream, which, in turn, carries this arousal neurotransmitter to all the tissues and organs of the body. The adrenal medulla receives preganglionic fibers primarily from the greater splanchnic nerves, but also from the lesser, and least splanchnic nerves (i.e., T5 through T12).

(glossopharyngeal) relay with postsynaptic neurons whose cell bodies are located in four discrete ganglia in the head. The arrangements and basic functions of these nerves are listed here.

The vagus nerve (CN10) and the sacral parasympathetics have relays on the surface of or within the organs they innervate and thus have no visible ganglia associated with them. Structures that these nerves innervate include the pharynx, larynx, and esophagus; the organs of the thoracic, abdominal, and pelvic cavities; and organs of the perineum.

VISCERAL AFFERENTS

Sensory information from visceral structures is conveyed to the CNS, mostly through small-diameter, slow-conducting neurons (C fibers). The cell bodies of these neurons are located in dorsal root ganglia and in ganglia associated with specific cranial nerves, most notably, the vagus (CN10, but also associated with other cranial nerves and sacral nerves 2 through 4). The parasympathetic afferent neurons primarily convey the sensation of stretch from the hollow organs (gut tube, bladder). The sympathetic afferents are associated with the cardiac and splanchnic nerves and almost exclusively convey pain. Therefore pain sensations from the organs of the thoracic and abdominopelvic cavities enter the spinal cord at segments T1 through L2. This arrangement is one reason why visceral pain is referred to somatic structures within these spinal cord segments (see later discussion). For example, pain from the heart is referred to the dermatomes, myotomes, and sclerotomes of segments T1 through T4. These structures include

PARASYMPATHETIC NERVE SUPPLY TO THE HEAD

Cranial Nerve	Relay Center	Function
Oculomotor (3)	Ciliary ganglion	Accommodation of the eye (for close vision)
Facial (7)	Pterygopalatine ganglion	Lacrimation, innervation of glands and vessels of the nasal and oral cavity
	Submandibular ganglion	Submandibular and sublingual salivary glands, innervation of glands of the tongue
Glossopharyngeal (9)	Otic ganglion	Parotid (salivary) gland

the left chest wall and medial left arm, spine and ribs, and muscles innervated by these segments.

REFLEXES

Reflexes are simple neuronal loops in which a stimulus and response occur as the result of a direct sensorimotor hookup. In neurologic terms, a stimulus activates a sensory neuron, which, in turn, directly activates a motor neuron (monosynaptic), producing a response (see Fig. 5-9). A reflex may also occur through an intervening neuron (disynaptic) or multiple neurons (polysynaptic). Neurons that mediate these signals within the spinal cord are referred to as *interneurons*. Some of these interneurons are excitatory; others are inhibitory. By combining the modulatory effects of these neurons, reflexes (as well as other activities mediated through the spinal cord) are rarely, if ever, all or none in terms of the response to a stimulus.

Under normal circumstances, most reflexes can be described as either somatic or visceral, in which both parts, or limbs (sensory and motor), of the reflex arc involve the same distribution (e.g., similar to a stretch reflex of a particular muscle or withdrawal reflex from a painful stimulus [somatic] or the stretch-void reflex of the bladder and rectum [visceral]). However, reflexes can also be described by the type of innervation that is present in the afferent limb of the reflex, followed by the efferent limb. Therefore these same types of reflexes can carry the terms **somatosomatic,** as the stretch reflex, or **viscero-visceral,** as the voiding reflex.

As might be imagined, reflexes can and do occur without the inclusion of the cerebral cortex, neither with the sensory component (consciousness) nor the motor component (intention). Thus reflexes are active and functional, even in the event of a spinal cord injury (with the exception, of course, of the injured segment).

As mentioned previously, sensory neurons collateralize and interact with more than one neuron in the spinal cord, as well as communicate with interneurons, which can also branch. One result of this collateralization and intercommunication is that somatosensory neurons can interact directly or indirectly with viscero-

motor neurons (i.e., those that will innervate the four types of tissues discussed earlier). The same can be said for visceral sensory neurons interacting with somatic motor neurons. This interplay between the somatic and visceral components of the spinal nerves creates two additional subclasses of reflexes, namely **somatovisceral** and **viscero-somatic.** Because of the distribution of the motor neurons of the sympathetic division of the autonomic nervous system, this type of interactivity is generally restricted to spinal cord segments T1 through L2 (within the limits of anatomic variation).

The implications of this phenomenon are significant to the practitioner of adjustive/manipulative procedures. Not only does this interactivity mean that visceral disease can exhibit, in part, as palpable, somatic hypertonicity, but also that correction of the dysfunctional somatic component may positively influence the ability of the body to combat and perhaps to rectify the problem. Conversely, allowing a chronic subluxation or segmental dysfunction (discussed later) to go uncorrected may negatively influence the function of the visceral structures associated with that segment and perhaps neighboring segments (Fig. 5-16).

PAIN (NOCICEPTION)

Pain is a protective function of the body. People who are unable to sense painful stimuli have a greatly increased risk of injury and tissue damage. Pain is sensed by free nerve endings that are functionally nonadaptive. This factor is important given that this feature of pain receptors allows the sensation of pain as long as the painful stimulus is active, giving the body accurate, up-to-the-moment information.

Nociceptors

Nociceptors (pain receptors) respond to three types of stimuli: mechanical, thermal, and chemical. Nonnociceptive mechanoreceptors normally respond to specific stimuli that are not painful. However, when the intensity of a mechanical stimulus begins to cause tissue damage, local nociceptors become activated. The

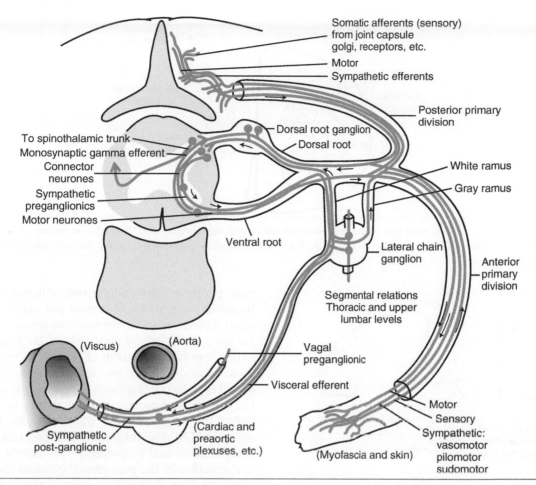

Fig. 5-16 Schéma of the spinal nerve showing several possible pathways of transmission. *(Courtesy of David Heilig, DO, FAAO.)*

same is true of tissue damage caused by extremes in temperature. The number of chemicals that will stimulate nociceptors, thereby causing pain, is fairly large. These substances include, but are not limited to, bradykinin and histamine (mediators of inflammation), serotonin (a neurotransmitter), potassium ions, and hydrogen ions (acids; this becomes important when thinking about the pain of muscle fatigue resulting from a buildup of lactic acid and how this phenomenon contributes to maintaining and exacerbating segmental dysfunction). Local tissue *ischemia* (lack of proper oxygen saturation) can also activate nociceptors, which can occur concomitant to muscle spasm.

Pathways of Pain Conduction

Pain is conducted peripherally and centrally by two distinct pathways, one fast and the other slow. Each of these pathways reaches different areas of the brain and is consequently perceived differently.

Fast Pain

The fast pain pathway, which responds to mechanical and thermal stimuli, is responsible for sharp, lancing, well-localized pain and begins with conduction through an A fiber, a

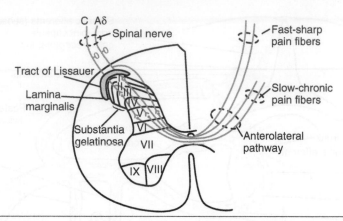

Fig. **5-17** Transmission of both fast-sharp and slow-chronic pain signals into and through the spinal cord on their way to the brain. *(From Guyton AC: Hall J: Textbook of medical physiology, ed 10, Philadelphia, 2001, WB Saunders.)*

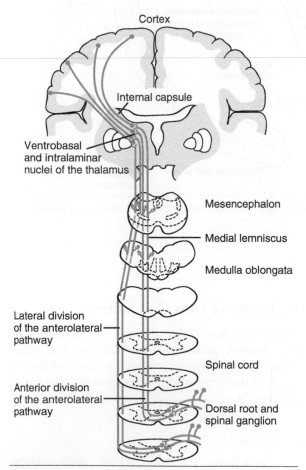

Fig. **5-18** Anterior and lateral divisions of the anterolateral pathway. *(From Guyton AC: Hall J: Textbook of medical physiology, ed 10, Philadelphia, 2001, WB Saunders.)*

thin, poorly myelinated neuron, which conducts impulses from 10 to 30 meters per second. The central processes of these neurons enter the dorsal horn of the spinal cord, where they synapse with a number of neurons (Fig. 5-17). One set of these secondary neurons transmits signals up the spinal cord to the thalamus. These neurons cross the midline and ascend to the thalamus in a tract called the spinothalamic tract or anterolateral system (ALS). The information is then relayed in the thalamus and projected to the cerebral cortex, specifically the postcentral gyrus of the parietal lobe (Fig. 5-18). This part of the cortex is somatotopically arranged so that specific body parts are represented in various locations of the gyrus (Fig. 5-19). This configuration allows the cortex to localize the pain to a very high degree (i.e., the individual can tell exactly where the pain is located). The ALS is a good example of the labeled line principle, in which multiple neurons form a pathway destined for a specific location in the CNS (Figs. 5-20 and 5-21).

The DRG neurons of the fast pain pathway will also synapse on other neurons that generate an appropriate response to the stimulus. One of these responses is the **withdrawal reflex,** in which alpha motor neurons are stimulated, resulting in almost immediate muscle contraction, thus allowing the organism to avoid the continued painful stimulus. The primary neurotransmitter for these neurons appears to be glutamate, which is relatively short acting (i.e., quickly extinguishes).

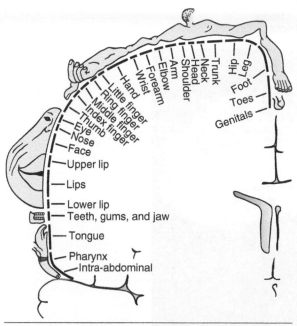

Fig. 5-19 Representation of the different areas of the body in somatosensory area I of the cortex. *(From Penfield W, Rasmussen T:* Cerebral cortex of man, a clinical study of localization of function, *New York, 1968, Hafner.)*

Slow Pain

Slow pain is the more long-lasting, poorly localized, deep, burning type of pain. Slow pain is conducted from the periphery by small unmyelinated C fibers, which conduct impulses at a rate as slow as 0.5 meters per second. These fibers are responsible for a more delayed perception and response to pain. Similar to the fast pain fibers, these neurons enter the cord through the dorsal horn and terminate on secondary neurons, which conduct the impulse up the spinal cord in the ALS. However, the vast majority of these secondary neurons, rather than projecting to the thalamus, terminate in the brainstem **reticular formation,** an extremely old part of the CNS. The reticular formation lies deep within the brainstem and is made up of neurons with relatively short axons. Extending the entire length of the brainstem and spinal cord, the reticular formation is responsible for a variety of functions. One function is to stimulate the organism to a state of increased alertness (the reticular-activating system), which certainly occurs during

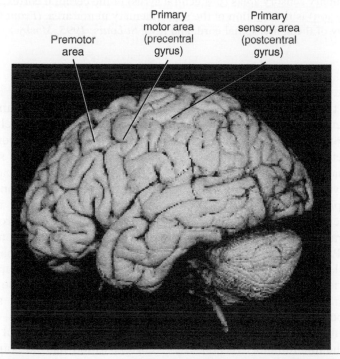

Fig. 5-20 Lateral view of the brain showing the primary motor (precentral gyrus), premotor, and primary sensory (postcentral gyrus) areas of the cerebral cortex. *(From Cramer GD, Darby SA:* Basic and clinical anatomy of the spine, spinal cord, and ANS, *St Louis, 1995, Mosby.)*

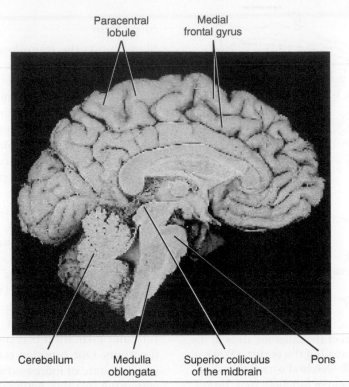

Paracentral
lobule

Medial
frontal gyrus

Cerebellum

Medulla
oblongata

Superior colliculus
of the midbrain

Pons

Fig. 5-21 Medial view of the brain. The paracentral lobule, which is the continuation of the primary motor area (precentral gyrus) and primary sensory areas (postcentral gyrus) of the cerebral cortex, is indicated. The medial frontal gyrus (posterior region) is the location of the supplementary motor area. *(From Cramer GD, Darby SA: Basic and clinical anatomy of the spine, spinal cord, and ANS, St Louis, 1995, Mosby.)*

the experience of pain. This increased vigilance is crucial to the future avoidance of pain. The reticular formation, in turn, projects to the limbic system, which governs emotional responses, as well as to the hypothalamus, which significantly influences the activity of the ANS. In addition, the reticular formation communicates with the periaqueductal gray of the midbrain, which projects back to the spinal cord to inhibit pain sensation (see later discussion).

The primary neurotransmitter for slow pain is the peptide **substance P,** the effects of which are considerably more long lasting than glutamate and is partially responsible for the chronicity of slow pain. Not only is substance P secreted at the central terminal of a C fiber, but it is also secreted at the peripheral end. Substance P has been shown to act as a cytokine in the inflammatory response. Another transmitter implicated in the pain pathway is calcitonin gene related peptide (CGRP).

Visceral Pain

Pain from the thoracic and abdominopelvic visceral organs is exclusively transmitted by substance P–producing C fibers. By comparison with the somatic nociceptive system, the number of pain fibers in the body cavities is relatively few. These nerves, as mentioned previously, are primarily associated with the sympathetics and enter the spinal cord from T1 to L2. As substance P–producing neurons, these neurons interact with the slow pain pathway secondary neurons, which project upward through the ALS (Fig. 5-22). Most of these neurons feed into the reticular formation, but some reach the thalamus. From the thalamus, third-order fibers project to either the parietal cortex, or the insular cortex, which has no somatotopic arrangement (Fig. 5-23). The insular cortex apparently deals in part with the relative sense of well being. As

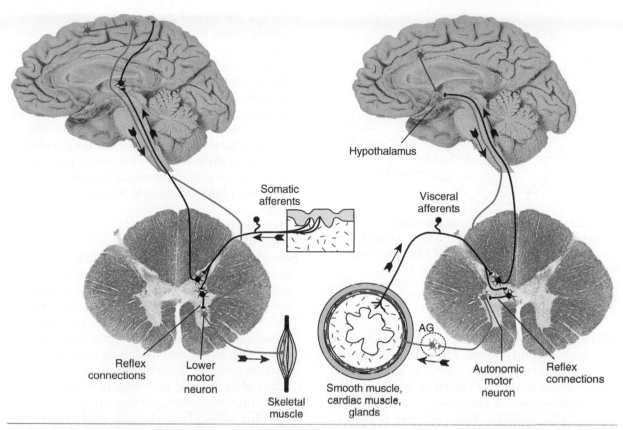

Fig. 5-22 Parallels between somatic and autonomic parts of the nervous system. Both parts involve specialized afferents and efferents, reflex connections, and ascending and descending pathways to and from higher levels of the central nervous system. In the case of the sympathetic and parasympathetic systems, however, the hypothalamus rather than the thalamus receives much of the ascending information, and the hypothalamus rather than the cerebral cortex is a major source of descending pathways. In addition, sympathetic and parasympathetic transmission to the periphery involves and intermediate synapse in an autonomic ganglion. *(From Nolte J: The human brain: an introduction to its functional anatomy, ed 5, St Louis, 2002, Mosby.)*

such, visceral pain primarily codes to consciousness as a sense of not feeling well, without a great deal of specificity (e.g., a stomachache). The relatively small number of fibers, coupled with the central distribution of C fibers (i.e., not many fibers reach the thalamus and thus the cortex) accounts for the poor localization of this type of pain. However, the nonadaptability of these neurons along with the activity of substance P is responsible for the relative severity and long lasting nature of visceral pain.

Inhibition of Pain

The pain pathway can be interrupted by an inhibitory system within the CNS. This pathway

originates in the midbrain and is known as the **periaqueductal gray** (PAG). These neurons project (send axons) to another area of the brainstem known as the raphe nuclei, where they relay. The raphe nuclei neurons, in turn, project to the dorsal horn of the spinal cord, secreting **endogenous opiates** as their primary neurotransmitter (the enkephalins and endorphins). This action effectively shuts off the transmission of pain information from the primary nociceptors to the secondary, ascending neurons of the ALS. The inhibition of pain is presumably a survival mechanism that allows the individual to function in spite of experiencing pain. The PAG cells receive input from the cerebral cortex, which explains the remarkable control some

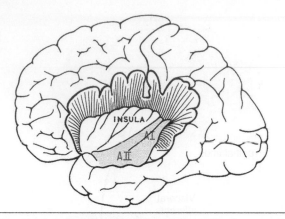

Fig. 5-23 Lateral surface of the left cerebral hemisphere showing the insular cortex. Parts of the temporal, parietal, and the frontal lobes have been removed. *(From Williams PL, editor:* Gray's anatomy, *ed 38, London, 1995, Churchill-Livingstone.)*

individuals demonstrate in tolerating otherwise extremely painful stimuli. The pain pathway can also be interrupted by certain activities or behaviors, as well as by electrical stimulation.

Stimulus-induced analgesia, or **afferent inhibition,** is an adaptive behavior that is used to distract the nervous system from the perception of pain. Examples include rubbing an elbow that has just been bumped, scratching an itch, shaking off a traumatized joint, and others. These behaviors are designed to bombard the CNS with additional strong stimuli so as to turn the attention of the system toward that stimulus and away from the pain. In the process, the individual becomes more aware of the behavior than the pain.

Other behaviors are designed to avoid pain:
Patient: "It hurts when I do that."
Clinician: "Then don't do that."

- As the person lies in bed asleep for extended periods, the pressure from the mattress can produce local tissue ischemia, which stimulates nociceptors. The response is to move away from the stimulus by turning over.
- As a weight-bearing joint begins to deteriorate from arthritis, the person develops a characteristic antalgic (pain-avoiding) gait to walk around or away from the painful joint surface (a limp).

- As the muscles of the low back respond to a minor tissue injury by contracting, over time, they become fatigued, resulting in an increase in local tissue pH. This stimulus activates nociceptors, causing more pain in the muscles, leading to additional guarding. The patient comes to the office and states that his or her back "went out." The patient exhibits a characteristic posture, which has developed to reduce the amount of perceived pain but which is usually mechanically inefficient, causing additional muscle fatigue and more pain.

Other responses to pain:
- Guarding or splinting

Splinting takes place when an injury to a joint occurs. The local tissue damage causes swelling and pain, which, in turn, activates nociceptors. These nociceptors interact with alpha and gamma motor neurons, creating hypertonicity of the muscles that move the joint. This hypertonicity (along with the tissue tension resulting from the swelling) has the effect of decreasing the range of motion of the joint, thus preventing further injury.

Guarding takes place when an injury to or inflammation of the abdominal **viscera** occurs. Guarding is an example of a **viscero-somatic reflex** arc. In this case, the pain from the viscera is transmitted to the spinal cord via C fibers, which enter the cord in the lower thoracic segments. These neurons stimulate alpha and gamma motor neurons that innervate the muscles of the abdominal wall, which become hypertonic. The contraction of these muscles not only helps prevent a repetition of the trauma, but also helps hold the organs in place, which also prevents further injury.

- Referred pain (Fig. 5-24)

This condition also occurs as the result of visceral organ involvement. Two phenomena are operative in this situation. The first is *convergence,* in which a visceral afferent converges on a secondary neuron of the ALS and activates it. This action sends a signal to the cortex, which interprets the information as pain coming from a somatic structure. Because the visceral afferents enter the cord at spinal cord segments T1 through L2, the patient will perceive pain within that somatic segment (i.e., dermatome, myotome, sclerotome). The second phenomenon is **neurotransmitter spillover.** As mentioned previously, nociceptors are nonadaptive; that is, as the pain persists, they will continue to fire. Substance P, characterized as a long-acting neurotransmitter, is therefore continuously secreted into the dorsal horn. Subsequently, more and more secondary ALS neurons (including those of the fast pathway) become involved in transmitting the pain. For example, the heart, which receives motor innervation from T1 through T4, will transmit pain back to those same cord segments. The patient will become aware of a vague tightness in the chest resulting the vagueness of the pain coded from the visceral afferents. However, as the pain persists and more substance P is secreted into the dorsal horn of the spinal cord, secondary ALS neurons become activated. The patient now complains of frank chest pain and pain running down the left arm (along the dermatomes of T1 through T4). Specific referred pain patterns exist for most organs, which is an important reason to carefully study the segmentation of the ANS (Fig. 5-25). The influx of substance P and the intersegmental collateralization of C fibers in the dorsal horn can also cause the spread of pain to adjacent segments, accounting for some patients' complaints of neck pain during a heart attack.

- The **allostatic response** (allostasis)

This reaction is an adaptive response, which can result from prolonged stress on the system

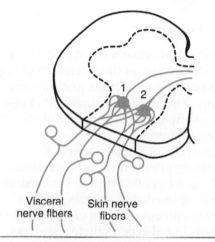

Fig. 5-24 Mechanism of referred pain and referred hyperalgesia. *(From Guyton AC: Hall J: Textbook of medical physiology, ed 10, Philadelphia, 2001, WB Saunders.)*

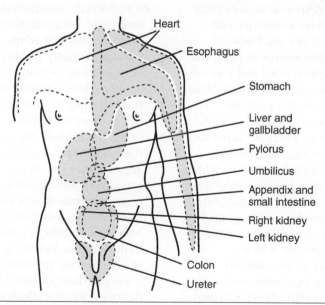

Fig. 5-25 Surface areas of referred pain from different visceral organs. *(From Guyton AC: Hall J: Textbook of medical physiology, ed 10, Philadelphia, 2001, WB Saunders.)*

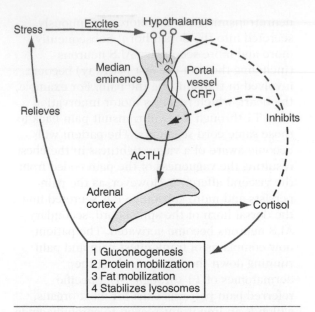

Fig. **5-26** Mechanism for regulation of glucocorticoid secretion. *ACTH,* Adrenocorticotropic hormone; *CRF,* corticotrophin-releasing factor. *(From Guyton AC: Hall J: Textbook of medical physiology, ed 10, Philadelphia, PA, WB Saunders, 2001).*

(Fig. 5-26). One such stressor, of course, is pain. Unfortunately, multiple inputs to this feedback loop (i.e., multiple stressors) may be present, which can exacerbate the condition. However, the allostatic response underscores the holistic nature of the interactivity and mobilization of several, if not all, body systems. Starting from the source of pain, the impulse travels to the spinal cord and ascends through the ALS via secondary neurons. Many of these neurons project to the reticular formation, which ascends through the brainstem to the hypothalamus. Stressful input to the hypothalamus causes the secretion of corticotropin-releasing hormone (CRH), which migrates through the hypophyseal portal system (the vascular system) to the anterior pituitary. CRH stimulates the synthesis and secretion of adrenocorticotrophic hormone (ACTH) into the bloodstream, which ultimately makes its way to the adrenal cortex. At this point, the synthesis and secretion of hormones is stimulated. Cortisol, which has a wide range of systemic effects, including suppression of the immune system,

is one of these hormones. Immune suppression is important in preventing **anaphylaxis** (a severe reaction to antigens or the allergic response). Aldosterone, which regulates kidney function, is another hormone produced by the adrenal cortex. A third hormone is androstenedione, a reproductive hormone.

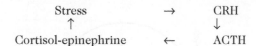

Therefore stress clearly has a global outreach in the body because of the interconnectivity of the nervous, endocrine, and immune systems. The somatic component of disease is easily extrapolated given its influence on the nervous system.

Unfortunately, ACTH also exerts a stimulatory effect on the adrenal medulla, which, as mentioned earlier, synthesizes and secretes epinephrine. Increased levels of serum epinephrine increase the state of alertness but also perpetuate the stress reaction-adaptive response caused by direct input to the reticular formation, the closure point of the loop.

• Facilitation and sensitization

As previously mentioned, nociceptors are considered nonadapting. On the contrary, not only do they not adapt, but they also have a unique property known as **sensitization.** Sensitization, synonymous with **facilitation,** occurs when a painful stimulus is applied over time. Rather than decreasing its rate of firing, the nociceptor actually *increases* its impulse rate. In addition, the excitation threshold of the nociceptor membrane becomes significantly lower, resulting in increased firing rates from subthreshold stimuli. This characteristic means that once a nociceptor is facilitated, a less than painful stimulus becomes painful, a condition known as **hyperalgesia.** Facilitation can also extend to the secondary neurons in the pain pathway, lowering their threshold for firing. This decrease causes **allodynia,** in which various normal stimuli become painful. Neuronal behavior of this kind in the trigeminal system

(CN 5) is responsible for the severity and duration of migraine headaches. Because of peripheral overlap of receptive fields, as well as central overlap of fields of distribution, entire spinal cord segments can become facilitated, leading to segmental dysfunction. This phenomenon was first elucidated by the physiologist Irvin Korr, Ph.D.

Note to the reader: Although all of the previously mentioned scenarios are real and potential, they are presented as the "worst case." The cybernetic loops that exist in the body enable it to maintain homeostasis under normal circumstances. When disruptions occur, the body is also able to compensate and self-correct through a number of healing processes.

SEGMENTAL DYSFUNCTION

Given all the information presented thus far, making a case for the existence of segmental dysfunction is relatively simple. Distillation of the concept to its most fundamental components would include initial perturbation (disturbance) of the segmental system, an attempt to self-correct, a destabilization of the system, and increased risk for further perturbation. However, the more one is aware of *all* the implications of the body segment, (the anatomy, physiology, pathology), the more one is equipped to diagnose and treat. *In addition, understanding of the visceral component as it relates to the segmentation and distribution of the ANS is of paramount importance.* As defined in Chapter 4, the segment includes the spinal nerve and *all* the tissues it innervates, both somatic and visceral.

Segmental dysfunction can have a variety of causes and expressions. By definition, the existence of the somatic component in disease is the defining factor, the understanding of which predisposes the chiropractor to a singularly useful set of manual tools for diagnosis and treatment. Also bearing in mind the nature of the musculoskeletal system as a tensegrity structure,

The Downward spiral

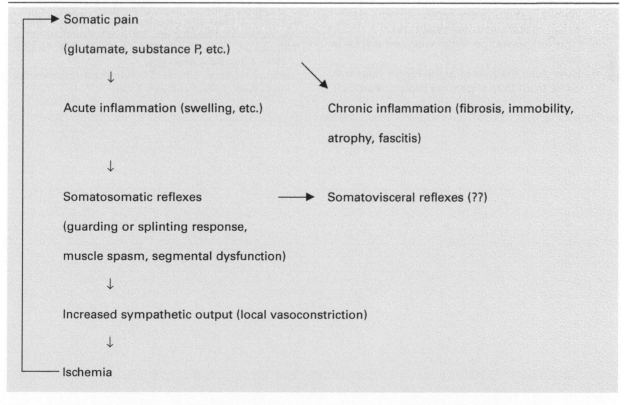

coupled with the prime directive of the equilibrial triad (consisting of the visual, proprioceptive, and vestibular systems as described in Chapter 4), maintaining an upright posture for visual acuity underscores the importance of holism in clinical practice.

Briefly stated, the relative balance of the body in space is routinely subjected to challenges to which the individual usually adapts and self-corrects. Indeed, some disruptions of the musculoskeletal system go untreated for years without any complaint from the individual. However, over time, the body gradually loses its capacity to withstand these challenges and begins to decompensate, which is usually when an individual becomes a patient.

Review *Questions*

1. Describe the basic structure of the neuron.
2. What is the relationship between the diameter of a nerve and the speed at which impulses are conducted by that nerve?
3. Explain the role of the dorsal root ganglion.
4. What are the primary types of exteroceptors and interoceptors?
5. How is knowledge of dermatomes useful in diagnosis?
6. How does the role of alpha motor neurons differ from that of gamma motor neurons?

7. Why is the diameter of the sciatic nerve substantially larger than the combined size of the nerve roots that comprise it?
8. What are the four types of tissue innervated by the ANS?
9. Describe the roles of the sympathetic and parasympathetic divisions of the ANS.
10. If the spinal cord's function is seen as information processing in a computer, what are the inputs and outputs?

Concept *Questions*

1. How can muscle hypertonicity or spasm contribute to maintaining the inflammatory state?
2. How can segmental dysfunction contribute to visceral disease?
3. How can visceral disease contribute to segmental dysfunction?

SUGGESTED READINGS

Cramer GD, Darby SA: *Basic and clinical anatomy of the spine, spinal cord, and ANS,* St Louis, 1995, Mosby.

Guyton AC, Hall JE: *Textbook of medical physiology,* ed 10, Philadelphia, 2001, WB Saunders.

Larsen WJ: *Anatomy: development, function, clinical correlations,* Philadelphia, 2002, WB Saunders.

Williams PL, editor: *Gray's anatomy,* ed 38, London, 1995, Churchill-Livingstone.

Zigmond MJ et al, editors: *Fundamental neuroscience,* San Diego, 1999, Academic Press.

CHAPTER 6

Basic Biomechanics

Joseph Morley, DC, PhD

Key Terms

ACCELERATION	HOOKE'S LAW	STRAIN
ANISOTROPIC	HYSTERESIS	STRESS
CHONDROCYTE	IMPULSE	TENSILE LOADING
COMPRESSION	INERTIA	TORSION
CREEP	KINEMATICS	TRANSLATION
DISPLACEMENT	LATERAL FLEXION	VELOCITY
DISTRACTION	NEWTON'S THREE LAWS OF	VISCOELASTICITY
ELASTICITY	MOTION	VISCOSITY
EXTENSION	PENNATE	WOLFF'S LAW
FLEXION	PLASTICITY	WORK
GROUND REACTION FORCES	SHEARING	

The human body is continually subjected to external and internal mechanical forces that tend to produce structural deformation of tissue. These forces, which include gravity, muscle activity, and **ground reaction forces** (i.e., the result of foot and ground interaction during locomotion) are resisted in the body by bone, muscle, and ligament, as well as other soft tissues. Loads, or external forces, can be individual or a combination of compression, torsion, translation (i.e., shearing), and tensile loading. Understanding these forces and the ways they affect the hard and soft tissues of the musculoskeletal system is essential for chiropractors, who are directly concerned with the restoration of balance and mobility to the spinal column and other musculoskeletal structures.

This chapter introduces the key terms and concepts of biomechanics that chiropractors deal with throughout their careers. It complements Chapter 4 (Spinal Anatomy), adding detail on the qualities and functions of the various tissues that make up the musculoskeletal system.

TYPES OF LOADING, STRESSES, AND STRAINS

Translation and Shearing

Translation occurs when all particles in a body move in parallel at a given time. When one body undergoes translation with respect to another adjacent body, **shearing** forces result. An example would be two adjacent vertebrae. If a load is applied to a structure and no rotation occurs, then shearing can result (Fig. 6-1).

For example, if the left hand is tightly wrapped around T12 and the right hand around L1 on a plastic model of the spinal column and an attempt is made to pull T12 while not allowing L1 to move, then a shearing force at the T12-L1 disk will occur. It is the sagittal orientation of the T12-L1 facets that permits this type of movement (Fig. 6-2). Shearing, which usually occurs in combination with other forces, can cause a fracture-dislocation. The orientation of the mid-cervical facets (Fig. 6-3) favors fracture-dislocation in car accidents involving violent forward flexion of the head. Fortunately, soft tissues such as the annulus fibers of the intervertebral disk contribute

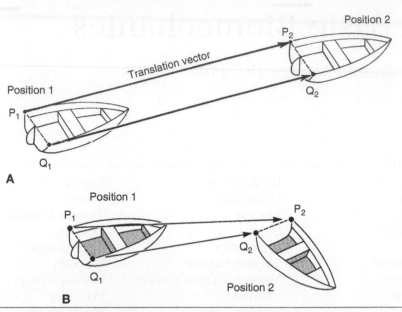

Fig. 6-1 A, Translation. When a body (boat) moves such that a line P_1Q_1 in it moves parallel to itself, the body is said to translate. Lines joining the same point on the body in two different positions (e.g., line P_1P_2 and Q_1Q_2) are called the translation vectors. The translation vectors of all points on the body are always equal and parallel to each other, indicating translation of the body. **B,** Rotation. A body is said to rotate when a line in it does not move parallel to itself. In the boat, the line P_2Q_2 is not parallel to P_1Q_1. *(From Panjabi MM, White AA:* Biomechanics in the musculoskeletal system, *New York, 2001, Churchill Livingstone.)*

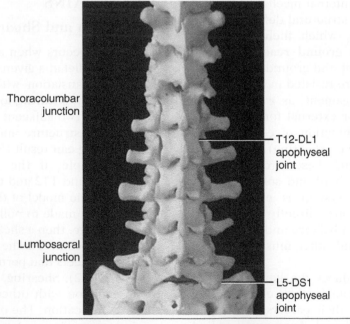

Fig. 6-2 Posterior view of the thoracolumbar and lumbosacral junctions. The transition in the orientation of the facet surfaces within the zygapophyseal joints between the two junctions is visualized. Compare sagittal orientation of T12-L1. *(From Neumann DA:* Kinesiology of the musculoskeletal system: foundations for physical rehabilitation, *St Louis, 2002, Mosby.)*

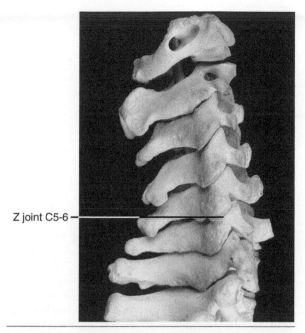

Fig. 6-3 Lateral view of the cervical spine. The angulation of the facets at the zygapophyseal joints is visualized. *(From Herzog W:* Clinical biomechanics of spinal manipulation, *Philadelphia, 2000, Churchill Livingstone.)*

Z joint C5-6

resistance to shearing forces and thus to the clinical stability of the spine.

Compression, Tensile Loading, and Distraction

Flexion is accompanied by compression of anterior structures and **tensile loading** (i.e., elongation or loading in the vertical axis) of posterior structures (Fig. 6-4). **Compression** in the spine resulting from flexion is possible and largely due to intervertebral disks that extend the height between the vertebrae. The spine is susceptible to compressive loads, either in single episodes involving high forces or by constant low-force compression. If flexion is violent, as in a car accident, then anterior compression injuries and posterior tearing of the restraining soft tissue is possible. Significant compression (loads greater than 600 pounds per square inch [psi]) of vertebral end plates and bodies can result in compression fractures or herniation of discal material through the vertebral end plate. **Distraction** and tensile loading are not common but can occur in an automobile accident when the seat belt restrains the trunk (Figs. 6-5 and 6-6).

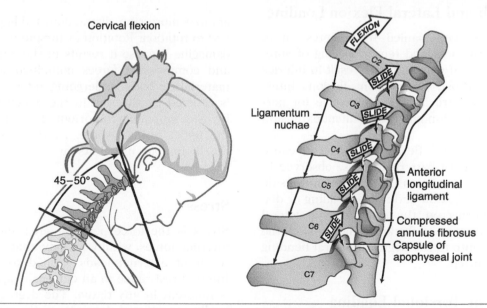

Cervical flexion

45–50°

FLEXION

C2

SLIDE

C3

Ligamentum nuchae

SLIDE

C4

SLIDE

C5

SLIDE

Anterior longitudinal ligament

C6

SLIDE

Compressed annulus fibrosus

Capsule of apophyseal joint

C7

Fig. 6-4 Flexion of the cervical spine. Flexion slackens the anterior longitudinal ligament and increases the space between the adjacent laminae and spinous processes. Elongated and taut tissues *(thin black arrows)* and slackened tissue *(wavy black arrow)* are indicated. *(From Neumann DA:* Kinesiology of the musculoskeletal system: foundations for physical rehabilitation, *St Louis, 2002, Mosby.)*

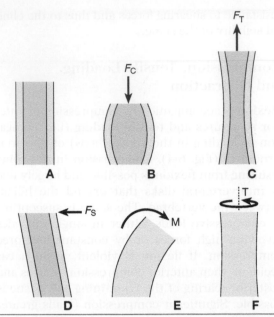

Fig. 6-5 Effects of different types of forces acting on a solid object. **A,** No forces acting; **B,** compressive force F_C; **C,** tensile force F_T; **D** shear force F_S; **E,** bending moment B; **F,** torsional moment, or torque T. *(From Adams MA et al: The biomechanics of back pain, Edinburgh, 2002, Churchill Livingstone.)*

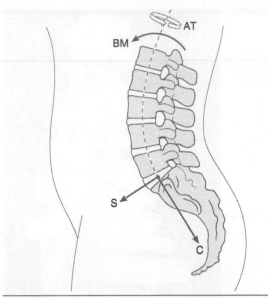

Fig. 6-6 Component forces acting on the lumbar spine. *C,* Compression; *S,* shear; *BM,* bending moment in the sagittal plane; *AT,* axial torque. In three dimensions a lateral shear force and lateral bending moment could also occur. *(From Adams MA et al: The biomechanics of back pain, Edinburgh, 2002, Churchill Livingstone.)*

Extension and Lateral Flexion Loading

Extension is accompanied by compression of posterior structures and tensile loading of anterior structures. If violent, it can result in injuries opposite to those observed in flexion. Intervertebral discs are largely responsible for permitting compression and the resultant extension (Fig. 6-7).

If forced, **lateral flexion** loading can cause injuries similar in pattern to those observed in forced flexion—compressive injuries on the side toward lateral flexion and tensile loading or distraction injuries on the side opposite lateral bending. As occurs in flexion and extension, the disks contribute to the degree of lateral bending that is permitted.

Rotation or Torsional Loading

Rotation or *torsional loading* occurs when all particles in a body move in concentric circles or arcs. The vertebral motion segment is far more resist-

ant to compression, distraction, and bending than it is to rotation. Rotation or **torsion** is potentially damaging because it results in shearing, tensile, and compressive forces combined within the material or body undergoing rotation. Torsion is resisted by the ribs in the dorsal spine and by the more sagittal-oriented facet joints in the upper lumbar spine. At the L5-S1 joints, the iliolumbar ligaments provide resistance to torsion.

Stress

Stress is the force per unit area and involves internal forces within a body that arise as a result of external loads applied to the body. Internal resistance to an externally applied load is inherent in any tissue. The degree to which loading is resisted depends on the material, its size, and the load applied. Low levels of tissue stress maintained over a long period or high levels of stress applied over a short period can result

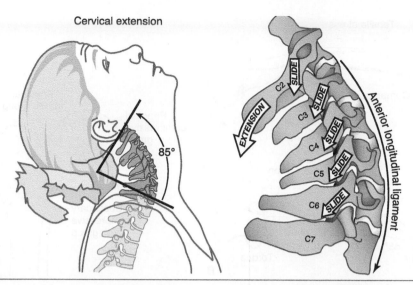

Fig. 6-7 Extension of the cervical spine. The extension stretches the anterior longitudinal ligament and decreases the space between the adjacent laminae and spinous processes. *(From Neumann DA:* Kinesiology of the musculoskeletal system: foundations for physical rehabilitation, *St Louis, 2002, Mosby.)*

in tissue damage. Stress can result in deformation of a body or **strain**. Deformation of a body can be temporary or permanent (Fig. 6-8).

Biologic materials are **anisotropic**; in other words, their response to loading varies with the direction of loading (Fig. 6-9). For example, bone resists compression differently than it resists tensile loading or shear loading; ligaments resist tensile loading differently than shear loading. **Hooke's law** states that deformation increases in proportion to the load that is applied; that is, strain increases in proportion to the body's internal stress that is resisting the applied load.

BIOMECHANICAL CHARACTERISTICS OF TISSUE

Elasticity is the tendency of tissue under load to return to its original size and shape after removal of the load. Rubber bands and ligaments are examples. Strain is instant. No energy is lost in deformation, and the tissue returns to its normal shape.

Plasticity is the property of a material that instantly deforms when a load is applied and does not return to its original shape when the load is removed. When the applied load is beyond the material's elastic limit, deformation results. Bone can alter its shape permanently, according to loads that are placed on it.

Viscosity is the property of a material that does not deform instantly when a load is applied. Stress develops but strain is delayed; consequently, deformation is related to time. Failure to return to the original shape when the load is removed is a property of pure viscosity. Energy is absorbed within the material.

Viscoelasticity, a combination of viscosity and elasticity, is the property of a material to deform slowly and nonlinearly when a load is applied and to return to its original size and shape slowly and nonlinearly when the load is removed. Articular cartilage and intervertebral disks exhibit viscoelasticity.

Creep is an increase in strain of a material that occurs during constant stress from loading. It is a deformation of a viscoelastic tissue to a constant, steadily applied load. In the body, the structure undergoing creep may or may not return to its original length or shape, depending on the load and whether the structure is damaged. A damaged intervertebral disk can deform when under a load in a shorter time than that of a normal disk.

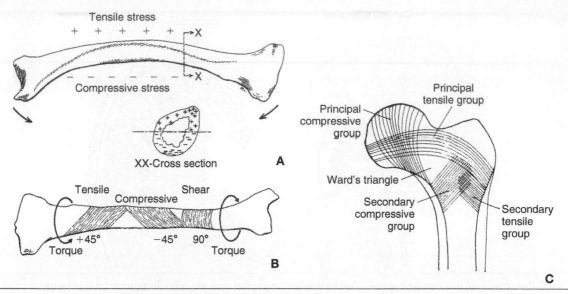

Fig. 6-8 Stresses on a long bone. When subjected to bending (**A**), the normal tensile stresses (+) are on the convex side, whereas the normal compressive stresses (-) are on the concave side of the bent bone. Torsion (torque) on a long bone (**B**) produces different types of stresses—tensile, compressive, and shear—at a point, depending on the direction chosen. **C**, Normal trabecular pattern of the proximal portion of the femur is shown. Four of the anatomic groups of trabeculae are indicated in this schematic drawing. Ward's triangle lies within the neutral axis, where compressive and tensile forces balance one another. (*A and B from Panjabi MM, White AA:* Biomechanics in the musculoskeletal system, *New York, 2001, Churchill Livingstone. C from Taylor JAM, Resnick D:* Skeletal imaging: atlas of the spine and extremities, Philadelphia, *2000, WB Saunders.*)

Hysteresis is an effect of repeated loading and unloading of a tissue. Although a tissue may resist one or more loads, the constant repetition of loading may cause the elastic limit to be exceeded. In the human body, hysteresis can be thought of as overuse. The material may not return to its original shape after many repetitions over a long period. Thus the loading and unloading characteristics are not the same. If a tissue is subject to fatigue or has a weakness in its internal architecture, repeated loading and unloading may result in damage. In the intervertebral disk and surrounding tissues, repetitive lifting in a forward-leaning position may result in repetitive axial loading with no opportunity for recovery, which may damage the annular fibers, ligaments, and muscles. If an articular joint has poor ligamentous support or if the muscles moving the joint are weak, then the articular cartilage may be damaged from repeated loading. Overuse combined with poor soft tissue support and protection can lead to damage.

QUALITIES OF MUSCULOSKELETAL TISSUES
Muscle

Muscle fibers aligned parallel to a tendon are able to transmit all their force to the tendon. Muscle fibers aligned in a pennate fashion to a tendon transmit less than 100% force to the tendon. A **pennate** arrangement occurs when the muscle fibers are at an angle to the direction of pull. A good example of this arrangement is the gastrocnemius muscle (Fig. 6-10).

Fascia

Muscle tissue is surrounded by connective tissue in the form of fascia. Thus muscular activity is dependent to a certain extent on the connective tissue sheath that surrounds it. Fascia responds favorably to tensile loading by improving its mobility; it also responds to inactivity by shortening.

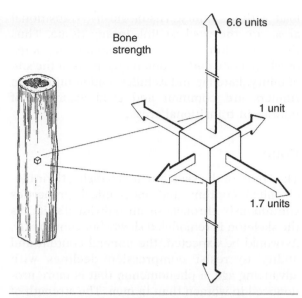

Fig. 6-9 Anisotropy of bone. The strength of bone material in the mid-diaphysis of a long bone varies in different directions. Generally, the axial strength is the greatest. *(From Panjabi MM, White AA:* Biomechanics in the musculoskeletal system, *New York, 2001, Churchill Livingstone.)*

Connective tissues are composed of collagen, elastin, ground substance, water, and minerals. These components vary with the type and age of connective tissue. Connective tissue tolerates tensile forces well, deforms with load, and recovers its shape when the load is removed.

Ligaments

Ligaments join bone to bone, stabilize joints, and prevent abnormal motion in joints. The fibers are parallel and directed along the axis of tensile loading. Similar to tendons, ligaments are composed of collagen and elastin; however, ligaments have a higher elastin content than do tendons. Ligaments are designed to resist tensile forces. The greater the cross-sectional area of a ligament, the greater the ability to tolerate the load. Exercise can result in hypertrophy of a ligament. In effect, the cross-sectional area can be increased within limits, thus offering increased resistance to failure or rupture. Conversely, disuse or immobilization results in a decrease in a ligament's mechanical properties.

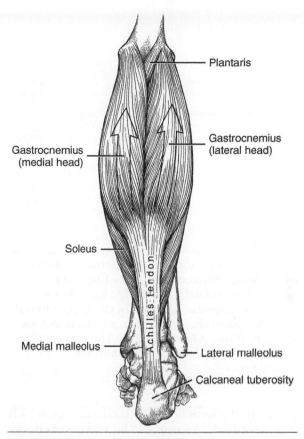

Fig. 6-10 The superficial muscles of the posterior compartment of the right leg are shown. The pennate arrangement of the fibers of the gastrocnemius muscle is visualized. *(From Neumann DA:* Kinesiology of the musculoskeletal system: foundations for physical rehabilitation, *St Louis, 2002, Mosby.)*

The mechanical properties of ligaments change with age, as do other body tissues. As expected, the ability to withstand tensile load decreases with age. The mechanism of ligament failure also changes as the body grows older, with avulsion (i.e., tearing away) of bone at the ligament site becoming more common than actual ligament rupture (Fig. 6-11).

Tendons

Tendons are joined to muscles and lie parallel to them; as a result, they bear the same load as the muscles. Tendons support muscle forces and deform minimally. They can store some potential

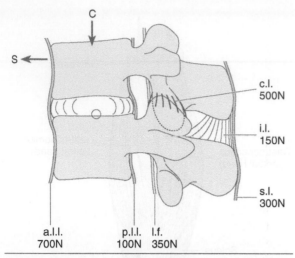

Fig. 6-11 Relative strength (in Newtons) of lumbar intervertebral ligaments (9.81 N = 1 kg). *a.l.l.,* Anterior longitudinal ligament; *l.f.,* ligamentum flavum; *c.l.,* capsular ligaments of the zygapophyseal joints; *i.l.,* interspinous ligament; *s.l.,* supraspinous ligament. *(From Adams MA et al: The biomechanics of back pain, Edinburgh, 2002, Churchill Livingstone.)*

energy in the form of elastic strain energy, which is evident in the kangaroo. The storage of energy also occurs in the quadriceps and gastrocnemius and soleus muscles in running humans. Immediately after heel strike, the quadriceps and gastrocnemius muscles act as brakes and contract while elongating. This contraction is eccentric, and this elongation of muscle under load is similar to the stretching of a rubber band. Energy is stored in the stretched muscle or rubber band. When the knee starts to flex and the ankle starts to plantar flex during the propulsive phase of stance, stored energy is returned, which makes running or walking more energy efficient.

Tendons must support large muscle forces with minimal deformation; as a result elastin content is less than it is in ligaments. The collagen fibers are arranged in parallel and run longitudinally. Tendons, similar to ligaments, are designed to resist tensile loads. As with other body tissues, tendon function decreases with age and disuse. Exercise results in a greater cross-sectional area as a result of hypertrophy. This gives the tendon the capacity to resist more of a

load without injury. Histologically, transitional areas are the weakest link in any tissue. Thus the area within which tendon and muscle merge or where bone and tendon merge is often the site of injury. Patellar and Achilles tendon injuries in runners are common and good examples of injuries in transitional areas.

Bone

The bones of the skeleton are changing their biochemical content and mechanical properties continuously throughout an individual's life, as the skeleton is remodeled slowly but continually. As would be expected, the mineral content and ability to resist compression declines with advancing age, a phenomenon that is more pronounced in women than in men. The strength of bone per unit area is similar in men and women, but because of hormonal changes, women have a greater tendency to lose bone with age; consequently, less unit area exists to resist loads and forces. Other factors that can contribute to bone loss are immobilization of a body part or a general lack of physical activity. According to **Wolff's law,** bone is shaped by the forces placed on it or the lack of force as in immobilization.

As noted earlier, bone is anisotropic, which means that its strength depends on the orientation of bone matrix with respect to the direction of the load. Bone is made up of 35% collagen and other proteins, 20% water, and 45% minerals, most notably calcium. The collagen imparts a degree of viscoelasticity, and the minerals impart strength and stiffness. The order of load resistance is least for shearing and greatest for compression, with tensile load resistance in between.

Diet, disease, and hormonal levels can affect osteoblastic and osteoclastic activity levels and thus the biochemical composition of bone. The change in biochemical content of bone alters its mechanical properties. This change is well demonstrated in osteoporosis, where a loss of calcium results in a decrease in the trabecular pattern and cortical diameter of bone, making it easier to fracture. Deficiency of vitamin D results in uncalcified osteoid that makes bone subject to mechanical deformities, which is observed in rickets.

Cartilage

Cartilage is a solid matrix of collagen embedded in a proteoglycan gel. Water is attracted by the proteoglycan gel. As water enters the gel, the gel swells. This swelling stretches the collagen fibers until their tensile stress balances the swelling force. This phenomenon occurs in the unloaded state. A compressive load applied to articular cartilage is immediately resisted and results in deformation of the cartilage. This deformation increases pressure within the cartilage. A creep response follows this increase in pressure if the load is maintained. During the creep response, fluid in the cartilage exits to an area of lower pressure. This fluid can aid in joint lubrication. Creep is time-delayed, depending on the viscosity of the fluid and is a viscoelastic property. It can be likened to the action of a shock absorber in a car.

The swelling of articular cartilage helps reduce surface defects and minimizes friction. Additionally, fluid exiting cartilage under load helps reduce contact between surfaces. This reduction of contact helps prevent or delay wear and tear. Articular cartilage is best designed to resist compressive loads and to distribute in an even manner the force caused by loading. Although damaged cartilage goes through a remodeling response that originates in the **chondrocytes,** cartilage has a small capacity to remodel and repair itself. The effects of trauma, wear and tear, and degeneration on body structures depend on various factors, including the mechanical properties of the structures. A normal flow of fluid in and out of articular cartilage supplies nutrients and removes waste, which can only be accomplished with physical activity. Immobilization can lead to the degeneration of articular cartilage.

KINEMATICS

The discipline of **kinematics** deals with motion of the body but not with the forces involved in that motion. Rather, it deals with the following variables:

Time. Time refers to the duration of an activity. For example, in gait analysis, how long is the foot in contact with the ground during a jog or during a sprint? The short contact time for the sprint means a high-loading rate for muscles and joints involved in sprinting and a higher chance of overuse injury.

Position. The position of a body or body part during an activity can give clues as to the nature of an injury. For example, a football player who is standing still and looking down field sustains an injury when another player hits the lateral aspect of his knee at a perpendicular angle.

Displacement. Displacement is the change in position of a body or body part. Instinctively, displacement is thought of in linear terms—pushing a book across a desk, walking down the street, moving an object from a high shelf to a lower one. Angular displacement also exists. A car speeding around a circular racetrack, an ice skater finishing off a routine with a series of rapid spinning moves, or a basketball player making a hook shot over a tall defender are all examples of angular displacements.

Linear displacement is easy to measure, but angular displacement requires a bit more thought. For example, eight runners, one in each lane, are lined up at the starting line on an eight-lane track that is perfectly circular. Obviously, the runner in the inside lane will cover less distance in a single lap than each of the other runners. The important factor is not the number of laps that are run but the radius from the center of the field to the specific lane. In circular terms, the runner in the outside lane subtends a greater arc of motion than the runner in the inside lane.

Velocity. Velocity is the change in position with respect to time. It has both magnitude and direction, whereas speed has only magnitude.

Acceleration. Acceleration is the change in velocity with respect to time. It is conventional to describe acceleration as meters per second squared (m/s^2). Acceleration can be constant, or it can grow at an increasing or a decreasing rate, or it can decline at an increasing or a decreasing rate. It can be described as positive when going in one direction (e.g., a ball thrown upward) or negative if going in the opposite direction (e.g., a ball falling toward the ground). Negative acceleration is called deceleration. As with velocity, acceleration can be linear or angular.

Acceleration is a major factor in sports injuries and automobile accidents. Rapid acceleration or deceleration of the head, shoulder, or any body part can result in tearing, fracture, or rupture of tissue. If a stationary football player is hit perpendicularly at the lateral aspect of his knee by a force of 4 g, then his knee will experience a force accelerating the knee at four times the acceleration caused by the force of gravity. In injuries caused by a car hitting a brick wall or another large object, acceleration is negative.

KINETICS

Kinetics is the study of forces producing motion and their effects. To understand kinetics, familiarity with certain force-related concepts is essential.

Mass. Mass is the quantity of matter within an object.

Inertia. Inertia is the property of a body to remain at rest or in uniform motion in a straight line unless acted on by an external force. This concept is called Newton's first law, or the law of inertia. Bodies tend to resist changes in motion. The mass of the body determines the magnitude of this resistance (Fig. 6-12).

Mass moment of inertia. Mass moment of inertia applies to rotating bodies that move at a constant angular velocity or bodies at rest that have a fixed axis. Such bodies tend to remain in motion or at rest unless acted on by an external force. This resistance to change is determined by the mass of the body and where the body lies on the axis of rotation (i.e., the radius squared).

Force. Force is a push or pull exerted on a body that tends to produce acceleration. Force gives rise to Newton's second law, which is that a force acting on a body causes an acceleration in the direction of the force.

Momentum. Momentum is an amount of motion. Momentum equals mass times velocity. Increasing either the mass of a body or its velocity will increase the momentum.

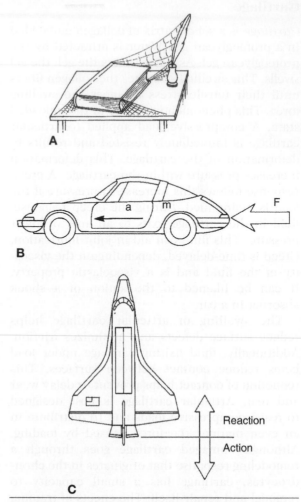

Fig. 6-12 **Newton's three laws of motion. A,** First law. A body remains at rest or in uniform motion until it is acted on by an external force. A book will remain on the table forever if it is not disturbed. **B,** Second law. Force equals mass time acceleration. Therefore the acceleration *(a)* of the car is inversely proportional to its mass *(m)* and directly proportional to the applied force *(F).* **C,** Third law. Reaction equals action. The thrust created by the engines of the shuttle pushes exhausted gases downward, which, as a reaction, pushes the rocket-plane upward. *(From Panjabi MM, White AA: Biomechanics in the musculoskeletal system, New York, 2001, Churchill Livingstone.)*

If a truck with a mass of 7000 kilograms (kg) (15,432 pounds) and a car with a mass of 400 kg (882 pounds) are traveling toward each other at a constant velocity of 20 kilometers per hour (km/hr) (12.4 miles per hour [m/hr]), the force that they exert on each other when they collide head on will be the same, but the momentum of each approaching the collision and the effect of the crash will be quite different. This is due to the different masses.

Center of mass and center of gravity. In physics or biomechanics, reducing the mass of a body to a single point and concluding that the body's mass is concentrated in this point is often a convenient presumption. The center of mass can be considered as the point about which the entire mass of the body is equally distributed. The center of mass of a flat plate is easy to find—it is at the origin. The plate would be able to balance if it were placed on a rod at its center of mass. The center of mass of irregularly shaped bodies, such as the human body, can be more difficult to locate, especially if the body is in an unusual position. For example, during a dive in which an Olympic diver is performing a forward flip, the center of mass will actually lie outside of the body, somewhere between the outstretched arms and legs. The center of gravity is often used interchangeably with center of mass; however, the point in a body through which the resultant force of gravity acts is the center of mass.

Moment. Moment of force is the product of force and distance through which the force acts. It tends to cause a twisting around the axis of rotation. A wrench or a long lever used to turn a wheel is an example of moments being generated.

Work. Work is force acting over a distance or force times displacement.

Power. Power is the rate of doing work.

Impulse. An impulsive force is the force that two colliding bodies exert on one another. This force usually acts over a very short period, such as during in an automobile collision.

APPLYING BIOMECHANICAL CONCEPTS

Whiplash Injuries

In whiplash injuries, acceleration or deceleration or both that involve substantial rotation and

KINETIC CHAINS

In an *open kinetic chain*, the most distal segment ends without attachment to any other structure. The head resting on the cervical spine is a good example, as is the hand. In a *closed kinetic chain*, the end segment is joined to another structure. In a closed kinetic chain, motion of one segment is related to the other segments in the chain. The pelvis is a good example, as is the leg when the foot is in contact with the ground. (For further discussion of kinetic chains, see Chapter 19.)

translation of various body parts can occur over very short periods. Croft[1] discusses the four different phases of the whiplash automobile injury. Automobile collisions are nonelastic, as opposed to elastic collisions such as billiard balls or a squash ball hitting a wall and rebounding. In nonelastic collisions, the vehicles involved strike each other and then assume the same velocity. For this to happen, the accident must result in a great deal of permanent deformity of the vehicles involved—a good example of plasticity.

As an example, a crash in which a car is struck from the rear is considered. In phase I the torso of the driver in the front vehicle is forced backward against the restraining seat. The head and neck remain stationary, and the vehicle accelerates forward, which creates high-tensile forces on the neck. In phase II the head is accelerated rapidly posteriorly, as a result of the events in phase I. This phase creates high-tensile loading on anterior neck structures and high-compressive loading on posterior neck structures. In phase III the head and torso are reaching their maximum posterior acceleration while the acceleration of the vehicle is decreasing. In phase IV the vehicle is not accelerating, and the head, neck, and torso rebound or decelerate forward. The seatbelt restrains forward deceleration of the torso; consequently, the head and neck bear the brunt. The weight of the head and the long lever arm of the cervical spine contribute to this whiplashing effect and associated soft tissue damage. Croft reports that the acceleration of the head can be 2.0 to 2.5 times the acceleration of the vehicle. In an automobile collision, each cervical motion segment contributes its acceleration to the segment above. Because the cervical spine has multiple motion segments, this acceleration effect at the distal or open end of the cervicocranial kinetic chain is considerable.

Throwing a Ball

A good example of the effects of one motion segment on acceleration and subsequent velocity is observed when comparing the velocity of a ball thrown by an elite fastball pitcher with the velocity of a ball thrown by an elite fast bowler in cricket. A cricket ball and baseball vary in mass by approximately 14 grams (g) (1/2 ounce), which is negligible. Both the elite fast-ball pitcher and the cricket fast bowler throw their respective balls at 150+ km/hr (93 m/hr). The baseball pitcher throws from a relatively stationary position on the mound. The cricket fast bowler takes a run up to 20+ meters (22 yards). The difference is that the cricket fast bowler must keep his elbow extended. Cricket regulations do not permit elbow flexion when launching the ball. The elimination of this one motion segment, the elbow, means that the cricket fast bowler must run 20 meters (22 yards) or more at a high speed to throw his ball with the same velocity of the relatively stationary baseball pitcher.

Review Questions

1. What structures in the body resist structural deformation of tissue?
2. In an automobile accident involving a violent flexion injury, tissues in which part of the vertebral motor unit are likely to undergo compression? Tissues in which part are most likely to tear?
3. What two types of structural damage can result from the application of compressive

loads of over 600 psi to the vertebral end plates and bodies?
4. Which structures in the dorsal and lumbar spine are best equipped to resist torsion?
5. How is the pennate form of muscle biomechanically advantageous? Give one example of such a muscle.
6. Describe the anisotropic property of bone.
7. How does the mechanism of ligament failure change with advancing age?
8. What are three factors that affect osteoblastic and osteoclastic activity levels and thus the biochemical composition of bone?
9. How does immobilization contribute to the degeneration of articular cartilage?
10. In biomechanical terms, what is the difference between stress and strain?

Concept Questions

1. Which biomechanical forces are involved in the various types of chiropractic adjustments?

BIBLIOGRAPHY

Adams MA et al: *The biomechanics of back pain*, Edinburgh, 2002, Churchill Livingstone.

Herzog W: *Clinical biomechanics of spinal manipulation*, Philadelphia, 2000, Churchill Livingstone.

Neumann DA: *Kinesiology of the musculoskeletal system: foundations for physical rehabilitation*, St Louis, 2002, Mosby.

Panjabi MM, White AA: *Biomechanics in the musculoskeletal system*, New York, 2001, Churchill Livingstone.

Taylor JAM, Resnick D: *Skeletal imaging: atlas of the spine and extremities*, Philadelphia, 2000, WB Saunders.

REFERENCE

1. Croft AC: Biomechanics. In Croft AC, Foreman SM, editors: *Whiplash injuries: the cervical acceleration/deceleration syndrome*, ed 3, Philadelphia, 2002, Lippincott–Williams & Wilkins.

CHAPTER

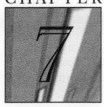

Vertebral Subluxation

Carl S. Cleveland III, DC

Key Terms

ADJUSTMENT	HARRISON MODEL	MOTION SEGMENT
ARTICULATION	HYPERMOBILITY	NEUROGENIC MOTOR-
ATONIA	HYPOMOBILITY	EVOKED POTENTIAL
ATROPHY	INTERVERTEBRAL	SPINAL MOTION SEGMENT
BIOMECHANICS	FORAMEN	SOMATOSENSORY-EVOKED
DEGENERATION	KENT MODEL	POTENTIALS
DISLOCATION	LANTZ MODEL	SUBLUXATION
DYSAUTONOMIA	MANIPULABLE SUBLUXATION	SUBLUXATION SYNDROME
DYSKINESIA	MANIPULATION	TETHERED CORD SYNDROME
DYSPONESIS	MANUAL THERAPY	TROPHIC
FAYE MODEL	MEDICARE	WORLD HEALTH
FIXATION	MOBILIZATION	ORGANIZATION

Vertebral subluxation is at the core of chiropractic theory, and its detection, management, and correction is at the heart of chiropractic practice. This central defining principle is simultaneously a source of debate within the profession.[1] In chiropractic's first century, **subluxation** was defined predominately in structural terms[2-7] and has evolved from a simplistic *static* concept, interpreted as a malpositioned spinal segment (bone out of place), to a contemporary model presented as a dynamic and complex biomechanical entity of multiple components. The components of the *dynamic* model include abnormal joint motion, muscular and connective tissue changes, and vascular, inflammatory, and biochemical changes. In addition, a most significant component of this entity, the associated neurologic manifestations, may result in symptoms either locally or at segmentally innervated anatomic levels (i.e., dermatomes, myotomes) far distant from the point of vertebral dysfunction. The orthopedist Jackson states that mechanical derangement or inflammation of these spinal joints may cause pain, sensory and motor disturbances, or both anywhere along the segmental distribution of the nerves.[8] The neurologic component of the vertebral subluxation complex (VSC) provides chiropractors the potential to move beyond symptomatic treatment of low back pain and other musculoskeletal ailments and to contribute to patient health, wellness, and enhanced function and quality of life.

The term *subluxation* comes from the Latin *sub*, meaning *under* or *less than*, and *luxation*, which means **dislocation**. *Stedman's Medical Dictionary* defines the term as "an incomplete luxation or dislocation; though a relationship is altered, contact between joint surfaces remains."[9] Contemporary interpretation embraces the concept of subluxation as a motion segment in which alignment, movement integrity, physiologic function, or any combination is altered, although contact between joint surfaces remains intact.[10]

Application of this term is fundamental to communication between chiropractors and their patients. For explaining the subluxation to laypeople, a good working definition is loss of proper motion or position of a vertebral joint that may affect proper nerve function[11]. In contrast, the term may be described technically as the vertebral subluxation complex and presented as a theoretical model of vertebral motion segment dysfunction that incorporates the complex interactions of pathologic changes in nerve, muscle, ligamentous, vascular, and connective tissue.[12] This latter model serves as a basis for communicating chiropractic concepts to the scientific community.

Classical and contemporary medical practitioners, osteopaths, and chiropractors have referred to the concept of subluxation extensively.[13] However, these professions differ on defining the term and interpreting its clinical significance. In the scientific literature, the terminology describing the functional or structural disorders of synovial joint structures has varied in name and description, ranging from the orthopedic context as a partial or incomplete dislocation to the chiropractic perspective that includes minor misalignment of articulations, hypomobile spinal segments, or both.[13] Box 7-1, from Peterson and Bergman,[14] provides an overview of contemporary terminology describing synovial joint dysfunction.

Rome,[15] in an extensive literature review, has identified over 296 synonyms (41 used to describe

---

Box **7-1**   TERMS DESCRIBING FUNCTIONAL OR STRUCTURAL DISORDERS OF THE
SYNOVIAL JOINTS

ORTHOPEDIC SUBLUXATION

This term is used to describe a partial or incomplete dislocation.

CHIROPRACTIC SUBLUXATION

This term is used to describe the alteration of the normal dynamic, anatomic, or physiologic relationships of contiguous articular structures; a motion segment in which alignment, movement integrity, or physiologic function is altered, although the contact between the joint surfaces remains intact; an aberrant relationship between two adjacent articular structures that may have functional or pathologic sequelae, causing an alteration in the biomechanical or neurophysiologic reflections of these articular structures or body systems that may be directly or indirectly affected by them.

SUBLUXATION SYNDROME

This term is used to describe an aggregate of signs and symptoms that relates to the pathophysiology or dysfunction of spinal and pelvic motion segments or to the peripheral joints.

SUBLUXATION COMPLEX

This term is used to describe a theoretic model of motion segment dysfunction (subluxation) that incorporates the complex interaction of pathologic changes in nerve, muscle, ligamentous, vascular, and connective tissues.

JOINT DYSFUNCTION

This term is used to describe joint mechanics that show area disturbances of function without structural change—subtle joint dysfunctions that affect quality and range-of-joint motion. Definition embodies disturbances in function that can be represented by decreased motion, increased motion, or aberrant motion.
    Joint hypomobility: Decreased angular or linear joint movement
    Joint hypermobility: Increased angular or linear joint movement; aberrant joint movements are typically not present
    Clinical joint instability: Increased linear and aberrant joint movement; the instantaneous axes of rotation (centroids) and patterns of movement that are disturbed

SOMATIC DYSFUNCTION

This term is used to describe impaired or altered function of related components of the somatic (body framework) system; skeletal, arthrodial, and myofascial structures; and related vascular, lymphatic, and neural elements.

Box 7-1 TERMS DESCRIBING FUNCTIONAL OR STRUCTURAL DISORDERS OF THE
SYNOVIAL JOINTS—CONT'D

OSTEOPATHIC LESION

This term is used to describe a disturbance in musculoskeletal structure or function, as well as accompanying disturbances of other biologic mechanisms. This term is also used to describe local stress or trauma and subsequent effects on other biologic systems (e.g., effects mediated through reflex nerve pathways, including autonomic supply of segmentally related organs).

JOINT FIXATION

This term is used to describe the state whereby an articulation has become temporarily immobilized in a position that it may normally occupy during any phase of physiologic movement; the immobilization of an articulation in a position of movement when the joint is at rest or in a position of rest when the joint is in movement.

From Peterson D, Bergman T: *Chiropractic technique: principles and procedures*, ed 2, St Louis, 2002, Mosby.

sacroiliac subluxation) and terms for the biomechanical condition known to chiropractors as *subluxation*. Such synonyms include manipulable spinal lesion, functional spinal lesion, dysfunctional segmental unit, somatic joint dysfunction, articular **dyskinesia,** joint blockage, hypomobile vertebral segment, and vertebral **fixation.** As an example, Seaman[16,17] proposes the term *joint complex dysfunction* to embrace pathologic and functional changes in a joint, including negative effects of hypomobility-immobility, functional imbalances of muscle tightening or shortening, and myofascial trigger points. Lack of uniform terminology, however, has created confusion and impeded interprofessional discussion.

One way to review the basic principles of spinal adjustment-manipulation is to look at the clinical characteristics of the entity to which the adjustment or manipulation is applied. Despite the various theoretical explanations for the mechanism of action of spinal adjustment/manipulation (see Chapter 8 for greater detail), substantial agreement exists on certain fundamental clinical characteristics of the manipulable lesion or joint subluxation.[18] This chapter explores various aspects of the theoretical models of vertebral subluxation.

SUBLUXATION: EARLY HISTORY

The earliest concepts of subluxation predate chiropractic by more than 200 years. Haldeman cites the earliest English definition of subluxation from Randle Holme in 1688,[19] who described it as, "dislocation or putting out of joynt."

Haldeman[13] and others[20-22] cite the following 1746 description from Joannes Herricus Hieronymus,[23] who wrote, "subluxation of joints is recognized by lessened motion of the joints, by slight change in position of the articulating bones and pain."

Terrett[24] cites an 1821 description by Edward Harrison:

When any of the vertebrae become displaced or too prominent, the patient experiences inconvenience from a local derangement in the nerves or the part. He, in consequence is tormented with a train of nervous symptoms, which are obscure in their origin as they are stubborn in their nature.

Harrison pursued the subject further, writing in 1824 that motion, as well as alignment, played a defining role in subluxation:

The articulating extremeties are only partially separated, not imperfectly disjoined . . . and . . . the articular motions are imperfectly performed, because the surfaces of the bones do not fully correspond.

Thomas Brown, writing in the *Glasgow Medical Journal* in 1828, coined the term *spinal irritation*.[25] Four years later, *The American Journal of Medical Sciences* began citing reports from European physicians about tenderness of vertebrae corresponding to diseased organs, with such observations taken as confirming a diagnosis of spinal irritation.[25]

Donald Tower[26] quotes physician J.E. Riadore's 1843 *Irritation of the Spinal Nerves* as follows: "[If] any organ is deficiently supplied with nervous energy or of blood, its functions immediately, and sooner or later its structure, becomes deranged." Riadore concluded that irritation of nerve roots resulted in disease and advocated treatment by manipulation. These conclusions regarding nerve irritation were published 2 years before the birth of D.D. Palmer.[21]

By 1874, Andrew Taylor Still, a medical physician who founded osteopathy 21 years before Palmer's discovery of chiropractic, developed his own concept and terminology. Still described the osteopathic lesion in terms of pressure applied by muscles to blood vessels coursing through and around these muscles, thereby shutting off the life force of the involved tissue.[27]

CHIROPRACTIC SUBLUXATION— EARLY CONCEPTS

Although the founder of chiropractic, D.D. Palmer, continued to modify his early concepts and explanations of chiropractic even until his death in 1913,[28] the sustaining, central Palmer hypothesis described *subluxation* as a "partial or incomplete separation, one in which the articulating surfaces remain in partial contact."[29] His hypothesis further proposed that such subluxations might impinge on spinal nerve roots as they exit through the intervertebral foramina. This action was postulated to obstruct flow of vital nerve impulses between the central nervous system and the periphery and to induce lowered tissue resistance and disease in the segmentally innervated tissues.[2,3,30] The founder later postulated that the primary cause of disease was interruption of normal tone resulting from subluxation, in which nerves became too taut (resulting in excess nerve energy) or too slack (producing too little nerve energy).[28-30]

In the December 1904 Palmer School of Chiropractic periodical, *The Chiropractor*, presented as "A monthly journal devoted to the interests of chiropractic—'KI-RO-PRAK-TIK, "[31] D.D. Palmer states:

Ninety-five percent of all deranged nerves are made by sub-luxations of vertebrae which pinch nerves to some one of the 51 joint articulations of the spinal column. Therefore to relieve the pressure upon these nerves means to restore normal action—hence, normal functions, perfect health.

This statement likely represents the earliest published mention of subluxation in the chiropractic literature. Significantly, the senior Palmer saw at least limited value (5%) in the adjustment of nonspinal articulations, stating that nerves related to nonvertebral joints may be *impinged* rather than pinched.

According to Gibbons,[32] *Modernized Chiropractic*,[33] by Smith, Langworthy, and Paxson, published in 1906, was the first chiropractic textbook to use the term *subluxation* and to relate it to the **intervertebral foramen.** This work was also the first to assert the supremacy of the nerves in relation to health and disease, in contrast to the osteopathic concept of supremacy of the blood. In chiropractic's early years, this citation often served as legal defense in arguing the distinction between the practice of chiropractic and that of osteopathy and medicine. In addition, chiropractic's focus on the importance of the nervous system and its emphasis on the correction of vertebral subluxation became key factors in defending chiropractors and in early attempts by the profession to gain separate licensure.

Langworthy and colleagues also were the first to characterize subluxation as a *fixation* and to describe the *field of motion* of a vertebra. This view of subluxation as a dysfunctional state of vertebral motion gradually fell into disuse until 1938, when the dynamic concept of subluxation was reintroduced with the motion palpation research of the Belgian chiropractors Gillet and Lichens.[34]

FOUNDER'S DEFINITION

In 1910, D.D. Palmer discussed subluxation in his text, *Science, Art and Philosophy of Chiropractic*,[2] as follows:

A vertebra is said to be displaced or a luxation when the joint surfaces are entirely separated. Sub-luxation is a partial or incomplete separation; one in which the articulation surfaces remain in partial contact. This later condition is so often referred to and known by chiropractors as sub-luxation. The relationship existing between bones and nerves are so nicely adjusted that any one of the 200 bones, more especially those of the vertebral column, cannot be displaced ever so little without impinging upon adjacent nerves. Pressure on nerves excites, agitates, creates an excess of molecular vibration, whose effects, when local are known as inflammation, when general, as fever. A subluxation does not restrain or liberate vital energy. Vital energy is expressed in functional activity. A subluxation may impinge against nerves, the transmitting channel may increase or decrease the momentum of impulses, not energy.

THE YOUNGER PALMER'S DEFINITION

By the early 1930s, B.J. Palmer had developed a concept of subluxation distinct from that of his father. The younger Palmer represented subluxation as restricted to a displaced upper cervical vertebra that created nerve impingement, resulting in interference with the transmission of vital nerve energy.[3] In his 1934 textbook, *The Subluxation Specific—The Adjustment Specific*, B.J. maintained that the only subluxation of significance was that of the atlas vertebra in relation to occiput or axis:

I reaffirm that no amount of "adjusting" upon any, many or all vertebrae below occiput, atlas, or axis, could or would directly ADJUST THE SPECIFIC three-direction torqued subluxation causing any, many or all sickness in a body. Any vertebra below atlas or axis MAY BE misaligned but CANNOT BE SUBLUXATED.[3] [Emphasis in original text.]

B.J. Palmer's delineation between simple misalignment and true subluxation is significant. Misalignment of a vertebra was described as no more than compensation to the major subluxation.

Thus in a span of 30 years, the Palmer School concept of subluxation and adjustment evolved from the founder's 1904 description of an entity affecting any of the 200 joints of the body, but primarily the joints of the spinal column, to the younger Palmer's insistence on exclusive adjustment of the full spinal column only and then later to his idea that subluxation was an entity limited only to the atlas vertebra in relation to the occiput and axis. This later concept, known as the *Hole in One Technique* (HIO), was developed in the early 1930s. For two decades, Palmer

College taught no adjusting methods except upper cervical specific technique. Not until 1956 did the school reintroduce instruction in adjusting techniques for the full spine (Himes HM, *Policy Talk*, unpublished letter, January 4, 1956).

STEPHENSON'S DEFINITION

According to Lantz,[35] the definition of subluxation most widely quoted by early chiropractors was from R.W. Stephenson's 1927 *Chiropractic Text Book*,[4] which states:

A subluxation is a condition of a vertebra that has lost its proper juxtaposition with the one above or the one below, or both; to an extent less that a luxation; which impinges nerves and interferes with the transmission of mental impulses.

Stephenson, a 1921 Palmer School graduate, insisted that nerve interference must exist to qualify the condition as a subluxation. Stephenson's definition served for decades as the preeminent expression of the static model (bone out of proper position or alignment) of vertebral subluxation.

DYNAMIC MODEL

Beginning with the writings of Gillet,[34] Illi,[36] and Mennell,[37] and continuing through the works of Sandoz,[38] Dishman,[39] and Faye,[40] the dynamic characteristics of joint subluxation moved to the forefront, with subluxation and joint integrity now described not solely in structural terms, but in functional terms as well with emphasis on altered joint motion. In this context, joint malposition became a potential sign of altered joint function, but not absolute confirmation.[14]

CONTEMPORARY DEFINITIONS

Contemporary definitions describe the subluxation as central to the principles of chiropractic science. Examples of policy statements regarding subluxation are the following:

State Statutes

The concept of subluxation is specifically identified in many U.S. state statutes defining the practice of chiropractic. After extensive review, Hendrickson[41] concluded that many state chiropractic statutes either directly or implicitly identify chiropractic with subluxation or the elements of subluxation complex and specify the doctor of chiropractic's responsibility for adjusting the spine and adjacent tissues for the purpose of eliminating nerve interference. An analysis by Hendrickson follows.

Examples of state statutes that expressly identify the detection of and caring for subluxations as the core of chiropractic practice include:

Arizona: *A doctor of chiropractic is a portal of entry health care provider who engages in the practice of health care that includes: the diagnosis and correction of subluxations, functional vertebral or articular dysarthrosis or neuromuscular skeletal disorders for the restoration and maintenance of health. Treatment by adjustment of the spine or bodily articulations and those procedures preparatory and complementary to the adjustment including physiotherapy related to the correction of subluxations.* (Arizona Revised Statutes Annotated, Title 32, Chapter 8, Article 2 32-925(a), No. 1, 3)

Connecticut: *The practice of chiropractic means the practice of that branch of the healing arts consisting of the science of adjustment, manipulation and treatment of the human body in which vertebral subluxations and other malpositioned articulations and structures that may interfere with the normal generation, transmission and expression of nerve impulse between the brain, organs and tissue cells of the body, which may be a cause of disease, are adjusted, manipulated or treated.* (Connecticut General Statutes Annotated, Title 20, Chapter 372, Section 20-24, (1))

District of Columbia: *"Practice of Chiropractic" means the detecting and correcting of subluxations that cause vertebral, neuromuscular, or skeletal disorder, by adjustment of the spine or manipulation of bodily articulations for the restoration and maintenance of health.* (District of Columbia Code 1981, Part 1, Title 2, Chapter 33, Subchapter I -2-3301.2(3)(A))

Delaware: *The practice of chiropractic includes, but is not limited to, the diagnosing and locating of misaligned or displaced vertebral subluxation complex.* (Delaware Code Annotated, Title 24, Chapter 7, 701 b.)

Florida: *"Practice of chiropractic" means a noncombative principle and practice consisting of the science, philosophy, and art of the adjustment, manipulation, and treatment of the human body in which vertebral subluxations and other malpositioned articulations and structures that are interfering with the normal generation, transmission, and expression of nerve impulse between the brain, organs, and tissue cells of the body, thereby causing disease, are adjusted, manipulated, or treated, thus restoring the normal flow of nerve impulse which produces normal function and consequent health by chiropractic physicians using specific chiropractic adjustment or manipulation techniques....* (Florida Statutes Annotated, Title XXXII, Chapter 460, Section 460.403 (8) (a))

Idaho: *"Adjustment" means the application of a precisely controlled force applied by hand or by mechanical device to a specific focal point on the anatomy for the express purpose of creating a desired angular movement in skeletal joint structures in order to eliminate or decrease interference with neural transmission and correct or attempt to correct subluxation complex.* (Idaho Code, Title 54 Chapter 7, 54-704 (1) (a))

Maine: *Chiropractic. "Chiropractic" means the art and science of identification and correction of subluxation and the accompanying physiological or mechanical abnormalities. The term subluxation, as utilized within the chiropractic health care system, means a structural or functional impairment of an intact articular unit. Chiropractic recognizes the inherent recuperative capability of the human body as it relates to the spinal column, musculoskeletal and nervous system.* (Maine Revised Statutes Annotated, Title 32, Chapter 9, Subchapter 1, Section 451 (1))

Massachusetts: *"Chiropractic," the science of locating, and removing interference with the transmission or expression of nerve force in the human body, by the correction of misalignments or subluxations of the bony articulation and adjacent structures, more especially those of the vertebral column and pelvis, for the purpose of restoring and maintaining health.* (Massachusetts General Laws Annotated Part I, Title XVI, Chapter 112, Section 89)

New York: *The practice of the profession of chiropractic is defined as detecting and correcting by manual or mechanical means structural imbalance, distortion, or subluxations in the human body for the purpose of removing nerve interference and the effects thereof, where such interference is the result of or related to distortion, misalignment or subluxation of or in the vertebral column.* (Consolidated Laws of New York, Chapter 16, Title VIII, Article 132, Section 6551 (1))

Other state statutes that define and identify the subluxation specifically include Kentucky, Nevada, New Jersey, Texas, Utah, Vermont, and Washington.

Medicare and Medicaid Definition

The U.S. government recognizes the detection and correction of subluxation as the primary function of the doctor of chiropractic.[41,42] The federal statutes governing the **Medicare** program, in which chiropractic services have been included since the early 1970s, defines chiropractic and reimbursable chiropractic services as:

A chiropractor who is licensed as such by the State (or in a State which does not license chiropractors as such, is legally authorized to perform the services of a chiropractor in the jurisdiction in which he performs such services), and who meets uniform minimum standards promulgated by the Secretary, but only for the purpose of subsections (s)(1) and (s)(2)(A) of this section and only with respect to treatment by means of manual manipulation of the spine (to correct a subluxation) which he is legally authorized to perform by the State or jurisdiction in which such treatment is provided. (42 USC Sec. 1395x (r) (5))

Medicare extends these concepts in the statute into the regulations governing the program with an express definition:

A chiropractor who is licensed by the State or legally authorized to perform the services of a chiropractor, but only with respect to treatment by means of manual manipulation of the spine to correct a subluxation. (42 CFR 482 Subpart B Section 482.12 (7) (c) (1) (v))

Federal statutes establishing chiropractic participation in the Medicaid program employ the same terminology as that in the general Medicare program. Federal employee health benefit programs recognize chiropractic on terms negotiated between representative committees of public employees and various insurance carriers, but the federal workers compensation program identifies and defines chiropractic, once again, very specifically to include chiropractors and chiropractic services as follows:

The term "physician" includes chiropractors only to the extent that their reimbursable services are limited to treatment consisting of manual manipulation of the spine to correct a subluxation.

Department of Veterans Affairs

In January 2002, President George W. Bush signed into law new provisions that established chiropractic services as a health care benefit for eligible military veterans in the United States. This law contains a specific passage referencing subluxation, which reads as follows[41]:

Program For The Provision of Chiropractic Care and Services to Veterans. (d) CARE AND SERVICES AVAILABLE. The chiropractic care and services available under the program shall include a variety of chiropractic care and services for neuro-musculoskeletal conditions, including subluxation complex. (United States Code, Title 38, 204 (d))

World Health Organization Classification

The **World Health Organization** (WHO), a multilateral health care agency of the United Nations, has accepted subluxation as a listing in the International Classification of Diseases,[43] referring to it as "M99.1 Subluxation complex (vertebral)." WHO also recognizes the classification "M99.0 Segmental and somatic dysfunction," a subtle variation.

Consortium for Chiropractic Research

The 1993 consensus definition of the nominal and Delphi panels of the Consortium for Chiropractic Research (CCR)[10] refers to subluxation as "...a motion segment in which alignment, movement integrity, and/or physiologic function are altered although contact between the joint surfaces remains intact."

American Chiropractic Association

The Indexed Synopsis of ACA Policies[44] describes subluxation as, "...[a] motion segment, in which alignment, movement integrity, and/or physiological function are altered although contact between joint surfaces remain intact."

ACA has also adopted the consensus definitions agreed on by the nominal and Delphi panels of the CCR[10,44]:

Subluxation is an aberrant relationship between two adjacent articular structures that may have functional or pathological sequelae, causing an alteration in the biomechanical and/or neurophysiological reflections of these articular structures, the proximal structures, and/or body systems that may be directly or indirectly affected by them.

The ACA-endorsed CCR definition[44] for subluxation complex is:

...[a] theoretical model of motion segment dysfunction (subluxation) which incorporates the complex interaction of pathological changes in nerve, muscle, ligamentous, vascular and connective tissues.

International Chiropractors Association

ICA Policy Statements[45] related to subluxation include the following:

Of primary concern to chiropractic are abnormalities of structure or function of the vertebral column known clinically as the vertebral subluxation complex. The subluxation complex includes any alteration of the biomechanical and physiological dynamics of contiguous spinal structures which can cause neuronal disturbances.... Directly or indirectly, all bodily function is controlled by the nervous system, consequently a central theme of chiropractic theories on health is the premise that abnormal bodily function may be caused by interference with nerve transmission and expression due to pressure, strain or tension upon the spinal cord, spinal nerves, or peripheral nerves as a result of displacement of spinal segments or other skeletal structures (subluxation).

The vertebral **subluxation syndrome** and/or complex and its component parts is any alteration of the biomechanical and physiological dynamics of the contiguous structures which can cause neuronal disturbances.[46]

The science of chiropractic deals with the relationship between the articulations of the skeleton and the nervous system and the role of this relationship in the restoration and maintenance of health. Of primary concern to chiropractic are abnormalities of structure or function of the vertebral column known clinically as the vertebral subluxation complex. The subluxation complex includes any alteration of the biomechanical and physiological dynamics of contiguous spinal structures which can cause neuronal disturbances.

According to the ICA Official Policy Handbook[45]:

Chiropractic is based on the premises that the relationship between structure and function in the human body is a significant health factor and that such relationships between the spinal column and nervous system are the most significant, since the normal transmission and expression of nerve energy is essential to the restoration and maintenance of health.

Association of Chiropractic Colleges

On July 1, 1996, presidents of all North American chiropractic colleges, as members of the Association of Chiropractic Colleges (ACC), seeking to clarify professional common ground and define chiropractic's role within the health care delivery system, generated a series of consensus position statements.[47] This effort represented the first time in the 100-year history of chiropractic education that all college presidents, representing schools with diverse institutional missions, have reached unanimous consensus on common core definitions fundamental to the principles of chiropractic. This paradigm is endorsed by the ACA, ICA, World Chiropractic Alliance, World Federation of Chiropractic, the Congress of Chiropractic State Associations, and most state chiropractic associations. This consensus therefore represents a common platform from which to communicate the unifying principles of this profession. Chapter 2, "The Chiropractic Paradigm," provides the ACC paradigm in its entirety.

ACC Consensus Definitions

On chiropractic:

Chiropractic is a health-care discipline which emphasizes the inherent recuperative powers of the body to heal itself without the use of drugs or surgery.

The practice of chiropractic focuses on the relationship between structure (primarily of the spine) and function (as coordinated by the nervous system) and how that relationship affects the preservation and restoration of health.

Doctors of Chiropractic recognize the value and responsibility of working in cooperation with other health care practitioners when in the best interest of the patient.

The ACC continues to foster a unique, distinct chiropractic profession that serves as a health care discipline for all. The ACC advocates a profession that generates, develops, and utilizes the highest level of evidence possible in the provision of effective, prudent and cost-conscious patient evaluation and care.

On subluxation:

A subluxation is a complex of functional, structural, and/or pathological articular changes that compromise neural integrity and may influence organ system function and general health.

A subluxation is evaluated, diagnosed and managed through the use of chiropractic procedures based on the best available rational and empirical evidence.

The preservation and restoration of health is enhanced through the correction of the subluxation.

CONTEMPORARY MODELS OF VERTEBRAL SUBLUXATION COMPLEX

As noted in the ACA and ICA definitions previously cited, the contemporary concept of sub-

luxation has been expanded beyond a joint phenomenon affecting nerve function to also include the role of muscular, connective, vascular, and biochemical components as part of a complex. This subluxation complex has been defined by Gatterman[20] as "a theoretical model of motion segment dysfunction (subluxation) that incorporates the complex interaction of pathologic change in nerve, muscle, ligamentous, vascular and connective tissues."

Although Janse,[48,49] Illi,[36] Gillet and Lichens,[34] and Homewood[50] provided an early foundation, Faye,[40] beginning in 1967, popularized the concept of the subluxation complex and organized a five-component model. Dishman[39] characterized the concept as *the chiropractic subluxation complex,* providing additional rationale for Faye's model. Lantz[22,35] modified the original five components of the VSC model by postulating three more components: connective tissue pathologic finding, vascular abnormalities, and the inflammatory response.

FIVE-COMPONENT MODEL OF VERTEBRAL SUBLUXATION COMPLEX (FAYE MODEL)

Building on the work of Gillet and Liekens,[34] as well as earlier pioneers such as Smith, Langworthy, and Paxson,[33] Faye[40] moved beyond the static "bone out of place" or "displaced vertebra" theory of subluxation, placing primary emphasis on dynamic vertebral joint motion. Basic movements of spinal segments include rotation about the longitudinal axis, right or left lateral flexion, anterior flexion, posterior extension, and long-axis distention. Factors inhibiting movement in one or more of these directions may cause abnormal translation and rotation, contributing to biomechanic and subsequent physiologic dysfunction and pathologic expressions.

Schafer and Faye[51] defined the term *fixation* as referring to any physical, functional, or psychologic mechanism that produces a loss of segmental mobility within its normal physiologic range of motion. As an example, ankylosis of a joint would be considered a 100% fixation. These authors state that clinically most fixations are in the 20%

to 80% range of normal mobility. According to Schafer and Faye, once the chiropractor has identified the **hypomobility**, adjustive procedures are used to mobilize the fixation. The therapeutic objective is to deliver a dynamic thrust, employing a specific contact and line of drive with the intention of freeing restricted vertebral joint motion altering specific symptomatology.

The **Faye model** of the vertebral subluxation complex (Fig. 7-1) presents subluxation as a complex clinical entity comprising one or more of the following components: neuropathophysiology, kinesiopathology, myopathology, histopathology, and a biochemical component. A central element of this concept is that subluxation results in pathophysiologic conditions, which can then lead to frank pathologic changes. Moreover, correction of a subluxation is considered to lead to the restoration of normal physiologic processes, thus allowing the reversal of reversible pathologic changes.

Specifics of Five-Component Model[51]

1. *Neuropathophysiologic component.*
   Biomechanical insult to nerve tissue is proposed to cause neural dysfunction in three forms, individually or in combination, to include:
   a. Irritation (sustained hyperactivity) of nerve receptors or nerve tissue. This irritation results in facilitating (lowering threshold of excitability) of afferent nerve cells (dysafferentation) and evoking activity of efferent neurons with nerve cell bodies located in the anterior horn of the spinal cord, which is exhibited as hypertonicity or spasm of muscles. Lateral horn cell irritation, which is exhibited as vasomotor changes, includes hypersympatheticotonic vasoconstriction. Irritation to the cells of the posterior horn is exhibited as sensory changes.
   b. Compression or mechanical insult (pressure, stretching, angulation, or distortion) to neural elements in or about the intervertebral foramina,

within fascial layers, or tonically contracted muscles. This compression results in **degeneration,** which is exhibited as muscular **atrophy,** anesthesia, and sympathetic **atonia,** to including hyposympathicotonic vasodilation and vascular stasis.
   c. Decreased axoplasmic transport affecting intraaxonal transport mechanisms for delivery of macromolecules (neurotrophic substances). This delivery is via the axon to end organs innervated by the nerve. Impediments to this microcellular transport mechanism may alter the development, growth, and maintenance of cells or structures that are dependent on this **trophic** (growth) influence expressed via the nerve.

2. *Kinesiopathologic component.* This component is described as hypomobility, diminished or absent joint play, or compensatory segmental kinematic **hypermobility.** Lack of appropriate joint motion is proposed to be associated with a variety of nociceptive and mechanoreceptive reflex functions that include proprioception. In addition, an early manifestation of a chronically fixated vertebral **articulation** is shortening of ligaments as an adaptation to limited range of motion.

3. *Myopathologic component.* This component may include spasm or hypertonicity of muscles as a result of compensation, facilitation, Hilton's Law, or any combination. (John Hilton, a nineteenth century English surgeon, stated that the nerve supplying a joint also supplies the muscles which move the joint and the skin covering the articular insertion of those muscles.)[9]

4. *Histopathologic component.* This component relates to inflammation, including pain, heat, and swelling, and can result from trauma, hypermobile irritation, or occur as part of the repair process. The component also includes osseous tissue changes in the joint

The Subluxation Complex

SUBLUXATION ——→ PATHOPHYSIOLOGY ——→ PATHOLOGY
AXIOM Ñ Correction of a subluxation restores normal processes and the reversible pathology reverses.
SUBLUXATION Ñ A complex clinical entity comprising one or more of the following:

1. NEUROPATHOPHYSIOLOGY
   - → Irritation ——→ Facilitation
     - → Anterior horn → Muscles hypertonic
     - → Lateral horn → Sympathetic vasmotor
     - → Posterior horn → Sensory
   - → Pressure ——→ Degeneration
     - → Atrophy
     - → Sympathetic atonia
     - → Anthesia
   - → Decreased axoplasmic flow

2. KINESIOPATHOLOGY
   - → Hypomobility — Ñ Fixation theory Ñ H. Gillet
   - → Hypermobility — Ñ Illi
   - → Loss of joint play — Ñ J. Mennel

   Compensation
   - → Hypermobility and hypomobility Ñ Normal
   - → Hypomobility and hypermobility can be in the same motion unit

   Change of axis of movement

3. MYOPATHOLOGY
   - → Spasm
     - → Compensation
     - → Facilitation → Visceromotor reflex
     - → HiltonÕs law
   - → Antonia

4. HISTOPATHOLOGY
   Cellular flow of inflammatory process
   Edema withln Intervertebral foramen, Impeding flow of circulating fluids

5. BIOCHEMICAL CHANGES
   - → L.A.S. (Selye) from local tissue damage or further G.A.S.
   - → Histamines
   - → Prostaglandins — Stress syndrome
   - → Kinines — ¥Proinflammatory

CHIROPRACTIC THERAPEUTIC APPROACH

Adjustive procedures ——→ Thrust, recoil, toggle, etc. → Produces a specific movement → Effects the movement component of a subluxation complex directly and others indirectly
Reflex technics
Exercise
Diet supplementation
Postural advice
Modalities
Socio-occupational advice
Other

Rationale for the adjustment
(A) Find the hypomobility; (B) use adjustive procedure to mobilize the fixation; (C) recheck to confirm that movement has improved.
Therapeutic approach is then applied to other components of the subluxation complex and their causes; therefore, a holistic, multicausal interdisciplinary approach for each patientÕs health problems. The prognosis depends on the reversibility of the pathology, the restoration of normal function, and the ability to keep the joints free of subluxation-fixations and other causes of malfunction.
Prevention Ñ Regular motion palpation examinations to discover early aberrant motion, especially fixations to prevent the subluxation complex from developing.

Reprinted with permission, 1986 L. John Faye and The Motion Palpation Institute

Fig. 7-1 Five-component (Faye) model of subluxation complex. *(From Schafer RC, Faye LJ:* Motion palpation and chiropractic technic: principles of dynamic chiropractic, *Huntington Beach, Calif, 1989, The Motion Palpation Institute, with permission.)*

that may be expressed according to the clinical principles of Weigert's law and Wolff's law. (Carl Weigert, a nineteenth century German pathologist, stated that loss or destruction of a part or element is likely to result in compensatory replacement and overproduction of tissue during the process of regeneration, repair, or both, as in the formation of callus when a fractured bone heals. Weigert's law is also known as the *over production* theory.)[9] Julius Wolff, a German anatomist of the same era, stated that every change in the form and the function of a bone, or in its function alone, is followed by certain definite changes in its internal architecture and secondary alterations in its external conformation.[9]

5. *Biochemical component.* Hormonal and chemical effects or imbalance related to the preinflammatory stress syndrome and the production of histamine, prostaglandin, and bradykinin. This component is a result of trauma or fixation of the spinal articulation and is proposed to affect nociceptive impulses, resulting in aberrant (deviating from the usual or normal) somatic afferent input into the segmental spinal cord.[51a]

Primary Clinical Approach

The primary therapeutic approach, related to the Faye model of VSC, is a specific dynamic adjustive thrust (e.g., toggle recoil, impulse) to release sites of fixation either directly or indirectly. In addition, supportive procedures designed to enhance the healing process, including exercise, rehabilitation, adjunctive procedures, and lifestyle counseling regarding posture, diet, and stress reduction, may be incorporated in clinical management of the patient.

NINE-COMPONENT MODEL (LANTZ MODEL)[22]

Lantz provides a more structured organization for the VSC model (Fig. 7-2) by describing a hierarchy of organization and a pattern of interrelatedness of the various components. In addi-

tion to the five components proposed by Faye, Lantz adds:

- Connective tissue pathologic finding
- Vascular abnormalities
- Inflammatory response
- Pathophysiologic finding

In an update to this nine-component model,[12] the term *pathoanatomy* has been substituted for *histopathology,* and reference to the suffix *pathology* has been changed in favor of more generic terminology. Thus *neurologic component* is used in place of neuropathology, *kinesiologic component* replaces kinesiopathology, and the *myology* is substituted for myopathology component.

A common denominator between the Faye and Lantz models is the focus on restricted motion of the manipulable subluxation. Such restriction or immobilization of the joint causes some degree of degenerative change in the musculoskeletal system and connective tissue that may adversely affect nerve system function. The early introduction of motion via adjustment or manipulation, mobilization, traction, and continuous passive motion may overcome these harmful effects.[52]

Kinesiologic Component

The kinesiologic component is represented at the apex of the Lantz VSC model (see Fig. 7-2), emphasizing the importance of motion and its interrelationship with other components. Positioned in the diagram beneath the kinesiologic component, but interconnected on the same level, are the neurologic, myologic, vascular, and connective tissue components. Lantz states:

Movement is affected by muscles (myologic component); guided, limited and stabilized by connective tissue; and controlled largely by the nervous system. The vascular system serves the essential nutritive and cleansing role for all tissues and is the conduit for the immediate stages of the inflammatory response (at least in vascularized tissues). These constitute the tissue-level components of the VSC and each works in coordination with the others to permit and sustain proper movement. Interference with any single component affects all others.

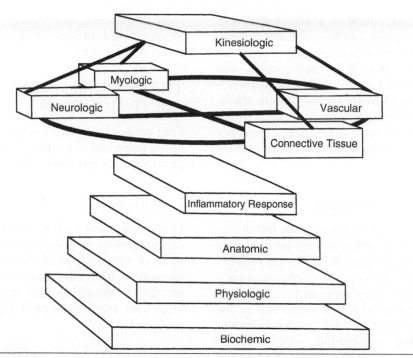

Fig. 7-2 Nine- component (Lantz) model of subluxation complex. *(Adapted from Lantz CA: The vertebral subluxation complex. In Gatterman MI, editor:* Foundations of chiropractic: subluxation, *St Louis, 1995, Mosby, with permission.)*

Neurologic Component

The neurologic component, as described by Lantz, includes the nerve roots, dorsal root ganglia, spinal nerve, recurrent meningeal nerve, and the articular neurology to include mechanoreceptors and nociceptors and related spinal reflex pathways (see Chapter 8).

Connective Tissue Component

Lantz' connective tissue component describes the impact of joint immobilization and connective tissue changes. This component includes bone, the intervertebral disks, articular cartilage, interspinous ligaments, and related supportive tissue elements. With connective tissue immobilization, synovial fluid undergoes fibrofatty consolidation, progressing to more adherent fibrous tissue and matrix development for the deposition of bone salts in the final stages of ankylosis.[53] In the immobilized joint, articular cartilage shrinks resulting from loss of proteoglycans.[54] This shrinkage leads to softening of cartilage, thus rendering the articulation more susceptible to damage by minor trauma.[55]

In the immobilized joint, adhesions form between adjacent connective tissue structures.[53] This action may occur between the nerve root sleeve and adjacent capsular and osseous structures in the intervertebral foramen, between tendons and articular capsules, or between other connective tissue structures. Forced motion creates a physical disruption of the adhesions, breaking intermolecular cross linkages, thereby improving joint mobility. Adjustment/manipulation is one means through which this may be accomplished.[56]

Vascular Component

The vascular component may also be affected by abnormal spinal **biomechanics.** A segmental artery passing through the intervertebral canal into the spinal canal supplies each vertebral motion segment. Through branching, this artery provides blood supply to the dorsal and ventral nerve roots. Each canal contains a segmental vein that drains the spinal canal and vertebral column. These blood vessels are susceptible to the same mechanical insults as nerve roots and may be compressed. Lantz[57] proposes that immobilization may lead to localized venous stasis, creating a negative relative pressure at the area of immobilization and that lack of proper venous drainage may lead to inflammatory states.

Inflammatory Component

Immobilization of a joint leads to an inflammatory response.[58] The inflammatory process may affect surrounding tissues and affect nerve function, as implied in the concept of chemical radiculitis.[59] This action may represent one example of how degeneration of spinal joints affects the neurologic component of VSC. Inflamed nerves are hyperexcitable and exhibit behavior different from normal nerve function.[60] The dorsal root ganglia (DRG) of normal nerves respond to mechanical stimulation by discharge of action potentials, which stops on cessation of the stimulation. In an inflamed DRG, the action potential discharge continues long after the mechanical stimulus has ceased.[59]

Although some authors consider the inflammatory component part of the vascular component of VSC, other authors such as Faye[40] and Dishman[39] discuss inflammation under the histopathology component of the five-part Faye VSC model. In addition, given the chemical nature of inflammation and tissue repair, inflammation cannot be considered independent of the VSC biochemistry component.

The model of the VSC represents the current state of the art concept of subluxation and provides a context bridging the basic science and clinical aspects of spinal function, dysfunction, and degeneration. This model offers a framework for discussion of the varied approaches to spinal manipulative therapy, the specific chiropractic vertebral adjustment, and adjunctive or rehabilitative management of the spine. Using this model in interaction with other health care providers may enhance interprofessional cooperation between chiropractors and others in co-management and referral of patients.

THREE-COMPONENT MODEL (KENT MODEL)[61]

Kent proposes a three-component model of vertebral subluxation to include the components of dyskinesia, **dysponesis,** and dysautonomia.

Dyskinesia

Dyskinesia refers to distortions of, difficulty with, or impairment of voluntary movement. Impairment of spinal range of motion may be reliably measured with inclinometry.[62] Alterations in segmental or regional ranges of motion are associated with the kinesiopathologic component of subluxation.[63]

Dysponesis

Dysponesis is described as a reversible pathophysiologic state consisting of unnoticed, misdirected neurophysiologic reactions to various agents (environmental events, body sensations, emotions, and thoughts) and the repercussions of these reactions throughout the organism. Kent proposes that these errors in energy expenditure, potentially capable of producing functional disorders, consist mainly of covert errors in action potential output from the motor and premotor areas of the cerebral cortex and include the consequences of that output. These neurophysiologic events result in aberrant muscle activity that may be evaluated through surface electrode techniques.[64]

Dysautonomia

The portion of the nervous system that controls visceral function of the body is the autonomic nervous system. Acquired **dysautonomia** may be associated with various functional abnormalities and is proposed as a manifestation of vertebral subluxation.[65-67] Dysautonomia may be evaluated through measurement of skin temperature differentials.[68] Normative values for skin temperature differences have been determined based on asymptomatic individuals. Uematsu[69] proposes that:

...these values can be used as a standard in assessment of sympathetic nerve function, and the degree of asymmetry is a quantifiable indicator of dysfunction.... [Further,] ...deviations from the normal values will all suspicion of neurological pathology to be quantitated and therefore can improve assessment and lead to proper clinical management.

Kent proposes that surface electromyography (EMG) recording and skin temperature measurements may be used to assess altered autonomic tone associated with vertebral subluxation and are useful in determining specific levels for application of spinal adjustive technique procedures.

Common clinical characteristics of the Faye, **Lantz**, and **Kent models** of subluxation complex identified in this discussion include the combined components of kinesiologic dysfunction and neurologic dysfunction.

POSTURAL MODEL OF SPINAL SUBLUXATION (HARRISON MODEL)

Harrison and colleagues[70-73] depart from the segmental models of vertebral subluxation, proposing a model related to altered spinal structure and biomechanics as observed with abnormal asymmetrical posture. Such postures over time result in degenerative changes in the muscles, ligaments, and bony structures.[74-78] Further proposals assert that asymmetric posture may also be directly or indirectly responsible for spinal pain syndromes.[79] An overview of Harrison's concepts follows.

Alterations in posture, especially in the sagittal plane, have direct and indirect effects on the central nervous system (CNS) and its associated structures.[80,81] Evidence supports the hypothesis that the static and dynamic deformations of the spinal column are directly transmitted to the CNS.[82-90] Understanding the stresses and strains within the CNS may lead to increased understanding of altered neural physiology, degenerative disorders, and acute or chronic pathologic processes occurring in the nervous system.

Spinal Canal Deformations Caused by Changes in Posture

Flexion and Extension

The spinal canal changes in length during physiologic movements or alterations in posture. Flexion and extension in the sagittal plane lead to the largest changes, but scoliosis, lateral bending, and axial rotation also lead to significant deformations of the spinal canal.[70-73] The axis of motion for single rotations is normally in the disk or vertebral bodies.[91] Consequently, during flexion of the spinal column, structures anterior to this axis of motion will shorten and be exposed primarily to compressive forces, while tissues posterior to the axis will lengthen and be exposed mainly to tensile forces. (See Chapter 6 for descriptions of these biomechanical forces.) The total change in length of the spinal column from extension to flexion was estimated by Breig[80] to be 5 to 7 cm, although Louis[92] suggested 5.0 to 9.7 cm. This change in length is greater at the posterior aspect of the canal because of its increased distance from the axis of motion. Thus the strain in the posterior portion of the spinal canal contents will be greater than the strain of the anterior structures.

Beginning in maximal extension and moving to maximal flexion, the anterior portion of the cervical canal increases in length 0% to 24%, and the posterior canal increases by 28% to 61%.[80,81] Because of the ribcage, the thoracic spinal canal has a decreased sagittal plane mobility, though an increased kyphosis will increase the length of the canal up to 3 mm.[92] Similar to the cervical spine, the lumbar canal has a relatively large increase in length during flexion. Here, the central axis of the canal increases in length by 20%.[80] Holmes and colleagues[93] measured spinal canal volume in neutral and flexion-extension of the lower cervical spines (C2 to C7) of 10 cadavers. The volume of liquid displaced increased with flexion and decreased with extension, but the average total change from extension to flexion amounted to only 1.9 ml.

Breig[80] noted that cervical flexion would affect not only the cervical cord and nerve roots, but also the hindbrain and cranial nerves V through VII. The significance being that certain cranial nerve symptoms may be derived from cervical kyphosis or head flexion posture. In addition, Breig noted that several patients with trigeminal neuralgia had axial head rotation postures.

Axial Rotation

Axial rotation of the spinal column, sets up a physiologic stress inside the pons-cord tract, although no overall lengthening of the bony canal occurs.[80,91] Depending on the segmental level, however, increases and decreases in the canal dimensions do occur. This action is a result of the segmental coupling patterns from axial rotation.

Lateral Bending

Lateral bending results in an increase in canal length on one side of the canal and a decrease on the opposite.

Combined Postural Loading

With combinations of postures, lateral flexion of the skull plus an axial rotation of the skull, the canal deformations may be much larger than simply the combination of the two loads, because a shift in the axis of rotation occurs with combined loads.[71]

Postural Deformations of the Intervertebral foramina

The dimensions of the intervertebral foramina (IVF) will also be affected with change in sagittal plane posture.[80,91] Brieg[80] showed that the IVF will decrease in vertical height by 33%, and the cross-sectional area of the space will decrease as a result of the impingement from the zygopophyseal joints on extension. Other authors have observed that the intervertebral space increased by 24% in flexion and decreased by 20% in extension.[91] The dimensions of the IVF change during rotation as well. The ipsilateral side decreases in total area while the contralateral side will increase slightly. Such rotational changes are not as significant as those observed with flexion and extension.[71]

Postural Changes and Neural Dysfunction

To what extent do changes in posture or spinal canal length impart enough stretch to the spinal cord to increase pressure and decrease blood flow and cord perfusion? Documented evidence suggests that distraction instrumentation, such as those used in surgery or traction devices, produces significant losses of lumbar and cervical curvatures.[94] Further, it is acknowledged that spinal column distraction results in a reduction of afferent and efferent impulse conduction, detected by **somatosensory-evoked potentials** and **neurogenic motor–evoked potential**.[95,96] Lew and colleagues[96] showed that the spinal cord elongation and displacement caused by traction forces are consistently less than that produced by cervical flexion. Breig's case studies[80] suggest that prolonged postural deformities, such as cervical kyphosis, may result in the same neuronal dysfunctions that occur with distraction instrumentation applied to the spine, spinal cord, or those that occur in **tethered cord syndrome.**

Physiologic changes are known to occur in astronauts exposed to microgravity conditions (space flight).[97] Under these conditions, the spine is decompressed, which results in height increases of up to 7 cm. This increase in spinal column length occurs as a result of straightening of the sagittal plane curves and an increase in disk height. This change, in turn, results in considerable longitudinal stress and strain of the spinal cord and was proposed as a mechanism to explain the neurologic dysfunctions found in astronauts, referred to as *microgravity-related physiologic phenomena* (MRPP). MRPP consists of nutritional, metabolic, cardiovascular, neurovestibular, and otolith-spinal reflex changes; sensory, motor, and autonomic dysfunctions such as hyperreflexia, back pain, paresthesia, and muscle atrophy were also associated.[71]

Several investigators[98-101] have studied spinal column-spinal cord distraction to clarify the relationship between tension and neuronal dysfunction. Fujita and Yamamoto[102] studied the effect of lumbosacral traction in 50 dogs. Traction was applied to the filum terminale externum, internum, dural tube, and conus medullaris. All areas where traction was applied showed an initial augmentation of spinal-evoked potentials, suggestive of early stages of cord impairment. Other researchers have shown and verified this finding.[104] The amplitude of spinal-evoked potentials changed earlier and were larger for the filum terminale internum traction than they were for filum terminale externum. Traction of the dural tube and the conus showed similar tendencies. Traction on these structures influenced the upper cervical cord function, and dysfunction was also found in the spinal nerve root potentials.

Yamada and colleagues[104,105] used humans and animals in an attempt to understand the effect of traction on the filum and lumbosacral cord and its relationship to the pathophysiology of tethered cord syndrome. The underlying mechanism of this disorder was determined to be a derangement of neural tissue metabolism caused by longitudinal tensile stress. The oxidative metabolism of the mitochondria was impaired. Neurons and glial cells rely entirely on energy derived from conversion of intramitochondrial adenosine diphosphate phosphorylation (ADP) to ATP. Any change in the metabolic efficiency of cellular mitochondria is proposed to lead to progressive neuronal dysfunction.[104,106]

The pons-cord tract (mesencephalon, pons, medulla oblongata, spinal cord, nerve roots, and associated cranial nerves V through XII) will develop increased intramedullary pressure, increased cerebrospinal fluid pressure, and increased intrafascicular pressure (inside the neural cell) resulting from stretch or tensile loads.[80,91,107-110]

Such increased pressure in or around the cord is known to cause a decrease of afferent and efferent impulse conduction and will increase the risk of damage to the neural and supporting tissues.[111-113]

Harrison and colleagues propose that abnormal postural rotations and translations cause altered stresses in static spinal positions and in dynamic spinal motions. These stress patterns in the spinal cord have been shown to correlate clinically with abnormal neurologic signs and symptoms following trauma and nonacute cord injuries.[92,114-116]

In relation to altered dimensions of the IVF, several experiments have reported on the effects of mechanical compression on the dorsal nerve roots. These effects include disturbance of blood flow,[117,118] change in impulse propagation,[119-121] inflammation,[122-124] increase in microvascular permeability,[125,126] and formation of an intraneural fibrotic scar.[127,128] Compression of the dorsal root ganglion has been associated with IVF encroachment. The positions and clinical relevance of the cervical and lumbar dorsal root ganglia have also been examined.[129-133]

Given the changes in spinal canal length and volume, and deformations of the IVF, at issue is the influence of altered posture, spinal alignment, and related mechanical forces on the structure and function of the CNS and related neural tissue.

Harrison states that prolonged flexion is the most offensive postural loading on spinal structures. Flexing the upper cervical spine alone results in a significant increase in the intramedullary cord pressure that is in the range, 10 to 20 mm Hg, required to reduce spinal cord blood flow and cord perfusion. Prolonged stresses of loading of neural tissue may result in impaired oxidative metabolism in the mitochondria. Kyphotic configurations of the cervical and lumbar curves are types of flexed spinal positions, that is, buckling modes.

In the context of this postural model of vertebral dysfunction, Harrison suggests that, in addition to symptomatic improvement or resolution, rehabilitative procedures should strive for an anatomic outcome of improved upright human posture in the anteroposterior and lateral views as a primary focus or goal of care.[134,135]

DEFINITIONS RELATED TO SUBLUXATION AND CLINICAL PROCEDURES

Other definitions related to subluxation and its management as presented by Gatterman[20] include:

Manipulable subluxation: A subluxation in which altered alignment, movement, or function can be improved by manual thrust procedures.

Motion segment: A functional unit made up of two adjacent articulating surfaces and the connecting tissues binding to them to each other.

Spinal motion segment: Two adjacent vertebrae and the connecting tissues binding them to each other.

Manual therapy: Procedures by which the hands directly contact the body to treat the articulations or soft tissues.

Mobilization: Movement applied singularly or repetitively within or at the physiologic range of joint motion, without imparting a thrust or impulse, with the goal of restoring joint mobility.

Manipulation: A manual procedure that involves a directed thrust to move a joint past the physiologic range of motion without exceeding the anatomic limit.

Adjustment: Any chiropractic therapeutic procedure that uses controlled force, leverage, direction, amplitude, and velocity directed at specific joints or anatomic regions.

EARLY STUDIES OF EFFECTS OF SPINAL MECHANICAL DERANGEMENT

The modern era of research on spinal manipulation began in 1975 as result of the 1974 Senate appropriation for the National Institute of Neurological and Communicable Diseases and Stroke (NINCDS) of the National Institutes of Health (NIH) and with the convening of the historic Workshop on the Research Status of Spinal Manipulative Therapy.[136]

It must be acknowledged, however, that early basic science laboratory investigation into the relationship between altered spinal structure and tissues or organ dysfunction may be traced back to the first part of the twentieth century in medical and osteopathic literature and as early as 1950 for the chiropractic profession.

Louisa Burns: Experimental Osteopathic Lesions in Animals

Early investigation of spinal reflexes by osteopath Louisa Burns from 1907[137] onward focused on effects of the osteopathic lesion.[138-140] Research at the A.T. Still Research Institute in Chicago conducted by Burns and colleagues[140] in 1948 investigated the pathogenesis of visceral disease following vertebral lesion. To study certain nervous reflexes and lesion-induced disturbances in distant visceral tissue, Burns and colleagues produced experimental lesions in a variety of animals, including rabbits, guinea pigs, cats, dogs, and goats. To induce a spinal lesion, the experimenter would twist and traction a spinal segment. Burns[140] describes, "when the limit of normal motion is reached, slight sudden additional pressure in the same plane is exerted, forcing the vertebra just beyond its normal range of movement and causing a slight strain of the tissue." The term *lesion* is defined as "a mechanical maladjustment of some sort which operates as one of the primary causes of disease." Early stages of the lesion demonstrated impairment of visceral circulation along with changes in smooth muscle function and glandular secretory function. Lesioned articular structures demonstrated changes in synovial fluid and later fibrotic changes. Later stages of the lesion involved circulatory congestion, denervation-related changes, and segmentally organized somato-autonomic reflex dysfunction, resulting in disturbed regulation of the viscera.

Henry Winsor: Spinal Curvatures and Visceral Disorders

In 1922, medical physician Henry K. Winsor,[141] using cadavers from the University of Pennsylvania, conducted necropsies to determine whether a connection existed between minor curvatures of the spine and diseased organs. Fifty bodies were examined. The anterior thoracic and abdominal wall was removed, the organs were removed and examined, and the anterior surfaces of the vertebral bodies were cleared for ease of examination for curvature. Forty nine of the fifty cadavers showed minor curvatures. Winsor reported,

[In] fifty cadavers with diseases in 139 organs, there was found curve of the vertebrae, belonging to the same sympathetic segments as the diseased organs 128 times, leaving an apparent discrepancy of ten, in which the vertebrae in the curve belonged to an adjacent segment to that which should supply the diseased organs with sympathetic filaments. However, the nerve filaments entering the cord or leaving it travel or have traveled up or down the cord for a few segments, accounting for all the apparent discrepancies.

Tabulation of Winsor's observations (Table 7-1) provides the following examples:

- Heart and pericardium disease was observed in 20 cases of the 50 cadavers. Minor spinal curvatures were identified in the upper five dorsal segments in 18 of the cases. Two cases involved neighboring segment C7 and D1.
- Stomach disease was identified in nine cases with eight of the nine demonstrating curvature in dorsal segments 5 through 9. In one case, curvature was found in a neighboring segment.
- Kidney disease was observed in 17 cases. Curvature was observed at dorsal segments 10 through 12 in 14 cases. One case demonstrated curvature at neighboring dorsal segments 5 through 9 and "few" at lumbar segment 1 and 2.

Winsor took these observations as "evidences of the association, in the dissected cadavers, of the visceral disease with vertebral deformities of the same sympathetic segments."

Carl Cleveland, Jr.: Experimental Subluxation Effects in Rabbits

In the early 1950s, Carl S. Cleveland, Jr.[142,143] in a pilot study investigated the effects of subluxation on the domestic rabbit. Misalignment of the intervertebral joint was produced by applying a spinal subluxation splint consisting of three adjustable metal pin clamps supported by a common suprastructure frame. With minimal surgical incision, the pin clamps were attached to the base of spinous processes of three contiguous vertebrae. Subluxation was produced by tightening Allen screws on the splint frame, thereby drawing the middle vertebra to the posterior and then laterally to produce misalignment. This procedure was accomplished under fluoroscopic assistance and verified by radiographs. Physiologic outcomes such as heart rate, blood pressure, and urinalysis were evaluated. Postmortem pathologic analysis was conducted on various organs and tissues. Findings included two cases of twelfth thoracic subluxation with subsequent kidney abnormalities. Other experimental subjects demonstrated "heart diseases, valvular leakages, paralysis, arrhythmias, vasomotor paralysis, dropsy, kidney conditions, and the formation of tumors." Vernon[143] cites this study as an innovative first attempt by chiropractic investigators to employ an animal model of spinal subluxation.

A RETROSPECTIVE

The forceful dynamic thrust as part of the application of spinal manipulation dates from the time of ancient Greece,[25,144] as identified by Withington's 1959 English translation of the writings of Hippocrates, circa 400 BC. Hippocrates recommended that with the patient lying prone on a wooden bed, combined extension and pressure should be exerted on the patient's spine, and

...[the] physician, or an assistant who is strong and not untrained, should put the palm of hand on the hump, and the palm of the other hand on that, to reduce it forcibly, taking into consideration whether the reduction should naturally be made straight downwards or towards the head or towards the hip.

References in this ancient writing to positioning of the hands and whether to direct the force downward or toward the head or the hip are strikingly similar to the fundamental components of toggle-type dynamic thrusts and the angle of drive (direction of thrust) found in contemporary chiropractic technique texts.

Table **7-1**   WINSOR'S CORRELATION OF SPINAL CURVATURES AND DISEASED ORGANS IN CADAVERS

Visceral Disturbances		Same Sympathetic Segment as Visceral Trouble		Neighboring Segment to Viscera		Sympathetic Connections between Vertebrae and Diseased Organ	Check System
Thymus diseased	2	C7 & D1 D2.3.4	1 1	None	0	Inferior cervical ganglia	2
Pleurae adherent	21	Upper dorsal	19	Lower dorsal	2	Upper dorsal ganglia Lower dorsal ganglia	19⎱21 2⎰
Lung diseases	26	Upper dorsal	26	Lower dorsal	0	Upper dorsal ganglia	26-26
Heart and pericardium cases	20	Upper five dorsal	18	C7 and D1	2	Upper dorsal ganglia Inferior cervical ganglia	18⎱20 2⎰
Stomach diseases	9	Dorsal 5-9	8		1	Greater splanchnic (dorsal 5-9)	8
Liver diseases	13	Dorsal 5-9	12		1	Greater splanchnic (dorsal 5-9)	12
Cholelithiasis cases	5	Dorsal 5-9	5		0	Greater splanchnic (dorsal 5-9)	5 5
Pancreas cases	5	Dorsal 5-9	3		0	Greater splanchnic (dorsal 5-9)	3
Splenic affections	11	Dorsal 5-9	10	Dorsal 10,11,12	1	Greater splanchnic (dorsal 5-9) Lesser and least Splanchnic	10⎱10 1⎰11
Inguinal diseases	2	Dorsal 12	2		0	Somatic nerve Ilio-inguinal	2
Kidney diseases	17	Dorsal 10, 11, 12	14	Dorsal 5-9 Lumbar 1 and 2	1 few	Least, lesser, and greater splanchnic Upper lumbar ganglia	17
Prostate and bladder diseases	8	Lumber 1, 2, 3	7	Dorsal 12 Sacral curve	1 1	Upper lumbar ganglia Last dorsal and sacral few	7 8
Uterus and adnexa	2	Lumbar Lordosis	2	0		Lumbar and sacral ganglia	2
Visceral diseases	139	Vertebral curve of same sympathetic segment as disease site	139	Vertebral curve of adjacent segment	10	Vertebral curve of segments not related to diseased site 1-5	138
			128				

The concept of spinal biomechanical dysfunction described and treated as the *hump* some 20 centuries earlier by Hippocrates reappeared in the medical literature some 300 years ago as the term *subluxation*.[19] Historical literature[23-25] records that spinal biomechanical dysfunction and its treatment by manipulation represented an area of substantive interest in the early nineteenth-century medical community. This approach later fell into disuse in North America as that profession moved toward the chemically focused allopathic model of patient care. This abandonment of manipulation by conventional medicine provided chiropractors the opportunity to progress with little competition from non-DC manual therapy practitioners and thus to become the most skilled practitioners of the spinal adjustment and manipulative procedures.

Maintaining this leadership role in conservative management of spinal function will depend on the chiropractic profession's ability to advance knowledge through research and clinical outcome assessment, especially regarding the effectiveness of chiropractic procedures in restoring and preserving health. The model of vertebral subluxation complex provides a common context bridging the basic science and clinical aspects of spinal function, dysfunction, and degeneration and may serve to enhance interprofessional cooperation between doctors of chiropractic and other health care providers participating in co-management and referral of patients.

Review *Questions*

1. What is the earliest known English definition of subluxation? In what year was this definition proposed?
2. What was D.D. Palmer's view of subluxation?
3. How did B.J. Palmer redefine subluxation?
4. What are the similarities and differences between Andrew Taylor Still's osteopathic concepts and the chiropractic concepts of D.D. Palmer?
5. What role did unique chiropractic nomenclature such as the term *subluxation* play in the struggle for separate licensure?

6. Which early chiropractors were the first to characterize subluxation as a *fixation* and to describe the *field of motion* of a vertebra?
7. Which two Belgian chiropractors developed the concepts of motion palpation?
8. In what ways are contemporary definitions of subluxation similar to, and different from, early definitions of the Palmers, Stephenson, and Langworthy?
9. What are the major characteristics of the five-component Faye model of vertebral subluxation complex?
10. What additional concepts are incorporated in the Lantz model?

Concept *Questions*

1. Why did it take until 1996 for the presidents of all North American chiropractic colleges to reach unanimous consensus on common core definitions fundamental to the principles of chiropractic? What intraprofessional divisions kept this consensus from occurring earlier?
2. What role does subluxation play in relation to visceral disease or dysfunction? What evidence supports this answer?
3. In considering various subluxation definitions that have evolved throughout the profession's history, identify examples that may be described as *static* or positional and those that more closely represent the *dynamic* concept or model of subluxation. Are there examples of subluxation definitions that would represent a blend or combination addressing both the concept of altered position, motion, or both?
4. Contrast the differences between the segmental models of subluxation and the postural model of spinal subluxation. Discuss in what ways these two concepts may interrelate.

REFERENCES

1. Nelson CL: The subluxation question, *J Chiropr Human* 7(1):46, 1997.
2. Palmer DD: *The science, art and philosophy of chiropractic*, Portland, 1910, Portland Printing House.
3. Palmer BJ: *The subluxation specific—the adjustment specific*, Davenport, Iowa, 1934, Palmer School of Chiropractic.

4. Stephenson RW: *Chiropractic text book,* Davenport, Iowa, 1948, Palmer School of Chiropractic.

5. Cleveland CS Jr: *Researching the subluxation on the domestic rabbit, Cleveland Chiropractic College monograph,* Kansas City, 1961, Cleveland College of Chiropractic.

6. Palmer DD, Palmer BJ: *The science of chiropractic: its principles and adjustments,* Davenport, Iowa, 1906, Palmer School of Chiropractic.

7. Sandoz R: Some critical reflections on subluxations and adjustment, *Ann Swiss Chiropr Assoc* 9:7, 1989.

8. Jackson R: *The cervical syndrome,* Springfield, Ill, 1976, Charles C Thomas.

9. *Stedman's medical dictionary,* ed 26, Baltimore, 1995, Williams & Wilkins.

10. Gatterman M, Hansen D: The development of chiropractic nomenclature through consensus, *J Manipulative Physiol Ther* 17:302, 1994.

11. Cleveland CS III: *Chiropractic 811, lecture notes,* Kansas City, 1995, Cleveland Chiropractic College.

12. Gatterman MI: *Foundations of chiropractic: subluxation,* St Louis, 1995, Mosby.

13. Haldeman SC: The pathophysiology of the spinal subluxation. In Goldstein M, editor: *The research status of spinal manipulative therapy,* HEW/NINCDS Monograph #15, Bethesda, 1975, U.S. Department of Health, Education and Welfare.

14. Peterson D, Bergman T: *Chiropractic technique: principles and procedures,* ed 2, St Louis, 2002, Mosby.

15. Rome PL: Usage of chiropractic terminology in the literature: 296 ways to say "subluxation": complex issues of the vertebral subluxation, *Chiropr Tech* 8(2):49, 1996.

16. Seaman D: Joint complex dysfunction, a novel term to replace subluxation/subluxation complex: etiological and treatment considerations, *J Manipulative Physiol Ther* 20:634, 1997.

17. Seaman R, Winterstein J: Dysafferentation: a novel term to describe the neuropathophysiological effects of joint complex dysfunction. A look at likely mechanisms of symptom generation, *J Manipulative Physiol Ther* 21(4):267, 1998.

18. Haldeman S et al: Spinal manipulative therapy. In Frymoyer JW, editor: *The adult spine: principles and practice,* vol 2, Philadelphia, 1997, Lippincott-Raven.

19. Holme R: *Academy of Armory,* printed in Chester by author, 1688, reprinted 1972 by the Scholar Press Limited, Menston, England.

20. Gatterman MI: What's in a word? In Gatterman MI, editor: *Foundations of chiropractic: subluxation,* St Louis, 1995, Mosby.

21. Leach RA: *The chiropractic theories-principles and clinical applications,* ed 3, Baltimore, 1994, Williams & Wilkins.

22. Lantz CA: The vertebral subluxation complex, *ICA Rev* 45:37, 1989.

23. Hieronymus JH: *De luxationibus et subluxationibus.* Thesis, Jena, Italy, 1746.

24. Terrett A: The search for the subluxation: an investigation of medical literature to 1985, *Chiropr Hist* 7:29, 1987.

25. Lomax E: Manipulative therapy: a historical perspective from ancient times to the modern era. In Goldstein M, editor: *The research status of spinal manipulative therapy,* HEW/NINCDS Monograph #15, Bethesda, 1975, U.S. Department of Health; Education and Welfare.

26. Tower D: Chairman's summary: Evolution and development of the concepts of manipulative therapy. In Goldstein M, editor: *The research status of spinal manipulative therapy.* HEW/NINCDS Monograph #15, Bethesda, 1975, U.S. Department of Health; Education and Welfare.

27. Wardwell WI: Before the Palmers: an overview of chiropractic's antecedents, *Chiropr Hist* 7(2):27, 1987.

28. Keating JC: "Heat by nerves and not by blood": the first major reduction in chiropractic theory, 1903, *Chiropr Hist* 15(2):70, 1995.

29. Vear HJ: *An introduction to the science of chiropractic,* Portland, 1981, Western States Chiropractic College.

30. Quigley WH: Chiropractic's monocausal theory of disease, *J Am Chiropr Assoc* 8(6):52, 1981.

31. Palmer DD: *The Chiropractor* 1(1):8, 1904.

32. Gibbons RW: Solon Massey Langworthy: keeper of the flame during the "lost years" of chiropractic, *Chiropr Hist* 1:15, 1981.

33. Smith O, Langworthy SM, Paxson M: *Modernized chiropractic,* Cedar Rapids, Iowa, 1906, American School of Chiropractic.

34. Gillet H, Liekens M: *Belgian chiropractic research notes,* Huntington Beach, Calif, 1981, Motion Palpation Institute.

35. Lantz CA: A review of the evolution of chiropractic concepts of subluxation, *Top Clin Chiropr* 2(2):1, 1995.

36. Illi FW: *The vertebral column: life line of the body,* Chicago, 1951, National College of Chiropractic.

37. Mennell J McM: *Joint pain diagnosis and treatment using manipulative techniques,* Boston, 1964, Little, Brown.

38. Sandoz R: Classification of luxations, subluxation and fixations of the cervical spine, *Ann Swiss Chiropr Assoc* 6:219, 1976.

39. Dishman R: Review of the literature supporting a scientific basis for the chiropractic subluxation complex, *J Manipulative Physiol Ther* 8:163, 1988.

40. Faye LJ: *Motion palpation of the spine,* Huntington Beach, Calif, 1983, Motion Palpation Institute.

41. Hendrickson RM: *The legislative establishment of subluxation as an element in chiropractic practice,* Arlington, Va, 2003, International Chiropractors Association.

42. Medicare Act, the United States Code Annotated, Title 42, The Public Health and Welfare, Section 10/395x, under (r)Physician, 1974.

43. World Health Organization: *International classification of diseases,* ed 10, Geneva, 1992, World Health Organization.

44. American Chiropractic Association: *Indexed synopsis of policies on public health and related matters,* Arlington, Va, 1995-1996.

45. International Chiropractors Association: *Membership referral directory,* ICA Policy Statements, Arlington, Va, 1986, International Chiropractors Association.

46. International Chiropractors Association: Minutes of Midyear Board of Directors Meeting, Universal City, Calif, January 21-24, 1988, Arlington, Va, 1988, International Chiropractors Association.

47. Association of Chiropractic Colleges: Minutes, Chicago, July 1, 1996.

48. Janse J, Houser RH, Wells BF: *Chiropractic principles and technic—for use by students and practitioners,* ed 2, Chicago, 1947, National College of Chiropractic.

49. Janse J, Hildebrandt RW, editor: *Principles and practice of chiropractic—an anthology,* Chicago, 1976, National College of Chiropractic.

50. Homewood AE: *The neurodynamics of the vertebral subluxation,* ed 3, St Petersburg, Fla, 1981, Valkyrie Press.

51. Schafer RC, Faye LJ: *Motion palpation and chiropractic technic: principles of dynamic chiropractic,* Huntington Beach, Calif, 1989, The Motion Palpation Institute.

51a. Seaman DR: *Chiropractic and pain control,* ed 3, Hendersonville, NC, 1995, DRS Systems.

52. Videman T: Connective tissue and immobilization, *Clin Orthop* 221:26, 1987.

53. Evans EB et al: Experimental immobilization and remobilization of rat knee, *J Bone Joint Surg* 42A:737, 1960.

54. Troyer H: The effect of short-term immobilization on the rabbit knee in joint cartilage, *Clin Orthop* 107:249, 1975.

55. Palmoski MJ, Colyer RA, Brandt KD: Joint motion in the absence of normal loading does not maintain normal articular cartilage, *Arthritis Rheum* 23:325, 1980.

56. Woo SL-Y et al: Connective tissue response to immobility: correlative study of biomechanical and biochemical measurements of normal and immobilized rabbit knees, *Arthritis Rheum* 18:257, 1975.

57. Lantz CA: The vertebral subluxation complex. In Gatterman MI, editor: *Foundations of chiropractic: subluxation,* St Louis, 1995, Mosby.

58. Davis D: Respiratory manifestations of dorsal spine radiculitis simulating cardiac asthma, *Ann Intern Med* 32:954, 1950.

59. Marshall LL, Thethewie ER, Curtain CC: Chemical radiculitis: a clinical, physiological and immunological study, *Clin Orthop* 129:61, 1977.

60. Howe JF, Loeser JD, Calvin WH: Mechanosensitivity of dorsal root ganglia and chronically injured axons: a physiological basis for radicular pain of nerve root compression, *Pain* 3:25, 1977.

61. Kent C: Models of vertebral subluxation: a review, *J Vertebral Subluxation Res* 1(1):11, 1996.

62. Saur PM et al: Lumbar range of motion: reliability and validity of the inclinometer technique in the clinical measurement of trunk flexibility, *Spine* 21(11):1332, 1996.

63. Blunt KL, Gatterman MI, Bereznick DE: Kinesiology: an essential approach toward understanding the chiropractic subluxation. In Gatterman MI, editor: *Foundations of chiropractic: subluxation,* St Louis, 1995, Mosby.

64. Whatmore GB, Kohi DR: Dysponesis: a neurophysiologic factor in functional disorders, *Behav Sci* 13(2):102, 1968.

65. Backonja M-M: Reflex sympathetic dystrophy/sympathetically mediated pain/causalgia: the syndrome of neuropathic pain with dysautonomia, *Semin Neurol* 14(3):263, 1994.

66. Goldstein DS et al: Sympathetic cardioneuropathy in dysautonomias, *N Eng J Med* 336(10):696, 1997.

67. Baron R, Engler F: Postganglionic cholinergic dysautonomia with incomplete recovery: a clinical, neurophysiological and immunological case study, *J Neurol* 243:18, 1996.

68. Korr IM: *The collected papers of Irvin M. Korr,* Indianapolis, Ind, 1979, American Academy of Osteopathy.

69. Uematsu S et al: Quantification of thermal asymmetry, *J Neurosurg* 69:552, 1988.

70. Harrison DE, Harrison DD, Troyanovich SJ: Three-dimensional spinal coupling mechanics. Part II: Implications for chiropractic theories and practice, *J Manipulative Physiol Ther* 21(3):177, 1998.

71. Harrison DE et al: A review of biomechanics of the central nervous system. Part I: spinal canal deformations due to changes in posture, *J Manipulative Physiol Ther* 22(4):227, 1999.

72. Harrison DE et al: A review of biomechanics of the central nervous system. Part II: strains in the spinal cord from postural loads, *J Manipulative Physiol Ther* 22(5):322, 1999.

73. Harrison DE et al: A review of biomechanics of the central nervous system. Part III: neurologic effects of stresses and strains, *J Manipulative Physiol Ther* 22(6):399, 1999.

74. Fukuyama S et al: The effect of mechanical stress on hypertrophy of the lumbar ligamentum flavum, *J Spinal Disord* 8:126, 1995.

75. Jones M, Pais M, Omiya B: Bony overgrowths and abnormal calcifications about the spine, *Radiol Clin North Am* 26:1213, 1988.

76. Zagra A et al: Posterior spinal fusion in scoliosis: computer-assisted tomography and biomechanics of the fusion mass, *Spine* 13:155, 1988.

77. Genaidy A, Karwowski W: The effects of neutral posture deviations on perceived joint discomfort ratings in sitting and standing postures, *Ergonomics* 36:785, 1993.

78. Beaman D et al: Substance P innervation of lumbar spine facet joints, *Spine* 18:1044, 1993.

79. Hiemeyer K, Lutz R, Menninger H: Dependence of tender points upon posture: a key to the understanding of fibromyalgia syndrome, *J Man Med* 5:169, 1990.
80. Breig A: *Adverse mechanical tension in the central nervous system. Analysis of cause and effect. Relief by functional neurosurgery*, New York, 1978, John Wiley & Sons.
81. Breig A, Turnbull I, Hassler O: Effects of mechanical stresses on the spinal cord in cervical spondylosis. A study on fresh cadaver material, *J Neursurg* 25:45, 1966.
82. Shacklock M: Neurodynamics, *Physiotherapy* 81:9, 1995.
83. Tencer AF, Allen BL, Ferguson RL: A biomechanical study of thoracolumbar spine fractures with bone in the canal. Part III: mechanical properties of the dura and its tethering ligaments, *Spine* 10:741, 1985.
84. Smith C: Changes in length and position of the segments of the spinal cord with changes in posture in the monkey, *Radiology* 66:259, 1956.
85. McCormick P, Stein B: Functional anatomy of the spinal cord and related structures, *Neurosurg Clin North Am* 1:469, 1990.
86. Kameyama T, Hashizume Y, Sobue G: Morphologic features of the normal human cadaveric spinal cord, *Spine* 21:1285, 1996.
87. Ruch WJ: *Atlas of common subluxations of the human spine and pelvis*, Boca Raton, Fla, 1997, CRC Press.
88. Reid J: Effects of flexion-extension movement of the head and spine upon the spinal cord and nerve roots, *J Neurol Neurosurg Psychiatry* 23:214, 1960.
89. Adams C, Logue V: Studies in cervical spondylotic myelopathy. Part I: movement of the cervical roots, dura and cord, and their relation to the course of the extrathecal roots, *Brain* 94:557, 1971.
90. Butler D: Adverse mechanical tension in the nervous system: a model for assessment and treatment, *Aust J Physiother* 35:227, 1989.
91. White A, Panjabi M: *Clinical biomechanics of the spine*, ed 2, Philadelphia, 1990, Lippincott.
92. Louis R: Vertebroradicular and vertebromedullar dynamics, *Anatomia Clinica* 3:1, 1981.
93. Holmes A et al: Changes in cervical canal spinal volume during in vitro flexion-extension, *Spine* 21:1313, 1996.
94. Peterson M et al: The effect of operative position on lumbar lordosis. A radiographic study of patients under anesthesia in the prone and 90-90 positions, *Spine* 20:1419, 1995.
95. Naito M et al: Effects of distraction on physiologic integrity of the spinal cord, spinal cord blood flow, and clinical status, *Spine* 17:1154, 1992.
96. Lew P, Morrow C, Lew A: The effect of neck and leg flexion and their sequence on the lumbar spinal cord, *Spine* 19:2421, 1994.
97. Wing P et al: Back pain and spinal changes in microgravity, *Orthop Clin North Am* 22:255, 1991.
98. Cusick J et al: Effects of vertebral column distraction in the monkey, *J Neurosurg* 57:651, 1982.
99. Dolan E et al: The effect of spinal distraction on regional blood flow in cats, *J Neurosurg* 53:756, 1980.
100. Naito M et al: Effects of distraction on physiologic integrity of the spinal cord, spinal cord blood flow, and clinical status, *Spine* 17:1154, 1992.
101. Yamada S et al: Pathophysiology of tethered cord syndrome, *Neurosurg Clin North Am* 6:311, 1995.
102. Fujita Y, Yamamoto H: An experimental study on spinal cord traction effect, *Spine* 14:698, 1989.
103. Hiraizumi Y et al: Differences in sensitivity between magnetic motor-evoked potentials and somatosensory-evoked potentials in experimental spinal cord lesions, *Spine* 21:2190, 1996.
104. Yamada S, Zinke D, Sanders D: Pathophysiology of tethered cord syndrome, *J Neurosurg* 54:494, 1981.
105. Yamada S et al: Pathophysiology of tethered cord syndrome, *Neurosurg Clin North Am* 6:311, 1995.
106. McCormick P, Stein B: Functional anatomy of the spinal cord and related structures, *Neurosurg Clin North Am* 1:469, 1990.
107. Jarzem P et al: Spinal cord tissue pressure during spinal cord distraction in dogs, *Spine* 17:S227, 1992.
108. Tachibana S et al: Spinal cord intramedullary pressure. A possible factor in syrinx growth, *Spine* 19:2174, 1994.
109. Kitahara Y, Lida H, Tachibana S: Effect of spinal cord stretching due to head flexion on intramedullary pressure, *Neurol Med Chir (Tokyo)* 35:285, 1995.
110. Lida H, Tachibana S: Spinal cord intramedullary pressure: direct cord traction test, *Neurol Med Chir (Tokyo)* 35:75, 1995.
111. Jarzem P et al: Spinal cord tissue pressure during spinal cord distraction in dogs, *Spine* 17:S227, 1992.
112. Breig A et al: Anatomic bases of medical and surgical techniques. Healing of the severed spinal cord by biomechanical relaxation and surgical immobilization, *Anat Clin* 4:167, 1982.
113. Francel P et al: Limiting ischemic spinal cord injury using a free radical scavenger 21-aminosteroid and/or cerebrospinal fluid drainage, *J Neurosurg* 79:742, 1993.
114. Harrison DE: Letter to the editor. [Konno S et al: Juvenile amyotrophy of the distal upper extremity: pathological findings of the dura mater and surgical management, *Spine* 22:486, 1997]; 22(21):2581, 1997.
115. Raynor RB, Koplik B: Cervical cord trauma. The relationship between clinical syndromes and force of injury, *Spine* 10:193, 1985.
116. O'Brien M, Sutterlin C: Occipitocervical biomechanics: clinical and biomechanical implications

for posterior occipitocervical stabilization and fusion, *Spine: State Art Rev* 10:281, 1996.

117. Olmarker K et al: Effects of experimental graded compression on blood flow in spinal nerve roots. A vital microscopic study on the porcine cauda equina, *J Orthop Res* 7:817, 1989.

118. Takahashi K et al: Double-level cauda equina compression: an experimental study with continuous monitoring of intraneural blood flow in porcine cauda equina, *J Orthop Res* 11:104, 1993.

119. Pedowitz RA et al: Effects of magnitude and duration of compression on spinal nerve root conduction, *Spine* 17:194, 1992.

120. Yoshizawa H, Kobayashi S, Morita T: Chronic nerve root compression. Pathophysiologic mechanism of nerve root dysfunction, *Spine* 20:397, 1995.

121. Kikuchi S et al: Increased resistance to acute compressive injury in chronically compressed spinal nerve roots. An experimental study, *Spine* 21:2544, 1996.

122. Matsui T et al: Quantitative analysis of edema in the dorsal nerve roots induced by acute mechanical compression, *Spine* 21(18):1931, 1998.

123. Olmarker K, Rydevik B, Nordborg C: Autologous nucleus pulposus induces neurophysiologic and histologic changes in porcine cauda equina nerve roots, *Spine* 18:1425, 1993.

124. Cornefjord M et al: Neuropeptide changes in compressed spinal nerve roots, *Spine* 20:670, 1995.

125. Kobayashi S et al: Vasogenic edema induced by compression injury to the spinal nerve root. Distribution of intravenously injected protein tracers and gadolinium-enhanced magnetic resonance imaging, *Spine* 8:1410, 1993.

126. Rydevik B et al: Effects of acute graded compression on spinal nerve root function and structure. An experimental study on the pig cauda equina, *Spine* 16:487, 1991.

127. Olmarker K, Rydevik B, Holm S: Edema formation in spinal nerve roots induced by experimental, graded compression. An experimental study on pig cauda equina with special reference to differences in effects between rapid and slow onset of compression, *Spine* 14:569, 1989.

128. Rydevik B et al: Pathoanatomy and pathophysiology of nerve root compression, *Spine* 9:7, 1984.

129. Lu J, Ebraheim NA: Anatomic considerations of C2 nerve root ganglion, *Spine* 23:649, 1998.

130. Cohen MS et al: Cauda equina anatomy II: Extrathecal nerve roots and dorsal root ganglion, *Spine* 15:1248, 1990.

131. Kikuchi S et al: Anatomic and radiologic study of dorsal root ganglia, *Spine* 19:6, 1994.

132. Sato K, Kikuchi S: An anatomic study of foraminal nerve root lesions in the lumbar spine, *Spine* 18:2246, 1993.

133. Yabuki S, Kikuchi S: Positions of dorsal root ganglia in the cervical spine. An anatomic and clinical study, *Spine* 21:1513, 1996.

134. Lennon J et al: Postural and respiratory modulation of autonomic function, pain and health, *AJPM* 4:36, 1994.

135. Kucherra M: Gravitational stress, musculoligamentous strain, and postural alignment, *Spine: State Art Rev* 9:463, 1995.

136. Wardwell WI: *Chiropractic: history and evolution of a new profession*, St Louis, 1992, Mosby.

137. Burns LA: Viscero-somatic and somato-visceral spinal reflexes, *J Am Osteopath Assoc* 7:51, 1907.

138. Burns LA: Effects of upper cervical and upper thoracic lesions, *J Am Osteopath Assoc* 22:266, 1923.

139. Burns LA: Laboratory proofs of the osteopathic lesion, *J Am Osteopath Assoc* 31:123, 1931.

140. Burns L, Chandler L, Rice R: *Pathogenesis of visceral diseases following vertebral lesions*, Chicago, 1948, American Osteopathic Association.

141. Winsor HK: Sympathetic segmental disturbances II, *Med Times* 49:267, 1922.

142. Cleveland CS Jr: Researching the subluxation on the domestic rabbit, *Sci Rev Chiropr* 1(4):5, 1965.

143. Vernon H: Basic scientific evidence for chiropractic subluxation. In Gatterman M, editor: *Foundations of chiropractic: subluxation*, St Louis, 1995, Mosby.

144. Cleveland CS III: The high-velocity thrust adjustment. In Haldeman S, editor: *Principles and practice of chiropractic*, East Norwalk, Conn, 1992, Appleton & Lange.

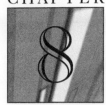

Neurobiologic Relations and Chiropractic Applications

Carl S. Cleveland III, DC

Key Terms

AFFERENT INHIBITION	IMPULSE-BASED NEURAL	PROPRIOCEPTION
AXOPLASMIC FLOW	MECHANISMS	REFLEX ARC
AXOPLASMIC	INTERPEDICULAR ZONE	SOMATOSOMATIC REFLEX
TRANSPORT	INTERVERTEBRAL FORAMINA	SOMATOVISCERAL REFLEX
CHRONIC CERVICAL	MORPHOLOGY	TRANSFORAMINAL
SYNDROME	NERVE COMPRESSION	LIGAMENTS
DYSAFFERENTATION	HYPOTHESIS	TROPHIC
DYSMENORRHEA	NERVE INTERFERENCE	VERTEBRAL SUBLUXATION
DYSPONESIS	NEURODYSTROPHIC	COMPLEX
END ORGAN	HYPOTHESIS	VISCERAL DISEASE
FACILITATION	NONIMPULSE-BASED NEURAL	SIMULATION
GATE CONTROL THEORY	MECHANISMS	VISCEROSOMATIC REFLEX

Chiropractic theory maintains that subluxation and adjustment/manipulation have important physiologic effects that include increasing range of joint motion, changes in facet joint kinematics, increased muscle strength, attenuation of alpha-motoneuron activity, enhanced **proprioception,** changes in beta-endorphins, and increased pain tolerance.[1] A common theme in each of the various conceptual models of vertebral subluxation is the expectation that spinal biomechanical derangement causes some form of nerve dysfunction or **nerve interference**. According to Vernon[2]:

This has come to be understood as either (1) some element of compression of the spinal nerves in the environs of the intervertebral foramen or (2) . . . initiation of pain in the spinal joints . . . capable of creating secondary aberrant reflex effects such as increases in motoneuron or sympathetic neural activity.

Harrison and colleagues[3-5] propose that prolonged alterations in posture or spinal canal length impart stretch, compression, or tensile forces to the spinal cord, especially in the sagittal plane (flexion and extension) and that such postures have direct and indirect effects on the central nervous system (CNS) and its associated structures.

For various reasons, including the increasing body of supportive research evidence, a rapid expansion of interest has occurred in spinal adjustive/manipulative procedures by medical physicians, physical therapists, osteopaths, and health care decision makers. Health providers who manage patients with low back pain and neck pain may find it rare not to have discussion on the topic of spinal manipulation and adjustment because a significant number of their patients are receiving or considering this form of health service. An understanding of the various theories and concepts related to the spinal adjustment, its mechanisms, clinical manifestations, and results is therefore increasingly necessary.[6] Various hypotheses have been advanced to explain the association of **vertebral subluxation complex** (VSC) with neuronal disturbance and related dysfunction and symptoms.[7-12] Meeker and Haldeman[1] identify at least five mechanical and neurologic mechanisms (Table 8-1).

The common hypotheses related to the neuropathophysiologic manifestations associated

Table **8-1**   PROPOSED MECHANISMS OF SPINAL MANIPULATION

Action	Mechanism
Mechanical-anatomic	Alleviation of an entrapped facet joint inclusion or meniscoid that has been shown to be heavily innervated[139–140]
Mechanical-anatomic	Repositioning of a fragment of posterior annular material from the intervertebral disk[140,141]
Mechanical-anatomic	Alleviation of stiffness induced by fibrotic tissue from previous injury or degenerative changes that may include adaptive shortening of fascial tissue[142,143]
Neurologic-mechanical	Inhibition of excessive reflex activity in the intrinsic spinal musculature or limbs or **facilitation** of inhibited muscle activity[144-146]
Neurologic-mechanical	Reduction of compressive or irritative insults to neural tissues[147]

From Meeker and Haldeman,[1] with permission.

Box **8-1**   NEUROBIOLOGIC RELATIONS OF SUBLUXATION COMPLEX

CONTEMPORARY HYPOTHESES

1. Nerve compression hypothesis
2. Aberrant spinal reflex hypotheses
   a. Somatosomatic
   b. Somatovisceral
   c. Viscerosomatic
3. Joint dysafferentation
4. Visceral disease simulation
5. Decreased axoplasmic transport
   a. Neurodystrophic hypothesis

with altered joint mechanics that represent the focus of this chapter appear in Box 8-1.

NERVE COMPRESSION HYPOTHESIS

From the beginnings of the chiropractic profession, the theory that nerves can become compressed through impingement from intersegmental spinal biomechanical derangements has been accorded biomechanical, functional, and clinical significance[13-21] and has even been proposed as a primary cause of disease.[13-21] Chiropractic authors emphasize the importance of the intervertebral foramen (IVF) and its anatomic contents—the spinal nerve, nerve roots, recurrent meningeal (sinuvertebral) nerves, blood vessels, lymphatics, and connective tissue—and devote much attention to

changes resulting from compression of the elements within the IVF.[13-18,20-26]

Although contemporary research[27-32] has demonstrated that other mechanisms of spinal biomechanical derangement may be responsible for inducing neuronal disturbances, the clinical significance of nerve compression should not be discounted.[21] Cramer and Darby[22] attribute much of the importance of the IVF to the fact that it provides an osteoligamentous boundary between the CNS and the peripheral nervous system.

The question is: To what extent are spinal nerves, nerve roots, and dorsal root ganglia vulnerable to compression or irritation by abnormal biomechanics affecting the IVF? The anatomy of the lumbar and thoracic spine suggests that sufficient room exists for spinal nerves to pass unimpeded through IVFs in these areas. However, the anatomic relationship of the spinal nerve to the cervical intervertebral foramen is significantly different.

Anatomy of the Cervical Intervertebral Foramen

Orthopedic surgeons DePalma and Rothman[23] describe the cervical spine **intervertebral foramina** as small ovoid canals with vertical diameters approximately 10 mm in height, with the anteroposterior diameter about one half the size of the vertical diameter. The authors state that the " . . . nerve roots and mixed spinal nerves completely fill the anteroposterior diameter of the intervertebral foramina. The upper one quarter of the canal is filled with areolar tissue and small veins" and "small arteries arising from the vertebra." DePalma and Rothman continue, "any space taking lesion which pinches the anteroposterior diameter of the intervertebral foramen might be expected to cause some compression of the nervous tissue elements traversing this limited space." In contrast, these authors describe the normal lumber IVF as five to six times the diameter of the spinal nerve, permitting relatively great freedom from constriction.

Jackson,[24] an orthopedist, in describing the boundaries of the cervical IVF, states:

[The] posterior walls of the canals are formed by the adjacent posterior articular processes, but primarily by the superior articulating process of the distal vertebrae. The anterior walls are formed by the lateral portion of the bodies of the adjacent vertebrae and the margins of the intervening interbody articulations. The anterior walls are of great significance from a mechanical standpoint, in as much as the nerve roots pass directly over and are in intimate contact with the margins of the lateral interbody joints. The gliding motion which occurs between these joints whenever the head and neck are turned or moved in any direction subjects the nerve roots to irritation if there is any mechanical derangement present.

Parallel to the conclusions of Rothman and DePalma, Jackson concludes:

The nerve roots lie on the floor of the canals and fill their anteroposterior diameter completely. The upper one-eighth to one-fourth of the foramina, or the canals, is filled with areolar and fatty tissues and small veins. Small spinal arteries which are branches from the vertebral artery pass back through the intervertebral foramina to enter the vertebral canal. Minute branches from the nerve trunks which are known as the recurrent meningeal nerve pass back through the intervertebral foramina anterior to the nerve roots.

Jackson notes that ventral nerve root fibers are in intimate contact with the margins of the lateral interbody joints. The posterior fibers, or posterior nerve roots, are in intimate contact with the posterior-superior articular processes of the adjacent distal vertebrae. Jackson explains:

[Because] of their close proximity to the anterior and posterior walls of the intervertebral foramina the cervical nerve roots are extremely vulnerable to compression or to irritation from any mechanical derangement or inflammatory condition in or about the foramina. Such irritation or compression may cause pain and/or sensory and motor disturbances anywhere along the segmental distribution of the nerves.

Jackson uses the term *cervical syndrome* to describe the group of symptoms and clinical findings resulting from irritation or compression of the cervical nerve roots in or about the IVF.[24] Lu and Ebraheim,[33] in dissections of the dorsal root ganglia of the second cervical nerve, found that the dorsal ganglia are all proximally placed and occupy most of the foramen. The cervical ganglia at this spinal level are confined within the foramina between the arch of the atlas and the lamina of the axis. These ganglia occupy 76% of the foramen height. Such anatomic relationships may render the second cervical dorsal ganglion vulnerable to entrapment. These authors further state that trauma with extreme rotation and extension, as occurs in whiplash injuries, at the C1-C2 joint has the potential to crush the second cervical ganglion between the arch of the atlas and the lamina of the axis and may be implicated in cervicogenic headache. Many patients with headache and or neck trauma have a history of motor vehicle accident typical of whiplash. Cervicogenic headache (see Chapter 24) may result from displacement, abnormal movements, or arthritic changes in the atlas-axis articulation, compromising the second cervical nerve root and ganglion. In addition, compressing or entrapping the second cervical ganglion involves fibers that contribute to the greater occipital nerve.

Crelin,[34] an anatomist, in a 1973 article frequently quoted by opponents of chiropractic, argued that nerve roots pass through *spacious intervertebral foramina* and that therefore exertion of pressure on a spinal nerve does not occur. However, a review of the study's methodology coupled with current research demonstrates that Crelin's conclusion is in error concerning the effects of joint subluxation.[35]

Seeking to "prove" that the theory of spinal nerve impingement is "impossible," Crelin[34] obtained vertebral columns from six individuals. Three columns were from full-term infants; the others were from adults ages 35, 73, and 76 years. The vertebral column of each was excised within 3 to 6 hours after death. The skull was disarticulated from the first cervical vertebra, and the fifth lumbar vertebra was disarticulated from the sacrum. Each spinal nerve was transected 8 cm after emerging from the IVF. Deep paraspinal musculature, ligaments, and joint capsules were left intact.

Two metal vises were clamped to a platform supported the vertebral column while it was subjected to compressive forces. Five vertebral segments of the newborn column and three of the adult columns were suspended between the vises. A Dillon force gauge was used to measure force of compression applied to the vertebra. A range of maximum compression forces, including twisting and flexion, were applied. The osseous boundary of the foramen did not come in contact with the nerve, and Crelin reported that there was never less than 1.5 mm of space completely surrounding the cervical nerves, 3 mm around the thoracic nerves, and 4 mm surrounding the lumbar nerves. Crelin explained that all spinal nerves emerging from their IVFs were exposed before testing and that gentle teasing with small forceps removed the flimsy areolar tissue surrounding the nerves to expose the border of the "spacious vertebral foramina."

However, this very tissue that Crelin removed contains important connective tissue elements that may be compressible[36] or, when irritated, may release chemicals having an adverse effect on nerve function.[37-41] Some critics of the nerve compression theory have neglected to recognize that spinal biomechanical derangements do not involve "hard bone on soft nerve." Instead, the key issue is the potential for altered interforaminal mechanics to affect vascular and connective tissue support structures, as well as the important neural components within the IVF.

Contemporary information describes the IVF as an extended interpedicular zone,[42] often containing transforaminal ligaments.[43-47] These anatomic factors, combined with current under-standing of spinal nerve root sensitivity to pressure[48-50] and irritation,[37-41,51] render Crelin's conclusions unsupportable.[52]

Interpedicular Zone

Giles[42] maintains that the IVF should no longer be conceptualized as a two-dimensional hole, but rather as a canal or tunnel through which the spinal nerve and other related structures pass. Giles maintains that "neural and associated vascular structures within the important **interpedicular zone** may well be compromised due to vertebral joint subluxation. This may result in chronic compression," adding, "The precise significance clinically... is yet to be determined."

Giles took nine randomly chosen sections of adult lumbosacral spinal tissue and examined them histologically for measurement of the L4-L5 and L5-S1 IVF canals. The zone between the pedicles of adjacent vertebrae was found to have a horizontal length of 8.2 to 12.2 mm. At a minimum, the distance between the nerve structures and the side of the IVF canal was 0.4 to 0.8 mm for both the L4-L5 and L5-S1 segments. Giles concludes that the Crelin study was "meaningless as a basis for consideration of the possible physiological and/or pathophysiological functions of spinal nerves beyond the intervertebral canal as he did not examine the important interpedicular zone." that contains the spinal nerve root and ganglion. Rather, he examined only "the relatively insignificant lateral border."

Transforaminal Ligaments—A Key Anatomic Structure

As described by Golub and Silverman,[43] **transforaminal ligaments** (TFL) are ligamentous bands crossing the IVF at any spinal level (Fig. 8-1). In dissections of 15 lumbar spines representing 150 IVFs, Bachop and Hilgendorf[44] found varying numbers of TFLs. Bakkum[45] determined that TFLs, once considered an abnormality, are normal and greatly reduce the functional compartment or space available for the spinal nerve. In Bakkum's study, four adult lumbosacral spines without visible pathology or degenerative changes

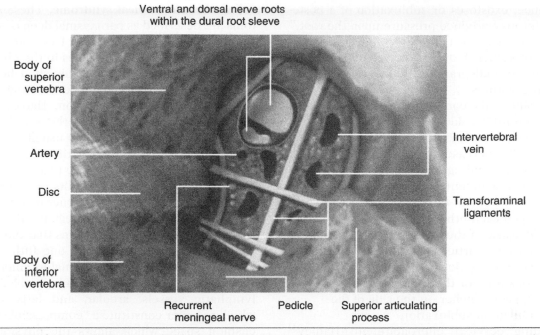

Fig. 8-1 Transforaminal ligaments. *(From Cramer G: Clinical anatomy of the lumbar region and sacroiliac joints. In Greenstein G, editor: Clinical assessment of neuromusculoskeletal disorders, St Louis, 1996, Mosby; with permission. Illustration by Dino Juarez, the National College of Chiropractic.)*

were examined, yielding the following results: 35 of the 49 IVFs examined (71%) had at least one TFL. More than one quarter (27%) had two TFLs, and 8% had three or four.

In the presence of TFLs, the superior-to-inferior dimension (height) of the functional compartment containing the ventral ramus of the spinal nerve was *significantly decreased*. The average height reduction was approximately one third (31.5%). In 12%, the reduction was at least 50% in the IVF containing a TFL, with one case being reduced by over two thirds (67.8%).

According to Bachop and Janse,[46] the higher the TFL is situated in the foramen, the less space remains for the spinal vessels. This anatomical relationship can conceivably lead to ischemia or venous congestion. On the other hand, the lower the TFL is located, the greater the possibility will be of sensory deficits, motor deficits, or both. In a study of accessory ligaments of the IVF, Amonoo-Kuoffi and colleagues[47] conclude that the spinal nerve, segmental veins and arteries, and the

recurrent meningeal nerve are held in place through the openings between the accessory ligaments within the IVF. In IVFs in which multiple TFLs are present, these nerves and vessels are literally threaded through a lattice created by the TFLs.

Hadley on Subluxation and the Intervertebral Formen

Hadley,[51] a medical radiologist, states that the importance of the IVF lies in the fact that, except for the first and second cervical nerves, each peripheral nerve must pass through one of these openings. The cervical region contains "a close five-way interrelationship between the foramen, the nerve root which passes through it, the vertebral artery contacting the root in front, the co-vertebral joint anteriorly and the posterior cervical articulation in back." Hadley also notes that arthrotic and degenerative changes involving these structures may become an important factor resulting in foraminal encroachment and that, "bulging disc substance, exostoses or subluxation of a poste-rior joint may produce pressure upon the root."

Hadley[51] goes on to state: "Subluxation (par-tial displacement) of the vertebral bodies . . . may present radiographically one or more of the following features:

1. Shift of the corresponding spinous process toward the side of the subluxation with the patient and film exactly centered
2. Slight increase in the size of the corresponding intervertebral foramen
3. Encroachment of the opposite foramen
4. Displacement of the articular surfaces upon each other
5. Because of the inclined plane of the posterior articulation, the side of the vertebra is elevated as it is carried forward. For that reason the disc appears thicker on the side of the unilateral subluxation."

Regarding cervical encroachment, Hadley[51] observes that, in addition to local and referred pain, patients can suffer from bizarre symptoms

Joint Restriction and Throat Inflammation

Hadley's observation of *spontaneous sublux-ation* associated with inflammation of the throat raises interesting questions from a chi-ropractic perspective. Is this inflammatory process truly a viscerosomatic reflex response, or are these symptoms a result of somatovis-ceral manifestations leading to lowered tissue resistance in the throat that contribute to the inflammation?

In a study of 76 children with chronic tonsil-litis, Czech physician and manual medicine specialist Lewit[53] observed, "The most striking and constant clinical finding was movement restriction at the craniocervical junction, in the great majority between occiput and atlas (70 cases or 92%)." Lewit concluded that "tonsillitis goes hand in hand with move-ment restriction... mainly between occiput and atlas, with little tendency to spontaneous recovery," adding, "our experience suggests that blockage (movement restriction) at this level increases the susceptibility to recurrent tonsillitis."

called **chronic cervical syndrome.** These symp-toms are described as paroxysmal deep or super-ficial pain in parts of the head, face, ear, throat, or sinuses; sensory disturbances in the pharynx; vertigo; and tinnitus, with diminished hearing. Vasomotor disturbances include sweating, flush-ing, lacrimation, and salivation. Hadley adds, "spontaneous subluxation at the C1-C2 level either unilateral or bilateral, is usually a sequel to an inflammatory process of the throat."

Commenting on the thoracic region, Hadley[51] states, "Since the thoracic roots are relatively small, compression of these structures does not occur in the foramina of this region." Regarding the lumbar region, Hadley affirms that the spinal nerve occupies approximately one fifth to one fourth the diameter of the normal foramen. The remainder of the space is taken up by blood and lymphatic vessels, areolar, and fatty tissue, which together constitute a "compressible safety cushion space which allows the physiological encroachment to occur without nerve compres-sion." Moreover, "any abnormal constriction in the size of a normal IVF if not actually causing nerve root pressure, nevertheless decreases the reserve safety cushion space surrounding that nerve and may predispose to pressure."

Effects of Degeneration

In a study of the kinematics of the lumbar IVF under normal physiologic spinal motions, Panjabi and colleagues[54] maintain that in cases of spinal degeneration, normal physiologic motion "may be enough to compromise the space around the nerve root to such a degree that very little safety margin is left." These authors further state:

[With] age and degeneration, the nerve loses its flexi-bility and develops adhesions with the IVF walls. It may not easily slip away from the compressing forces. The result may be a chronic threat of compression and mechanical irritation leading to inflammation of the nerve root.

Panjabi, discussing the research of Sunderland,[48] agrees that "in contrast to the thicker connec-tive tissue covering of the peripheral nerve, the anatomical and mechanical weakness of the spinal nerve root more easily causes interneural fibrosis and adhesions to the surrounding IVF tissues."

Muscular Influences on Nerves

Korr,[55] a physiologist and osteopathic researcher, observes that much of the pathway taken by nerves as they emerge from the cord is through skeletal muscle. The contractile forces of this muscle along with associated chemical changes exert profound influences on the metabolism and excitability of neurons. In such an environment, neurons are subject to considerable mechanical insult (compression and torsion), as well as chemical influences. Nerve sheaths, which are extensions of the meninges surrounding the spinal cord, extend distally along the spinal nerve roots, providing a root sleeve that allows the nerves to slide smoothly in and out without friction during a wide range of vertebral column movement. Over time, however, slight mechanical stresses may produce adhesions, constrictions, and angulations. From a chiropractic prospective, this vulnerability of nerve trunks represents effects associated with the myologic component of the VSC and also relates to its inflammatory and biochemical components.

Vascular and Sympathetic Influences

Vascular structures pass through the IVF and provide blood supply to both the bony vertebral column and the spinal cord.[56] Ischemia of the nerve cells within the dorsal root ganglia may lead to progressive loss of sensory function, including proprioception. Edematous pressure from even slight congestion of venous drainage may affect nerve conduction.[56] Such relationships are associated with the vascular and neurologic components of VSC. Olmarker and colleagues,[56a] in studying the effects of experimental compression on intraneural capillary and venular blood flow through tracking the intraneural transport of tracer-labeled glucose, determined that as low as 10 mm Hg pressure applied to the dorsal roots reduced nutritional transport to the peripheral axons to 20% to 30%.

Sympathetic ganglia in the highly mobile neck area and the cervical chain of ganglia positioned against the vertebral column are subject to stress imposed by motion. This stress may exert profound influence on the physiology of sympathetic nerve cells. Furthermore, the mechanical disturbances or somatic insults previously described by Korr exert slight forces resulting in slight tissue changes within the IVF and in paraspinal structures. This condition may adversely affect nerve function. A further proposal asserts that disorders of muscle tension, tissue texture, and visceral and circulatory function are reflected at the body surface as observable diagnostic elements.[49,50]

Neurophysiologic Effects of Nerve Compression

Spinal nerve roots, as compared with peripheral nerves, have a less abundant protective epineurium, no branching fasciculi, and poor lymphatic drainage.[56-58] These facts imply that the nerve root is more susceptible to injury by mechanical forces.[59] Panjabi and colleagues[54] state that "the nerve root is constrained in the intervertebral foramen and may be easily compressed or mechanically irritated under adverse conditions of degeneration and movement." In consideration of the effects on nerve function by subluxation or spinal biomechanical impairment, questions arise regarding possible pathophysiologic mechanism associated with compression or mechanical irritation of nerves.

Sharpless,[60] in a study to determine the susceptibility of spinal nerve roots to compression, concluded:

[Pressure] of only 10 mm Hg produced a significant conduction block, the potential falling to 60% of its initial value in 30 minutes. After such a small compressive force is removed, nearly complete recovery occurs in 15 to 30 minutes. With higher levels of pressure, we have observed incomplete recovery after many hours of recording.

Rydevik[61] determined:

Venous blood flow to spinal roots was blocked with 5-10 mm Hg pressure. The resultant retrograde venous stasis due to venous congestion is suggested as a significant cause of nerve root compression. Impairment of nutrient flow to spinal nerves is present with similar low pressure.

Konno and colleagues[62] reported that compression of cauda equina nerve roots decreased action potentials with as little as 10 mm Hg of pressure. Hause[63] proposed a mechanism of progression in which mechanical changes lead to circulatory changes, after which inflammatogenic agents produce chemical radiculitis. This action, in turn, leads to disturbed flow of cerebrospinal fluid, with defective fibrinolysis and subsequent cellular changes. In addition, the influence of the sympathetic system may result in synaptic sensitization of the central and peripheral nerves, creating a *vicious circle*, resulting in radicular pain. Hause also proposes that compressed nerve roots can exist without causing pain.

Mechanical Tension and the Muscle-Dural Connection

Mechanical tension on the pain-sensitive dura mater may contribute to headache. Hack and colleagues[64] found that the rectus capitis posterior minor muscle extends from the occiput to the posterior arch of the atlas vertebra and connects via a bridge of connective tissue to the spinal dura. This connection may resist inward folding of the dura, which may compromise cerebrospinal fluid flow when the neck is extended. The dura is extremely sensitive, and tension applied during surgery is felt as headache. The muscle-dura connection may transmit forces from the neck muscles to the pain-sensitive area of the dura. This muscle-dura connection may represent an anatomic basis for the effectiveness of manipulation/adjustment, which may decrease muscle tension and reduce pain by reducing the forces between C1 and C2 involving the rectus capitis posterior major and oblique capitis inferior muscles (see Fig. 23-5, p. 479).

ABERRANT SPINAL REFLEX HYPOTHESES

A basic chiropractic hypothesis holds that abnormal spinal biomechanics and muscle dysfunction have effects, via the nervous system, throughout the body and that the chiropractic adjustment is applied not only to restore range of motion and alignment, but also to cause or relieve reflex effects in the nervous system. In this respect, the chiropractor functions not only as an engineer (correcting joint function), but also as a telecommunications specialist (influencing spinal reflexes and nerve function).[35]

Except for skilled movements, body functions are largely reflexive. Examples include heartbeat, respiratory movements, digestive activity, and postural adjustments. Reflexive responses to stimuli include muscular contraction and glandular secretion. These spinal reflexes, which are involuntary responses to stimuli, are purposeful and exist to regulate physiologic functions, including somatic, autonomic, and endocrinologic processes. A **reflex arc** consists of a stimulus-activated receptor, transmission over an afferent pathway to an integration center, transmission over an efferent pathway to the effector, and induction of a reflex response[65] (Fig. 8-2).

Reflexes can be divided into four types based on the contributions of somatic and autonomic nerves to the efferent and afferent pathways of the reflexes. These reflexes include (from Sato[65]):

1. **Somatosomatic:** Reflexes whose afferents and efferents are somatic nerve fibers

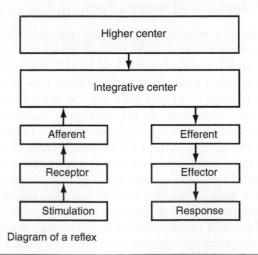

Fig. 8-2 Diagram of a reflex. (*From Haldeman S: Principles and practice of chiropractic, ed 2, East Norwalk, Conn, 1992, Appleton & Lange; with permission.*)

2. **Viscerovisceral**: Reflexes whose afferents and efferents are visceral sensory fibers and autonomic nerve fibers
3. **Somatovisceral** (also termed somatoautonomic): Reflexes whose afferents are somatic sensory fibers and whose efferents are autonomic efferent fibers
4. **Viscerosomatic** (also termed visceromotor reflexes): Reflexes whose afferents are visceral sensory fibers and whose efferents are somatic motor nerve fibers

It is proposed that joint subluxation or biomechanical impairment can, however, alter these reflexes adversely. Korr[27,28,66-68] conducted much of the basic clinical research demonstrating that prolonged nerve excitability, sustained hyperactivity of afferent receptors, and reflex response were associated with movement restriction in the spine. Korr reported evidence of heightened reflexive reactivity at spinal cord levels associated with palpable osteopathic lesions and observed reliable increases in galvanic skin response (GSR) readings at specific cord levels that he termed *facilitation*, the *facilitated segment*, or the *facilitated lesion*.

A fundamental hypotheses of both osteopathy and chiropractic is that locally altered somatovisceral reflexes associated with traumatized spinal joints evoke a vicious cycle of altered afferent and efferent impulse traffic, therefore leading to a facilitated or hyperactive spinal segment.[27,28,66-69]

As presented by Dhami and DeBoer,[70] this hyperactivity is proposed to further alter neural activity, both segmentally and centrally, within the cord, resulting in increased local somatic tissue changes with altered joint function and tissue texture, along with muscle splinting, tenderness, and temperature changes. This facilitated segment at a specific spinal level is proposed to lead to altered sympathetic and parasympathetic outflow affecting local vascularity and ongoing neural and visceral activity.[71]

Spinal adjustment, manipulation, mobilization, and pressure point therapy are proposed by Korr[55] to influence these sustained and facilitated spinal reflexes in the following ways:

1. *Directly*, as a reflex therapy in itself, in that the adjustive/manipulative or mechanical intervention introduces a stimulus to joint and muscle receptors producing a reflex response that modifies or inhibits the current facilitated reflex activity, thus reducing pain and causing relaxation of paraspinal muscles
2. *Indirectly*, in that the manual procedure normalizes joint mechanics, thereby removing spinal joint and muscle dysfunction that produces abnormal levels of spinal reflex activity that resulted in the facilitated lesion at a given spinal segment

Akio Sato,[65] a medical physician and researcher in the area of spinal reflex physiology, states:

Manipulation performed by chiropractors excites somatic afferent fibers in the musculoskeletal structures of the spine. These afferent excitations may, in turn, provoke reflex responses affecting skeletal muscle, autonomic, hormonal, and immunologic functions. An understanding of spinal reflex physiology is, therefore, fundamental to comprehending the effects of manipulation.

VARIETIES OF SPINAL REFLEXES

Three major types of spinal reflexes—somatosomatic, somatovisceral, and viscerosomatic—are referred to extensively in chiropractic, osteopathic, and medical literature. The order in which the root words are combined indicates the origin of the reflex and the site of its effect, respectively. For example, *somatovisceral* denotes that the initial stimulus or insult to the nervous system was a somatic receptor as in a spinal joint and that the efferent reflexive manifestation or response is expressed in a visceral tissue or organ.

Aberrant Somatosomatic Reflex Hypothesis

In Greek, *soma* means "body." In the **somatosomatic reflex** hypothesis, stimulus at one level of the soma or musculoskeletal system produces reflex activity in the nervous system, which is then exhibited elsewhere in the musculoskeletal system. The knee-jerk reflex is an example of a somatosomatic reflex. A light tap on the patellar ligament activates stretch receptors located within that ligament and in the tendon of the quadriceps muscle, which inserts on the patella. Impulses are conducted by sensory (afferent) neurons to the CNS, specifically at the intersegmental L3 and L4 levels, where these neurons synapse with motor neurons in the gray matter of the spinal cord. Without conscious involvement of the brain, impulses are then conducted by motor (efferent) neurons back to the quadriceps muscle. The muscle contracts in response to the impulses traveling along its motor nerve.

In this example, a stimulus was applied to a receptor in a somatic structure, eliciting a response in another somatic structure. Similarly, stimuli to receptors in spinal structures, whether from abnormal joint or muscle tension or from chiropractic adjustment[72] or manipulative treatment[30,31,73,74] to relieve it, cause various spinal reflex responses in the musculoskeletal system.

The interneurons of the dorsal horn are proposed to be involved in pain inhibition. As an example, strong tactile stimulation, as in skin rubbing, has long been known to diminish sensations of dull aching or sharp pain originating from an injured area. This decreased sensation is the result of the effect of **afferent inhibition** or the **gate control theory**. The mechanical intervention of rubbing activates the large, fast-conducting tactile-or touch-responsive A-alpha fibers (mechanoreceptors), which, in turn, inhibit the synaptic transmission of the pain signals by blocking the synaptic *gates* normally used by the smaller C-fibers that convey pain signals, therefore suppressing the signals of pain.

Wyke[30-32] suggested that spinal manipulation stretches mechanoreceptors in the joint capsule and that this stimulus has an inhibitory effect, mediated through spinal cord interneurons, on nociceptive activity. Increased mechanoreceptive input from increased joint motion reduces, or closes, the gate on pain signal transmission. This proposed mechanism is an adaptation of Wall's *gate control theory*.[75]

A subcomponent of the somatosomatic reflex model, referred to as the *proprioceptive insult* hypothesis[26,76,77] suggests that receptors in the highly innervated soft tissue in and around joints

may become irritated, leading to reflex modifications in postural tone and neural integration of postural activities. The proprioceptive insult hypothesis has been described in chiropractic writings[78,79] as undue irritation and stimulation of sensory receptors (including **proprioceptors**) located in the articular structures and in the parasegmental spinal ligaments. This irritation may result when structures are under stress from derangement of the intervertebral motor units caused by subluxation. Janse[26] proposes that the afferent barrage of impulses into the nervous system may disturb equilibrium, create somatosomatic reflexes, and cause aberrant somatovisceral and somatopsychic reflexes.

Reflex muscle spasm is another example of a somatosomatic reflex.[80] This reflex has been associated with the facilitated segment, in which muscle spasm may result from and contribute to proprioceptive irritation. Theories[80] suggest that the spinal cord segments in the vicinity of a spinal fixation have a lower threshold for firing and therefore are neurologically hyperexcitable. Korr refers to this concept as the *facilitated lesion*.[81,82]

Aberrant Somatovisceral Reflex Hypothesis

The Latin meaning of *viscera* is *internal organ*. In this concept, a stimulus to nerves or receptors related to spinal structures produces reflexive responses influencing function in the visceral organs, such as those in the digestive, cardiovascular, or respiratory systems. Alternate terms for this form of spinal reflex are *somatosympathetic* and *somatoautonomic*.

Lewit,[53] in a review of vertebrovisceral relations in a variety of cases, cites an example in which changes in spinal function (joint blockage or hypomobility) are linked to tachycardia. Therefore when mobility of the spinal column is normalized, heart rhythm also becomes normal and remains so as long as no relapse occurs in spinal column dysfunction. Lewit states that "although direct evidence of disturbed motor function causing organic heart disease is lacking, it would seem reasonable to grant it the role of a possible risk factor." Lewit uses the term *blockage* to describe spinal movement restriction, noting that the characteristic pattern of spinal hypomobility in ischemic heart disease is "blockage affecting the thoracic spine from T3 to T5, most frequently between T4 and T5, movement restriction being most noticeable to the left, and at the cervicothoracic junction." Of historical relevance is that as early as the 1920s, chiropractic authors such as Vedder[83] and Firth[84] recommended adjustment of *Heart Place*, identified as the second and third dorsal vertebral segments, for treating tachycardia.

Somatovisceral Studies—Hypertension, Dysmenorrhea, Infantile Colic, and Female Infertility

In a 1988 randomized controlled trial involving 21 hypertensive patients, Yates and colleagues[85] observed significant short-term (1-10 minutes) decreases in systolic and diastolic blood pressure in the chiropractic adjustment group, although no significant change was noted in the placebo and control groups. Adjustive procedures were applied to the T1 through T5 spinal levels. Kokjohn and colleagues,[87] in a study of 45 subjects, including experimental and *sham* manipulation control groups, concluded that spinal manipulative therapy may be an effective and safe nonpharmacologic alternative for relieving the pain and distress of primary **dysmenorrhea**.

Hondras and colleagues,[139] in a larger follow-up to Kokjohn and colleagues' dysmenorrhea study, failed to find significant differences in pain (as measured by visual analog scales), disability (as measured by questionnaire), or serum prostaglandin levels of patients with dysmenorrhea receiving side posture manipulation versus patients receiving a sham procedure. Patients in both the manipulation and sham groups demonstrated mild improvement. (See Chapter 25 for more detailed discussion of this and other chiropractic research studies on somatovisceral disorders.)

In a prospective study of 316 cases of infantile colic treated by chiropractors, Klougart and colleagues[87] found satisfactory results in 94% of cases within 14 days from the start of chiropractic care. The authors found that chiropractic

treatment resulted in "both a reduction of the daily length of colic periods and a reduction of the number of colic periods per day." Because recovery began between 5.7 and 7.7 weeks of age, the authors maintained that this finding provided substantial evidence that the improvement might not be attributed strictly to "natural cessation of colic symptoms."

In a 1999 study, Wiberg, Nordsteen, and Nilsson[88] found that "spinal manipulation has a positive short-term effect on infantile colic." Researchers randomly placed otherwise healthy, colicky infants into either a chiropractic treatment or a dimethicone medication group. Parents maintained a diary of symptoms and behaviors before and during the trial. Both groups received 2 weeks of treatment. The infants in the chiropractic group exhibited a "reduction of 67% on day 12" of daily hours with colic (nearly identical to the study by Klougart and colleagues[87]). The "dimethicone group only had a reduction in daily hours with colic of 38% by day 12." The authors noted:

[Manipulation] is normally used in treatment of musculoskeletal disorders, and the results of this trial leave open two possible interpretations. Either spinal manipulation is effective in treatment of the visceral disorder infantile colic or infantile colic is, in fact, a musculoskeletal disorder, and not as normally assumed, visceral.

Volejnikova,[59] in concert with Karel Lewit, conducted a randomized trial involving women referred for medical rehabilitation for infertility. The study population consisted of 166 women between the ages of 22 and 30, with normal sperm partners and patency of the fallopian tubes. The women in all groups had received unsuccessful infertility treatment for an average of 4 years. These women were randomly allocated to five different groups. Two treatment groups received procedures termed Majzisova's Protocol, directed to the lumbar spine and pelvis, which included stretching and relaxation of lumbar and pelvic musculature, postisometric relaxation of the gluteal and pelvic floor muscles, and other exercises. In the first half of the menstrual cycle, a physiotherapist performed mobilization of hypomobile areas of the sacroiliac joints, lumbar spine, and ribs. Home exercises were also prescribed.

Typical symptoms other than infertility were painful menstruation, bleeding with clots, dyspareunia (painful coitus), back pain, and headache. On examination, frequent structural and somatic manifestations included bad posture, scoliosis, sacroiliac dysfunction, asymmetry of the intergluteal line, gluteal and levator ani muscle weakness, and tenderness of coccyx, sacroiliac joints, and lumbar erector spinae. The course of treatment ended after six visits and was considered successful if pregnancy occurred within the study period. Other subject groups were assigned active and passive exercises or other nontreatment interventions. The two treatment groups experienced 34.3% and 27.4% success rates for pregnancy, compared with 8% to 9% success rate for each of the three minimal or nonintervention control groups.

Pikalov Study on Duodenal Ulcers

Going beyond the consideration of visceral dysfunction and observing the effects of spinal adjustment or manipulation on structural visceral pathology, Pikalov and Vyatcheslav[90] in a 1994 study demonstrated improved remission rates of actual pathologic conditions in patients with observable duodenal ulcer. The statistically significant results suggest that spinal somatic dysfunction predisposes the duodenum to disease and is a cause of the true visceral disease and pathologic conditions. Andrei Pikalov, who conducted this study, is a medical physician and physiology researcher, formerly of the Medical Research Institute at the Russian Ministry of Internal Affairs in Moscow and a former member of the research faculty of Cleveland Chiropractic College, Kansas City.

In this study, 35 adults attending the Gastroenterological Department at Moscow Central Hospital with acute, uncomplicated duodenal ulcer confirmed by endoscopic examination were examined for vertebral subluxation. Twenty three participants demonstrated characteristics of subluxation, that is, displacement, spinous process tenderness, restricted motion, contracture, and painful paravertebral muscles. Spinal segments T9 through T12 were the most

frequently affected. This finding again coincides with the writings of chiropractors Vedder[84] and Firth,[84] who in 1920 associated duodenal ulcer with subluxation of T9.

In the Pikalov study, patients were assigned to either a standard medical management group or a spinal manipulation group. Patients in the medical group received standard drug therapy and dietary regime over 4 to 7 weeks. For the other group, a course of spinal manipulation up to 14 treatments over a 3-week period was undertaken along with the standard dietary regime. Remission or healing took an average of 16.4 days in the manipulation group, approximately 9 days or 40% faster than the 25.7-day average in the medical group. The principal outcome, confirmed by endoscopic examination, was full clinical remission of the ulcer in terms of smooth healing of the lining of duodenum (epithelialization) or healing by scar formation (cicatrization). Pain resolved in 3.8 days on average in the manipulation group. The authors speculate that possible mechanisms to explain their results include "normalization of the action of the autonomic nervous system which influences both cellular metabolism and the vasomotor dynamics of the stomach and duodenum" and "stimulation of the endogenous opiate system."

These patients did not have simulated or pseudoulcer (visceral disease simulation is discussed later in this chapter) but actually exhibited endoscopically observable duodenal ulcers, confirmed by photographs. The manipulation applied to relieve somatic or spinal dysfunction not only relieved the pain, but also apparently provided a healing effect significantly superior to that obtained from standard drug therapy.

Aberrant Viscerosomatic Reflex Hypothesis

The **viscerosomatic reflex** is, logically, the opposite of the somatovisceral reflex. Respiratory or digestive dysfunction such as asthma or colic may cause reflex disturbances in the spine leading to muscle tension and joint subluxation or dysfunction.[52] Margaret Wislowska[91] of the Institute of Clinical Medicine in Warsaw, in a study on the contribution of pain to rotation of vertebrae in the origin and pathogenesis of lateral spinal curvature, determined that irritation of the nervous system resulting in pain in the abdominal cavity may reflexively cause symptomatic rotation of the lumbar vertebrae. In this study, 30 patients with radiographically confirmed nephrolithiasis (kidney stone) were examined, 15 with calculi in the right kidney, 15 with calculi in the left kidney. Radiographs were made during acute paroxysms of nephrolithiasis. In most cases, rotation of lumbar vertebrae was observed. For comparison, 15 patients with other kidney diseases were also examined. Angles of vertebral rotation were observed in anteroposterior radiographs by measuring the relationship of the pedicle to the lateral edge of the vertebral body. Wislowska states that ". . . in 70% of the patients with nephrolithiasis studied there is rotation of vertebrae towards the affected kidney." A proposed mechanism is that a viscerosomatic reflex (via visceral afferent nerves) in the kidney resulted in the muscle contraction (via somatic efferents) at segmental spinal levels correlated with sympathetic segmental innervation of the affected organ (kidney).

Danish gastroenterologists Jorgensen and Fossgreen[92] concluded, based on a controlled study, that a high correlation exists between back pain and functional gastrointestinal pain. A *functional ailment* is described as having "symptoms that are persistent, painful, and real," but where "no underlying organic problem can be found." Researchers examined the patients' spines segmentally, testing for tenderness, skin sensibility, and range of motion. Of the patients with back pain, 75% showed physical abnormalities during back examination, especially skin sensibility. Most of the spinal abnormalities were localized to the thoracic and thoracolumbar segments, "the same segments that innervate the upper gastrointestinal tract." According to Jorgensen and Fossgreen, "This suggests the existence of a connection between abdominal pain and back pain."

Jorgensen and Fossgreen suggest two possible pathophysiologic mechanisms: (1) stimulation of receptors in trigger areas of the abdomen, via nerve communication to the spinal cord, causing corresponding changes in the back (viscerosomatic reflex), or (2) irritation of nerve roots at the intervertebral foramina leading to changes in the gut (somatovisceral reflex). One may also speculate that given the *functional* nature of these clinical observations, the vertebral column is causing symptoms that are mistaken for visceral disease.

JOINT DYSAFFERENTATION

The intervertebral motion segment is richly supplied with mechanoreceptive and nociceptive structures.[93-97] For this reason, theories suggest that spinal biomechanic dysfunction may result in the alteration of normal nociception, mechanoreception, or both. Kent[98] proposes that, "aberrated afferent input to the CNS may lead to dysponesis." To use the contemporary jargon of the computer industry, "garbage in-garbage out." **Dysponesis** is reversible physiopathologic state consisting of unnoticed, misdirected neurophysiologic reactions to various agents (environmental events, body sensation, emotions, and thoughts) and the repercussions of these reactions throughout the organism. A similar concept once known by the outdated term, *spill over hypothesis*, has been used within the chiropractic profession to imply that aberrant sensory input (i.e., undue irritation of receptors) after reaching the segmental spinal cord level may *spill over* and evoke an aberrant efferent response.

Seaman[99-101] proposes that restoration of afferent input is the probable mechanism by which the chiropractic adjustment affords symptom relief and health improvement. The author asserts that joint restriction or dysfunction reduces large diameter afferent nerve fiber input from the mechanoreceptors in the articular capsule and from intrinsic muscles (intertransversarii and rotatores) of the spine, resulting in functional deafferentation.

The prefix *dys-* is used to describe activity that is abnormal, difficult, or disordered. In this context, Seaman proposes use of the term *dysafferentation* to describe the abnormal afferent input associated with joint complex dysfunction.

- *Afferentation* refers to the transmission of afferent nerve impulses.

- *Deafferentation* is defined as the elimination or interruption of afferent nerve impulses and is typically reserved for conditions in which peripheral nerves are either damaged or completely severed or avulsed.
- *Dysafferentation* refers to an imbalance in afferent input such that an increase in nociceptor input and a reduction in mechanoreceptor input occur.[100]

Standard texts in neurology identify two categories of somatic receptors: nociceptors and mechanoreceptors.[102,103] Research indicates that abnormal joint complex function can alter the activity of nociceptors[104] and mechanoreceptors[105] such that nociceptive activity increases and mechanoreceptive activity decreases. Hooshmand[105] illustrates that restricted joint mobility results in decreased firing of large diameter mechanoreceptor axons (A-beta fibers) and increased firing of nociceptive axons (A-delta and C-fibers). The term *altered somatic afferent input theory* has been presented by Henderson[106] to classify the neurophysiologic theory of chiropractic subluxation. Henderson further proposes that chiropractic adjustive intervention may normalize articular afferent input and reestablish normal nociceptive and kinesthetic reflex thresholds.

Wyke[30] demonstrates that the results obtained from spinal manipulation are reflexogenic and depend on adequate stimulation of articular mechanoreceptors. Also addressing reflexogenic effects, Seaman[72] states that "nociceptive reflexes promote the development of various components of subluxation complex." Seaman's concept of *joint dysafferentation* describes abnormal afferent input as a result of joint restriction, involving a functional decrease in the activity of large diameter mechanoreceptor afferent fibers and a simultaneous functional increase in activity of nociceptive afferent nerve fibers. Slosberg[107] has used the phrase *altered articular input* to describe this condition.

Along these lines, Lewit[53] states:

[Changes] of mechanical function alone do not cause clinical symptoms (pain). They constitute, however,

the nociceptive stimulus which produces reflex changes in the segment (muscle spasm, hyperalgesic zones, etc.). If these are of sufficient intensity to pass the pain threshold, pain is felt. The most likely nociceptive stimulus is increased tension.

Seaman[108] proposes that nociceptors are irritated by mechanical insult (trauma or injury, including joint restriction) and chemical irritants (toxins) (Fig. 8-3). Seaman further proposes that the associated nociceptive axons (A-delta and C-fibers) enter the spinal cord, conveying signals that excite interneurons originating in the dorsal horn, producing autonomic symptoms and pain and also exciting visceral afferent neurons (producing sympathetic vasoconstriction) and somatic efferent neurons (producing reflex muscle spasm). The potential end result is local tissue vasoconstriction and muscle spasm, which play a role in reducing joint mobility. Local nociceptors may be further irritated by this muscle spasm and sympathetic discharge into the area of injury, creating even greater spasm and vasoconstriction. Seaman states, "As the joint in question becomes more hypomobile, it is likely that the various pathologic components of subluxation complex (histopathology, inflammation, etc.) will become more pronounced and further irritate local nociceptors." (See Chapter 9 for further detail on nociception.)

He further suggests:

The adjustment serves to reduce the kinesiopathological component of the subluxation complex and as a result, most likely reduces mechanical and chemical irritation of articular nociceptors. Thus the restoration of joint motion, with consequently reduced mechanical and chemical irritation, appears to be the direct effect the adjustment has on the subluxation complex.[108]

Seaman describes the process:

The reflex effects of mechanoreceptor stimulation include the inhibition of pain, relaxation of spasmed muscles, and reduction of vasoconstriction. Thus, the adjustment appears to inhibit muscle spasm and vasoconstriction, which are known to cause general mechanical and chemical irritation of extra-articular nociceptors . . . . The adjustment directly reduces mechanical and chemical irritation of articular tissues

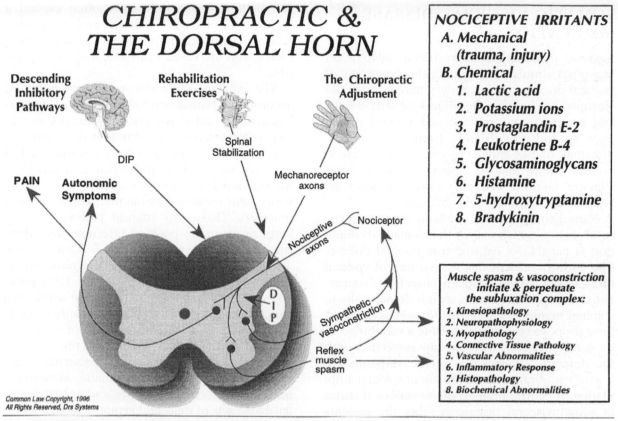

CHIROPRACTIC & THE DORSAL HORN

Descending Inhibitory Pathways

Rehabilitation Exercises

The Chiropractic Adjustment

DIP

Spinal Stabilization

Mechanoreceptor axons

PAIN   **Autonomic Symptoms**

Nociceptive axons

Nociceptor

D I P

Sympathetic vasoconstriction

Reflex muscle spasm

NOCICEPTIVE IRRITANTS
A. *Mechanical (trauma, injury)*
B. *Chemical*
1. *Lactic acid*
2. *Potassium ions*
3. *Prostaglandin E-2*
4. *Leukotriene B-4*
5. *Glycosaminoglycans*
6. *Histamine*
7. *5-hydroxytryptamine*
8. *Bradykinin*

Muscle spasm & vasoconstriction initiate & perpetuate the subluxation complex:
1. *Kinesiopathology*
2. *Neuropathophysiology*
3. *Myopathology*
4. *Connective Tissue Pathology*
5. *Vascular Abnormalities*
6. *Inflammatory Response*
7. *Histopathology*
8. *Biochemical Abnormalities*

Fig. 8-3 Chiropractic and the dorsal horn. *(From Seaman DR: Chiropractic and pain control, ed 3, Hendersonville, NC, 1995, DRS Systems; with permission.)*

by restoring motion to restricted joints. The adjustment indirectly reduces mechanical and chemical irritation of extra-articular tissue by causing a reflex inhibition of muscle spasm and vasoconstriction. The adjustment also stimulates afferent input which drives propriospinal pathways, spinocerebellar tracts and the dorsal column system.

Descending inhibitory pathways, according to Seaman,[108] can influence the pathogenesis of the subluxation complex as descending fibers from higher centers of the nervous system stimulate the same inhibitory interneurons, as does the chiropractic adjustment. Seaman further proposes that positive emotions can influence neural pathways such that pain and sympathetic hyperactivity (vasoconstriction) are inhibited. Conversely, he presents the possibility that negative emotions and depression can have the opposite effect on these neurons, in a contemporary restatement of D.D. Palmer's idea that *auto-suggestion* is one possible cause of subluxation. If these assumptions are correct, therapies such as stress management and biofeedback may have a role in case management of the subluxation complex.[108]

Limited joint motion or hypomobility may be associated with effects identified in Box 8-2.[37]

Box **8-2**   RESULTS OF JOINT FIXATION

- Degenerative changes
- Pain
- Excitation of alpha-motoneurons: myospasm
- Excitation of preganglionic sympathetic neurons: vasoconstriction, nociceptive reflexes
- Deafferentation of propriospinal tract, dorsal columns, spinocerebellar tracts

SOMATIC VISCERAL DISEASE SIMULATION

Somatic dysfunction or vertebral subluxation can often simulate, or mimic, the symptoms of visceral disease. Such mimicry may mislead the diagnostician because the clinical patterns of signs and symptoms for somatic and visceral causes may be indistinguishable from one another. Alternate names applied to this concept include pseudovisceral disease, organ disease mimicry, somatic visceral disease mimicry syndromes, and somatic simulation syndromes.

Nansel and Szlazak[109] challenge the somatovisceral theory, which claims that somatic dysfunction is capable of causing true visceral disease. The authors present instead the idea of **visceral disease simulation** to explain patients with apparent visceral disease that responds dramatically to a spinal manipulative thrust. Numerous authors* have proposed theories regarding a vertebrogenic or vertebrovisceral relationship associated with the dramatic changes in visceral symptoms following vertebral joint adjustment or spinal manipulation. A central premise of the various theories of somatovisceral disease is "that the patients involved in these rather 'miraculous' clinical situations were really suffering from true visceral disease."[109]

After an extensive literature review, Nansel and Szlazak propose that somatic pain, combined with the complex patterns of symptoms and signs, often is "virtually identical to and, therefore, easily mistaken for those induced by primary visceral disease." Such *pseudo* or *simulated* visceral disease syndromes may often result in misdiagnoses. These somatic visceral disease mimicry syndromes, as proposed, may account for perceived miraculous "cures" of presumed visceral disease in response to spinal manipulation.

Somatically induced visceral disease was described in the 1930s work of Lewis and Kellgren,[113] in which hypertonic saline was injected into deep somatic paraspinal structures. This action resulted in diffuse, regional pain referral patterns identical to those characteristic of certain internal organ diseases. This noxious

*References 13-20, 49, 53, 83-87, 110-112.

stimulation of somatic tissues often evoked a variety of associated somatic and autonomic reflexes, including hyperalgesia, reflex muscle spasm, and increased heart rate and blood pressure.

The explanation for visceral disease mimicry, according to Nansel and Szlazak, is that (1) phylogenetically primitive visceral afferent nerves transmit nociceptive information from internal organs, and (2) equally primitive somatic afferents are involved in transmitting nociceptive information from deep connective tissue (e.g., bone, joint capsules, ligaments, tendons, fascia muscles). These two afferent pathways, "converge on common pools of interneurons within the spinal cord and brainstem." With somatic afferent and visceral afferent signals subsequently transmitted into common CNS pathways, afferent neuronal convergence within the spinal cord may lead to clinical manifestations that are difficult to identify as being of visceral or somatic origin. That is, facilitating the common neuronal pool by either visceral or somatic inputs results in common sets of somatic, autonomic, and neuroendocrine responses leading to indistinguishable sets of signs and symptoms (Fig. 8-4).

Melzack and Wall[114] and Milne and colleagues[116] have shown that nociceptive stimuli from all structures in a segment converge to cells in the lamina V of the basal spinal nucleus of the spinal cord. This result also applies to pain signals from receptors in the zygopophyseal joints, as well as pain receptors in the walls of blood vessels. Lewit[53] therefore proposes that the locomotor system (spinal column) "can readily simulate visceral pain, and vice versa, and that this constitutes an important aspect to be taken into account in differential diagnosis."

An illustrated synopsis of segmentally related pain referral patterns observed by various investigators is presented in Fig. 8-5.[81] From a historic perspective, these pain patterns are in part similar (at least with respect to cutaneous pain distribution) to early chiropractic observations[2,9] from *nerve tracing*, an early chiropractic palpation procedure.[84] In nerve tracing, the chiropractor palpated along the path of tenderness over *impinged nerves* efferently or afferently (e.g., from the spinal tissues to the site of symp-

SIMULATED VISCERAL DISEASE MODEL

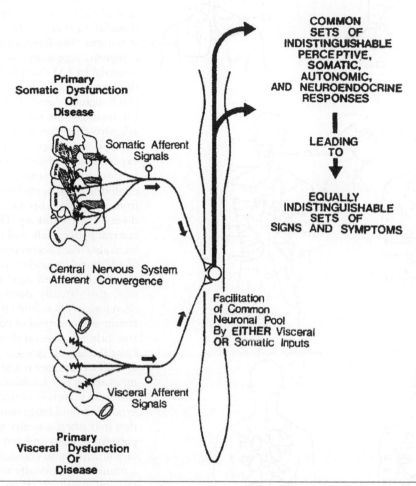

Fig. 8-4   Schematic depiction of the basic neurologic mechanism by which dysfunction confined to purely somatic structures is capable of producing signs and symptoms that are identical to those typically associated with primary dysfunction involving various internal organs. It is now well-established that afferent fibers that transmit nociceptive information from deep somatic structures converge on the same central neuronal pools as do the independent afferent fibers that transmit noxious stimuli from regionally related visceral structures. It presents a challenge for the diagnostician that subsequent relaying of either of these two sources of afferent information by this convergent pool of neurons into other common central pathways can often result in overt patterns of signs and symptoms that may be virtually indistinguishable with respect to their somatic versus visceral etiologies. The fact that somatic dysfunction can often mimic, or simulate, the symptoms of visceral disease (and be easily mistaken for it), is supported by an impressive amount of experimental and clinical scientific data. *(From Nansel D, Szlazak M: Visceral disease simulation,* J Manipulative Physiol Ther *18(6):379, 1995; with permission.)*

toms and vice versa). Nerve tracing, the tracing of tenderness from a point of emergence from the spine to a point at the periphery, was an outgrowth of the meric system[89] (see Chapter 25 for further discussion of the meric system). Early chi-

ropractic writings[9] considered such tenderness the *cry of nature* or *innate intelligence,* indicating that a nerve was affected. The early practitioners considered nerve tracing not only to be a valuable clinical tool, but also "very convincing to the

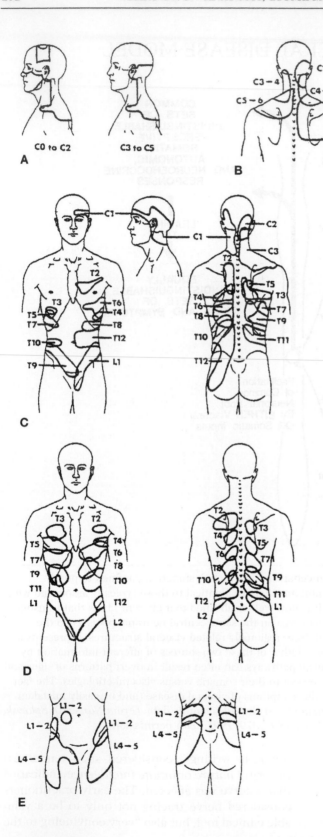

Fig. 8-5 Segmentally related referred pain patterns observed over the years by a number of independent investigators immediately after the experimental noxious stimulation over purely somatic paraspinal structures. The illustrations shown here are composite representations of results obtained by (A) Campbell and Parsons;[115] (B) Dwyer et al;[117] (C) Feinstein et al;[118] (D) Kellgren;[114] and (E & F) McCall et al.[116] Interestingly, the intensity, distribution and affective characteristics of the pain perceptions induced in these normal experimental subjects were often found to be astonishingly similar to those typically exhibited by patients known to be suffering from a variety of primary internal organ diseases or conditions. The diffuse pain referral patterns elicited in these subjects were also often accompanied by a number of additional secondary regional and/or global reflex-based signs and symptoms that were also virtually identical to (and therefore easily mistaken for) those commonly observed in patients harboring true primary visceral disease (see Fig. 8-4). Over the last 50 years, a significant amount of both experimental and clinical information has accumulated in the scientific literature concerning somatic pain syndromes and basic neuronal mechanisms that may often conspire to create overt patterns of signs and symptoms that mimic or simulate those classically associated with a number of regionally related primary visceral disorders. (From Nansel D, Szlazak M: Visceral disease simulation, J Manipulative Physiol Ther 18(6):379, 1995; with permission.)

patient, for the patient is the only one who can distinguish between nerves that are tender or affected and those that are not."[9]

Nansel and Szlazak take the position that primary dysfunction of somatic structures of the spinal column cannot cause regionally or segmentally related visceral (internal organ) disease and that no clinical evidence supports the notion of a regionally or segmentally induced *somatovisceral disease* connection. Further, the authors assert that the autonomic nervous system does not seem capable of inducing frank tissue disease in any organ it innervates. A well-referenced list developed by these authors (Table 8-2) presents a correlation of regionally related patterns of signs and symptoms that often result from primary somatic dysfunction, together with a collection of primary visceral conditions that such patterns of signs and symptoms have been shown to mimic or simulate.

Table **8-2**   Some Somatically Induced Symptoms and the Visceral Disorders That They Simulate or Mimic

Signs and Symptoms	Simulated Visceral Disorders
Referred head, face, eye, ear, sinus, mouth, dental, throat pain and/or hyperesthesias and/or dysesthesias	Pseudomigraine and cluster headache, pseudo–temporal arteritis, pseudo–trigeminal neuralgias, pseudo-Menier's, pseudo–otitis media, pseudoptosis, pseudosinusitis or rhinitis, pseudopharyngitis, pseudolaryngitis, pseudo–cranial nerve involvement
Narrowing of the palpebral fissure	
Vertigo/dizziness, blurred vision, light or sound intolerance, tinnitus, diminished/muffled hearing, difficulty swallowing, sense of object in throat, hoarseness, dysphonia	
Erythemia, sweating, nausea, vomiting, sinus congestion, and runny nose (coryza)	
Referred chest, breast, shoulder, arm pain and/or hyperesthesias, and/or dysesthesias	Pseudo–cardiac angina, pseudo–breast disease, pseudo asthma, pseudo pleurisy
Difficulty breathing/dyspnea	
Sweating, pallor, cardiac palpitations and arrhythmias, anomalous resting and/or treadmill electrocardiographic findings	
Abdominal pain and/or hyperesthesias and/or dysesthesias and/or cramping, pyrosis, intestinal colic, epigastric discomfort after meals (dyspepsia)	Pseudo–peptic ulcer, pseudo–duodenal ulcer, pseudo–gastric ulcer, pseudocholelithiasis, pseudocholycystitis, pseudoappendicitis, pseudoabdominal/intestinal disorders
Food intolerance, irritable bowel	
Sense of abdominal fullness (bloating)	
Hyperperistalsis of intestines (borborygmus)	
Nausea, vomiting, belching, flatulence, constipation, diarrhea	
Urinary urgency/irritable bladder, renal, loin, urethral, pelvic, perineal/groin/rectal pain and/or hyperesthesias and/or dysesthesias, urge for defecation, dysmenorrhea, dyspareunia, dysuria	Pseudorenal and urinary tract disorders, pseudoendometriosis, pseudosalpingitis, pseudo–pelvic inflammatory disease, pseudo–pelvic disorders
Stress incontinence	

From Nansel and Szlazak,[109] with permission.

Nansel and Szlazak affirm that afferent nociceptive signals generated from dysfunctional deep somatic structures can often result in the referred pain patterns, along with a number of equally misleading autonomic reflex responses. These reflex responses have been shown to simulate (rather than cause) true visceral disease because of their convergence on the same pools of CNS neurons that also receive afferent input from regionally related internal organs.

The concept of somatic visceral disease simulation provides a sound alternative explanation for the apparent effectiveness of a variety of somatic therapeutic interventions in patients with presumed true visceral disease. Nansel and Szlazak conclude that the existence of these somatic visceral disease mimicry syndromes justifies cooperation between medical physicians and health care providers such as chiropractors who specialize in the evaluation and treatment of primary somatic dysfunction.

DECREASED AXOPLASMIC TRANSPORT

The consequences of vertebral subluxation or spinal biomechanical impairments include pain and other sensory manifestations, as well as motor and autonomic disturbances. Manifestations discussed thus far have related to disturbances in excitation and conduction of nerve impulses. The impulse-based mechanisms underlying these clinical manifestations seem to be initiated through either direct insult to nerves and nerve roots or altered sensory input from affected joints, ligaments, tendons, and muscles.

Another component of neural function, also proposed to be affected by vertebral subluxation and related musculoskeletal problems, is **axoplasmic transport**. This component is a nonimpulse mechanism based not on transmission of signals along the surface of the neuron's neurolemma, but rather on the intraaxonal transport and exchange of macromolecular materials. This action involves a neurotrophic relationship between neurons and **end organs** or target cells.[56] Terms such as *end organs*, *target cells*, and *postsynaptic cells* refer to organs supplied or affected by a nerve.

It is now well established[116-123] that macromolecular substances are synthesized in the nerve cell body, packaged by Golgi apparatus, and transported within the axon to the terminal ending of the neuron. These substances are released at the synapse and then exert a subtle influence to maintain proper vitality and function of the target tissues. The axoplasmic transport system may convey material at a rate up to 400 mm/day.[120,121] Chemicals transported by this process are collectively known as **trophic** substances, and have been found to be essential for the maintenance of proper tissue function and **morphology** (structure or framework).[116-127]

Within the context of this discussion, *trophic* means *relating to growth*. In the neuroscience literature,[119] trophic influence on the peripheral nervous system refers to (1) the influence of the nervous system on differentiation and development of structures into mature end organs and (2) the role of trophic function in maintenance of end organs.

To distinguish trophic function from the neuron's function of conducting nerve impulses to the end organ, Guth's[127,128] definition of trophic function—"those interactions between nerves and other cells which initiate or control molecular modification in the other cell."—is most appropriate. This definition may be restated as follows: trophic function influences the development and maintenance of chemical changes in cells supplied by the nerve.

The nerve impulse is a fast acting *nerve membrane phenomenon* (120 m/sec), in contrast to the much slower (up to 400 mm/day, +/– 50)[120,121] intracellular or intraneuronal transport mechanism conveying trophic influences to target end organs.

Swartz[116] describes the complex transport systems that have evolved to carry large molecules formed in the nerve cell body. These chemicals are carried the full length of the axon to the terminals, after which materials from the terminals are returned to the cell body for reprocessing. Two forms of intracellular transport are identified. The slower kind, **axoplasmic flow,** conveys materials only from the cell body toward the nerve fiber terminals; the faster form, axonal transport, carries materials in both directions (Fig. 8-6).

Studies by Weiss and colleagues in 1948, as described by Swartz,[116] first proved experimentally that substances originating in the neuronal cell body move at a steady rate along the axon (Fig. 8-7). The experimental procedure involved surgical constriction of branches of the sciatic nerve in rats, chickens, and monkeys. After several weeks, examination of the region just above (proximal to) the constricted axon demonstrated swelling, suggesting that "axoplasm had accumulated behind the blockade." Furthermore, "the portion of the axon beyond (distal) the constriction had degenerated." Weiss removed the constriction, timed the movement of material, and observed that, "the accumulated axoplasm progressed down the regenerating fibers at a constant rate of one or two millimeters a day."[116]

Chiropractors may note a similarity between this observation and B.J. Palmer's simplified *foot on hose* analogy, historically presented to the public as a description of the effects of nerve compression.

Trophic Influences on End Organ Growth and Function

Examples of trophic influences on target tissues as adapted from Korr[55] include:

1. **Atrophy of denervation.** An example is the atrophy skeletal muscle undergoes after denervation. Apparently, the integrity of the connection between the nerve and

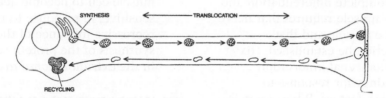

Fig. 8-6 Life cycles of vesicles and other membranous organelles involved in the transmission of nerve signals at a synapse (the specialized region of contact between a nerve terminal and another neuron or a muscle cell) begins with their synthesis in the cell body. Organelles move outward along the axon by fast axonal transport. Some of the material is deposited along the axon to maintain the axolemma, the external membrane along which the electrical cells are propagated, and some, including the synaptic vesicles, is delivered to the terminal. The material is then returned to the cell body in retrograde movement, also by fast transport, and there it is either restored or destroyed. *(From Schwartz JH: The transport of substances in nerve cells,* Sci Am *242:152, 1980; with permission. Illustration by Alan D. Iselin.)*

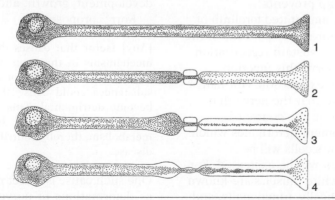

Fig. 8-7 Constriction experiments done at the University of Chicago in 1948 by Paul A. Weiss and his colleagues demonstrated that material from the cell body of a neuron moves along the axon at a steady rate. The experiment is depicted here schematically for a single mature nerve fiber (*1*), with the cell body at the left and the axon leading away from it to the nerve terminal at right. A constricting cuff was applied to the fiber (*2*). After several weeks the axon was swollen above the constriction (*3*) and reduced in size below it, showing that the axoplasm (the material from the cell body) had been dammed up by the constriction. It flowed again (*4*) when the cuff was taken off. *(From Schwartz JH: The transport of substances in nerve cells,* Sci Am *242:152, 1980; with permission. Illustration by Alan D. Iselin.)*

muscle, rather than the impulses to the muscle, is the critical factor. When observing the effects of removing the nerve supply from the sensory organ, the connectedness between two kinds of cells has been demonstrated to be the crucial issue. Sensory organs are the initiators of the nerve impulses, not receivers. In the case of gustatory organs (taste buds), these structures undergo trophic changes or even complete dedifferentiation on denervation.[122,123] Recovery or restoration of the taste buds follows soon after reinnervation.[119]

2. **Morphogenetic influences.** In embryonic development, complete differentiation and development of muscle requires that nerve supply reach the muscle and that a myoneural junction be established. Hix[124] demonstrated that renal innervation prepares the kidney for response to circulating growth factors. When a pup is deprived of that preparation by denervation in the first few days of postnatal life, kidney development is arrested.

3. **Role of nerve in regeneration.** Certain amphibians are capable of regenerating entire limbs and tails after amputation. Singer[125] has demonstrated that denervation of the fibers coursing towards the amputated stump prevents regeneration of the amputated forelimb of the newt. Furthermore, only portions of the fibers are required to sustain regeneration and sensory fibers serve this function.

4. **Regulation of genic expression.** Gutman[126] and Guth[127] propose that the nerve that grows into a muscle in the course of embryonic development determines which genes of that muscle's cells will be repressed and which will be expressed. For example, red and white muscles are known to differ morphologically, functionally, and chemically. Their chemical differences include those related to proteins, enzymes, and metabolic pathways.[128] Surgical section of nerves and cross-reinnervation of red and white muscles are followed by a high degree of cross transformation. Korr[55] interprets this metabolic transformation to be an expression of neurally mediated genetic influence, in which the nerve instructs the muscle what kind of muscle to become.

5. **Nerve-to-muscle transmission.** Another example of neurally influenced genic expression and repression occurs in the transmission from nerve to muscle at the myoneural junction. Receptor molecules for acetylcholine, which is released by the nerve terminals, are normally restricted to the area of the muscle surface where the myoneural junction is located.[55] Cutting the nerve causes the entire surface of muscle cell to become acetylcholine sensitive, in response to removal of the repressive influence of the nerve on the synthesis of the protein receptor molecules in the *extrajunctional areas*.[129]

CLINICAL IMPLICATIONS OF AXOPLASMIC TRANSPORT

According to multiple authorities,[116-129] peripheral nerves not only conduct impulses to or from nonneuronal cells and tissues that they innervate, but they also exert long-term influences on these end organs through trophic or neurotrophic influences that are essential for their development, growth, and maintenance.

Korr[55] proposes:

[Any] factor that causes derangement of transport mechanisms in the axon or that chronically alters the quality or quantity of the axonally transported substances could cause the trophic influences to become detrimental. This alteration in turn would produce aberrations of structure, function, and metabolism, thereby contributing to dysfunction and disease.

One such cause is direct mechanical insult, such as deformations of nerves and roots, including compression, stretching, angulation, and torsion, "that occur commonly and that . . . disturb the intraaxonal transport mechanisms, intraneural microcirculation." Moreover, "neural structures are especially vulnerable in their passage over highly mobile joints, through bony canals, intervertebral foramina; fascial layers, and tonical contracted muscles."

An additional factor, also biomechanic in origin is, "sustained hyperactivity of peripheral neurons (sensory, motor, and autonomic) related to those portions of the spinal cord associated with intervertebral strain or other types of somatic dysfunction."[130] Korr concludes:

[Sustained] high rates of impulse-discharge place increased energy demands on the affected neurons thus affecting their metabolism and... their synthesis and turnover of proteins and other macromolecules... such intense activity does impair axonal transport, and... trophic interchange with other cells.

NEURODYSTROPHIC HYPOTHESIS

Neurodystrophy is the proposition that neural dysfunction is stressful to viscera and other body structures, which may modify immune responses and alter the trophic function of involved nerves.[131,132] In its most basic form, the concept may be reduced to D.D. Palmer's assertion that "lowered tissue resistance is the cause of disease."[13] According to the **neurodystrophic hypothesis,** spinal biomechanical insult to nerves may affect intraneural axoplasmic transport mechanisms and, in turn, affect the quality of neurotrophic influence and molecular (chemical) changes in the cells. This decrease in trophic factors is understood to render innervated structures vulnerable to dysfunction or disease.

CLINICAL CONSIDERATIONS

This text has now examined a variety of hypotheses that seek to explain the cause-and-effect relationship between altered spinal biomechanics and clinical manifestations, dysfunction, and disease. How may these hypotheses be conceptually applied so as to enhance the chiropractor's understanding in a particular clinical situation?

Lewit presents the following explanations of *vertebrovisceral correlations* in his text, *Manipulative Therapy in the Rehabilitation of the Locomotor System:*[53]

1. The vertebral column (locomotor system) is causing or mimicking symptoms that are mistaken for visceral disease.
2. The visceral disease is causing a reflex reaction, resulting in the hypomobility or fixation of the corresponding vertebral segment.
3. The visceral disease that reflexively caused restricted segmental mobility has subsided, but the hypomobility remains, causing symptoms simulating visceral disease (as in item 1).
4. Disturbance of the vertebral locomotor segment is causing visceral disease.

Readers may consult Lewit's text for an expanded presentation on a variety of visceral disorders and their associated segmental spinal relationships.

Keeping Lewit's four choices in mind, the following clinical experience presented by Chapman-Smith[35] in *The Chiropractic Report* might be considered:

Mr. A.T., a 56 year old dairy farmer complaining of chest pain that feels like "a tire around my chest," is referred by his family physician to a cardiologist. Examinations including imaging, ECGs, and exercise stress tests, reveal many classic signs and symptoms of myocardial ischemia—deep chest and arm pain, paleness, sweating, cardiac dysrhythmia, and coronary arteriosclerosis.

Mr. A.T. is told he has a heart problem and is treated accordingly. He is advised to stop strenuous physical work and change his occupation. However, the medications prescribed, nitrates, then beta-blockers, are ineffective. Faced with the sale of his farm and anxious to find something that might help, he seeks the advice of a chiropractor.

Chiropractic examination reveals joint subluxation, with restricted joint range of motion and muscle tension in the lower cervical and upper thoracic spine. Palpation of the two top segments in the thoracic spine reproduces the cardiac pain. Radiographs show marked narrowing of the intervertebral foramina at C6/C7.

Following a short course of spinal manipulation, designed to restore normal function to the spinal segments and paraspinal muscles and to relieve irritations of the spinal nerve roots, joint function is normal and pain relieved. Mr. A.T. returns to his normal farm work and lifestyle, and has no further symptoms.

Chapman-Smith adapted this case from one cited by Kunert, a German cardiologist. In his paper, "Functional Disorders of the Internal Organs Due to Vertebral Lesions"[133] Kunert states:

[We] have records of numerous cases similar to the one described here, in which a definite connection appears to exist between a functional disorder in an internal organ and a spinal lesion . . . lesions of the spinal column are perfectly capable of simulating, accentuating, or making a major contribution to (organic) disorders. There can, in fact, be no doubt that the state of the spinal column does have bearing on the functional status of the internal organs.

Chapman-Smith then applies Lewit's vertebrovisceral correlations as possible explanations for Mr. A.T.'s case. The author proposes these possibilities:

1. The spinal or somatic problem (subluxation) is simulating or mimicking heart disease.
2. Heart disease and pain have caused a reflex reaction in the spine and paraspinal muscles. The resulting spinal dysfunction (subluxation) then exaggerates or mimics cardiac pain.
3. Heart disease has reflexively caused subluxation as in (2), the underlying disease has now subsided, and the spinal lesion gives symptoms simulating continuing heart disease.
4. Spinal subluxation is causing heart disease, maybe through altered somatovisceral reflexes that, either alone or together with other stressors, cause ischemia and disease.

In view of the explanations proposed previously regarding patients such as Mr. A.T., cardiologists and other health practitioners must be educated regarding the possible role of subluxation or spinal biomechanical lesion and its potential role in presumed cardiac pain and other visceral manifestations.

OVERVIEW OF BIOMECHANICAL AND NEUROPHYSIOLOGICAL MECHANISMS OF SPINAL ADJUSTMENT/MANIPULATION

Various hypotheses proposing explanation for the apparent effects associated with subluxation and nerve system function have been presented in the chapter. A close interface between spinal biomechanics and nerve function has been established.[53,55,134-137] The nervous system has been identified as a major and central mediator of the clinical effects of spinal manipulative therapy, chiropractic adjustment, or both.[55,130,137] Gutziet, as cited by Lewit,[53] characterizes the spinal column as the *initiator, provoker, multiplier,* and *localizer* of the pathogenesis of certain diseases. Lewit[53] maintains that any disturbance of function in a single motor segment will have repercussions throughout the body axis and must be compensated and that once the lesion becomes painful, the nervous system determines how intensely the spinal segment will manifest clinically.

Symptoms resulting from biomechanical impairments of the musculoskeletal system that are responsive to spinal manipulative therapy or spinal adjustment encompass sensory manifestations, including pain, as well as motor and autonomic disturbances.* Spinal biomechanic dysfunction (vertebral subluxation) and concomitant nervous system manifestations appear to be associated with and affect both the impulse-based and nonimpulse-based mechanisms of nerve function.[55]

Impulse-Based Neural Mechanisms

Insult to the impulse-based neural mechanisms occurs through:

- Direct insult to the nerves and nerve roots resulting from compression, torsion, stretching, or angulation resulting from adhesions[54] or foraminal encroachment.† Neural structures are vulnerable in their passage over highly mobile joints, intervertebral foramina, fascial layers, and tonically contracted muscles.‡
- Altered sensory input (sustained hyperactivity) from affected muscles, tendons, ligaments, and joints produces aberrant somatosomatic and somatovisceral spinal reflexes.§ Undue irritation to

*References 27, 53, 55, 63, 66-68, 130, 134-137.
†References 13-18, 20-24, 51.
‡References 48, 51, 54, 55, 59, 62.
§References 27, 50, 55, 75, 108.

nociceptors in visceral organs is proposed to contribute to aberrant sensory input at intersegmental spinal levels, resulting in abnormal viscerosomatic reflexes and changes in paraspinal musculature that may contribute to spinal joint hypomobility, subluxation, or both.[19,55,80,108] Given that somatic afferent and visceral afferent signals converge equally into common central nervous system pathways at intersegmental spinal levels, vertebral subluxation or spinal dysfunction may simulate or mimic symptoms of visceral disease, potentially misleading diagnosticians in all health professions.[110,113]

Nonimpulse-Based Neural Mechanisms

Interference with nonimpulse-based neural mechanisms results in decreased axoplasmic transport of neurotrophic factors to the terminal ending of the nerve.[55] Such trophic factors influence chemical changes at the molecular level, which affects the development, growth, and maintenance of end organs in tissue supplied by the nerve.[117-131] This mechanism is not based on the transmission of nerve impulses. Rather, it is based on the transport and exchange of macromolecular materials via intraaxonal transport and neurotrophic relationships between neurons and the postsynaptic or target cells.* The sustained high rates of impulse discharge proposed to result from altered joint function place increased energy demands on the affected neurons, thus affecting synthesis and the turnover of proteins and other macromolecules, as well as impairing axonal transport and trophic interchange with other cells. The intraaxonal transport mechanisms may be affected either by direct deformation of the nerve through mechanical insult or by altered activity or sustained hyperactivity of sensory receptors. This alteration may, in turn, produce aberrations of structure, function, and metabolism, thus contributing to dysfunction and disease.

*References 55, 116-118, 127, 128.

Fig. 8-8 outlines the theoretical progression of joint complex dysfunction's effects on neural mechanisms associated with the neuropathophysiologic component of vertebral subluxation complex.

The neurophysiological and biomechanical mechanisms underlying the effects of spinal manipulation/adjustment are reviewed by Pickar[148,149] and conceptualized in the theoretical model presented in Fig. 8-9.

Pickar proposes that structural dysrelationships between vertebral segments may hypothetically produce biomechanical overloads and stimulate the receptive endings of mechanically or chemically sensitive neurons in the paraspinal tissues. Sustained afferent input could result in abnormal or aberrant neural reflexes. Pickar[149] states the following:

These changes in sensory input are thought to modify neural integration either by directly affecting reflex activity and/or by affecting central neural integration within motor, nociceptive and possibly autonomic neuronal pools. Either of these changes in sensory input may elicit changes in efferent somatomotor and visceromotor activity. Pain, discomfort, altered muscle function or altered visceromotor activities comprise the signs or symptoms that might cause patients to seek spinal manipulation. Spinal manipulation, then, theoretically alters the inflow of sensory signals from paraspinal tissues in a manner that improves physiological function.

In addition, endogenous metabolites such as bradykinin, substance P, and related inflammatory mediators may result from joint dysfunction. These substances are noxious stimuli that likely activate paraspinal afferents.[99-101, 148]

Altered vertebral segment mechanics may result in *compression* of nerve roots within the intervertebral foramen. It is known that spinal nerve roots and the dorsal root ganglia are more susceptible to the effects of mechanical compression than the axons of peripheral nerves[60-63] and that mechanical compression of the dorsal roots and dorsal root ganglia may alter both impulse-based and non–impulse-based neural mechanisms.[54,55,149]

Pickar examines the neurophysiological basis for the effects of manual procedure, presenting a theoretical model describing the relationships

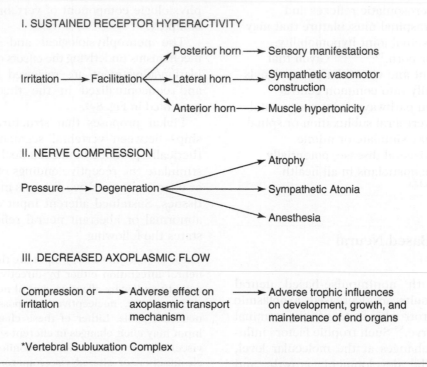

NEUROPATHOPHYSIOLOGY OF VSC*

I. SUSTAINED RECEPTOR HYPERACTIVITY

Irritation ⟶ Facilitation ⟶ Posterior horn ⟶ Sensory manifestations

Lateral horn ⟶ Sympathetic vasomotor construction

Anterior horn ⟶ Muscle hypertonicity

II. NERVE COMPRESSION

Pressure ⟶ Degeneration ⟶ Atrophy

Sympathetic Atonia

Anesthesia

III. DECREASED AXOPLASMIC FLOW

Compression or irritation ⟶ Adverse effect on axoplasmic transport mechanism ⟶ Adverse trophic influences on development, growth, and maintenance of end organs

*Vertebral Subluxation Complex

Fig. 8-8 Neuropathophysiology of vertebral subluxation complex (VSC). *(Adapted by Carl S. Cleveland III, DC from Faye model of VSC. From Schafer RC, Faye LJ: Motion palpation and chiropractic, technic principles of dynamic chiropractic, Huntington Beach, Calif, 1989, The Motion Palpation Institute, with permission.)*

between spinal manipulation/adjustment, segmental biomechanics, the nervous system, and end-organ function (see Fig. 8-9).

As conceptualized through this model, the biomechanical changes influenced by spinal manipulation are thought to have physiological consequences by means of their effects on inflow of sensory information (via paraspinal sensory receptors, see Fig. 8-9, *1*) into the central nervous system. Muscle spindle afferents and Golgi tendon organ afferents are stimulated by spinal manipulation and smaller-diameter sensory nerve fibers are likely activated.

Mechanical and chemical changes in the intervertebral foramen (see Fig. 8-9, *2*) may result from a herniated intervertebral disc affect-

ing the dorsal roots and dorsal root ganglia. Whereas the direct effect of manipulation on these changes is not understood, individuals with herniated lumbar discs have shown clinical improvement in response to spinal manipulation/adjustment.

The phenomenon of central facilitation or central sensitization (see Fig. 8-9, *3*) that is described as an increased excitability of dorsal horn neurons within the spinal cord due to persistent aberrant afferent input, is known to increase the receptive field of central neurons, enabling either subthreshold or nonnoxious stimuli access to central pain pathways. It is known that spinal adjustment/manipulation increases pain tolerance and/or threshold of excitation.

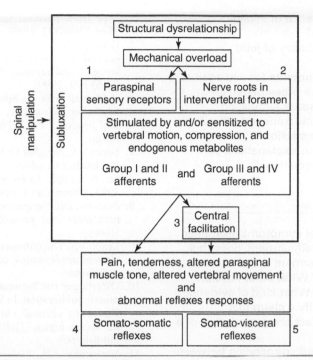

Fig. 8-9 A theoretical model showing components that describe the relationships between spinal manipulation, segmental biomechanics, the nervous system, and physiology. The neurophysiological effect of spinal manipulation could be mediated at any of the numbered boxes.

A mechanism underlying the effectiveness of manipulation may be the effect of altering central sensory processing by removal of subthreshold mechanical or chemical stimuli from the paraspinal tissues.

Spinal manipulation/adjustment is proposed to affect reflex neural outputs in both muscle (see Fig. 8-9, *4*) and visceral organs (Fig. 8-9, *5*). Such manual procedures evoke paraspinal muscle reflexes and alter motorneuron excitability producing both excitatory and inhibitory effects. Whereas it is known that sensory input, especially noxious irritants, from paraspinal tissues may reflexively elicit sympathetic neural activity, the understanding regarding the effect of manipulation/adjustment on somato-visceral reflexes and visceral end-organ function is limited.

It is difficult to know which operational models or combination of hypotheses provides the most plausible explanation for the effects of manual adjustive procedures in a given clinical situation. What is known is that a close interface exists between spinal biomechanics and nerve function and that additional basic and clinical research will assist in understanding the mechanisms affected through the intervention of spinal manipulation and the adjustive techniques.

Review *Questions*

1. Discuss the anatomic differences among the intervertebral foramina in the cervical, dorsal, and lumbar regions. How do these differences influence the relevance of the **nerve compression hypothesis** for these three areas?
2. What was a flaw in Crelin's attempt to refute chiropractic claims regarding spinal nerve pressure?
3. How might the presence of transforaminal ligaments affect the course of a back pain patient's recovery?
4. Discuss the knee-jerk reflex as an example of a somatosomatic reflex.
5. Identify two studies that provide clinical support for the assertion that chiropractic adjustments effect somatovisceral reflex responses.

6. What is the significance of Pikalov's study on duodenal ulcers?
7. Discuss Seaman's theory of joint dysafferentation.
8. What are some arguments for and against Nansel and Szlazak's presentation on somatic visceral disease simulation?
9. How does axoplasmic transport differ from nerve impulse transmission?
10. What are Lewit's four explanations of vertebrovisceral correlations?

Concept *Questions*

1. If a patient's visceral symptoms disappear after a chiropractic adjustment, does this mean that the adjustment cured or relieved a visceral disorder? What other possible explanations exist? What kind of evidence is necessary to justify a claim that chiropractic did in fact bring resolution of a visceral disorder?
2. How might enhanced cooperation between chiropractors and medical physicians benefit patients with visceral symptoms?
3. In the Wiberg, Nordsteen, and Nilsson study on infantile colic, the authors noted that ". . . manipulation is normally used in treatment of musculoskeletal disorders, and the results of this trial leave open two possible interpretations. Either spinal manipulation is effective in treatment of the visceral disorder infantile colic or infantile colic is, in fact, a musculoskeletal disorder, and not as normally assumed, visceral." Of the theories discussed in this chapter, which may best describe the observations in this study?

REFERENCES

1. Meeker WC, Haldeman S: Chiropractic: a profession at the crossroads of mainstream and alternative medicine, *Ann Int Med* 136(3):217, 2002.
2. Vernon H: Basic scientific evidence for chiropractic subluxation. In Gatterman M, editor: *Foundations of chiropractic: subluxation*, St Louis, 1995, Mosby.
3. Harrison DE et al: A review of biomechanics of the central nervous system. Part I: spinal canal deformations due to changes in posture, *J Manipulative Physiol Ther* 22(4):227, 1999.
4. Harrison DE et al: A review of biomechanics of the central nervous system. Part II: strains in the spinal cord from postural loads, *J Manipulative Physiol Ther* 22(5):322, 1999.
5. Harrison DE et al: A review of biomechanics of the central nervous system. Part III: neurologic effects of stresses and strains, *J Manipulative Physiol Ther* 22(6):399, 1999.
6. Haldeman S et al: Spinal manipulative therapy. In Frymoyer JW, editor: *The adult spine: principles and practice*, vol 2, Philadelphia, 1997, Lippincott-Raven.
7. Lopes MA, Plaugher G: Vertebral subluxation complex. In Plaugher G, editor: *Textbook of clinical chiropractic: a specific biomechanical approach*, Baltimore, 1993, Williams and Wilkins.
8. Peterson DH, Bergmann TE: *Chiropractic technique: principles and procedures*, ed 2, St Louis, 2002, Mosby.
9. Leach RA: *The chiropractic theories, principles and clinical applications*, ed 3, Baltimore, 1994, Williams & Wilkins.
10. Osterbauer PJ: Technology assessment of the chiropractic subluxation. In Mootz RD, Hansen DT, editors: *Topics in clinical chiropractic series, chiropractic technologies*, Gaithersburg, Md, 1999, Aspen Publishers.
11. Marsarsky CS, Todres-Masarsky M: Subluxation and the special senses. In Marsarsky CS, Todres-Masarsky M, editors: *Somatovisceral aspects of chiropractic: an evidence-based approach*, Philadelphia, 2001, Churchill Livingstone.
12. Lantz CA: A review of the evolution of chiropractic concepts of subluxation, *Top Clin Chiropr* 2(2):1, 1995.
13. Palmer DD: *The science, art and philosophy of chiropractic—the chiropractor's adjuster*, Portland, 1910, Portland Printing House.
14. Palmer BJ: *The science of chiropractic—its principles and philosophies*, vol 1, Davenport, Iowa, 1906, Palmer School of Chiropractic.
15. Beatty HG: *Anatomical adjusting technique*, ed 2, Denver, 1937, (self-published).
16. Firth JN: *A textbook on chiropractic symptomatology*, Rock Island, Ill, 1914 (self-published).
17. Forster AL: *Principles and practice of spinal adjustment for the use of students and practitioners*, Chicago, 1915 (self-published).
18. Loban JM: *Technic and practice of chiropractic*, Davenport, Iowa, 1912 (self-published).
19. Janse J, Houser R, Wells B: *Chiropractic principles and technic*, Chicago, 1947, National College of Chiropractic.
20. Cleveland CS Sr: *Chiropractic principles and practice—outline*, Kansas City, 1950, Cleveland Chiropractic College.
21. Kent C: Models of vertebral subluxation: a review, *J Vertebral Subluxation Res* 1(1):11, 1996.
22. Cramer G, Darby S: Anatomy related to spinal subluxation. In Gatterman M, editor: *Foundations of chiropractic: subluxation*, St Louis, 1995, Mosby.

23. DePalma AF, Rothman RF: *The intervertebral disc,* Philadelphia, 1970, WB Saunders.

24. Jackson R: *The cervical syndrome,* Springfield, Ill, 1976, Charles C. Thomas.

25. Herbst R, editor: *Gonstead chiropractic science and art: the chiropractic methodology of Clarence S. Gonstead,* Mt Horeb, Wisc, Sci-Chi Publications (undated).

26. Janse J: History of the development of chiropractic concepts: chiropractic terminology. In Goldstein M, editor: *The research status of spinal manipulative therapy,* HEW/NINCDS Monograph #15, Bethesda, Md, 1975, U.S. Department of Health Education and Welfare.

27. Korr IM, Thomas PE, Wright HM: A mobile instrument for recording electrical skin resistance patterns of the human trunk. In Korr IM, editor: *The collected papers of Irvin M. Korr,* Colorado Springs, Colo, 1979, American Academy of Osteopathy.

28. Korr IM: The concept of facilitation and its origins. In Korr IM, editor: *The collected papers of Irvin M. Korr,* Colorado Springs, Colo, 1979, American Academy of Osteopathy.

29. Denslow J, Korr IM, Krems A: Quantitative studies of chronic facilitation in human motoneuron pools. In Korr IM, editor: *The collected papers of Irvin M. Korr,* Colorado Springs, Colo, 1979, American Academy of Osteopathy.

30. Wyke BD: Articular neurology: a review, *Physiotherapy* 58:94, 1972.

31. Wyke BD: Articular neurology and manipulative therapy. In Glasgow EF et al, editors: *Aspects of manipulative therapy,* ed 2, Melbourne, 1985, Churchill Livingstone.

32. Kirkaldy-Willis HK: *Managing low back pain,* New York, 1983, Churchill Livingstone.

33. Lu J, Ebraheim N: Anatomic considerations of C2 nerve root ganglion, *Spine* 23(6):649, 1998.

34. Crelin ES: A scientific test of the chiropractic theory, *Am Sci* 61:574, 1973.

35. Chapman-Smith D: Chiropractic research in the centennial year—part II, *Chiropr Rep* 9:1, 1995.

36. Plaintiff Exhibit 1483A. Handwritten letter from ES Crelin to Ray Sullivan of Connecticut State Medical Society, January 4, 1974. Anti-trust exhibit provided by McAndrews G in *Wilk v. AMA.*

37. Seaman DR: *Chiropractic and pain control,* ed 3, Hendersonville, NC, 1995, DRS Systems.

38. Lantz CA: The vertebral subluxation complex. In Gatterman MI, editor: *Foundations of chiropractic: subluxation,* St Louis, 1995, Mosby.

39. Davis D: Respiratory manifestations of dorsal spine radiculitis simulating cardiac asthma, *Ann Intern Med* 32:954, 1950.

40. Marshall LL, Thethewie ER, Curtain CC: Chemical radiculitis: a clinical, physiological and immunological study, *Clin Orthop* 129:61, 1977.

41. Howe JF, Loeser JD, Calvin WH: Mechanosensitivity of dorsal root ganglia and chronically injured axons:

a physiological basis for radicular pain of nerve root compression, *Pain* 3:25, 1977.

42. Giles LFG: A histological investigation of human lower lumbar intervertebral canal (foramen) dimensions, *J Manipulative Physiol Ther* 17(1):4, 1994.

43. Golub B, Silverman B: Transforaminal ligaments of the lumbar spine, *J Bone Joint Surg* 51:947, 1969.

44. Bachop W, Hilgendorf C: Transforaminal ligaments of the human lumbar spine (abstract), *Anat Rec* 99(4):14a, 1981.

45. Bakkum BW: The effects of transforaminal ligaments on the sizes of T11-L5 human intervertebral foramina, *J Manipulative Physiol Ther* 17(8):517, 1994.

46. Bachop W, Janse J: The corporotransverse ligament at the intervertebral foramen (abstract), *Anat Rec* 205(3):13a, 1983.

47. Amonoo-Kuoffi HS et al: Ligament associated with lumbar intervertebral foramina. 1. L1 to L4, *J Anatomy* 156:177, 1988.

48. Sunderland S: Meningeal-neural relations in the intervertebral foramen, *J Neurosurg* 40:756, 1974.

49. Korr IM: *The physiological basis of osteopathic medicine,* New York, 1970, Postgraduate Institute of Osteopathic Medicine and Surgery.

50. Greenman PE: *Principles of manual medicine,* ed 2, Baltimore, 1996, Williams & Wilkins.

51. Hadley LA: *Anatomico-roentgenographic studies of the spine,* Springfield, Ill, 1976, Charles C Thomas.

52. Chapman-Smith D: Chiropractic research in the centennial year—part II, *Chiropr Rep* 9:1, 1995.

53. Lewit K: *Manipulative therapy in rehabilitation of the locomotor system,* ed 2, Oxford, 1991, Butterworth-Heinemann.

54. Panjabi M, Takata M, Goel V: Kinematics of the lumbar intervertebral foramen, *Spine* 8(4):348, 1983.

55. Korr IM: The spinal cord as organizer of disease processes IV. Axonal transport and neurotrophic function in relation to somatic dysfunction, *J Am Osteopath Assoc* 80:451, 1981.

56. Adams W: The blood supply of nerves: II. The effects of exclusion of its regional sources of supply on the sciatic nerve of the rabbit, *J Anat* 77:243, 1943.

56a.Olmarker et al: Compression-induced changes on nutritional supply to the porcine cauda equina, *J Spinal Disord* 3:25-29, 1990.

57. Sunderland S: *Nerves and nerve injuries,* Baltimore, 1968, Williams & Wilkins.

58. Sunderland S, Bradley L: Stress-strain phenomena in human spinal nerve roots, *Brain* 84:120, 1961.

59. Rydevik B, Lundborg G, Bagge U: Pathoanatomy and pathophysiology of nerve root compression, *Spine* 9:7, 1984.

60. Sharpless SK: Susceptibility of spinal roots to compression block. In Goldstein M, editor: *The research status of spinal manipulative therapy,* HEW/NINCDS Monograph #15, Bethesda, 1975, U.S. Department of Health Education and Welfare.

61. Rydevik BL: The effects of compression on the physiology of nerve roots, *J Manipulative Physiol Ther* 15(1):62, 1992.

62. Konno S et al: Intermittent cauda equina compression, *Spine* 20(1):1223, 1995.

63. Hause M: Pain and the nerve root, *Spine* 18(14):2053, 1993.

64. Hack GD et al: *1998 Medical and health annual,* Chicago, 1997, Encyclopedia Britannica.

65. Sato A: Spinal reflex physiology. In Haldeman S, editor: *Principles and practice of chiropractic,* ed 2, East Norwalk, Conn, 1992, Appleton & Lange.

66. Korr IM, Goldstein MJ: Abstract: Dermatomal autonomic activity in relation to segmental motor reflex threshold. In Korr IM, editor: *The collected papers of Irvin M. Korr,* Colorado Springs, Colo, 1979, American Academy of Osteopathy.

67. Korr IM, Wright HM, Thomas PE: Effects of experimental myofascial insults on cutaneous patterns of sympathetic activity in man. In Korr IM, editor: *The collected papers of Irvin M. Korr,* Colorado Springs, Colo, 1979, American Academy of Osteopathy.

68. Korr IM: Sustained sympathicotonia as a factor in disease. In Korr IM, editor: *The collected papers of Irvin M. Korr,* Colorado Springs, Colo, 1979, American Academy of Osteopathy.

69. Patterson MM, Steinmetz JE: Long-lasting alterations of spinal reflexes: a basis for somatic dysfunction, *Man Med* 2:38, 1986.

70. Dhami MSI, DeBoer KF: Systemic effects of spinal lesions. In Haldeman SC, editor: *Principles and practice of chiropractic,* ed 2, East Norwalk, Conn, 1992, Appleton & Lange.

71. Haldeman SC, editor: *Modern developments in the principles and practice of chiropractic,* New York, 1980, Appleton-Century-Crofts.

72. Seaman DR: The subluxation complex: nutritional considerations, *J Am Chiropr Assoc* 30(3):77, 1993.

73. Suter E et al: Reflex responses associated with manipulative treatment of the thoracic spine, *J Neuromusculoskel Sys* 3:124, 1994.

74. Chapman-Smith DA: *The chiropractic profession, its education, practice, research and future directions,* West Des Moines, Iowa, 2000, NCMIC Group.

75. Wall PD: The gate control theory of pain mechanism: a re-examination and a re-statement, *Brain* 101:1, 1978.

76. Mootz R: Theoretic models of chiropractic subluxation. In Gatterman MI, editor: *Foundations of chiropractic: subluxation,* St Louis, 1995, Mosby.

77. Homewood AE: *The neurodynamics of the vertebral subluxation,* ed 3, St Petersburg, Fla, 1979, Valkyrie Press.

78. Hayes S: The chiropractic subluxation: a new hypothesis for consideration, *J Natl Chiropr Assoc* 27:9, 1957.

79. Hviid H: A consideration of contemporary chiropractic theory, *J Natl Chiropr Assoc* 25:17, 1955.

80. Korr IM: Proprioceptors and the behavior of lesioned segments. In Stark EH, editor: *Osteopathic medicine,* Acton, Mass, 1975, Publication Sciences Group.

81. Korr IM, editor: *The neurobiologic mechanism in manipulative therapy,* New York, 1978, Plenum Press.

82. Korr IM: *The collected papers of Irvin M. Korr,* Colorado Springs, Colo, 1979, American Academy of Osteopathy.

83. Vedder HE: *Analysis guide,* Kansas City, Cleveland Chiropractic College (undated).

84. Firth JN: *Chiropractic symptomatology,* Davenport, Iowa, 1925 (self-published).

85. Yates RG et al: Effects of chiropractic treatment on blood pressure and anxiety: a randomized, controlled trial, *J Manipulative Physiol Ther* 11(6):484, 1988.

86. Kokjohn K et al: The effect of spinal manipulation on pain and prostaglandin levels in women with primary dysmenorrhea, *J Manipulative Physiol Ther* 15(5):279, 1992.

87. Klougart N, Nilsson N, Jacobsen J: Infantile colic treated by chiropractors: a prospective study of 316 cases, *J Manipulative Physiol Ther* 12(4):281, 1989.

88. Wiberg JMM, Nordsteen J, Nilsson N: The short-term effect of spinal manipulation in the treatment of infantile colic: a randomized controlled clinical trial with a blinded observer, *J Manipulative Physiol Ther* 22(1):13, 1999.

89. Volejnikova H: Female infertility: a study of physical treatment by the method of L. Mojzisova for functional disturbance of the pelvic region, *J Orthop Med* 23(2):47, 2001.

90. Pikalov AA, Vyatcheslav VK: Use of spinal manipulative therapy in the treatment of duodenal ulcer: a pilot study, *J Manipulative Physiol Ther* 17(5):310, 1994.

91. Wislowska M: A study of the contribution of pain to rotation of vertebrae in the etiology and pathogenesis of lateral spinal curvature, *J Man Med* 4:161, 1989.

92. Jorgensen L, Fossgreen J: Back pain and spinal pathology in patients with functional upper abdominal pain, *Scand J Gastroenterol* 25:1235, 1990.

93. Bogduk N, Tynan W, Wilson A: The nerve supply to the human lumbar intervertebral disc, *J Anat* 132:39, 1981.

94. Bogduk N, Twomey L: *Clinical anatomy of the lumbar spine,* ed 2, Melbourne, 1991, Churchill Livingstone.

95. Bogduk N, Windsor M, Inglis A: The human lumbar dorsal rami, *J Anat* 134:383, 1982.

96. Fielding J, Burstein A, Frankel V: The nuchal ligament, *Spine* 1:3, 1976.

97. Bogduk N: The clinical anatomy of the cervical dorsal rami, *Spine* 7:319, 1982.

98. Kent C: Beyond back pain, *Calif Chiropr Assoc J* 21(8):45, 1996.

99. Seaman DR: *Chiropractic and pain control,* Hendersonville, NC, 1995, DRS Systems.

100. Seaman D: Joint complex dysfunction, a novel term to replace subluxation/subluxation complex: etiological and treatment considerations, *J Manipulative Physiol Ther* 20:634, 1997.

101. Seaman DR, Winterstein JF: Dysafferentation: a novel term to describe the neuropathophysiological effects of joint complex dysfunction. A look at likely mechanisms to symptom generation, *J Manipulative Physiol Ther* 21(4):267, 1998.

102. Guyton A: *Basic neuroscience*, ed 2, Philadelphia, 1991, WB Saunders.

103. Willis W, Coggeshall R: *Sensory mechanisms of the spinal cord*, ed 2, New York, 1991, Plenum Press.

104. Schaible H, Grubb B: Afferent and spinal mechanisms of joint pain, *Pain* 55:5, 1993.

105. Hooshmand H: *Chronic pain: reflex sympathetic dystrophy, prevention and management*, Boca Raton, Fla, 1993, CRC Press.

106. Henderson C: Three neurophysiologic theories on chiropractic subluxation. In Gatterman M, editor: *Foundations of chiropractic: subluxation*, St Louis, 1995, Mosby.

107. Slosberg M: Effects of altered afferent articular input on sensation, proprioception, muscle tone and sympathetic reflex response, *J Manipulative Physiol Ther* 11(5):400, 1988.

108. Seaman DR: A physiological explanation of subluxation and its treatment, *Calif Chiropr Assoc J* 21(3):32, 1996.

109. Nansel D, Szlazak M: Visceral disease simulation, *J Manipulative Physiol Ther* 18(6):379, 1995.

110. Burns LA: Effects of upper cervical and upper thoracic lesions, *J Am Osteopath Assoc* 22:266, 1923.

111. Burns LA: Laboratory proofs of the osteopathic lesion, *J Am Osteopath Assoc* 31:123, 1931.

112. Burns L, Chandler L, Rice R: *Pathogenesis of visceral diseases following vertebral lesions*, Chicago, 1948, The American Osteopathic Association.

113. Lewis T, Kellgren JH: Observation relating to referred pain, visceromotor reflexes and other associated phenomena, *Clin Sci* 4:47, 1939.

114. Melzack R, Wall PD: Pain mechanisms, *Science* 150:974, 1965.

115. Milne RJ et al: Convergence of cutaneous and pelvic visceral nociceptive inputs onto primate spinothalamic neurons, *Pain* 11:163, 1981.

116. Swartz JH: The transport of substances in nerve cells, *Sci Am* 242(4):152, 1980.

117. Lubinska L: On the arrest of regeneration of frog peripheral nerves at low temperatures, *Acta Biol Experiment* 16:65, 1952.

118. Guth L: Trophic effects of vertebrate neurons, *Neurosci Res Prog Bull* 7:1, 1969.

119. Werner JK: Trophic influence on nerves on the development and maintenance of sensory receptors, *Am J Phys Med* 53(3):127, 1974.

120. Ochs S, Ranish N: Characteristics of the fast transport in mammalian nerve fibers, *J Neurobiol* 1:247, 1969.

121. Ochs S: A brief review of material transport in nerve fibers. In Goldstein M, editor: *The research status of spinal manipulative therapy*, HEW/NINCDS Monograph #15, Bethesda, 1975, U.S. Department of Health, Education and Welfare.

122. Zalewski AA: Regeneration of taste buds after reinnervation by peripheral or central fibers of vagal ganglia, *Exp Neurol* 25:429, 1969.

123. Zalewski AA: Combined effects of testosterone and motor, sensory or gustatory nerve reinnervation on the regeneration of taste buds, *Exp Neuro* 24:285, 1969.

124. Hix EL: An apparent trophic function of renal nerves [abstract], *Fed Proc* 21:428, 1962.

125. Singer M: Trophic function of the neuron. Part 6: other trophic systems; neurotrophic control of limb regeneration in the newt, *Ann NY Acad Sci* 228:308, 1974.

126. Gutman E: Neurotrophic relations, *Ann Rev Physiol* 38:177, 1976.

127. Guth L: "Trophic" influences of nerve on muscle, *Physiol Rev* 48:645, 1968.

128. Guth L: The effects of glossopharyngeal nerve transection on the circumvallate papilla of the rat, *Anat Rec* 128:715, 1957.

129. Fernandez HL, Ramirez BV: Muscle fibrillation induced by blockage of axoplasmic transport in motor nerves, *Brain Res* 79:385, 1974.

130. Korr IM: Discussion. Papers of Sidney Ochs and David E. Pleasure. In Goldstein M, editor: *The research status of spinal manipulative therapy*. HEW/NINCDS Monograph #15, Bethesda, 1975, U.S. Department of Health, Education and Welfare.

131. Lantz CA: The vertebral subluxation complex, *ICA Rev* 45(5):37, 1989.

132. Lantz CA: A review of the evolution of chiropractic concepts of subluxation, *Top Clin Chiropr* 2(2):1, 1995.

133. Kunert W: Functional disorders of the internal organs due to vertebral lesions, *CIBA Symposium* 13(3):85, 1965.

134. Korr IM: *The neurobiologic mechanisms in manipulative therapy*, New York, 1978, Plenum Press.

135. Korr IM: The spinal cord as organizer of disease processes. Some preliminary perspectives, *J Am Osteopath Assoc* 76:35, 1976.

136. Korr IM: The spinal cord as organizer of disease processes II. The peripheral autonomic nervous system, *J Am Osteopath Assoc* 79:82, 1979.

137. Korr IM: The spinal cord as organizer of disease processes III. Hyperactivity of sympathetic innervation as a common factor in disease, *J Am Osteopath Assoc* 79:232, 1979.

138. Hondras MA, Long CR, Brennan PC: Spinal manipulative therapy versus a low force mimic maneuver

for women with primary dysmenorrhea: a randomized, observer-blinded, clinical trial, *Pain* 81:105, 1999.

139. Giles LG, Harvey AR: Immunohistochemical demonstration of nociceptors in the capsule and synovial folds of human zygapophyseal joints, *Br J Rheumatol* 26:3624, 1987.

140. Bogduk N, Jull G: The theoretical pathology of acute locked back: a basis for manipulative therapy, *Man Med* 23:77, 1985.

141. Bogduk N, Tynan W, Wilson AS: The nerve supply to the human lumber intervertebral discs, *J Anat* 132:39, 1981.

142. Arkuszewski Z: Joint blockage: a disease, a syndrome, or a sign, *Man Med* 3:132, 1988.

143. Lantz CA: The vertebral subluxation complex. In Gatterman MI, editor: *Foundations of chiropractic: subluxation,* St Louis, 1995, Mosby.

144. Bolton PS: Reflex effects of vertebral subluxations: the peripheral nervous system. An update, *J Manipulative Physiol Ther* 23:101, 2000.

145. Budgell BS: Reflex effects of subluxations: the autonomic nervous system, *J Manipulative Physiol Ther* 23:104, 2000.

146. Suter E et al: Conservative lower back treatment reduces inhibition in knee–extensor muscles: a randomized controlled trail, *J Manipulative Physiol Ther* 23:7680, 2000.

147. Haldeman S: Neurological effects of the adjustment, *J Manipulative Physiol Ther* 23:112, 2000.

148. Pickar JG: Health care in the 21st century . . . neurophysiologic issues of the subluxation lesion, *Top Clin Chiropr* 8(1):9-15, 2001.

149. Pickar JG: Neurophysological effects of spinal manipulation, *The Spine J* 2:357-371, 2002.

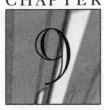

Nociceptors, Pain, and Chiropractic

Geoffrey M. Bove, DC, PhD, Rand S. Swenson, DC, MD, PhD

Key Terms

AFFERENT	LONG-TERM DEPRESSION	ONGOING ACTIVITY
ALLODYNIA	LUMBAR FACET	OPIATES
AXON REFLEX	SYNDROME	ORTHOPEDIC TESTS
CONDUCTION VELOCITIES	MICRONEUROGRAPHY	PAIN
EFFERENT	NERVE SHEATH	PLASMA EXTRAVASATION
ENDOGENOUS OPIATES	NERVI NERVORUM	RADIATING PAIN
ENDORPHIN	NEURITIS	RADICULOPATHY
GROUP III NOCICEPTOR	NEUROGENIC INFLAMMATION	RECEPTIVE FIELDS
GROUP IV NOCICEPTOR	NOCICEPTION	REFERRED PAIN
HYPERALGESIA	NOCICEPTIVE	SENSITIZATION
LONG-TERM	NOCICEPTOR	WINDUP
POTENTIATION	NOXIOUS STIMULUS	

Pain and its relief are critical to the chiropractic profession. Chiropractic doctors and students need a strong background in the basic concepts of the neurophysiology underlying pain. The purpose of this chapter is to present and clarify issues related to the basic science of pain and to direct the reader to more complete works on the major issues in pain physiology and control. All of the information in this chapter is clinically relevant, although it may not seem so on first reading. If the reader perseveres, the final section will be very rewarding, because the concepts presented will aid in understanding the reasons patients seek care and will also provide a clinical rationale for chiropractic treatment.

First, pain and several associated terms are defined. Subsequent discussion considers the neural elements involved in pain, describing them anatomically and functionally. An overview of the changes in the central nervous system after noxious stimuli is provided, and an introduction to the psychology of pain is offered.

Finally, an example is given that demonstrates how these basic scientific concepts fit with the day-to-day practice of chiropractic.

DEFINITIONS

Taxonomy is important for any discipline, and discussions of pain are most fruitful when appropriate terms are used. The following terms have been defined by a committee of experts from diverse specialties, in association with the International Association for the Study of Pain (IASP), and the definitions are used with permission.[1]

Pain. An unpleasant sensory and emotional experience associated with actual or potential tissue damage, or described in terms of such damage.

Biologists agree that pain is a sensation; however, because it is unpleasant, it is also emotional. Thus the foundation of this definition is that pain is always subjective and may or may not have an objective component. It is possible to have pain without peripheral noxious stimuli; the definition purposely avoids linking pain to any specific stimulus. Therefore each individual defines pain on the basis of his or her experiences, usually related to injury. However, a report of pain in the absence of apparent cause cannot be dismissed, because central mechanisms, including psychologic factors, are often sufficient to cause pain.

Nociception. Activity in a neural structure considered capable of leading to or contributing to a sensation of pain.

Nociception is objective because the activity in nociceptive neurons and axons can be measured, at least in the laboratory. Nociception does not necessarily lead to pain, especially when the nociceptor activity is found in the peripheral nervous system. To cause pain, the nociceptor activity must be of sufficient intensity or frequency to activate central elements of the nociceptive pathways.

Noxious stimulus. Noxious is defined as *harmful*, and a noxious stimulus is defined as a stimulus that damages, or even potentially damages, normal tissue. Unfortunately, there are stimuli that are noxious by this definition that are not painful, such as radiation injury and cutting the wall of a normal small intestine, but there is no descriptive term for this subset of noxious stimuli.

Nociceptor. A receptor preferentially sensitive to a noxious stimulus or to a stimulus that would become noxious if prolonged.

A nociceptor is a sensory structure that senses noxious stimuli; in response, it generates neural activity to communicate to the central nervous system that a potentially harmful stimulus has occurred. Terms like *pain sensor* or *pain receptor* have been applied to nociceptors, but they should be avoided. Some nociceptors have been reported to respond to nonnoxious stimuli as well, but this discussion falls outside the scope of this text.

Nociceptive. Although not defined by the IASP, this adjective is often misused to modify *stimulus*. A stimulus cannot be nociceptive, but it can be noxious. However, a nociceptor is considered to be nociceptive when activated.

Allodynia. Pain due to a stimulus which does not normally provoke pain.

Pain as a result of a stimulus that does not normally cause pain is termed *allodynia*. Allodynia is the loss of specificity of any sensory modality, such as light touch or thermal sensitivity, with the final perception being pain. Examples of mechanical allodynia are the pain of light brushing when the skin is sunburned and the pain caused by lightly squeezing a muscle the day after unaccustomed exercise.

Hyperalgesia. An increased or prolonged response to a stimulus which is normally painful.

Hyperalgesia is distinct from allodynia. With allodynia, the modality of stimulus (such as light touch), differs from the perceptual modality (pain). In hyperalgesia the modalities are the same, but the intensity of the perception is greater. Both hyperalgesia and allodynia are commonly experienced simultaneously. Indeed, clinically, the use of the term *hypersensitivity* is often more appropriate to avoid possible mechanistic implications of hyperalgesia versus allodynia. Although rare, certain conditions may destroy pain nerve fibers in an area while leaving touch and pressure sensors intact. In such cases, the patient may not be sensitive to pinprick stimulation that is commonly used to test the pain pathways, but a simple touch may produce an intensely unpleasant sensation. The most common clinical example of this occurs in rare cases of postherpetic neuralgia (most cases have both hyperalgesia and allodynia).

Radiating, referred, and radicular pain. These terms are often used incorrectly, perhaps because published definitions are rare. A requirement of **radiating pain** is that the symptom is perceived to radiate away from the site of the pathology or the site of presumed pathology. Radiating pain can follow pathology of any component of the nervous system. *Radicular pain* is reserved for pain due to pathology of one or more nerve roots (the Latin word for nerve root is *radix*, hence the word *radicular*). Radicular pain is perceived distal to the pathology and is thus a subset of radiating pain. Radicular pain has also been termed *projected pain*, because the pain is perceived to be specifically localized to the distal segmental distribution of the affected nerve root (Fig. 9-1).

Referred pain is reserved for symptoms that occur in portions of the body that are not directly innervated by damaged nerves or nerve roots. Thus the arm pain that often occurs with angina is referred; the cause of the arm pain is thought to be that the sensory nerve from the heart muscle and arm project to similar areas in the central nervous system; thus under some circumstances, an inappropriate "spillover" of neuronal activation occurs. Clinicians are urged to use the term *referred pain* sparingly, unless they are confident that there is no pathology in the peripheral nervous system.

NOCICEPTORS

Primary Afferent Nociceptors

Nociceptors serve a primordial function for an organism, providing information about harmful or potentially harmful events that may cause loss of function or life. Even simple organisms essentially have nociceptive function. For example, protochordates display the *coiling reflex*, a withdrawing from a noxious stimulus.[2] Through evolution, this defense mechanism was conserved and refined, although the basic function of signaling harmful events remained unchanged. The importance of nociceptors is revealed in rare cases in which children have been born without nociceptors. These children are constantly being injured and often die from complications of minor infections or trauma. Similarly, rats whose nociceptors have been destroyed by neonatal treatment with capsaicin have a short life span and are always bruised and incautious.

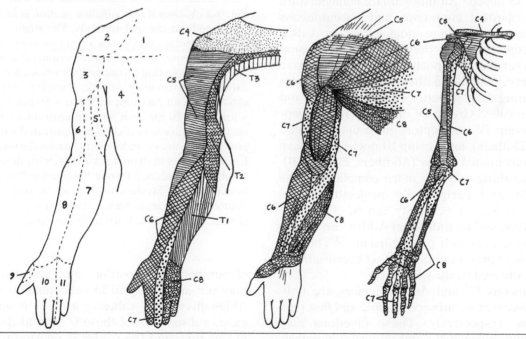

Fig. 9-1 Innervation patterns *(left to right)* of peripheral nerves, dermatomes, myotomes, and sclerotomes are compared. Symptom descriptions by patients, including depth of sensation and location, are invaluable to diagnosis. *1 and 2,* Supraclavicular nerves; *3,* axillary; *4,* intercostobrachial and intercostals; *5,* medial brachial cutaneous; *6,* posterior brachial cutaneous; *7,* medial antebrachial cutaneous; *8,* lateral antebrachial cutaneous; *9,* radial; *10,* median; *11,* ulnar. *(Dermatomes from Foerster O: The dermatomes in man, Brain 56:1-39, 1933. Myotomes and sclerotomes redrawn and used with permission. Inman VT, Saunders JBdM: Referred pain from skeletal structures, J Nerve Ment Dis 99:660-667, 1944.)*

On a moment-to-moment basis, nociceptors signal that a stone that needs removing is in a shoe, that the time to go to the dentist has arrived, or the time has come to shift from a position that may cause a leg to "go to sleep" (possible beginnings of sciatic or peroneal neuropathy). Inflammation causes pain that is perceived, in part, through activity of nociceptors responding to chemical mediators released by the process. In general, nociceptors exist where it makes sense for them to be, which is anywhere that the organism may be subjected to harmful stimuli.

Nociceptors in the peripheral nervous system are pseudounipolar dorsal root ganglion neurons with unmyelinated or thinly myelinated axons (Fig. 9-2, *A*). The unmyelinated axons are referred to as C-fibers, with **conduction velocities** of less than 2.5 m/sec; and the thinly myelinated axons are referred to as Aδ-fibers, with conduction velocities of 2.5 to approximately 15 m/sec.[3] An unfortunate nomenclature exists regarding cutaneous and noncutaneous nociceptors. Cutaneous nociceptors are called *C-nociceptors* when they have unmyelinated (C-fiber) axons or Aδ-nociceptors when they have thinly myelinated (Aδ-fiber) axons. Nociceptors innervating deep structures such as muscle and joint are called **Group IV** or **Group III nociceptors.** Group IV nociceptors have unmyelinated axons (C-fibers), and Group III nociceptors have thinly myelinated axons (Aδ-fibers, Fig. 9-2, *B*). To make things slightly more complicated, the centrally and peripherally projecting axons from a nociceptor cell body can be of a different caliber, and an individual A-fiber can thin to a C-fiber caliber as it passes distally.[4,5] This terminology is presented in this text because it will be encountered in the literature.

Cutaneous C- and Aδ-nociceptors are typically discussed as subserving *slow* and *fast* pain function, respectively. These functions may have some physiologic and clinical differences, with C-nociceptor activity being more likely to give rise to burning or aching sensations and Aδ-nociceptor activation to better-localized sharp, stabbing, or pricking pain. However, significant overlap in function occurs. Furthermore, this differentiation was determined from studies

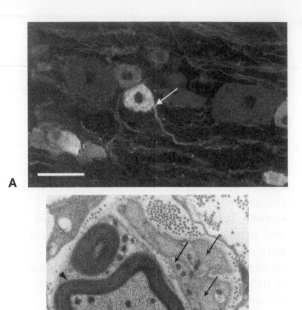

Fig. 9-2 A, Dorsal root ganglion section is labeled with a sodium channel antibody. The single pseudounipolar axon leaves a primary afferent neuron *(arrow)* to branch into peripheral and centrally projecting processes *(not on section)*. This axon is approximately 4 μm in diameter and thus classified as an Aδ axon; scale bar = 50 μm, section 8 = μm thick. **B,** Electron photomicrograph of a cross-section of a nerve branch is demonstrated within the cranial dura mater. Individual C-axons *(arrows)* are less than 1 μm in diameter and are, with their neighbors, combined by one Schwann cell into a Remak bundle. Myelin sheath of an Aδ axon is demonstrated *(arrowhead)*; scale bar = 2 μm. *(Image courtesy Dr. Andrew Strassman.)*

of cutaneous innervation, and this distinction may not apply to pain in subcutaneous tissues. Although several subcategories of nociceptors exist, a discussion of these is beyond the scope of this text, and the reader is referred to excellent reviews by Cervero, Kumazawa, Mense, and Schaible.[6-9] For the purposes of this text, all subcategories of nociceptors are considered together under the heading *nociceptor*.

The distal projection of nociceptive neurons terminates in what has historically been called a *free-nerve ending.* This unfortunate term implies a nonspecialized structure. The anatomic specialization of these terminals remains elusive, especially for C-fiber nociceptors. However, the terminals are sufficiently specialized to discriminate among mechanical, chemical, and thermal stimuli, or they may respond to all these stimuli, depending on the type of nociceptor. The terminals of cutaneous nociceptors usually split into numerous small branches in the skin, yielding one or more very small (<1 mm²) points on the skin surface at which they respond most strongly. A zone of lesser sensitivity usually surrounds these points. The **receptive fields** of nociceptors in subcutaneous tissues have similar properties but branch more freely, thereby having more complex receptive fields.[10] These fields could be partially responsible for the relative difficulty in localizing deep, painful stimuli (Fig. 9-3).

As implied by the preceding definitions, the simple anatomic presence of small nerve fibers ending in free-nerve endings does not prove that the structure is a nociceptor; a number of procedures are needed for confirmation, discussed briefly below. It should be kept in mind that axons belonging to the autonomic nervous system are also unmyelinated (C-fiber), but they have purely **efferent** functions. **Afferent** fibers that are intermingled with autonomic nerves, such as those accompanying splanchnic nerves, are not part of the autonomic nervous system; they are simply following a convenient path to their innervation target. For the most part, their cell bodies reside in a dorsal root ganglion, and they are part of the peripheral nervous system. Some of these neurons are probably nociceptors.

The skin is the largest organ in the body and most subject to external stimuli. It follows that the skin is heavily innervated by nociceptors and by sensory nerve fibers subserving other modalities, such as touch, pressure, and temperature. The densest nociceptive innervation is in the cornea, perhaps pointing to its importance and vulnerability to injury. Muscles, joint capsules, periosteum, and most viscera are also innervated by nociceptors, though less densely. This may be caused by the lesser vulnerability of these tissues. Blood vessels are known to have a rich innervation, consisting of somatic afferent and autonomic fibers; indeed these structures are painful when stimulated.[11] Recently, **nerve sheaths** and their accompanying blood vessels have been shown to have nociceptive nerve fibers as part of their **nervi nervorum** (the intrinsic innervation of nerves).[10] Because blood vessels and nerves travel to virtually every tissue in the body, the nervi nervorum may provide a major source of nociceptive input. The paraspinal tissues, including the muscles, joints, and periosteum, are innervated by small diameter nerve fibers,[12-15] and even small inclusion bodies (intraarticular meniscoids) of the zygapophyseal joint can be innervated.[16]

Small caliber nerve fibers can be microscopically identified using numerous staining techniques. They can also be labeled using antibodies to various peptide neurotransmitters. Knowledge of the peptide functions provides insight into the function of the cell. However,

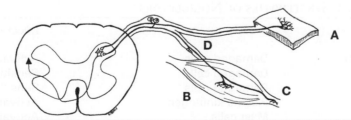

Fig. 9-3 Schematic of primary afferent innervation pattern. Two neurons are depicted, one innervating skin (**A**) and the other innervating deep structures. The cutaneous neuron extends to one area of the skin, and the deep neuron branches extend to innervate muscle (**B**), tendon (**C**), and even the nerve in which it passes (**D**). Both neurons are depicted as extending to a single neuron in the dorsal horn, which would be termed a *wide dynamic range* neuron.

functional testing using specific stimuli is usually necessary to prove that the nerve fiber or neuron is indeed nociceptive. Knowledge of nociceptors for different tissues varies. For instance, much is known about the nociceptors innervating skin; less is known about subcutaneous and visceral nociceptors. Interestingly, functional information on the innervation of paraspinal tissues is scarce. Only relatively recently have studies shown a substantial nociceptor population, supporting these structures as potential pain sources.[10,12,17]

How Nociceptors Are Studied

Nociceptors can be studied in a variety of ways in humans and animals. In humans, testing can be as simple as applying a stimulus and getting a subjective report from the subject. However, because the stimuli that are known to evoke responses from nociceptors also evoke responses from mechanoreceptors and often thermoreceptors, the results are somewhat nonspecific. Capsaicin, the hot ingredient in peppers, has gained popularity for use in experimental studies because it is fairly specific for activating nociceptors. Numerous studies of the psychophysical parameters of pain have used subdermal injections of capsaicin to activate nociceptor terminals. In animals, the selective response of a nociceptor terminal to application of this chemical has been used as evidence that the receptor is a nociceptor.

Studying the response of individual nociceptors is possible in both animals and humans. In animals, a nerve can be exposed and small nerve filaments (5 to 15 µm) can be carefully teased apart and placed over electrodes connected to amplification and recording devices. This procedure isolates a small population of axons, with the process being repeated until only one neuron or axon is found to be active. The receptive field(s) and sensitivities of this neuron or axon are then determined. In humans, a similar process, called **microneurography,** can be performed. Fine needle electrodes are placed into nerves, and the receptive fields of identified axons are characterized. Yet another process in animals uses microelectrodes to record from individual cells in ganglia. In this case, a fine electrode is advanced into the ganglion, and used to record the electrical activity of individual cells. Much of the information that follows was gathered using methods similar to these.

Nociceptor Function

In normal, undisturbed tissue, very little (<0.5 Hz) or no activity in nociceptors is usually observed.[18] By definition, nociceptors respond to damaging or potentially damaging stimuli, and neurons are characterized as nociceptors if they respond to noxious mechanical, thermal, or chemical stimuli. Various chemical stimuli have been found to activate nociceptors, including components found in the inflammatory milieu, neurotransmitters, and tissue metabolites (Table 9-1).[19] Some of these substances directly activate nociceptors, some only sensitize them to other compounds, and some will only activate

Table **9-1**   CHEMICAL SENSITIVITIES OF NOCICEPTORS

Substance	Source	Effect on Nociceptor
Acid and potassium	Damaged cells	Activation and sensitization
Prostaglandins	Damaged cells	Sensitization
Leukotrienes	Damaged cells	Sensitization
Bradykinin	Plasma kininogen	Activation
Histamine	Mast cells	Activation
TNF-α	Immune cells	Activation and sensitization
Serotonin	Platelets (neurotransmitter)	Activation
Substance P	Nociceptors	Sensitization

TNF-α, Tumor necrosis factor-alpha.

nociceptors that have already sustained some injury. These substances have been tested on animal and human nociceptors in a variety of preparations[20] and can evoke discharge from individual nociceptors, cause behavioral changes, and evoke reports of pain. Among the cytokines, the best studied are tumor necrosis factor–alpha (TNF-α) and interleukin 1-β, which are released from numerous cells during immune-mediated inflammation. When injected into the skin, these chemicals are noxious.[21] When TNF-α is placed on a peripheral nerve, nociceptors develop ongoing discharge,[22] and rat feet demonstrate allodynia.[23] Although individual chemicals will elicit responses from varying populations of nociceptors, the combination of mediators, found *in vivo*, is most effective.

In diseased or damaged tissue, the properties of nociceptors may change. In a phenomenon called **sensitization**, they develop **ongoing activity,** along with a decrease in the thresholds to noxious stimuli and an increase in the size of receptive fields. The effect can occur with even a brief stimulus and can last for hours.[24] In skin, this effect is observed in response to burns, even a small-sized burn. The spontaneous pain and increased sensitivity of the damaged area is mediated by sensitized nociceptors, though other types of receptor may also be active and play a role during injury. Sensitization has been shown to occur in both nociceptors from cutaneous and deep tissues, but the full mechanism of the process remains poorly understood.

Stimulation of sympathetic nerves can affect nociceptors in certain situations. Normally, nociceptors may be sensitized by sympathetic stimulation,[25,26] but they do not directly respond to increased sympathetic activity or to the application of norepinephrine.[27,28] However, during chronic inflammation or after nerve injury, sympathetic stimulation can directly activate C-fiber nociceptors.[29-33] Pain and psychologic stressors increase sympathetic discharge, leading to increased levels of norepinephrine.[34-36] This well-known response provides at least a partial explanation for the clinical observations that reducing psychologic stress responses may decrease pain and facilitate a more rapid recovery.

At the beginning of the twentieth century, it was discovered that electrical stimulation of dorsal roots caused cutaneous vasodilation and **plasma extravasation** whenever the stimulus intensity was high enough to excite unmyelinated fibers.[37] This response was termed the **axon reflex.** Later, this neurally controlled and reflexive release of initiators and inflammatory mediators was termed the *nocifensor system*.[38] More recently, the nerves contributing to the axon reflexes were found to be nociceptors,[39] strongly suggesting that nociceptors have both sensory and efferent functions. Calcitonin gene-related peptide (CGRP) and substance P (SP), which are co-localized in the nociceptor terminal (Fig. 9-4), are the two most important mediators that these nerves release.[40-42] Substance P and CGRP are potent vasodilators, and CGRP potentiates the effects of SP.[43-48] Moreover, SP contributes to nociceptor sensitization[49] and is thought to participate in the immune response.[50] Electrical stimulation of nociceptor axons anywhere along their course will cause the release of these peptides from distal terminals, resulting in a focal inflammation, termed **neurogenic inflammation.**

Nociceptors may be essential for an animal to mount an inflammatory response through neurogenic inflammation. For example, it has been shown that the development of peripheral experimental arthritis is at least in part dependent on the presence of afferent innervation.[51] Additionally, the severity of experimental arthritis is reduced in animals depleted of nociceptors through neonatal injection of capsaicin.[52] Finally, the increased cerebral blood flow as a result of meningitis is greatly attenuated by denervation of the primary afferents innervating the intracranial structures.[53] These lines of evidence support a critical role of nociceptors in the organism's response to injury.

Although the role of nociceptors in neurogenic inflammation is undisputed, less is known about the role of the sympathetic nervous system in this process. However, sympathetic nerves are clearly important to the generation of experimental immune arthritis. They are also known to participate in the localized edema that occurs in certain models of chronic neuropathic

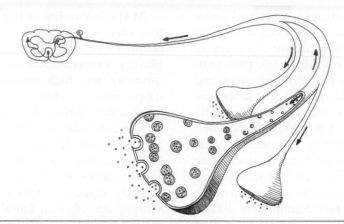

Fig. 9-4 Release of substance P and calcitonin gene-related peptide (CGRP) by primary afferent nociceptors. When an appropriate stimulation elicits an action potential, the action potential is propagated to the central nervous system and to other branches of the neuron *(arrows)*. Simultaneously, the endings release substance P and CGRP *(small closed and open symbols)* from the terminals, which are co-localized in vesicles that are transported from the cell body. This process is thought to occur in terminals that are invaded by the action potential even when they are not directly stimulated. Substance P and CGRP cause plasma extravasation and vasodilation, respectively, which are necessary components of the inflammatory response. This process is termed *neurogenic inflammation.*

pain. This participation may explain why stressful situations may exacerbate inflammatory conditions and increase pain.

Differences between Deep and Cutaneous Nociceptors

Although most studies of nociceptors have been performed on skin, few clinically important pain conditions exist that primarily affect the skin. Even among conditions felt in the skin, most are *neuropathic* (the term *neuropathic* refers to a nerve pathology or functional disturbance of a nerve or some axons within a nerve) and may not involve cutaneous nociceptors at all. Cutaneous neuropathic pain is very possibly mediated by sensitization of neurons that are normally not responsive to noxious stimuli, such as neurons that respond to light touch. Recently, the authors of this chapter interviewed 25 people with diagnoses of lumbar **radiculopathy** (i.e., radiating pain due to a pathology of one or more dorsal roots). The participants were asked to identify the perceived location of the radiating leg pain. In every case, the pain at rest and the pain evoked during a straight leg raise test were reported to be "deep" rather than "on the skin."

Thus studies of cutaneous nociceptors may not be fully applicable to deep nociceptors. Indeed, studies that have compared nociceptor sensitivity by innervated structure have shown critical differences. The response to pinch was found to be dramatically greater after a stimulus delivered to a muscle nerve rather than to a cutaneous nerve.[54] Deep nociceptor axons also seem to respond differently to inflammation. During **neuritis,** or nerve inflammation, axons of deep nociceptors become mechanically sensitive, whereas cutaneous nociceptor axons do not.[55] The percentage of deep nociceptors that develop ongoing activity during neuritis is also greater than their cutaneous counterparts. After axonal damage, recordings from nociceptors in muscle nerves reveal ongoing discharge more often than do recordings from cutaneous neurons.[56,57] These data point to fundamental differences in deep versus cutaneous nociceptor physiology.

Neuronal Response to Injury

When their peripheral axons are injured, the central projections of myelinated and unmyelinated dorsal root neurons can sprout into wider territories in the spinal cord.[58,59] The sprouting of presumably nociceptive terminals in the superficial dorsal horn could explain hyperalgesia, because the discharge of an individual sensory axon would be transmitted to more second-order neurons, with their sum predictably leading to an increased perception of pain. The sprouting of larger fibers, usually nonnociceptive, into the laminae (layers) of the spinal cord, which is usually reserved for nociceptor input, may explain allodynia, because their discharge may now activate nociceptive neurons. Indeed, possibly the allodynia that often accompanies chronic regional pain syndromes is mediated by myelinated fibers.[60,61]

Spinal Cord Projections of Nociceptors

Nociceptive dorsal root ganglion neurons project into the dorsolateral portion of the spinal cord where they branch T-wise, sending branches 1 through 5 segments rostral and caudal (1 to 2 for C-fiber nociceptors, 1 through 5 for Aδ-nociceptors).[62] The region of the spinal cord white matter located adjacent to the dorsal horn that contains these ascending and descending fibers has been termed the *Lissauer's zone*. C-fiber nociceptors ultimately terminate in the dorsal horn in the most dorsal part of the dorsal horn, termed *laminae I and II*,[63] whereas Aδ-nociceptors additionally project to *laminae V and X*.[64] Most dorsal horn neurons are classified as *wide dynamic range*, which means they respond to both noxious and innocuous stimuli, with more intense and widespread stimuli producing greater activation (see Fig. 9-3). A smaller percentage of dorsal horn neurons, particularly located within the most superficial laminae of the dorsal horn, are nociceptive specific. It is believed that the nociceptive specific neurons are more important to signal the presence of pain and its precise location, whereas the wide dynamic range neurons are more important to the recognition of intensity of pain. Nociceptors from the limbs terminate ipsilaterally. However, paraspinal tissue nociceptors project bilaterally to dorsal horn neurons.[65,66] This projection predicts the typically poorly defined nature of back pain and emphasizes the need for bilateral spinal examination.

Molecular Changes in the Spinal Cord Related to Nociception

When nociceptors are stimulated, their central terminals release SP, CGRP, and glutamate onto spinal cord neurons. Besides transmitting information to these high-order neurons, genes in second and higher order neurons increase their expression of some proteins. With even a brief stimulus, some genes are known to be *upregulated*. The c-fos and c-jun genes have been intensely studied, and their protein products can be visualized indirectly using immunohistochemical techniques. Studies using these techniques have confirmed the projection of the nociceptive primary afferents, though the stimuli used are not usually specific for nociceptors.[67-69]

The protein products of c-fos and c-jun initiate a cascade of biochemical reactions in the neurons, resulting in the production of enkephalins and dynorphin (**endogenous opiates**) in the central nervous system (see the following text).[70] Enkephalin is an inhibitor of dorsal horn cells, but dynorphin is known to have variable responses, inhibiting one third of neurons, sensitizing one third of neurons, and increasing the receptive fields of many spinal cord neurons.[71] This effect could also contribute to hyperalgesia and to chronic pain, as well as to their modulation.

The generation of neuronal action potentials requires the opening and closing of numerous ion channels. An electrical charge passing through these channels changes the membrane potential, and if this is changed enough, the neuron will generate an action potential (for details, see any neurophysiology text). Alteration in the number and type of ion channels will change the resting potential and excitability of the neuron. For instance, an increase of tonically open sodium channels or a decrease of tonically open potassium channels would be expected to depolarize the membrane. A depolarized membrane requires less additional depolarization to induce an action potential; a neuron that had such changes in ion channels could be considered *facilitated*.

Evidence is building that in pathologic states, dorsal root ganglion cells undergo numerous changes in the expression of ion channels, especially sodium channels. Sodium channel expression has been reported to change after axonal injury and during inflammation (reviewed by Waxman et al.[72]), and some of these channels have also been linked to pain.[73-76] Increased cation channel production may lead to increased insertion in axonal membranes and axonal hyperexcitability. Such changes were proposed to account for the recovery of mechanical sensitivity in the tips of previously cut mechanoreceptive axons.[77,78] Increased cation channel production was also proposed to lead to ongoing activity in sensory neurons from muscle, but not from skin, after damage to neighboring axons.[57]

Central Mechanisms Related to Nociception

Nociceptors are not the only neurons active in response to painful stimuli. In a classic study, Adriaensen and colleagues[79] demonstrated that sustained pinch of the skin led to increasing reports of pain with time, whereas the neural discharge from nociceptors supplying the area actually decreased. Explaining this paradox is difficult, but other nociceptors are probably recruited and the spinal cord and higher centers are changing their "gain" (i.e., amplifying the signal) in response to the input from the nociceptors.

Substantial evidence suggests that peripheral noxious stimulation leads to changes in the central nervous system, collectively called *spinal cord plasticity* (for reviews, see Coderre,[80] Woolf,[81] and Chen et al.[82]). These changes lead to sensitization of central nervous system neurons and may result in hyperalgesia, allodynia, and spontaneous discharge of neurons. Under some conditions, these symptoms may be sustained even if the sensory input from the original source is terminated. All of the characteristics of stimuli that are capable of producing these changes are not yet known, although some experimental models, such as ligating the sciatic nerve, readily produce long-term sensory facilitation. Additionally, because spinal cord neurons have receptive fields that converge from many tissue types (sometimes bilaterally),[65] allodynia and hyperalgesia may be perceived very broadly from uninjured and even rather remote tissues.

Indeed, these symptoms are observed among the plethora of acute and chronic back pain presentations; central nervous system plasticity could help explain these variable presentations.

Concepts of Plasticity

The principal concepts of spinal cord plasticity include **windup, long-term potentiation** (LTP), and **long-term depression** (LTD). A brief presentation of these processes follows, and further details can be found in a review by Pockett.[83] *Windup* is a term that was coined for the phenomenon of increasing the response of a spinal cord neuron to repeated stimuli.[84] When depolarized by the primary afferent neuron, dorsal horn neurons do not always fully recover their resting potential before the arrival of another volley from the primary afferent neuron. Therefore the threshold for firing of the neuron is lower (facilitated). This process typically lasts seconds to minutes. LTP is similar to windup, but it lasts much longer; indeed, some consider LTP to be permanent. This process requires a high-frequency conditioning discharge from the primary afferent neuron[85] and results in increased synaptic efficiency mediated by activation of a specific type of glutamate receptor, the N-methyl-D-aspartate (NMDA) receptor. It differs from windup in that the increased synaptic efficiency is not related to a change in the resting membrane potential of the postsynaptic cells; rather, it involves complicated changes within the postsynaptic dorsal horn neurons that can best be described as a type of memory. For example, there are changes in postsynaptic receptor properties and possibly numbers.[86] These changes are accompanied by alterations in the expression of messenger ribonucleic acid (RNA), as well as in the expression of specific gene products. Once established, there is nothing known that will reverse LTP, except the induction of LTD. LTD can be established by both high- and low-frequency conditioning stimuli, and it involves a long-lasting decrease in synaptic efficacy (thus it is the mirror image of LTP). Repeated episodes of windup may possibly induce LTP or LTD, but this response has not been studied.

Hypothetically, LTP is at least partially responsible for chronic pain; and, if so, LTD induction by stimulating an appropriate nerve may relieve it.[83] This mechanism may be behind the anecdotal effectiveness of various forms of clinical electrical stimulation, but it remains to be demonstrated.

Several additional mechanisms may be important to the changes that occur in the sensitivity of spinal cord pathways in pain syndromes. For example, the expression of inflammatory cytokines by the glial cells of the spinal cord increase during an experimental model of nerve injury.[87] Indeed, the interactions between the two great communication systems in the body, the immune system and the nervous system, are substantially more complex and bidirectional than had been previously appreciated.[88,89] However, it must be remembered that the role of long-term changes that occur after experimental injuries, and indeed whether they occur in clinical problems in humans, remain to be determined. However, painful stimuli can have potent and long-lasting effects on the functions in the spinal cord and other levels of the nervous system.

Descending Modulation of Nociception

The ability to perceive pain is critical to the survival and general well being of the individual. However, it is also important to be able to modulate pain. An example taken from common experience is the ability to "shake off" an injury that produces severe tissue damage until any immediate threat is past. At that time the pain may become severe or even immobilizing, although the injury itself has not changed. What, then, explains this ability to modulate pain transmission and processing?

The earliest hints as to the mechanisms behind pain modulation arose from studies of the most potent pain-suppressing drugs, the opiates.[90] Receptors for opiates have been localized to several brain regions (notably the periaqueductal gray [PAG], dorsal horn of the spinal cord, ventral medullary raphe nuclei, and basal ganglia). Electrical stimulation of some of these regions (notably the PAG and raphe nuclei) was found to inhibit nociceptive responses in animals and produce analgesia in humans.[91]

Of course, the presence of these receptors begs the question of why the nervous system would have specific receptors (opiate receptors) for an exogenous compound (opium) derived from a Middle Eastern poppy. Investigation of this question led to the discovery of a group of transmitters contained in small interneurons that bind to these receptors and activate them. These "endogenous opiates" consist of a family of very small peptides (enkephalins) that are synthesized in small neurons of the central nervous system, as well as a larger compound **(endorphin)** that is found in the region of the pituitary gland and is released into the circulation. Injection of these compounds into portions of the nervous system that have opiate receptors produces powerful analgesia. As previously discussed, these compounds are also directly produced by spinal cord neurons after intense activity of primary afferent neurons.

It became apparent that some of the enkephalin neurons directly inhibit the pain transmission neurons in the dorsal horn of the spinal cord. For example, intense nociceptive input results in the release of enkephalin from the dorsal horn, providing at least a partial explanation for the inhibition of pain that can occur shortly after the onset of a powerful noxious stimulus. However, that does not adequately explain the role of opiates at the level of the PAG, because the endogenous opiate containing neurons do not have axons that leave the PAG and also because the PAG does not have direct neuronal connection with the pain pathway. Further investigation revealed that the influence of PAG on pain transmission is rather complex, involving excitatory projections from the PAG to the caudal medulla. These projections, in turn, excite descending projections to the dorsal horn that release norepinephrine and serotonin from their terminals in the spinal cord dorsal horn.

Norepinephrine and serotonin, called monoamine transmitters, have complex effects at the dorsal horn, both by directly affecting the pain transmission neurons and by activating other neurons at the spinal level (e.g., small enkephalinergic interneurons). Of course, in understanding this system the regions that connect with and thereby influence the PAG became important considerations. Many brain regions connect with the PAG, including the frontal and insular cortex, amygdala, hypothalamus, reticular formation, locus ceruleus, and collateral branches of the spinothalamic tract. This connection illustrates the diverse brain regions that can play a part in regulating pain transmission. This descending system, based on the endogenous opiates and monoamines, has become the best-known inhibitory circuit for pain modulation. It defines the analgesic effects of opiates, such as morphine, but it also explains at least some of the role that serotonin and norepinephrine play in pain control. Despite the fact that descending inhibition is the best characterized of all pain-suppression mechanisms (notwithstanding the known effects of various drugs on this system), less well known mechanisms are other physiologic factors that are capable of activating this potent pain-suppression mechanism.

Although, undoubtedly, endogenous opiates play a powerful role in controlling pain, other inhibitory systems are also found in the nervous system. For example, gamma aminobutyric acid (GABA) is the most common inhibitory neurotransmitter in the central nervous system.[92] Activation of GABAergic interneurons appears to be at least one important mechanism of analgesia provoked by the stimulation of large diameter sensory nerve fibers (e.g., proprioceptive nerve fibers).[93] Glycine, another neurotransmitter, has a significant inhibitory influence at the spinal cord level with at least some of its effect produced by inhibition of excitatory neurotransmission through NMDA receptors.[94] This effect may be important not only in inhibiting the initial signal but also in preventing the kind of LTP that can accompany activation of NMDA receptors. Recent studies have shown that activation of spinal facet joint receptors can powerfully inhibit the reflex effects of noxious stimulation of the spine.[95] Although the mechanisms of this inhibition are not known, the inhibitory transmitters in the spinal cord represent prime candidates for investigation.

Psychology and Nociception

Why is it that two individuals can be injured in exactly the same manner, with dramatically different results (at least in terms of pain and suffering)? Although, undoubtedly, some of these different results are the result of the differences in the peripheral pain systems and the pain transmission systems in the central nervous system, the experience of pain goes well beyond the mere activation of a nociceptor and the conduction of an impulse to the cerebral cortex.

Pain is defined as an unpleasant sensory *and emotional* experience. In addition, the issue of suffering, which is the behavioral and psychologic component that is reflected in the patient's outward affect, is expressed. The patient typically describes his or her suffering as the consequence of the painful disorder. Although all of the mechanisms involved in suffering or in the psychologic ramifications of pain are not understood, several lines of evidence indicate that the frontal lobes of the cerebral cortex are critical in this regard. The first hints of this conclusion arose from the clinical evaluation of patients with frontal lobe injuries and those who had been subjected to frontal lobectomy. Patients with frontal lobe damage can describe the intensity of a painful stimulus, indicating that the principal transmission pathways are intact; however, they do not appear to suffer in proportion to the degree of pain. In such patients, both behavioral and autonomic responses to pain are blunted. Evidence suggests that some of the analgesic effects of some sedatives and antianxiety drugs may have their primary effect at the level of the frontal lobe rather than (or in addition to) affecting pain transmission through nociceptive pathways.

Other lines of investigation have also directed attention to areas of the frontal lobe. These include experimental pain models that have been shown on functional magnetic resonance imaging to activate selectively specific portions of the frontal lobes.[96] Additionally, it has been shown that patients with pain who were effectively hypnotized to block the unpleasantness, but not the intensity of their pain, showed changes in the anterior cingulate cortex (i.e., the medial portion of the frontal lobe).[97] It is interesting to note that similar areas of the medial frontal lobes, particularly in the areas of the anterior cingulate and subcallosal gyri, have been shown to be metabolically altered in certain affective disorders, particularly depression. It is well known that a complex interaction between depression and pain exists, and it would appear that at least some physiologic basis for this interaction is evident. Although much has been written about the capacity of depression to magnify pain, some evidence also suggests that effective treatment of chronic pain is capable of ameliorating depression.[98]

Most of the interest in cortical mechanisms of pain has been focused on the issue of suffering rather than pain perception, and there is reason to believe that behavioral factors might have some influence over pain transmission as well. For example, several studies indicate that placebo analgesia is real and is probably mediated via endogenous opiate mechanisms.[99] Certainly, the connections between the frontal cortex and PAG (among other places) might provide the substrate for this effect, though the precise mechanisms remain unknown. Overall, there is good reason to believe that cortical mechanisms play a role in analgesia, and excellent evidence suggests that suffering is a cortical phenomenon that is largely based in the frontal lobes. These findings provide some theoretical underpinning for behavioral interventions in pain management.

SOURCES OF PAIN

Local Tissue Damage

Of course, local tissue damage can lead to pain through direct activation of the peripheral nervous system. Acute activation is usually secondary to direct activation of nociceptor terminals. Persistent pain can be the result of continued direct activation, the result of chemical excitation by inflammatory mediators, or in some cases, maintained at least in part by the central nervous system.

A few common sources of somatic pain need mentioning. First, the intervertebral disk has been blamed for most spinal pain, usually sec-ondary to its ability to compress nerve roots when herniated. However, compression alone is not painful, and patients can recover from so-called compressive radiculopathy without resolution of the compression.[100] The source of pain is inflammation induced by the discal pathology; when the inflammation subsides with healing, the pain also subsides. The inner part of the intervertebral disk is called the *nucleus pulposus* and contains TNF-α.[101] When released from the disk, this substance promotes an immune-mediated inflammation, which generates more local noxious chemicals. Persistent pain from discal herniation probably means that the disk is still releasing noxious material, maintaining sufficient inflammation to sensitize the nociceptors in the neighboring tissues. Additionally, in older people the nucleus pulposus dries and therefore cannot herniate; consequently, the prevalence of disk-related pain also decreases with age.

Chronic muscle pain also presents a problem. Two familiar incidences of muscle insult that lead to pain are considered: (1) injury as a result of excessive stretch during an automobile accident, and (2) pain after the overload of muscle during unaccustomed exercise. Although the acute stretch during an automobile accident is at least transiently painful, pain during unaccustomed exercise is not common. In both cases, symptoms start within 12 to 24 hours and render the muscle allodynic. Why, then, does the pain of an injury often persist, whereas the pain after exercise resolves rapidly and without incident? In the case of accidental injury, nerves are damaged through stretch. In the case of normal exercises, nerve injuries are far less likely to occur. This major difference between these two scenarios appears to be the cause of the different results. Afferent activity of damaged or even intact but injured axons would be perceived as coming from the target muscle. This could even be responsible for maintaining a low-grade inflammation in the region through the neurogenic mechanisms previously outlined. The authors of this chapter propose that persistent pain probably requires a source of persistent nociceptor activity, called a *peripheral generator*.

Indeed, many cases of persistent severe pain will follow nerve injuries, especially stretch injuries.

Although a complicated layering of connective tissues protects the axons within nerves, the nerves can be damaged by direct trauma or stretch. (For further reading, see Sunderland.[102]) Such damage leads to mechanical, chemical, and thermal sensitivity at the cut and regrowing terminal. However, it is not necessary for the axon to be completely interrupted for axonal injury and inflammation to lead to action potential generation.

Radiating Pain Mechanisms

Nerve injury and inflammation result in the perception of radiating pain (radicular pain, if the nerve roots are involved). Neurobiology texts present sensory neurons as having a transducer or receptor in the periphery, an axon, a cell body, another axon, and a synaptic terminal in the spinal cord (Fig. 9-5, *A*). The axons are presented as simple electrical conduits. Normal sensation occurs when the transducer is sufficiently stimulated by touch, generating, for example, an action potential that is propagated to the spinal cord for possible transmission to higher centers. If perceived, the sensation will be in the area of the original transducer.

When the axon has been cut, no possibility of action potential conduction is left from the transducer. The regenerating tip of the severed axon can become chemically and mechanically sensitive. Touching this tip will generate action potentials (Fig. 9-5, *C*). These action potentials will be perceived as coming from the tissue that contains the now dead transducer, because the signal will follow pathways that originally conducted impulses from that tissue. This mechanism is the likely cause of "phantom" sensations that often follow limb amputation. The only exception would be if the nervous system reorganizes to accommodate the amputation. More recently, it has been shown that at least some injured axons can develop ongoing activity and mechanical sensitivity without interrupting their normal conduction, secondary to inflammation (Fig. 9-5, *B*).

Neurons thus have two potential sources of action potential generation—their receptors in the innervated tissue and their axon. It is critical to remember that activity generated at either site will be perceived as coming from the tissue innervated and will probably be difficult or impossible for the patient to distinguish. Such ectopic activity can also arise in injured axons in the dorsal root ganglion and will be similarly perceived as coming from the innervated tissue. For example, inflammation within the intervertebral foramen or TNF-α applied to the dorsal root ganglion causes hyperalgesia of the foot, as well as ongoing activity localized to the dorsal root ganglia.[103,104] These data further support that the radiating or projected pain associated with discal

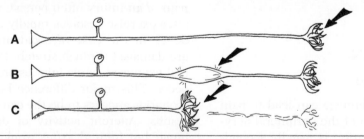

Fig. 9-5 **A,** Typical representation of primary afferent neuron, with *(right to left)* a receptor, a peripherally projecting axon, the cell body, a centrally projecting axon, and a terminal in the dorsal horn of the spinal cord. Sufficient stimuli of the receptor lead to the generation of action potentials, which are propagated along the axon to the central nervous system. **B,** The axon is an alternate source of action potential generation for slowly conducting neurons innervating deep tissues. Importantly, any sensation arising from stimulation of the axon at such a sensitive site will be perceived as coming from the distal receptive area, not from the site of action potential generation. **C,** A damaged and regrowing axon is another source of action potentials. If numerous axons are cut, the regrowth can cause a mass called a neuroma. Regrowing axons are very sensitive to chemical and mechanical stimuli. As in **B,** sensations arising from such stimuli would also be perceived as coming from the innervated tissue.

herniation probably arises as a result of ectopic activity of the dorsal roots or ganglia and therefore is not referred.

Referred Pain Mechanisms

A common human experience is the perception of pain radiating into the scapula, posterior head, or upper limb after pressure over so-called "trigger points" in the muscles of the shoulder girdle. Of course, if this pressure were to be placed on nerve trunks (e.g., upper brachial plexus), the explanation would have to consider radiating pain as described in the preceding section.

However, because most of the stimuli that produce such pain do not directly activate the nerve trunks projecting to these areas, what can explain this perception of pain? Referred pain is the perception of pain in locations other than the site of generation and not localized to the distribution of a damaged nerve.[105] It is a direct result of activation of nociceptive endings in somatic tissues or internal organs. The process depends on the activation of nociceptors that project to the wide dynamic range neurons that receive highly convergent input from the many sites that make input to that particular part of the spinal cord. These projection neurons seem to be primarily designed to relate the intensity rather than the location of a painful stimulus. Typically, the nervous system relies on other clues as to the origin of pain and, in the absence of adequate clues, often "paints" the pain on the body in a manner that may be at some distance from the actual site of pain generation. Because activity in the wide dynamic range neurons is usually perceived as a deep aching or burning sensation, referred pain is rarely sharp, even though it can be both intense and very unpleasant. Additionally, it is not well localized and has indistinct borders that overlap the distribution of several nerves and nerve roots.

CLINICAL RELEVANCE

Lumbar Facet Syndrome

The preceding sections have described physiologic mechanisms for the initiation and maintenance of nociception and pain. However, how are these principles relevant to a patient's condition? This section describes how these mechanisms may apply to a common clinical condition, the lumbar facet syndrome.

Lumbar facet syndrome is described as a sprain of the zygapophyseal joints and can be either acute or chronic. The acute form can follow an excessive movement in any plane or combination of planes of motion and more likely involves pinching or excessive stretching of the articular capsule. Although this structure is relatively small, why can the pain be hard to localize and difficult to manage?

Assuming that the injury is restricted to the left L5-S1 joint and is, in fact, from pinching of the joint capsule itself or an intraarticular meniscoid arising from the capsule, the joint capsules are innervated by nociceptors,[17,66] which respond to noxious mechanical stimulation with a high-frequency discharge. This injury leads to mast cell degranulation, releasing histamine that can amplify the neural response and can also lead to the recruitment of macrophages to clear the damaged tissue. Macrophages produce a multitude of proinflammatory cytokines that can directly elicit discharges from nociceptors and their axons.[22] The activated primary afferent neurons release SP and CGRP into the surrounding tissue. The end result is an inflammatory reaction in the joint and perhaps in other surrounding tissues. Increased concentrations of noxious chemicals and reduced pH, which are also effective stimuli for nociceptors, are also present in the inflammatory milieu.[106]

At the same time, nociceptors that have been damaged or sensitized may now respond to products of increased sympathetic activity; indeed, the inflammation may be affecting the sympathetic axons directly, though no data exist to support this possibility. These pain fibers relay through nociceptive specific neurons in the dorsal horn of the spinal cord (to signal the presence and location of pain) and through wide dynamic range neurons (to signal its intensity). Although the majority of pain will be felt in the region and on the side of the injured facet, the divergence of nociceptive afferent input over several spinal cord segments and the bilateral input of some nociceptors from axial tissues, such as paraspinal muscles and zygapophyseal joints, will mean that the aching component of pain will probably be perceived over a broader area.

The preceding scenario describes the generation of acute pain after a noxious incident. However, in the absence of continued or maintained noxious input, the inflammation is expected to subside and the injury is expected to heal. Indeed, in most cases, the acute injury and pain do resolve. Subsequently, why do many patients have what appears to be chronic facet syndrome with the addition of other typically poorly defined symptoms extending to other areas? Two possible explanations exist, explanations that are not mutually exclusive. First, the symptoms may continue because of continued activity of the nociceptor. This explanation would imply some ongoing mechanical or inflammatory process that continually irritates the nociceptor. In this case, the job of the clinician is to determine the peripheral generator of the afferent discharge and to do whatever is necessary to reduce or terminate the neuronal activity. This might occur if the joint capsule was being intermittently impinged by bony structures, with movement reinforcing or worsening the damage. Interventions that remove the impingement would be expected to remove the source of afferent discharge, allowing the inflammation and the pain to subside. One possible mechanism of action of spinal adjustment and manipulation is the removal of such impingements.

Second, and more problematic, would be the persistence of pain symptoms in the apparent absence of afferent discharge. In this case, the practitioner is always urged to continue the search for a peripheral generator, because this represents the more easily correctable problem. Only after a diligent search should it be assumed that the central pain transmission pathways have been facilitated and are now responsible for the prolonged pain. Persistent pain, hyperesthesia, or allodynia would be expected if LTP has resulted in prolonged sensitization. Unfortunately, no available diagnostic tests are currently available to determine the role of such central mechanisms in pain. When all other options have been exhausted, the clinician may have to rely on the previously described (and clinically hypothetical) mechanisms to explain the persistence of symptoms. However, it is proposed that spinal adjustment and manipulation may be an effective source of high-frequency neural discharge that could conceivably reverse LTP.

As previously discussed, nociceptor activity stimulates neurons in the central nervous system; otherwise, there would be no perception at all. The innervation of the facet joint in question is predominantly through the posterior ramus of the spinal nerve from L4-S1, though there is some evidence from animal studies for even greater spread via sensory fibers that follow lumbar sympathetic nerves. The nociceptive nerve fibers likely synapse with neurons over at least the cord levels L2-S2, with most but certainly not all terminating in the ipsilateral spinal cord dorsal horn. This anatomy has two possible effects: (1) spinal cord neurons receive convergent input from many structures, contributing to poor localization of the pain; and (2) axon reflexes may be propagated to any tissue innervated by these levels. As mentioned, these axon reflexes cause the release of SP and CGRP by antidromic mechanisms, with the development of at least some degree of neurogenic inflammation. Paraspinal, gluteal, and even leg pain are common and might be explained by these mechanisms in cases where facet joint syndrome is diagnosed.

These two theories of chronic pain are often regarded as mutually exclusive, and a great deal of controversy remains regarding the relative importance of ongoing nociceptor activation versus plastic changes in pain systems in chronic pain. However, these theories are not mutually exclusive and, even in cases with clear sensitization of the central nervous system, evidence also typically suggests ongoing peripheral impulse generation.[107] Importantly, until the processes of sensitization are clearly understood and until such time as there are methods for expediting the reversal of such sensitization, therapy will be predominantly directed at the peripheral pain generators. To the extent that central sensitization has occurred, slower improvement in the condition would, of course, be anticipated.

Diagnosis of the facet syndrome is based, at least partially, on orthopedic testing. **Orthopedic tests** are simple motions that are designed to isolate particular tissues to determine whether these tissues are responsible for the symptom. In the case of pain, the test is considered positive if it reproduces the pain. (*Note:* Production of a new or different pain does not help in the diagnosis.) Unfortunately, in the case of the spine, no motions isolate a single tissue. Therefore orthopedic tests of the spine must be carefully interpreted. Nonetheless, in the case of the patient with facet syndrome, motions that place a load or a stretch on the injured joint would be likely to reproduce the pain, aiding in diagnosis. However, it must be remembered that if significant facilitation of pain pathways exists, activation of sensory nerve fibers that are not nociceptive may be capable of provoking pain by the mechanisms previously described for allodynia. By this mechanism, the initial injury may have left the patient with hypersensitive tissues, and normally innocuous movements could reinitiate or aggravate the processes, which gives further justification for care in interpreting orthopedic tests, particularly in patients with severe or chronic pain.

Despite pain with movement, not all movements are bad. For example, substantial evidence suggests that stimulating mechanoreceptors inhibits nociceptor activity, at least in the acute situation. Therefore movement may be beneficial to the control of pain. In addition, movements that place normal stresses on an injured tissue are important for directing the proper orientation of collagenous tissue during repair. Such interventions could include spinal adjustment and manipulation, mobilization, and exercise.

Neurogenic Inflammation

The issue of neurogenic inflammation as a factor prolonging pain is not settled, particularly in the deeper tissues that are less accessible to direct observation. Nonetheless, neurogenic inflammation is probably important in many cases of prolonged pain, as witnessed by the number of patients who receive at least some relief from powerful antiinflammatory medications.

Historically, some changes in tissue texture and consistency and in temperature and sweating patterns associated with various musculoskeletal lesions (e.g., vertebral subluxation complex) have been observed. At least some of these observations could be explained by neurogenic inflammation. However, this process would require significantly more investigation before anything more than speculative explanations could be offered.

Unanswered Questions about Chronic Pain

The previous sequence of events describes the pain-dysfunction cycles so often used to illustrate musculoskeletal disease processes. It is thought that clinical efforts directed at breaking these cycles will help the patient's recovery. However, most musculoskeletal injuries do get better on their own, probably through the gradual spontaneous resolution of the events described. One major problem with this theory is that it does not explain the significant population of musculoskeletal pain sufferers with chronic pain in the absence of detectable pathology. In many cases these patients are thought to have suffered permanent plastic changes in their central nervous system, leading to the perception of spontaneous pain thought to be originating from a peripheral site. However, it seems likely that in the majority of cases, there is at least some persistent peripheral pathology that has remained undetected and maintains the peripheral noxious input and associated pain. It also seems likely that the persistent peripheral generator is arising from damaged nerve tissue.

CONCLUSION

Pain and nociception are related but different events. The neural events leading to pain usually involve activation of nociceptors innervating a threatened or damaged tissue. Once activated, nociceptors transmit information to the spinal cord for processing and may also participate in the generation of the inflammatory reaction. The response properties of nociceptors are plastic, and they can become sensitized by continued stimulation. This sensitization also occurs in the central nervous system, evidenced by the development of windup and LTP. Several mechanisms in the central nervous system can suppress pain transmission. These have been best studied at the level of the spinal cord, although similar mechanisms probably exist at higher levels, such as the thalamus. The high degree of convergence of nociceptors from various parts of the body on projection neurons in the spinal cord provides a substrate for referred pain. Additionally, axon reflexes from nociceptive neurons are capable of producing neurogenic inflammation in tissues that are not involved in the initial injury. The neural basis for the affective (emotional) components of pain and suffering are localized to the frontal lobes, in areas known to be affected in depression and anxiety disorders. This is the physiologic substrate for the common and complex clinical interaction between pain and mood.

Review *Questions*

1. What is the difference between pain and nociception?
2. What is the conduction velocity of the neurons that subserve nociception?
3. What is an axon reflex? How is it related to neurogenic inflammation?
4. Where are nociceptors located?
5. Damage to nociceptor axons leads to what anatomic changes?
6. To what levels of the spinal cord can a C-fiber nociceptor projecting through the L4 dorsal root project?
7. What is a possible clinical effect of long-term potentiation?
8. Describe the nervi nervorum.
9. What nociceptors are likely to be activated during a positive straight-leg raise?
10. How can light brushing cause pain?

Concept *Questions*

1. A local herbalist gives you a poultice that he claims reduces the pain of sprains. You use it on the next patient that you see and not only does the patient report less pain within 30 minutes but also you observe that local redness and swelling are reduced. Being familiar with nociceptor physiology, you think that it may be affecting them directly. How would you investigate your hypothesis?
2. A patient presents with bilateral foot pain. The symptoms started on the right; after an exacerbation 2 weeks ago, the left side also started hurting. Your examination indicates a biomechanical lesion on the right, but a normal left foot, although it is somewhat tender to palpation. You make a diagnosis of right plantar fasciitis. Why does the patient have symptoms on the left? Do you treat the left foot?

REFERENCES

1. Merskey H, Bogduk N: *Classification of chronic pain*, Seattle, 1994, IASP.
2. Carew TJ et al: Classical conditioning in a simple withdrawal reflex in Aplysia californica, *J Neurosci* 1(12):1426, 1981.
3. Lawson SN: Phenotype and function of somatic primary afferent nociceptive neurones with C-, A delta- or A alpha/beta-fibres, *Exp Physiol* 87(2):239, 2002.
4. Duclaux R et al: Conduction velocity along the afferent vagal dendrites: a new type of fiber, *J Physiol* 260(2):487, 1976.
5. Morrison JFB: Splanchnic slowly adapting mechanoreceptors with punctate receptive fields in the mesentery and gastrointestinal tract of the cat, *J Physiol* 233:349, 1973.
6. Cervero F: Sensory innervation of the viscera: peripheral basis of visceral pain, *Physiol Rev* 74:95, 1994.
7. Kumazawa T: Functions of the nociceptive primary neurons, *Jpn J Physiol* 40(1):1, 1990.
8. Mense S: Nociception from skeletal muscle in relation to clinical pain, *Pain* 54:241, 1993.
9. Schaible HG, Grubb BD: Afferent and spinal mechanisms of joint pain, *Pain* 55:5, 1993.
10. Bove GM, Light AR: Unmyelinated nociceptors of rat paraspinal tissues, *J Neurophysiol* 73:1752, 1995.
11. Bazett HC, McGlone B: Note on the pain sensations which accompany deep punctures, *Brain* 51:18, 1928.
12. Cavanaugh JM et al: Sensory innervation of the soft tissues of the lumbar spine of the rat, *J Orthop Res* 7:378, 1989.
13. El-Bohy A et al: Localization of substance P and neurofilament immunoreactive fibers in the lumbar facet joint capsule and supraspinous ligament of the rabbit, *Brain Res* 460:379, 1988.
14. Giles LG et al: Human zygapophyseal joint synovial folds, *Acta Anat* 126:110, 1986.
15. Giles LG, Harvey AR: Immunohistological demonstration of nociceptors in the capsule and synovial folds

of human zygapophyseal joints, *Br J Rheumatol* 26: 362, 1987.

16. Giles LG, Taylor JR: Intra-articular synovial protrusions in the lower lumbar apophyseal joints, *Bull Hosp Jt Dis Orthop Inst* 42:248, 1982.

17. Yamashita T et al: Mechanosensitive afferent units in the lumbar facet joint, *J Bone Joint Surg* 72-A:865, 1990.

18. Lundberg LE et al: Intra-neural electrical stimulation of cutaneous nociceptive fibres in humans: effects of different pulse patterns on magnitude of pain, *Acta Physiol Scand* 146:41, 1992.

19. Reeh P: Chemical excitation and sensitization of nociceptors. In Urban L, editor: *Cellular mechanisms of sensory processing*, Berlin, 1994, Springer-Verlag.

20. Handwerker HO, Reeh PW: Nociceptors in animals. In Besson JM et al, editors: *Peripheral neurons in nociception: physiopharmacological aspects*, Paris, 1994, John Libbey Eurotext.

21. Watkins LR et al: Mechanisms of tumor necrosis factor-alpha (TNF-alpha) hyperalgesia, *Brain Res* 692(1-2):244, 1995.

22. Leem JG, Bove GM: Mid-axonal tumor necrosis factor-alpha induces ectopic activity in a subset of slowly conducting cutaneous and deep afferent neurons, *J Pain* 3(1):45, 2002.

23. Sorkin LS, Doom CM: Epineurial application of TNF elicits an acute mechanical hyperalgesia in the awake rat, *J Peripher Nerv Syst* 5(2):96, 2000.

24. Perl ER et al: Sensitization of high threshold receptors with unmyelinated (C) afferent fibers, *Prog Brain Res* 43:263, 1976.

25. Sanjue H, Jun Z: Sympathetic facilitation of sustained discharge of polymodal nociceptors, *Pain* 38:85, 1989.

26. Koltzenburg M et al: The nociceptor sensitization by bradykinin does not depend on sympathetic neurons, *Neuroscience* 46:465, 1992.

27. Shea VK, Perl ER: Failure of sympathetic stimulation to affect responsiveness of rabbit polymodal nociceptors, *J Neurophysiol* 54(3):513, 1985.

28. Barasi S, Lynn B: Effects of sympathetic stimulation on mechanoreceptive and nociceptive afferent units from the rabbit pinna, *Brain Res* 378:21, 1986.

29. Devor M, Jänig W: Activation of myelinated afferents ending in a neuroma by stimulation of the sympathetic supply in the rat, *Neurosci Lett* 24:43, 1981.

30. Sato J, Perl ER: Adrenergic excitation of cutaneous pain receptors induced by peripheral nerve injury, *Science* 251:1608, 1991.

31. Koltzenburg M et al: Receptive properties of nociceptors in a peripheral neuropathy, *Soc Neurosci Abstr* 19:325, 1993.

32. Sato J et al: Adrenergic excitation of cutaneous nociceptors in chronically inflamed rats, *Neurosci Lett* 164:225, 1993.

33. Bossut DF, Perl ER: Effects of nerve injury on sympathetic excitation of a delta mechanical nociceptors, *J Neurophysiol* 73(4):1721, 1995.

34. Cannon WB: *Bodily changes in pain, hunger, fear, and rage*, New York, 1929, D. Appleton.

35. Ecker A: Norepinephrine in reflex sympathetic dystrophy: an hypothesis, *Clin J Pain* 5:313, 1989.

36. Selye H: The general adaptation syndrome and diseases of adaptation. In Karsner HT, Sanford AH, editors: *The 1950 year book of pathology and clinical pathology*, Chicago, 1950, Year Book Publishers.

37. Bayliss WM: On the origin from the spinal cord of the vaso-dilator fibers of the hind limb, and on the nature of these fibers, *J Physiol Lond* 26:173, 1900.

38. Lewis T: The nocifensor system of nerves and its reactions, *BMJ* 1:431, 491, 1937.

39. Kenins P: Identification of the unmyelinated sensory nerves which evoke plasma extravasation in response to antidromic stimulation, *Neurosci Lett* 25:137, 1981.

40. Alvarez FJ et al: Presence of calcitonin gene-related peptide (CGRP) and substance P (SP) immunoreactivity in intraepidermal free nerve endings of cat skin, *Brain Res* 442:391, 1988.

41. Gulbenkian S et al: Ultrastructural evidence for the coexistence of calcitonin gene-related peptide and substance P in secretory vesicles of peripheral nerves in the guinea pig, *J Neurocytol* 15:535, 1986.

42. Gibbins IL et al: Co-localization of calcitonin gene-related peptide-like immunoreactivity with substance P in cutaneous, vascular and visceral sensory neurons of guinea pigs, *Neurosci Lett* 57:125, 1985.

43. Brain SD et al: Potent vasodilator activity of calcitonin gene-related peptide in human skin, *J Invest Dermatol* 87:533, 1986.

44. Holzer P: Peptidergic sensory neurons in the control of vascular functions: mechanisms and significance in the cutaneous and splanchnic beds, *Rev Physiol Biochem Pharmacol* 121:49, 1992.

45. Kenins P et al: The role of substance P in the axon reflex in the rat, *Br J Derm* 111:551, 1984.

46. LeGreves P et al: Calcitonin gene-related peptide is a potent inhibitor of substance P degradation, *Eur J Pharmacol* 115:309, 1985.

47. Ishida-Yamamoto A, Tohyama M: Calcitonin gene-related peptide in the nervous tissue, *Prog Neurobiol* 33:335, 1989.

48. Uddman R et al: Calcitonin gene-related peptide (CGRP): perivascular distribution and vasodilatory effects, *Regul Pept* 15:1, 1986.

49. Cohen RH, Perl ER: Contributions of arachidonic acid derivatives and substance P to the sensitization of cutaneous nociceptors, *J Neurophysiol* 64:457, 1990.

50. Mantyh PW: Substance P and the inflammatory and immune response, *Ann N Y Acad Sci* 632:263, 1991.

51. Rees H et al: Do dorsal root reflexes augment peripheral inflammation? *Neuroreport* 5:821, 1994.

52. Levine JD et al: Contribution of sensory afferents and sympathetic efferents to joint injury in experimental arthritis, *J Neurosci* 6:3423, 1986.

53. Weber JR et al: The trigeminal nerve augments regional cerebral blood flow during experimental bacterial meningitis, *J Cereb Blood Flow Metab* 16:1319, 1996.

54. Wall PD, Woolf CJ: Muscle but not cutaneous C-afferent input produces prolonged increases in the excitability of the flexion reflex in the rat, *J Physiol* 356:443, 1984.

55. Bove GM et al: Neuritis induces ectopic mechanical sensitivity in nociceptor axons with deep but not cutaneous receptive fields, *Soc Neurosci Abstr* 27:928.3, 2001.

56. Li L et al. Effect of lumbar 5 ventral root transection on pain behaviors: a novel rat model for neuropathic pain without axotomy of primary sensory neurons, *Exp Neurol* 175(1):23, 2002.

57. Michaelis M et al: Axotomized and intact muscle afferents but no skin afferents develop ongoing discharges of dorsal root ganglion origin after peripheral nerve lesion, *J Neurosci* 20(7):2742, 2000.

58. Cameron AA et al: Evidence that fine primary afferent axons innervate a wider territory in the superficial dorsal horn following peripheral axotomy, *Brain Res* 575:151, 1992.

59. Woolf CJ et al: Peripheral nerve injury triggers central sprouting of myelinated afferents, *Nature* 355:75, 1992.

60. Campbell JN et al: Myelinated afferents signal the hyperalgesia associated with nerve injury, *Pain* 32:89, 1988.

61. Price DD et al: Psychophysiological observations on patients with neuropathic pain relieved by a sympathetic block, *Pain* 36:273, 1989.

62. Light AR: Normal anatomy and physiology of the spinal cord dorsal horn, *Appl Neurophysiol* 51:78, 1988.

63. Sugiura Y et al: Central projections of identified, unmyelinated (C) afferent fibers innervating mammalian skin, *Science* 234:358, 1986.

64. Light AR, Perl ER: Spinal termination of functionally identified primary afferent neurons with slowly conducting myelinated fibers, *J Comp Neurol* 186:133, 1979.

65. Gillette RG et al: Characterization of spinal somatosensory neurons having receptive fields in lumbar tissues of cats, *Pain* 54:85, 1993.

66. Gillette RG et al: Spinal projections of cat primary afferent fibers innervating lumbar facet joints and multifidus muscle, *Neurosci Lett* 157:67, 1993.

67. Bullitt E: Somatotopy of spinal nociceptive processing, *J Comp Neurol* 312:279, 1991.

68. Bullitt E: Induction of c-fos-like protein within the lumbar spinal cord and thalamus of the rat following peripheral stimulation, *Brain Res* 493:391, 1989.

69. Menétrey D et al: Expression of c-fos protein in interneurons and projection neurons of the rat spinal cord in response to noxious somatic, articular, and visceral stimulation, *J Comp Neurol* 285:177, 1989.

70. Iadorola MJ et al: Enhancement of dynorphin gene expression in spinal cord following experimental inflammation: stimulus specificity, behavioral parameters and opioid receptor binding, *Pain* 35:313, 1988.

71. Hylden JLK et al: Effects of spinal kappa-opioid receptor agonists on the responsiveness of nociceptive superficial dorsal horn neurons, *Pain* 44:187, 1991.

72. Waxman SG et al: Sodium channels and pain, *Proc Nat Acad Sci USA* 96(14):7635, 1999.

73. Akopian AN et al: The tetrodotoxin-resistant sodium channel SNS has a specialized function in pain pathways, *Nature Neurosci* 2(6):541, 1999.

74. Matzner O, Devor M: Hyperexcitability at sites of nerve injury depends on voltage-sensitive Na+ channels, *J Neurophysiol* 72(1):349, 1994.

75. Novakovic SD et al: Distribution of the tetrodotoxin-resistant sodium channel PN3 in rat sensory neurons in normal and neuropathic conditions, *J Neurosci* 18(6):2174, 1998.

76. Tanaka M et al: SNS Na+ channel expression increases in dorsal root ganglion neurons in the carrageenan inflammatory pain model, *Neuro Rep* 9(6):967, 1998.

77. Koschorke GM et al: Ectopic excitability of injured nerves in monkey: entrained responses to vibratory stimuli, *J Neurophysiol* 65(3):693, 1991.

78. Koschorke GM et al: Cellular components necessary for mechanoelectrical transduction are conveyed to primary afferent terminals by fast axonal transport, *Brain Res* 641(1):99, 1994.

79. Adriaensen H et al: Nociceptor discharges and sensations due to noxious mechanical stimulation—a paradox, *Hum Neurobiol* 3:53, 1984.

80. Coderre TJ et al: Contribution of central neuroplasticity to pathological pain: review of clinical and experimental evidence, *Pain* 52(3):259, 1993.

81. Woolf CJ: Recent advances in the pathophysiology of acute pain, *Br J Anaesth* 63:139, 1989.

82. Chen R et al: Nervous system reorganization following injury. *Neuroscience* 111(4):761, 2002.

83. Pockett S: Spinal cord synaptic plasticity and chronic pain, *Anesth Analg* 80(1):173, 1995.

84. Mendell LM: Physiological properties of unmyelinated fiber projection to the spinal cord, *Exp Neurol* 16:316, 1966.

85. Randic M et al: Long-term potentiation and long-term depression of primary afferent neurotransmission in the rat spinal cord, *J Neurosci* 13:5228, 1993.

86. Bliss TVP, Collingridge GL: A synaptic model of memory: long-term potentiation in the hippocampus, *Nature* 361:31, 1993.

87. Hunt JL et al: Repeated injury to the lumbar nerve roots produces enhanced mechanical allodynia and persistent spinal neuroinflammation, *Spine* 26(19):2073, 2001.

88. DeLeo JA, Yezierski RP: The role of neuroinflammation and neuroimmune activation in persistent pain, *Pain* 90(1-2):1, 2001.

89. Watkins LR, Maier SF: The pain of being sick: implications of immune-to-brain communication for understanding pain, *Ann Rev Psychol* 51:29, 2000.

90. Sandkuhler J: The organization and function of endogenous antinociceptive systems, *Prog Neurobiol* 50(1):49, 1996.

91. Fields HL, Basbaum AI: Central nervous system mechanisms of pain modulation. In Wall PD, Melzack R, editors: *Textbook of pain*, New York, 1994, Churchill Livingstone.

92. Malcangio M, Bowery NG: GABA and its receptors in the spinal cord, *Trends Pharmacol Sci* 17(12):457, 1996.

93. Lundeberg T et al: Pain alleviation by vibratory stimulation, *Pain* 20(1):25, 1984.

94. Dickenson AH et al: The pharmacology of excitatory and inhibitory amino acid-mediated events in the transmission and modulation of pain in the spinal cord. [Review], *Gen Pharmacol* 28(5):633, 1997.

95. Indahl A et al: Interaction between the porcine lumbar intervertebral disc, zygapophysial joints, and paraspinal muscles, *Spine* 22(24):2834, 1997.

96. Rainville P: Brain mechanisms of pain affect and pain modulation, *Curr Opin Neurobiol* 12(2):195, 2002.

97. Rainville P et al: Pain affect encoded in human anterior cingulate but not somatosensory cortex, *Science* 277(5328):968, 1997.

98. Wallis BJ et al: Resolution of psychological distress of whiplash patients following treatment by radiofrequency neurotomy: a randomised, double-blind, placebo-controlled trial, *Pain* 73(1):15, 1997.

99. ter Riet G et al: Is placebo analgesia mediated by endogenous opioids? A systematic review, *Pain* 76(3):273, 1998.

100. Garfin SR et al: Compressive neuropathy of spinal nerve roots: a compressive or biological problem? *Spine* 16:162, 1991.

101. Olmarker K, Larsson K: Tumor necrosis factor-alpha and nucleus-pulposus-induced nerve root injury, *Spine* 23(23):2538, 1998.

102. Sunderland S: *Nerve injuries and their repair*, Edinburgh, 1991, Churchill Livingstone.

103. Song XJ et al: Mechanical and thermal hyperalgesia and ectopic neuronal discharge after chronic compression of dorsal root ganglia, *J Neurophysiol* 82(6):3347, 1999.

104. Homma Y et al: A comparison of chronic pain behavior following local application of tumor necrosis factor-alpha to the normal and mechanically compressed lumbar ganglia in the rat, *Pain* 95(3):239, 2002.

105. Lundeberg T, Ekholm J: Pain—from periphery to brain, *Disabil Rehabil* 24(8):402, 2002.

106. Steen KH et al: A dominant role of acid pH in inflammatory excitation and sensitization of nociceptors in rat skin, in vitro, *J Neurosci* 15:3982, 1995.

107. Gracely RH et al: Painful neuropathy: altered central processing maintained dynamically by peripheral input, *Pain* 51:175, 1992.

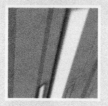

PART THREE

SPINAL ANALYSIS AND DIAGNOSTIC PROCEDURES

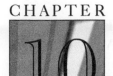

Palpation: The Art of Manual Assessment

John G. Scaringe, DC, DACBSP, Leonard John Faye, DC

Key Terms

ACCESSORY JOINT MOVEMENT	END-PLAY ZONE	ORTHOGONAL
ACCESSORY MOTION	FIXATION	ORTHOPEDIC SUBLUXATION
ACTIVE MOTION	HYPERMOBILE	OSTEOPATHIC LESION
ADJUSTIVE LESION	HYPERMOBILITY	PARTS
ALGOMETRY	HYPERTONIC	PASSIVE MOVEMENTS
ANATOMIC BARRIER	HYPOMOBILE	PATHOLOGIC BARRIER
ANKYLOSIS	INSPECTION	PHYSIOLOGIC BARRIER
ANTALGIC	JOINT DYSFUNCTION	PINCER PALPATION
AUSCULTATION	JOINT FIXATION	SOMATIC DYSFUNCTIONS
CHIROPRACTIC SUBLUXATION	(RESTRICTION)	SPRINGY END FEEL
DYNAMIC PALPATION	JOINT PLAY	STATIC PALPATION
EFFUSION	LAYER PALPATION	TACTILE PALPATION
END PLAY	LINE OF DRIVE	TENDERNESS
	MOTION PALPATION	TRIGGER POINTS

Palpation is a cornerstone of manual adjusting procedures. Many hours of practice and concentration are necessary to master this art. Manual palpation is the chiropractor's primary evaluative intervention and is used in combination with other diagnostic methods of chiropractic case management. The very core of adjusting lies in the ability to identify contact landmarks, contracted muscles, inflammation, restrictions of movement, and hard end-feel resistance. This chapter describes different forms of palpation and the best methods of learning these skills.

Aside from its unsurpassed value in enabling the chiropractor to determine the most advantageous adjustive strategies, palpation can serve as a powerful doctor-patient communication tool, helping the patient understand the importance of following through on a recommended treatment plan. Patients can feel pain and resistance as the chiropractor palpates. In response to chiropractic care, patients feel diminished pain and restriction, *often before their symptoms abate*. Through skilled palpation, the focus subtly shifts away from an overemphasis on symptoms toward awareness of the changes the chiropractor is palpating and monitoring from one office visit to the next.

The reliability of palpating landmarks and decreased range of motion is not on a par with reading a thermometer, but it is comparable to cardiac auscultation and the reading of radiographs.[1-5] Quantifying a manual art is difficult because of the lack of a standard for comparison. Palpation is a skill that develops over time and must be nurtured. Tissues become warm, muscles atrophy and or go into spasm, joints block or become **hypermobile,** and *these conditions can be felt.* How well the chiropractor will be able to feel them depends on how seriously he or she chooses to practice the various palpation procedures described in this chapter.

IDENTIFYING THE ADJUSTIVE/ MANIPULATIVE LESION

All professions that perform adjustment/ manipulation involving the spine, an extremity, or both, describe the same phenomenon, using different nomenclature (Box 10-1). Traditionally,

Box **10-1**   DEFINITION OF TERMS DESCRIBING FUNCTIONAL OR STRUCTURAL DISORDERS OF THE SYNOVIAL JOINTS

Orthopedic subluxation: Partial or incomplete dislocation

Chiropractic subluxation: Aberrant relationship between two adjacent structures that may have functional or pathologic sequelae

Joint dysfunction: Joint mechanics showing functional disturbances without structural changes

Somatic dysfunction: Impaired or altered function or related components of the body framework (somatic system)

Osteopathic lesion: Disturbance of musculoskeletal structure, function, or both, as well as accompanying disturbances of other biologic mechanisms

Joint fixation (restriction): Temporary immobilization of a joint in a position that it may normally occupy during any phase of normal movement

Adapted from Peterson DH, Bergmann TF: *Chiropractic technique: principles and procedures*, ed 2, St Louis, 2002, Mosby.

chiropractors have used the term *subluxation complex* to encompass all the mechanical, inflammatory, and neurobiologic components of this neuromusculoskeletal entity. The adjustive/manipulative lesion is the component to which chiropractic techniques are applied so as to impose a demand for increased function. When this procedure is successful, the body responds by restoring function to the joints adjusted. From this perspective, a dysfunction of the joint is involved, not a "bone out of place" misalignment. It is true that joints that regain movement can change their resting position, but an important point to recognize is that adjustment affects the joint's ability to function in all its ranges of motion. Enhanced function changes the neurobiologic mechanisms and leads to the reduction of the inflammatory process. For these reasons, to identify when, where, why, and how often to adjust a patient, chiropractors need to be able to work with the following procedures and feel what is occurring specifically in each patient.

COMPONENTS OF THE ADJUSTIVE/MANIPULATIVE LESION

As with other aspects of patient examination, the doctor of chiropractic uses observation, palpation, percussion, and auscultation when identifying the adjustive/manipulative *lesion*. Using the acronym *PARTS* modified from the osteopathic profession to identify **somatic dysfunctions**,[6,7] Bergmann and Finer[8] describe five diagnostic criteria (**P**ain and tenderness; **A**symmetry; **R**ange-of-motion abnormality; **T**issue tone, texture, and temperature abnormality; and **S**pecial tests) for identifying joint subluxation or dysfunction.

Pain and Tenderness

Pain is the localized sensation of discomfort, distress, or agony reported by an individual.[9] By contrast, **tenderness** is defined as abnormal sensitivity to touch or pressure.[9] Although these reports are *subjective signs*, a skilled and experienced doctor can feel the tissue changes that correspond with patients' feeling pain and tenderness. Identifying whether the pain lingers after the pressure of palpation is removed is significant. Pressure over inflamed tissues causes a lingering pain. Pressure and challenging the end resistance of a dysfunctional but noninflamed joint will hurt only while the pressure is applied. As a general rule, inflamed joints should not be adjusted until the inflammation has subsided and the postinflammatory pattern of **joint dysfunction** has appeared. Pain can occur with *vibration*, such as placing a tuning fork over a bone fracture. *Traction* and *compression* can elicit pain that is mild at rest; once again, whether it lingers is significant. The chiropractor can use various reliable and valid tools to measure and quantify pain. These tools include self-administered pain and functional questionnaires, **algometry** (the measurement of pressure or painful stimuli) visual analog scales (VAS), pain scales, pain diagrams, and pain drawings.

Asymmetry

Antalgic (leaning to avoid pain) and asymmetric postures are common in acute presentations but are often within normal limits in mildly symptomatic patients. Therefore asymmetries and misalignments can occur on a segmental or a regional level. Observation of posture and gait often shows a gross distortion of the patients' pelvis, spinal column, shoulders, knees, feet, and ankles. The forward displacement of a lumbar *spondylolisthesis* will be observed and palpated as a dimple *(step defect)*, with the patient in a side-lying position. The spine is not normally perfectly symmetrical, and the chiropractor is unlikely to be able to palpate a displacement of a few millimeters based on the location of the spinous processes. As the spinal connective tissues degenerate, the resulting displacement is visualized on x-rays and other diagnostic imaging methods by placing patients in full flexion and extension suggestive of excessive intersegmental movement **(hypermobility)** or instabilities.

Range of Motion

Gross range of joint motion can be measured by using an inclinometer, protractor, ruler, plumb line, and various computerized methods. Ultrasound and motion x-ray studies have been used to observe and measure the complex intersegmental movement of spinal and extremity joints. Various systems of **motion palpation** have been described, and until an article by Marcotte and colleagues,[10] interexaminer reliability has been a major concern. Joints move, and the chiropractor can palpate that movement, but agreeing on which joints are not moving fully and by what degree of dysfunction has been a challenge. Many chiropractors use motion palpation to determine the joints to be adjusted and the **line of drive** (direction of dynamic thrust) they introduce into the joint complex. Other chiropractors simply use these records of the ranges of joint motion for evaluating a patient's progress.

Active gross movement (the range-of-joint motion possible through the patient's voluntary effort) is tested first. *Passive gross movement* is then tested, with the doctor pressing the range a little further. Accessory joint movements are tested at the end of the passive range of motion by springing further to see if a little elasticity is present, called the **springy end feel.** Intersegmental motion of spinal joints is well described in texts on biomechanics. The goal for all doctors of chiropractic is to be able to assess these rotations around the **orthogonal** axes to determine the correct adjustments to restore normal active, passive, and joint play movement. Many chiropractors use motion palpation to determine the specificity of the thrust into the directions of resisted end feel in a spinal motion unit or extremity joint. This procedure is demonstrated later in this chapter.

Tissue Tone, Texture, and Temperature

Tissue tone is determined by palpation, observation, instrumentation, and tests for the length and strength of muscles. The doctor should be able to palpate nodules to determine if they are loose or attached to bone, ligament, or tendon. In some areas, nerves are palpable, such as the ulnar nerve in the forearm. Classical diagnosis considers the liver palpable when it is enlarged, as are the lymph nodes, arterial pulses, and some hernias. The biceps tendon can be palpated when it slips out of the biceps groove of the humerus.

None of these skills are natural to a student, and perseverance is needed to become a professional. Soft, skillful hands convey an important sense of confidence to a patient, which promotes relaxation and minimizes guarding resistance to being adjusted. Short or **hypertonic** muscles will restrict the joint motion of the agonist, and these shortened antagonists will often be full of palpable nodules that need specific treatment before normal, active ranges of motion can be attained. A hamstring or quadriceps can feel similar to a ridged washboard because of these adhesions from past tears. Tissue swelling is easy to visualize, but by using palpation, the doctor can determine whether pitting edema is present. The fluids drawn into the legs by gravity in certain heart and kidney diseases causes pitting after pressure is applied. Joint **effusion** is a tight swelling and is quite painful when tested for pitting. Palpation of the deep muscles in the neck will often reveal a knotted feeling in the specific muscle responsible for a patient's cervicogenic headache (see Chapter 24). These very common headaches often disappear when corrected by joint adjustment/ manipulation and soft tissue procedures targeted at the chronic muscle spasm that has been identified through skilled palpation. Identifying normal and abnormal tissue characteristics is an art worth practicing and mastering.

Special Tests

Special tests include additional physical examination, laboratory procedures, or both, which aid in the differential diagnosis of joint dysfunction. Examples include orthopedic and neurologic tests, diagnostic imaging procedures, blood and urine testing, and electrodiagnosis. Testing procedures specific to a technique system, such as leg-length assessment, specific radiographic marking techniques, and particular muscle testing procedures, should also be considered.

DEFINITION AND CLASSIFICATION OF PALPATION PROCEDURES

Inspection, auscultation, and palpation are the three basic diagnostic methods used in conventional clinical medicine.[11] However, in an age of rapidly advancing technology with sophisticated diagnostic and laboratory equipment, palpation is underused in conventional medicine and is slowly becoming a lost art. To the contrary, palpation is recognized as an essential skill by chiropractors, osteopaths who use manipulation, and physical and manual therapists and is the most important tool that doctors of chiropractic can use to identify the manipulative/adjustive lesion. An important point to note is that, after a well-executed history, palpation provides the first direct physical contact with the patient.[12] The quality of this contact may strengthen existing trust or nullify positive rapport established between clinician and patient.

The foundations of palpatory literacy are knowledge of anatomy (cognitive) and the acute ability to touch and feel (psychomotor)[12] (Box 10-2). Although anatomic knowledge is primarily cognitive in nature, the development of psychomotor skill is a complex phenomenon that must be obtained by experience and practice. Thus developing good palpation skills requires many hours of practice and concentration. The skillful palpator who develops both tactile and kinesthetic sensation will also find the art of adjustment/manipulation easier to master.

Palpation procedures are commonly divided into static and dynamic assessments (Box 10-3). Static palpation is usually performed with the patient in a stationary position and includes bony (joint structures) and soft tissue assess-

---

Box **10-2**   STATIC PALPATION TIPS

1. Use the least pressure possible. (Touch receptors are designed to respond only when not pressed too firmly.)
2. Concentrate on the area, structure, or both, which are to be palpated.
3. Try not to cause pain if possible. (Pain may induce protective muscle splinting and make palpation more difficult.)
4. Carefully penetrate to deeper structures. (Brisk progress may induce reflex muscle spasm.)
5. Try not to lose skin contact before completing the palpation of the area.
6. Use broad contacts whenever possible.
7. Close sight to increase palpatory perception.

Modified from Peterson DH, Bergmann TF: *Chiropractic technique: principles and procedures*, ed 2, St Louis, 2002, Mosby.

Box **10-3**   TYPES OF PALPATION

Static palpation
  Bony
  Soft tissue
Dynamic (motion) palpation
  Active
  Passive
    Joint play
    End play (end feel)
    Accessory

ment. **Dynamic palpation,** or motion palpation, is commonly performed to assess abnormal vertebral or extremity joint motion and is performed with the patient in a variety of positions.[13-18]

Static Palpation

Static palpation of bony landmarks of the spine and pelvis includes assessment of spinous, transverse, and mammillary processes of the vertebrae and of the posterior superior iliac spine (PSIS), ischial tuberosities, and iliac crest contours of the innominate bones. Bony landmarks such as femoral condyles, olecranon processes, and greater trochanters are examples of bony landmarks commonly palpated around extremity joints. The evaluator should note any asymmetries or anomalies while keeping in mind that positional faults are unreliable and should be confirmed with additional evaluation procedures.

Palpatory tenderness has been shown to be a reliable method for identifying the **adjustive lesion.**[19-23] However, a difference exists between palpation of pain and tenderness and tactile palpation. **Tactile palpation** provides thermal and mechanical information that aids in structural assessment and may correlate with previous examination and historical findings. Tenderness palpation, on the other hand, may help distinguish healthy from unhealthy tissues.[12] Healthy tissues can usually tolerate greater pressure than can injured or diseased tissues. In the absence of a destructive lesion, these tissue changes are important indicators of joint subluxation or dysfunction that may respond to manual treatment procedures.

Layer palpation is a systemic method of assessing the mobility and condition of myofascial and other soft tissue structures.[24] Palpation begins with the most superficial structures and proceeds to deeper tissues. Light palpation with the pads of the fingers is used to assess superficial tissues (Fig. 10-1). Deeper structures require increased pressure and should be performed in a firm but gentle manner. Anatomic landmarks commonly palpated are listed in Table 10-1.

On palpating the paraspinal tissues and myofascial structures of the extremities, areas of

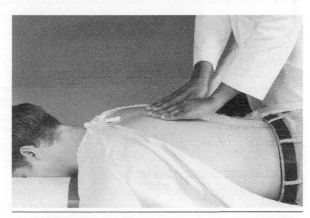

Fig. 10-1 Light palpation with the pads of the fingers over the transverse processes of the thoracic spine.

Table **10-1** SURFACE ANATOMY AND OSSEOUS LANDMARKS OF SPINE AND PELVIS

Landmark	How to Locate	Clinical Significance
CERVICAL SPINE		
EOP	*Posterior.* Midline projection of posterior aspect of skull at junction of head and neck.	Used as a reference landmark. Adjustive contact points lateral to EOP are commonly used with occipital (C0-C1) dysfunctions (subluxations).
C2 spinous process	*Posterior.* First bony point palpated in midline inferior to EOP.	Commonly used as an adjustive contact point and reference land mark. Tender with spinal fractures, infections, sprain or strains, neoplasia, and dysfunctions (subluxations).

Continued

Table **10-1**   SURFACE ANATOMY AND OSSEOUS LANDMARKS OF SPINE AND PELVIS—CONT'D

Landmark	How to Locate	Clinical Significance
CERVICAL SPINE—cont'd		
C6 spinous process	*Posterior.* Moves (anteriorly) away from palpating finger during cer-vical extension; easily palpated in cervical flexion.	Commonly used as an adjustive contact point and reference landmark. Tender with spinal fractures, infections, sprain or strains, neoplasia, and dysfunctions (subluxations).
C7 spinous process	*Posterior.* Most prominent spinous process in this region (T1 may be the most prominent in some individuals); C7 moves on T1 during cervical flexion and extension; C7 palpated throughout cervical flexion and extension.	Commonly used as an adjustive contact point and reference land-mark. Tender with spinal fractures, infections, sprain or strains, neoplasia, and dysfunctions (subluxations).
Cervical facet joints	*Posterior.* Palpated 1.5-2.0 cm lateral to spinous process.	Commonly used as an adjustive contact point. Soft tissues over these areas are commonly tender to palpation with facet joint sprains or strains, and dysfunctions (subluxations).
C1 transverse process	*Lateral.* Palpated between mastoid process (prominence of temporal bone posterior to ear) and angles of the jaw.	Used as an adjustive contact point. Tender with common conditions such as spinal dysfunctions (subluxations), sprains or strains, and postural syndromes.
THORACIC SPINE AND RIBS		
T1 spinous process	*Posterior.* May be most prominent spinous process in this region; C7 moves on T1 during cervical flexion and extension; also located at the level of acromioclavicular joint.	Commonly used as an adjustive contact point and reference landmark. Tender with spinal fractures, infections, sprain or strains, neoplasia, and dysfunctions (subluxations).
T3 spinous process	*Posterior.* Lies at the middle of a line drawn between medial aspects of spine of scapulae.	Commonly used as an adjustive contact point and reference landmark. Tender with spinal fractures, infections, sprain or strains, neoplasia, and dysfunctions (subluxations).
T7-T8 spinous process	*Posterior.* Lies at the middle of a line drawn between inferior borders of scapulae.	Commonly used as an adjustive contact point and reference landmark. Tender with spinal fractures, infections, sprain or strains, neoplasia, and dysfunctions (subluxations).

Table **10-1**   SURFACE ANATOMY AND OSSEOUS LANDMARKS OF SPINE AND PELVIS—CONT'D

Landmark	How to Locate	Clinical Significance
THORACIC SPINE AND RIBS—cont'd		
T1-T4 transverse process	*Posterior.* Palpated one interspinous space above spinous process lateral to midline.	Commonly used as an adjustive contact point and reference landmark. Tender with spinal fractures, infections, sprain or strains, neoplasia, and dysfunctions (subluxations).
T5-T8 transverse process	*Posterior.* Palpated two interspinous spaces above spinous process lateral to midline.	Commonly used as an adjustive contact point and reference landmark. Tender with spinal fractures, infections, sprain or strains, neoplasia, and dysfunctions (subluxations).
T9-T12 transverse process	*Posterior.* Palpated one interspinous space above spinous process lateral to midline.	Commonly used as an adjustive contact point and reference landmark. Tender with spinal fractures, infections, sprain or strains, neoplasia, and dysfunctions (subluxations).
Second rib	*Posterior.* Palpated at superior border of scapula.	Serves as a reference landmark.
Seventh rib	*Posterior.* Palpated at inferior border of scapula.	Serves as a reference landmark.
LUMBAR SPINE AND PELVIS		
L4 spinous process	*Posterior.* Lies at the middle of a line drawn between the highest points of iliac crests.	Commonly used as an adjustive contact point and reference landmark. Tender with spinal fractures, infections, sprain or strains, neoplasia, and dysfunctions (subluxations).
L4-L5 intervertebral disk	*Posterior.* Lies at the middle of a line drawn between the highest points of iliac crests.	Serves as a reference landmark. Soft tissues over this area are tender to palpation with intervertebral disk injury and syndromes.
Lumbar facet joints	*Posterior.* Palpated one interspinous space above spinous process and lateral approximately 1-1$\frac{1}{2}$ in.	Commonly used as an adjustive contact point. Soft tissues over these areas are commonly tender to palpation with facet joint sprains or strains, and dysfunctions.
S2 spinous process (sacral tubercle)	*Posterior.* Lies at the middle of a line drawn between PSIS.	Serves as a reference landmark and as a contact point for adjustments.
PSIS	*Posterior.* Skin dimples superior and lateral (approximately 4 cm from midline) to intergluteal cleft.	Commonly used as a reference landmark and as a contact point for sacroiliac adjustments. Tender to palpation with sacroiliac dysfunctions (subluxations) and sprains.

EOP, External occipital protuberance; *PSIS,* posterior superior iliac spine; *ASIS,* anterior superior iliac spine.

Continued

Table **10-1** SURFACE ANATOMY AND OSSEOUS LANDMARKS OF SPINE AND PELVIS—CONT'D

Landmark	How to Locate	Clinical Significance
LUMBAR SPINE AND PELVIS—cont'd		
Tip of coccyx	*Posterior.* Lies at the middle of a line drawn between ischial tuberosities (approximately 2.5 cm postero-superior to anus).	Tender with fractures, sprains, and dysfunctions (subluxation) of the coccyx.
Ischial tuberosity	*Posterior.* Palpated in the inferior part of buttock when hip is flexed.	Commonly used as a contact point for sacroiliac adjustments. Tender to palpation with conditions such as apophyseal injuries, fractures, bursitis, and hamstring tendinopathies
ASIS	*Anterior.* Palpated by tracing iliac crest anterior and inferior; easier to palpate with the person seated when muscles attachments are relaxed.	Serves as the superior attachment site for the inguinal ligament.
Iliac tubercle	*Anterior.* Palpated 5-6 cm posterior to the ASIS. Represents the widest point of iliac crest.	Tenderness along the iliac tubercle and crest may occur with muscle strains of the muscles inserting onto this area and from contusions ("hip pointer").
Pubic symphysis	*Anterior.* Palpated in midline, approximately a hand's width inferior to umbilicus.	Tenderness may indicate osteitis pubis or pubic joint dysfunction (subluxation). Sacroiliac dysfunctions may also cause a tender pubic symphysis when palpated.
Pubic tubercle	*Anterior.* Approximately 2.5 cm anterior and lateral to pubic symphysis.	Important landmark when palpating the superficial inguinal ring (superolateral to pubic tubercle) in diagnosing inguinal hernias. Also serves as the inferior attachment site for the inguinal ligament.

EOP, External occipital protuberance; *PSIS,* posterior superior iliac spine; *ASIS,* anterior superior iliac spine.

focal irritation with discrete palpable thickening or muscle contraction are commonly felt. These taut and tender fibers, or **trigger points,** can be found in the long paraspinal muscles, shoulder girdle muscles (infraspinatus, supraspinatus, trapezius, rhomboid, and levator scapulae), the pelvis (iliopsoas, piriformis, quadratus, gluteal, and tensor fascia lata), and extremity muscles (extensor carpi radialis, vastus medialis, and soleus).[25-27]

Myofascial trigger points can be identified by flat or **pincer palpation.**[27] During flat palpation, the palpator's fingertips move the patient's sub-cutaneous tissue and skin across the taut muscle fibers. Pincer palpation is performed by grasping the muscle belly between the thumb and fingers while gently squeezing the tissues with a back-and-forth motion to locate taut bands. Fig. 10-2 demonstrates pincer palpation of the common wrist extensor muscle group.

Dynamic (Motion) Palpation

A widely held view on the primary effect of the adjustment is that it increases the range of

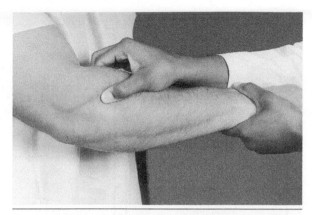

Fig. 10-2 Pincer palpation of the patient's common wrist extensor muscle group.

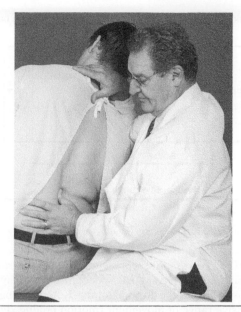

Fig. 10-3 Motion (dynamic) palpation assessment for right lateral flexion of the L2 vertebra (L2-L3 motor unit) in the seated position.

motion of a joint.[13,15,17,28] The location and characteristics of the altered or restricted joint movement (**fixation**) must therefore be determined before an adjustment/manipulation can be performed. The primary technique for this evaluation is the dynamic (motion) assessment of the various joints of the spine, pelvis, and extremities. Specific techniques for palpating motion in joints can be divided into active, passive, and accessory movements (see Box 10-3).

Normally a joint will move through a certain range of **active motion.** The patient performs active movements while the examiner guides the patient through a particular motion. The patient's voluntary muscle contraction causes the joint to move, and the clinician evaluates associated periarticular soft tissues for tension and resiliency. At the end of active motion, the clinician can passively push the bony lever (e.g., spinous process), thereby further assessing the quality of resistance, called **end play** or *end feel.* Springing of the joint and the determination of end play are an integral part of the examination preceding adjustment/manipulation (Fig. 10-3).

Joint play assessment "is the qualitative evaluation of the joint's resistance to movement when it is in a neutral position."[13] Joint play exists because the articular surfaces do not perfectly fit. The incongruent articular surfaces also prevent a fixed axis of rotation from occurring during joint motion. The joint capsules and ligaments remain somewhat lax to allow for rolling and gliding of the articular surfaces to accommodate for the changing axis of rotation around these irregular surfaces. The joint demonstrates joint play in the neutral position, when it is under the least amount of stress, with the joint capsule and ligaments in the position of greatest laxity (Fig. 10-4). An active range of motion produced by voluntary muscle contraction follows this joint play near the neutral position. The end point of the active range of motion is called the **physiologic barrier**[7] (see Fig. 10-4).

If active range of motion is under the control of the musculature, **passive movements** are involuntary. Passive range of motion is defined as "movements carried through by the operator (clinician) without the conscious assistance or resistance of the patient."[13] The passive range of motion can be greater than the range of active joint movement (see Fig. 10-4). During active movements, the muscles move the joint to the physiologic barrier. Further movement past this barrier, into the **end-play zone,** is produced by additional overpressure performed by the examiner (see Figs. 10-3 and 10-4). The end-play zone, or increase in passive resistance, is thought to result from the elastic properties of the joint capsule and periarticular soft tissues. If

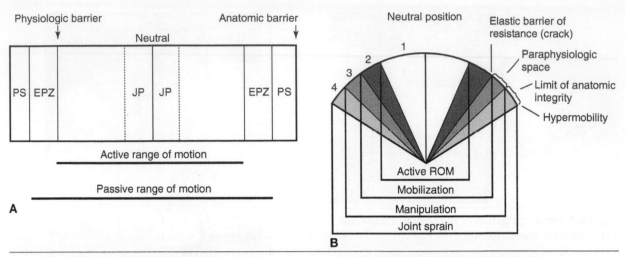

Fig. 10-4 Two graphic representations of joint range of motion. **A,** Active and passive components of joint motion. *PS,* Paraphysiologic space; *EPZ,* end-play zone; *JP,* joint play. **B,** Sandoz chart. Four stages of range of movement in diarthrodial joints: *1,* Active range of movement (motion produced by muscular action). *2,* Passive range of movement (motion produced by traction or springing the joint/joint play, up to the elastic barrier or resistance); characterizes mobilization. *3,* Paraphysiologic range of movement (motion beyond the elastic barrier of resistance up to the limit of anatomic integrity produced by adjustment/ manipulation and accompanied by an audible release). *4,* Pathologic movement (motion beyond the limit of normal anatomic integrity, which damages ligaments and capsule, resulting in joint hypermobility). Adjustment/manipulation that is too forceful may move the joint beyond the limit of anatomic integrity, creating or perpetuating joint instability. *(From Gatterman MI:* Foundations of chiropractic: subluxation, *St Louis, 1995, Mosby.)*

the examiner were to release the pressure while stressing the tissues in the end-play zone, the joint would spring back to its physiologic barrier. Movement beyond the end-play zone is typically associated with an audible "cracking" noise followed by slight increase in the range of motion and has been referred to by Sandoz[29] as the *paraphysiologic space.* Movement into the paraphysiologic space is within the normal boundaries of the joint and does not cause joint injury. At this point, another barrier is encountered, called the **anatomic barrier.** Further movement beyond this point will damage anatomic structures associated with the joint (see Fig. 10-4).

To illustrate this point, the reader is instructed to actively flex the right index finger at the metacarpophalangeal (MCP) joint as far as possible (active movement to the physiologic barrier). With a finger from the left hand, additional pressure is applied to flex the right MCP

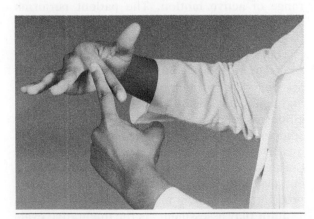

Fig. 10-5 Passive movement into the end-play zone of the metacarpophalangeal joint (index finger).

joint further (passive movement into the end-play zone) (Fig. 10-5). The quality of this resistance (increased, decreased, or normal) in the end-play zone is that which the examiner evaluates during end play palpation. Now, the next step is to release the overpressure caused by the left finger, noting how the right finger springs back toward the physiologic barrier (elastic properties of the capsule and periarticular soft tissues).

Accessory joint movements are small specific movements independent of voluntary muscle action.[13,20,28,30] Normal voluntary muscle action depends on their character. If integrity of accessory movement is lacking, the active range of joint motion is decreased. Accessory movements are evaluated when performing joint play and end-play procedures. As previously stated, joint play involves the qualitative assessment of resistance from the neutral joint position, and end play is resistance near the end of passive motion at the end-play zone.[13] The goals of **accessory motion** testing are to evaluate[30]:

- Aspects of tissue compliance
- Amount of available range of motion
- Change in resistance relative to the range of motion
- Degree of resistance to motion

Information gained from accessory motion testing should be used with the history and other physical examination findings to establish a clinical impression (working diagnosis) and treatment plan. As a diagnostic tool, however, accessory motion is primarily performed to determined relative joint resistance or stiffness (normal, hypermobility, or hypomobility). In the abnormal joint, an increased resistance (restriction) of movement in one or more directions occurs forming a **pathologic barrier** (*dysfunctional barrier*). This resistance can vary in severity: it may be minor so that the range of movement is only slightly less than normal, or it may be major so that only a small range of joint movement remains.

One way to illustrate the qualitative assessment of joint play and end play would be to separate the thumb and index finger while having them wrapped with a single rubber band (Fig. 10-6). The resistance felt with a single rubber band represents the normal tension and resiliency of a joint. Placing additional rubber bands around the fingers would represent the increased resistance felt with joint dysfunctions or restrictions.

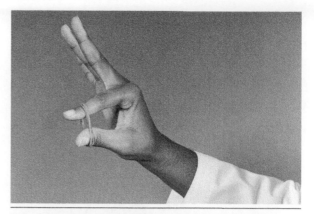

Fig. 10-6 A rubber band is wrapped around the index finger and thumb to illustrate the qualitative resistance felt during joint end play assessment.

PALPATION OF ACUTE AND CHRONIC SUBLUXATIONS OR DYSFUNCTIONS

Acute Spinal Subluxations or Dysfunctions

In acute cases, a history of a recent onset of symptoms is usually present, often involving an injury or specific triggering event. Palpation of the skin and subdermal layer (subcutaneous adipose tissue, fascia, nerves, and blood vessels)[13] may be warmer than the surrounding tissues and appear red or inflamed with increased moisture. The dorsum (back) of the hand is commonly used when palpating the skin for temperature and moisture changes. The skin and deeper tissues directly over the subluxation or dysfunction may be tender with light to slightly firmer palpation pressure. Mobility of the dermal and subdermal layers usually appears normal but may palpate as sluggish over the involved area with the skin rolling technique. Deeper palpation of the *functional layer* (muscles, tendons, tendon sheaths, bursae, ligaments, and fascia)[13] may detect a local increase in muscle tone and a boggy, congested texture as a result of swelling in the deep periarticular tissues. Dynamic (motion) intersegmental palpation reveals increased resistance in one or more directions when assessing end play.

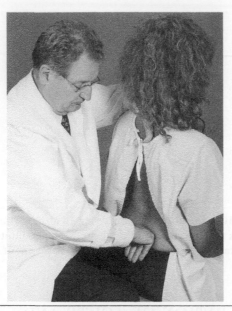

Fig. **10-7** Doctor and patient positions for the general quick scan of the sacrum. The sacral scan is performed with the back of the hand and fingers parallel to the SI joints. The examiner pushes forward gently over the center of the sacrum and then over the individual SI joints to ascertain the springy feel of normal joint play or a blocked feeling with joint restrictions.

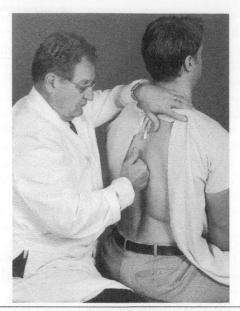

Fig. **10-8** The quick scan of the thoracic spine is performed with the back of the hand and fingers perpendicular to the spinous processes. The patient is held in the neutral-sitting posture, and a series of gentle pushes are performed.

Chronic Spinal Subluxations or Dysfunctions

In contrast to acute subluxations or dysfunctions, chronic subluxations have a long-standing history of symptoms, functional limitations, or both. Palpation may uncover evidence of many chronic tissue changes. The skin may appear pale and feel cool, while the subdermal layer may be less mobile and palpate fibrotic and ropy, with less elasticity. The functional layer may actually palpate with decreased muscle tone, and the periarticular soft tissues may feel thickened and stringy. Tenderness over the dysfunctional tissue is present and is usually described by the patient as dull and achy. Intersegmental joint challenge into the end-play zone during dynamic (motion) palpation reveals restricted movement in one or more directions. In advanced stages of degeneration, soft tissue and ligamentous contractures may restrict the quality of motion considerably to include joint anky-

losis. Somatovisceral effects thought to be caused by subluxations or dysfunctions are more likely to be associated with chronic subluxations or dysfunctions than they are with acute subluxation syndromes.[31]

Dynamic (Motion) Palpation Procedures

To obtain an integrated view of a patient's overall spinal dynamics, a general quick scan of the whole spine may precede motion palpation procedures at a specific spinal motion unit. The patient sits on a stool, and the doctor sits on another stool, behind the patient. The doctor places the patient in a neutral upright posture by draping his or her hand and elbow over the patient's shoulders. Using the back of his or her free hand, the doctor can gently apply posterior-to-anterior springing movements to the spine, gliding from sacrum to the occiput, to feel for blocked areas (Figs. 10-7 and 10-8). A smooth, rhythmic motion should be applied during the quick scan, and the doctor must avoid hyperex-

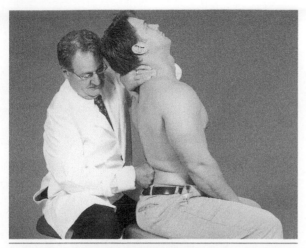

Fig. 10-9 Motion palpation end play assessment for extension of the L2-L3 motion unit using a thumb contact over the L2 spinous process.

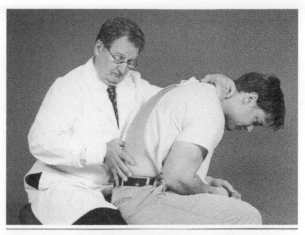

Fig. 10-10 Motion palpation assessment for flexion of L2-L3 feeling for the separation between the spinous processes of L2 and L3.

tending the spine. The blocked areas are palpated specifically for flexion, extension, right and left rotation, and right and left lateral flexion, as now described.

Dynamic (Motion) Palpation of a Lumbar Motion Unit[17]

Extension and Flexion

With the left elbow on the patient's left shoulder and the left hand on the patient's right shoulder, the doctor, who is sitting on a stool behind the patient (who is sitting on another stool), pushes the spinous processes forward as the patient is pulled back into slight extension. The doctor feels the normal springy end feel or a resisted, blocked feeling of **hypomobile** extension (Fig. 10-9). In the same position, the doctor's right thumb is placed between two spinous processes, and the patient is flexed forward from the level of the doctor's thumb. The spinous separation will be felt in a normal motion unit (Fig. 10-10).

Lateral Flexion

For lateral flexion, the doctor's right thumb is placed to the left side of the spinous process. As the doctor pushes the spinous to the right, the patient is bent to the left in lateral flexion from the level of the doctor's thumb. The spinous is prevented from rotating to the left, and the doc-

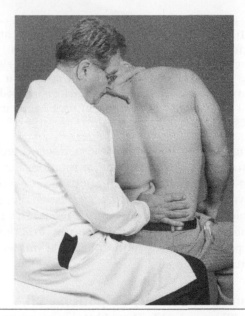

Fig. 10-11 Motion palpation end play assessment for left lateral flexion of L2-L3. The doctor's thumb is on the left side of the L2 spinous process.

tor feels a springing movement as the right posterior spinal joints open on the right side. The doctor's arms and hands are reversed to test for right lateral flexion (Fig. 10-11).

Rotation

For rotation from posterior to anterior on the right, the right is pushed with the thumb just to the right of the spinous process. Once again, a

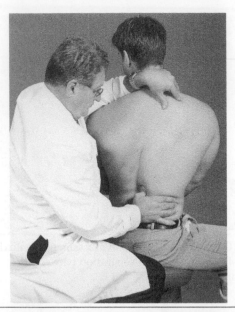

Fig. **10-12** Motion palpation end play assessment for left rotation of L2-L3. The doctor's thumb is contacting over the mammillary process to the right of the L2-L3 interspinous space while applying a posterior-to-anterior force. An alternative method would be to contact the left side of the L2 spinous process.

springy feeling is normal, and a blocked feeling is a fixation or hypomobility of rotation. For the left posterior-to-anterior rotation, the procedure is reversed (Fig. 10-12). In all cases, challenging the blocked motions will cause a temporary pain to the patient. Adjustment into the direction of this painful blocked motion is made unless the elicited pain lingers.

Dynamic (Motion) Palpation of a Thoracic Motion Unit[17]

The thoracic motion unit is not a three-joint complex because of the presence of the costo-transverse and costo-vertebral joints. A point to remember is that a single vertebra cannot be adjusted, but instead, the joints between the vertebrae can be. Thoracic spine adjustments involve not only the zygapophyseal joints, but also the joints with the ribs. Therefore feeling all of these motions is essential.

Flexion and extension of the thoracic spine is similar to the lumbars except that the extension

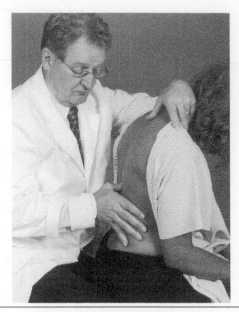

Fig. **10-13** Motion palpation assessment for flexion of T8-T9 feeling for the separation between the spinous processes of T8 and T9. Note that spinal flexion occurs above the point of contact with the lumber spine maintained in a relatively neutral position.

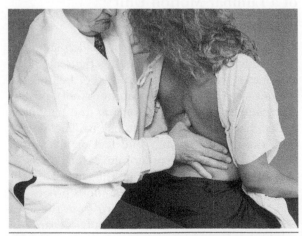

Fig. **10-14** Motion palpation end play assessment for extension of T8-T9 using a thumb contact over the T8 spinous process.

and flexion movements are repeated a second time out by the costo-transverse joints (Figs. 10-13 and 10-14). *Lateral bending and rotation are also the same as for the lumbars except that*

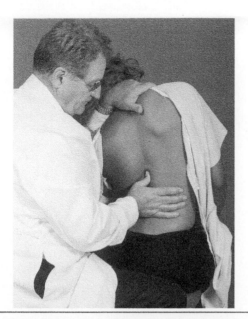

Fig. 10-15 Motion palpation end play assessment for left lateral flexion of T8-T9. The doctor's thumb is on the left side of the T8 spinous process. Note that the lumbar spine is kept in a neutral position while the thoracic spine is laterally flexed above the point of contact.

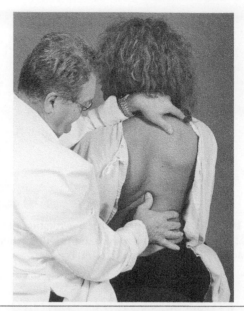

Fig. 10-16 Motion palpation end play assessment for left rotation of T8-T9. The doctor's thumb is contacting the right transverse process of T8 while applying a posterior-to-anterior force. An alternative method would be to contact the left side of the T8 spinous process and push laterally to induce left rotation. Assessment of the costo-transverse joints is performed in the same manner except the examiner contacts lateral to the transverse process on the rib and applies a posterior-to-anterior force at end range.

the movements are repeated a few inches laterally, where the rib can be felt (Figs. 10-15 and 10-16). Springy end feel is normal. A blocked feeling is abnormal.

Dynamic (Motion) Palpation of the Cervical Spine[17]

For the *atlantooccipital* articulation, the space between the atlas and the mandible is palpated while the patient's head is guided forward (chin parallel to floor) with the opposite hand. The doctor should avoid excessive flexion and extension of the head when gliding the occiput forward (Fig. 10-17).

For *posterior-to-anterior rotation* of the C1-C2 articulation, the doctor's palpating hand is pronated with the palm facing anteriorly. The doctor contacts the posterior arch with the middle or index finger of the palpating hand while the opposite hand rotates the patient's head. A gentle posterior-to-anterior force is applied to the posterior arch of atlas (Fig. 10-18).

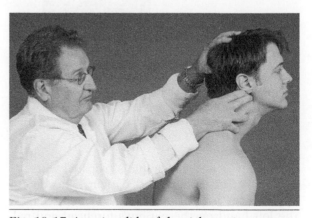

Fig. 10-17 Anterior glide of the right occiput on atlas. Note that the chin is protruded forward (chin parallel to floor) without hyperextending or flexing the head.

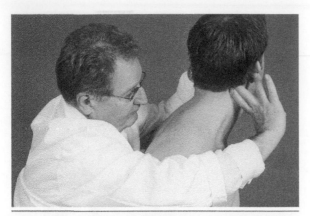

Fig. **10-18** Left posterior-to-anterior rotation of C1 on C2. Note the palm forward hand position when contacting the posterior arch of atlas.

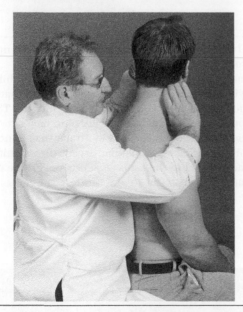

Fig. **10-19** Motion palpation end play assessment for left rotation (posterior to anterior) of C3-C4. The doctor contacts the right articular pillars with the finger pads of the index and middle fingers (palm facing forward) while applying a posterior-to-anterior force at end range of motion.

The lower cervical spine is palpated with the doctor sitting behind the patient. The doctor controls the patient's head movement by placing the left hand on the patient's forehead and palpating the right side over the articular pillars (Fig. 10-19). The palpating hand is facing palm forward, with fingertips pushing the articular

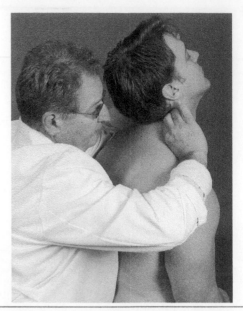

Fig. **10-20** Motion palpation end play assessment for extension of C3-C4. With the patient's head positioned in extension, the doctor contacts the right articular pillars with the finger pads while applying posterior-to-anterior force at end range. The procedure is repeated on the opposite side by contacting the left articular pillars with the doctor's left hand.

pillars posterior to anterior for *rotation* (see Fig. 10-19), into extension for *extension* (Fig. 10-20), and laterally for *lateral flexion* (Fig.10-21). For *flexion* (Fig. 10-22) and *anterior-to-posterior rotation* (Fig. 10-23) the hand is placed with the palm facing posterior, and the palpating finger is placed in front of the articular pillar and pull backward, very gently in flexion and anterior-to-posterior rotation. These palpations are directly over the cervical sympathetic ganglion chain and often elicit a positive *doorbell sign* (reproduction or exaggeration of symptoms) to the shoulder, chest, and arm.

Dynamic (Motion) Palpation of the Sacroiliac Joint

The sacroiliac joints are palpated with the patient standing while holding onto something (such as a doorknob or a rail attached to a wall) to maintain balance. The doctor places one

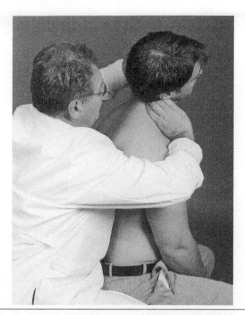

Fig. 10-21 Motion palpation end play assessment for right lateral flexion of C3-C4. With the patient's head positioned in right lateral flexion, the doctor contacts the right articular pillars with the finger pads (palm facing forward) while applying a lateral-to-medial force at end range.

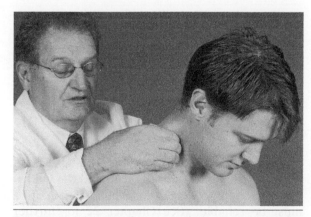

Fig. 10-22 Motion palpation end play assessment for flexion of C3-C4. With the patient's head positioned in flexion, the doctor contacts the anterior aspect of the right articular pillars with the pads of the index or middle fingers (palm facing toward the doctor) while applying a very gentle anterior-to-posterior and slightly superior force. This procedure should be repeated on the opposite side to assess anterior-to-posterior gliding of the left C3-C4 articulation.

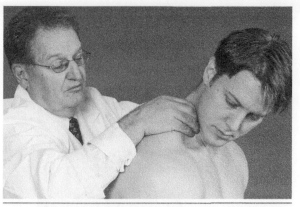

Fig. 10-23 Motion palpation end play assessment for right anterior to posterior rotation of C3-C4. The doctor contacts the anterior aspect of the right articular pillars with the pads of the index or middle fingers (palm facing toward the doctor) while applying a very gentle anterior-to-posterior force at the end of right rotation.

thumb on the PSIS and the opposite thumb on the second tubercle of the sacrum. In a normally moving joint, the thumb on the PSIS should glide inferior as the patient lifts his or her leg to 90 degrees of hip flexion (Fig. 10-24). If the thumbs do not separate, a sacroiliac flexion restriction may be present. Holding the same contacts while the patient flexes the opposite leg assesses sacroiliac extension. In a normally moving joint, the thumb on the sacrum should move inferior. The sacroiliac assessment is continued by moving the thumbs to each side of the lowest palpable borders of the inferior sacroiliac (SI) joint (Fig. 10-25) and then repeating the right and left leg raises. Both processes on the opposite side are repeated, reversing the contacts.

Dynamic (Motion) Palpation of the Wrist

Palpation of the extremities is a very gentle and subtle art, most easily experienced by palpating the wrist. To feel the joint play movement of *anterior-to-posterior glide* and *posterior-to-anterior glide*, one hand is placed over the distal end of the radius and ulna bones and the other hand over the proximal end of the metacarpals on the posterior aspect (Fig. 10-26).

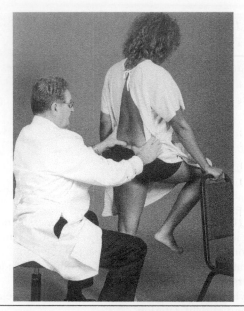

Fig. **10-24** Motion palpation assessment of the right sacroiliac joint while the patient flexes her femur to 90 degrees. The doctor's right thumb is contacting the patient's right posterior superior iliac spine and his left thumb is contacting the second sacral tubercle.

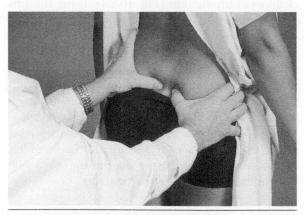

Fig. **10-25** Hand position for palpation of the lower aspect of the patient's right sacroiliac joint. The doctor's left thumb contacts the patient's sacral apex and the right thumb contacts the adjacent ischium.

The clinician pushes and pulls alternately, keeping the both hands from flexing or extending the wrist but instead feeling the gliding motion. This motion is present normally when tested but cannot be performed actively by a patient. The loss

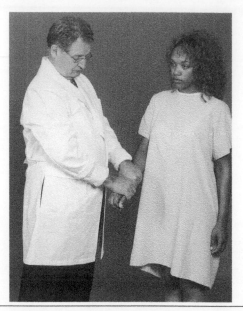

Fig. **10-26** Motion palpation assessment of anterior-to-posterior and posterior-to-anterior glide of the right intercarpal joint. Doctor stands on the affected side and grasps the distal radius with one hand and the proximal metacarpals with the other. Stress the intercarpal joints by applying and anterior-to-posterior stress with one and a posterior-to-anterior force with the other.

of this gliding motion causes pain and dysfunction of the active ranges of motion. Many other specific motions can be tested for in the wrist, all of which were described originally by Mennell.[28]

RELIABILITY: A BRIEF REVIEW OF THE PALPATION LITERATURE

Reliability refers to the consistency of data. In essence, reliability is the accuracy and precision of a measurement. Both the data and the instrument used to collect and evaluate such data must be reliable. (See Chapter 22 for further discussion of reliability.) When chiropractors use tests and instruments to measure outcomes, the consistency of such data is extremely important in clinical decision-making. When palpation or visual observation of clinical subjects is the "instrument," the presence of a "human factor" must be assumed, indicating that individuals will be expected to demonstrate some degree of inconsistency. Thus any observed value has both the true value and an error component (observed value = true value + error). The difference between the true value and the observed value is the measurement error. Therefore reliability equals the true variance divided by the total variance:

Reliability = True Variance ÷ (True Variance + Error)

The reliability testing for palpation is usually performed to determine the consistency between and within examiners. Interexaminer reliability compares the results between two or more examiners, and intraexaminer reliability tests how consistent the same examiner can reproduce the same results. Several statistical methods are used in literature to estimate reliability. (See Appendix I for further detail on these methods.)

Summary of Research Data

Reliability testing for static and dynamic (motion) palpation procedures has demonstrated varied results.* (Table 10-2). Interexaminer reliability for palpation has demonstrated poor results, and intraexaminer findings are generally more reliable. Although reliability measures for static and dynamic (motion) palpation demonstrate poor to moderate results, palpation for bony and soft tissue tenderness reveals acceptable reliability. Breaking out the subsets of the data further reveals that interexaminer reliability for bony static palpation and detection of muscle tension has demonstrated poor results.† However, palpation of tenderness of bony processes and paraspinal soft tissues reveals good to excellent interexaminer reliability.‡ As with static palpation, the level of interexaminer reliability for dynamic (motion) palpation is poor, with slightly higher reliability values in the cervical spine.§

*References 10, 19-23, 30, 32, 33-65.
†References 23, 33, 37, 38, 41.
‡References 3, 19-22, 33, 35
§References 10, 36, 45, 47, 59, 61, 62.

Context for Evaluating Palpation Research

An important point to remember is that reliability measures in research studies are not the same as clinical acceptability. Reliability testing is best evaluated by using more than one statistic and considering questions about possible confounding factors in the research process. Some authors[11,13] have suggested that the poor interexaminer reliability of some measures of palpation may be the result of the relatively small quantitative and qualitative changes in the degree of restricted joint motion that are being measured. Additionally, other theories suggest that most follow-up visits for chiropractic care are with the same doctor, thus moderate *intraexaminer* reliability values may demonstrate clinical utility for motion palpation as an outcome measure for the adjustive/manipulative lesion.

Perhaps most significantly, the very process of manual examination and palpation may itself alter joint mobility, so that subsequent motion palpation of the same patient, even when accurate, will yield different results.[66] Until these crucial methodologic questions are resolved, caution is advisable before reaching any definitive conclusions about the reliability of palpation.

The results of studies on dynamic (motion) palpation procedures are thus far inconclusive, and discontinuing their use in the routine examination of patients would be premature. *This is especially true in light of the fact that "acceptable" standard medical diagnostic procedures such as x-ray interpretation[2,4,5] and cardiac auscultation[1,3] produce similar reliability results* (Table 10-3). Currently, efforts toward improving standards for teaching dynamic (motion) palpation procedures, as demonstrated by Marcotte and colleagues,[10] are progressing and may yield greater interexaminer and intraexaminer reliability.

Health care is an art, as well as a science. Evidence-based health care requires that the best documented procedures be used. In cases in which the evidence supporting the best available procedures is not strong, practitioners in all

Text continued on p. 234.

Table **10-2**   INTEREXAMINER AND INTRAEXAMINER AGREEMENT FOR PALPATION SKILLS

Reference	Interexaminer Agreement	Intraexaminer Agreement	Subjects	Examiners	Comments
STATIC AND TENDERNESS PALPATION					
Boline et al[21]	Osseous pain = Moderate to excellent (k) Soft tissue pain = Moderate to good (k)	—	28	Two	Lumbar spine; symptomatic subjects and asymptomatic subjects
Boline et al[33]	Pain = Moderate (k) Spasm = Poor (k)	—	50	Two	Thoracic and lumbar spines; 23 symptomatic and 27 asymptomatic
Byfield et al[34]	55%-81% agreement	39%-62% agreement	42	Two chiropractors	Lumbar spine palpation in sitting and prone positions; asymptomatic subjects
Christensen et al[35]	Paraspinal tenderness = Good (k)	Paraspinal tenderness = Good (k)	85	Three chiropractors	Thoracic spine; two chiropractors examined asymptomatic and symptomatic subjects for interexaminer reliability; one chiropractor examined 29 asymptomatic and symptomatic subjects for intraexaminer reliability
DeBoer et al[36]	Pain = Poor to moderate (k_w)	Pain = Fair to moderate (k_w)	40	Three chiropractors	Cervical spine; asymptomatic students
French et al[41]	Static = Poor to fair (k)	Static = Moderate (k)	29	Five chiropractors	Lumbar spine and sacroiliac joints; symptomatic subjects
Hubka and Phelan[19]	Pain = Good (k)	—	30	Two chiropractors	Cervical spine; symptomatic subjects
Keating et al[23]		Static = Poor (k) Pain = Fair to good (k) Temp. = Poor (k) Muscle tension = Poor (k)	46	Three	Thoracic and lumbar spine; 21 symptomatic and 25 asymptomatic
Maher and Adams[20]	Pain = Poor to moderate (k_w)	—	30	Six physical therapists	Lumbar spine; symptomatic subjects
O'Haire and Gibbons[37]	Static = Poor (k_g)	Static = Poor to moderate (k_g)	10	10 osteopathic students	Sacroiliac joint; asymptomatic subjects

Study	Reliability	Reliability	N	Examiners	Subjects
Richter and Lavall[22]	Pain = Moderate (k)	Fair to good ⟨k⟩	35	Five medical physicians	Lumbar spine; symptomatic subjects
Spring et al[38]	Poor (k)	Poor (k)	10	10 osteopaths	Lumbar spine; asymptomatic subjects
Van Suijlekom et al[39]	Joint tenderness = Poor to fair (k)	—	24	Two neurologists	Cervical spine; headache patients
DYNAMIC (MOTION) PALPATION					
Bergstrom and Courtis[40]	65%-81% agreement	93.0%-99.3% agreement	100 interexaminers; 20 intraexaminers	Two senior students	Lumbar spine; asymptomatic chiropractic students
Boline et al[33]	Poor to fair (k)	—	50	Two	Thoracic and lumbar spine; 23 symptomatic and 27 asymptomatic
Brinkley et al[30]	Poor (ICC)	—	18	Six physical therapists	Lumbar spine; symptomatic subjects
Bronemo et al[65]	84.4%-84.8% agreement	88.2%-94.7% agreement	102	Two senior students	Cervical spine; asymptomatic students
Carmichael[64]	Poor (k)	Fair (k)	53	Two	Sacroiliac joint; asymptomatic subjects
Christensen et al[35]	Poor (k)	Good (k)	85	Three chiropractors	Thoracic spine; two chiropractors examined 56 asymptomatic and symptomatic subjects for interexaminer reliability; one chiropractor examined 29 asymptomatic and subjects for intraexaminer reliability
Cibulka et al[42]	Excellent (k)	—	26	Two physical therapists	Sacroiliac joint; symptomatic subjects; high agreement scores when several test results combined
DeBoer et al[36]	Poor to moderate (k_w)	Poor to substantial (k_w)	40	Three chiropractors	Cervical spine; asymptomatic students

k, Kappa; k_w, weighted kappa; k_g, generalized kappa; *ICC*, intraclass correlation coefficient; *r*, Pearson's *r*. (See Appendix I for further description of these measurements.)

Continued

Table **10-2** INTEREXAMINER AND INTRAEXAMINER AGREEMENT FOR PALPATION SKILLS—CONT'D

Reference	Interexaminer Agreement	Intraexaminer Agreement	Subjects	Examiners	Comments
DYNAMIC (MOTION) PALPATION—cont'd					
Fjellner et al[43]	Poor to moderate (k-k_w)	—	47	Two physical therapists	Cervical and upper thoracic spines; first rib mobility
Haas et al[44]	Poor (k)	Moderate (k)	73	Two chiropractors	Thoracic and lumbar spines; symptomatic and asymptomatic students
Hanten et al[45]	Poor to excellent (k)	Poor to excellent (k)	40	Three	Cervical spine; two examiners palpated 20 symptomatic subjects for interexaminer reliability; one examiner palpated 20 symptomatic subjects for intraexaminer reliability
Inscoe et al[46]	48.6% agreement	66.7%-75.0% agreement	Six	Two physical therapists	Lumbar spine; symptomatic subjects
Jull et al[47]	Excellent (k)	—	40	Seven physical therapists	Cervical spine; symptomatic and asymptomatic
Jull and Bullock[48]	Excellent relationship (r) 86.0% agreement	Excellent relationship (r) 87.5% agreement	10 interexaminers; 20 intraexaminers	Two physical therapists	Lumber spine; asymptomatic students
Keating et al[23]	Poor (k)	—	46	Three	Thoracic and lumbar spines; 21 symptomatic and 25 asymptomatic
Lewit and Rosina[49]	Good (k)	—	33	Two	Sacroiliac joint; symptomatic subjects
Love and Brodeur[50]	Insignificant reliability (r)	Significant reliability (r)	32	Eight chiropractic students	Thoracolumbar spine; asymptomatic student volunteers
Maher and Adams[20]	Poor (*ICC*)	—	30	Six physical therapists	Lumbar spine; symptomatic subjects
Maher et al[51]	Good (*ICC*)	—	27	Two physical therapists	Lumbar spine; asymptomatic subjects

Study			Number	Examiners	Spine/Joint; Subjects
Marcotte et al[10]	Fair to good (k)	—	12	24 trained students and chiropractors	Cervical spine; subjects with history of neck pain; standardization of motion x palpation procedure increased kappa scores from 0.35-0.68
Meijne et al[52]	Poor (k)	Poor (k)	37	Two physical therapy students	Sacroiliac joint; symptomatic and asymptomatic subjects
Mior et al[53]	Poor (k)	Poor to perfect (k)	15	74 senior students and experienced chiropractors	Sacroiliac joint
Mior et al[54]	Poor (k)	Poor to moderate (k)	59	Two senior students	Cervical spine; asymptomatic students
Mootz et al[55]	Poor (k)	Poor to moderate (k)	60	Two	Lumbar spine; asymptomatic students
Nansel et al[56]	Poor (k)	—	76 seated; 88 supine	Three	Cervical spine; asymptomatic students
Phillips and Twomey[57]	Poor (k_w)		72	Two physical therapists	Lumbar spine; symptomatic subjects
Richter and Lawall[22]	Poor to moderate (k)	Fair to good (k)	35	Five medical physicians	Lumbar spine; symptomatic subjects
Riddle et al[58]	Poor (k)	Poor (k)	65	34 physical therapists	Sacroiliac joint; symptomatic subjects
Schoensee et al[59]	Poor to good (k)	Good (k)	Five interexaminers; 10 intraexaminers	Two physical therapists	Cervical spine; five headache patients; 10 asymptomatic subjects
Schoeps et al[60]	Poor (k) = Mobility Moderate (k) = Pain	—	20	Five medical physicians	Cervical spine; asymptomatic volunteers
Smedmark et al[61]	Poor to moderate (k)	—	61	Two physical therapists	Cervical spine; symptomatic subjects
Smith et al[62]	Poor to moderate (k)	Poor to perfect (k)	27	Three physical therapists	Cervicothoracic spine; upper-quarter disorders
Vincent-Smith and Gibbons[63]	Poor (k)	Moderate (k)	9	Nine	Sacroiliac joint (standing flexion test); asymptomatic subjects

k, Kappa; k_w, weighted kappa; k_g, generalized kappa; ICC, intraclass correlation coefficient; r, Pearson's r. (See Appendix I for further description of these measurements.)

Table **10-3** RELIABILITY OF OTHER COMMON EXAMINATION PROCEDURES

INTERPRETATION OF RADIOGRAPHS

Meade et al[2]	Fair to moderate (*k*)
Melbye and Dale[4]	Moderate to good (*k*)
Norgaard et al[5]	Poor to moderate (*k*)

CARDIAC AUSCULTATION

Gaskin et al[1]	Poor (*k*)
Lok et al[3]	Poor (*k*)

k, Kappa.

professions rely on the best available objective evidence coupled with clinical skill in patient assessment. Examples of clinical assessment requiring skillful clinical assessment include auscultation, observation, and palpation. As long as no superior forms of diagnosis arise to replace these methods, they will remain core methods of diagnosis.

CONCLUSION

Palpation is an art, not an exact science, and time is required for development of psychomotor skills. Some individuals are gifted in this area; others have to practice hard to acquire the basic skills in the manual arts. A thorough understanding of the basic and applied clinical sciences, along with many hours of practice and concentration, are necessary for the student and practitioner to master this art.

Historically, static palpation has been used to identify the adjustive/manipulative lesion. Recently, many doctors of chiropractic have adopted a more contemporary, multimodal (PARTS) assessment model, including dynamic (motion) palpation, to identify this lesion. Worthy of note is that the adjustive/manipulative lesion should not be viewed as "moving or not moving" but instead as a continuum from normal joint motion to severe ankylosis. Therefore the qualitative precision of end-feel assessment should be mastered to facilitate the most advantageous adjustive strategies. The responsibility of the chiropractic student and practitioner lies in their willingness and ability to develop and maintain the necessary cognitive and psychomotor skills to practice and master the art of manual assessment successfully.

Review *Questions*

1. Identify the four methods of examination employed by chiropractors to identify the adjustive lesion.
2. Using the acronym PARTS, describe the diagnostic criteria used for identification of joint dysfunction.
3. To what other diagnostic procedures is the reliability of motion palpation statistically comparable?
4. Briefly describe the difference between static and motion palpation.
5. What are active, passive, and accessory joint motions?
6. Describe the difference between an anatomic barrier and a pathologic barrier with regard to joint movement.
7. What role can palpation play in encouraging patients to follow through with a recommended treatment plan?
8. Name several synonyms for *subluxation*.
9. Based on the current research literature, what can be said about the reliability of palpation?
10. A step defect noted in palpation is indicative of what clinical problem?

Concept *Questions*

1. Are objective signs always, sometimes, or never more useful than subjective signs?
2. In both the medical and chiropractic professions, to what extent is high-technology diagnostic procedures expected to replace palpation in the next 50 years?

REFERENCES

1. Gaskin P et al: Clinical auscultation skills in pediatric residents, *Pediatrics* 105(6):1184, 2002.
2. Meade MO et al: Interobserver variation in interpreting chest radiographs for the diagnosis of acute respiratory distress syndrome, *Am J Resp Crit Care Med* 161(1):85, 2000.
3. Lok CE, Morgan CD, Ranganathan N: The accuracy and interobserver agreement in detecting the "gallop

sounds" by cardiac auscultation, *Chest* 114:1283, 1998.

4. Melbye H, Dale K: Interobserver variability in the radiographic diagnosis of adult outpatient pneumonia, *Acta Radiologica* 33(1):79, 1992.

5. Norgaard H et al: Interobserver variation in the detection of pulmonary venous hypertension in chest radiographs, *Eur J Radiology* 11(3):203, 1990.

6. DiGiovanna EL: Somatic dysfunction. In DiGiovanna EL, Schiowitz S, editors: *An osteopathic approach to diagnosis and treatment*, ed 2, Philadelphia, 1997, Lippincott-Raven.

7. Greenman PE: *Principles of manual medicine*, ed 2, Baltimore, 1996, Williams and Wilkins.

8. Bergmann T, Finer B: Joint assessment—PARTS, *Topics Clin Chiropr* 7(3):1, 2000.

9. *Dorland's illustrated medical dictionary*, ed 26, Philadelphia, 1981, WB Saunders.

10. Marcotte J, Normand MC, Black P: The kinematic of motion palpation and its effect on the reliability for cervical spine rotation, *J Manipulative Physiol Ther* 25:7, 2002.

11. Lewit K, Liebenson C: Palpation: problems and implications, *J Manipulative Physiol Ther* 16:586, 1993.

12. Eder M, Tilscher H: *Chiropractic therapy: diagnosis and treatment*, Gaithersburg, Md, 1990, Aspen.

13. Peterson DH, Bergmann TF: *Chiropractic technique: principles and procedures*, ed 2, St Louis, 2002, Mosby.

14. Kaltenborn FM: *The spine: basic examination and treatment techniques*, ed 2, Minneapolis, Minn, 1993, Orthopedic Physical Therapy Products.

15. Maitland GD: *Peripheral manipulation*, ed 3, London, 1991, Butterworth-Heinemann.

16. Kaltenborn FM: *Manual mobilization of the extremity joints: basic examination and treatment techniques*, ed 4, Minneapolis, Minn, 1989, Orthopedic Physical Therapy Products.

17. Schafer RC, Faye LJ: *Motion palpation and chiropractic technique: principles of dynamic chiropractic*, Huntington Beach, Calif, 1989, The Motion Palpation Institute.

18. Maitland GD: *Vertebral manipulation*, ed 5, London, 1990, Butterworth-Heinemann.

19. Hubka MJ, Phelan SP: Interexaminer reliability of palpation for cervical spine tenderness, *J Manipulative Physiol Ther* 17(9):591, 1994.

20. Maher C, Adams R: Reliability of pain and stiffness assessments in clinical manual lumbar spine examination, *Phys Ther* 74:801, 1994.

21. Boline PD et al: Interexaminer reliability of eight evaluative dimensions of lumbar segmental abnormality: part II, *J Manipulative Physiol Ther* 16(6):363, 1993.

22. Richter T, Lawall J: Zur zuverlassigkeit manualdianostischer befunde, *Man Med* 31:1, 1993.

23. Keating JC et al: Interexaminer reliability of eight evaluative dimensions of lumbar segmental abnormality, *J Manipulative Physiol Ther* 13(8):463, 1990.

24. Cantu RI, Grodin AJ: *Myofascial manipulation: theory and clinical application*, Gaithersburg, Md, 1992, Aspen.

25. Hammer WI: *Functional soft tissue examination and treatment by manual methods: the extremities*, ed 2, Gaithersburg, Md, 1999, Aspen.

26. Haldeman S et al: Spinal manipulative therapy. In Frymore JW, editor: *The adult spine: principles and practice*, ed 2, Philadelphia, 1997, Lippincott-Raven.

27. Travell JG, Simons DG: *Myofascial pain and dysfunction: the trigger point manual*, Baltimore, 1983, Williams and Wilkins.

28. Mennell J McM: *The musculoskeletal system: differential diagnosis from symptoms and physical signs*, Gaithersburg, Md, 1992, Aspen.

29. Sandoz R: Some physical mechanisms and affects of spinal adjustments, *Ann Swiss Chiropr Assoc* 6:91, 1976.

30. Brinkley J, Stratford PW, Gill C: Interrater reliability of lumbar accessory motion mobility testing, *Phys Ther* 75:786, 1995.

31. Kappler RE: Palpatory skills: an introduction. In Ward RC, editor: *Foundations for osteopathic medicine*, Baltimore, 1997, Williams and Wilkins.

32. Huijbregts PA: Spinal motion palpation: a review of reliability studies, *J Man Manipulative Ther* 10(1):24, 2002.

33. Boline PD et al: Interexaminer reliability of palpatory evaluations of the lumbar spine, *Am J Chiropr Med* 1:5, 1988.

34. Byfield D, Humphreys K: Intra- and inter-examiner reliability of bony landmark identification in the lumbar spine, *Euro J Chiropr* 72:13, 1992.

35. Christensen et al: Palpation of the upper thoracic spine: an observer reliability study, *J Manipulative Physiol Ther* 25:285, 2002.

36. DeBoer KF et al: Reliability study of detection of somatic dysfunctions in the cervical spine, *J Manipulative Physiol Ther* 8:9, 1985.

37. O'Haire C, Gibbons P: Inter-examiner and intra-examiner agreement for assessing sacroiliac anatomical landmarks using palpation and observation: pilot study, *Man Ther* 5(1):13, 2000.

38. Spring F, Gibbons P, Tehan P: Intra-examiner and inter-examiner reliability of a positional diagnostic screen for the lumbar spine, *J Osteopath Med* 4(2):47, 2001.

39. Van Suijlekom HA et al: Interobserver reliability in physical examination of the cervical spine in patients with headache, *Headache: J Head Face Pain* 40(7):581, 2001.

40. Bergstrom E, Courtis G: An inter- and intraexaminer reliability study of motion palpation of the lumbar spine in lateral flexion in the seated position, *Euro J Chiropr* 34:121, 1986.

41. French SD, Green S, Forbes A: Reliability of chiropractic methods commonly used to detect manipulable lesions in patients with chronic low-back pain, *J Manipulative Physiol Ther* 23:231, 2000.

42. Cibulka MT, Delitto A, Koldehoff RM: Changes in innominate tilt after manipulation of the sacroiliac joint in patients with low back pain: an experimental study, *Phys Ther* 68:1359, 1988.

43. Fjellner A et al: Interexaminer reliability in physical examination of the cervical spine, *J Manipulative Physiol Ther* 22:511, 1999.

44. Haas M et al: Reliability of manual end-play palpation of the thoracic spine, *Chiropr Tech* 7:120, 1995.

45. Hanten WP, Olson SL, Ludwig GM: Reliability of manual mobility testing of the upper cervical spine in subjects with cervicogenic headache, *J Manipulative Physiol Ther* 10(2):76, 2002.

46. Inscoe et al: Reliability in evaluating passive intervertebral motion of the lumbar spine, *J Man Manipulative Ther* 3: 135, 1995.

47. Jull G et al: Interexaminer reliability to detect painful upper cervical joint dysfunction, *Aust J Physiother* 43:125, 1997.

48. Jull G, Bullock M: A motion profile of the lumbar spine in an aging population assessed by manual examination, *Physiother Pract* 3:70, 1987.

49. Lewit K, Rosina A: Why yet another diagnostic sign of sacroiliac movement restriction? *J Manipulative Physiol Ther* 22:154, 1999.

50. Love RM, Brodeur RR: Inter- and intra-examiner reliability of motion palpation for the thoracolumbar spine, *J Manipulative Physiol Ther* 10:1, 1987.

51. Maher CG, Latimer J, Adams R: An investigation of the reliability and validity of posteroanterior spinal stiffness judgments made using a reference-based protocol, *Phys Ther* 78:829, 1998.

52. Meijne W et al: Intraexaminer and interexaminer reliability of the Gillet test, *J Manipulative Physiol Ther* 22:4, 1999.

53. Mior SA, McGregor M, Schut B: The role of experience in clinical accuracy, *J Manipulative Physiol Ther* 13(2):68, 1990.

54. Mior SA et al: Intra- and interexaminer reliability of motion palpation in the cervical spine, *J Canadian Chiropr Assoc* 29:195, 1985.

55. Mootz RD et al: Intra- and interobserver reliability of passive motion palpation of the lumber spine, *J Manipulative Physiol Ther* 12:440, 1989.

56. Nansel DD et al: Interexaminer concordance in detecting joint-play asymmetries in the cervical spines of otherwise asymptomatic subjects, *J Manipulative Physiol Ther* 12:428, 1989.

57. Phillips DR, Twomey LT: A comparison of manual diagnosis with a diagnosis established by a uni-level lumbar spinal block procedure, *Man Ther* 2:82, 1996.

58. Riddle DL, Freburger JK: Evaluation of the presence of sacroiliac joint region dysfunction using a combination of tests: a multicenter intertester reliability study, *Phys Ther* 82(8):772, 2002.

59. Schoensee SK et al: The effect of mobilization on cervical headaches, *J Orthop Sports Phys Ther* 21:184, 1995.

60. Schoeps P, Pfingsten M, Siebert U: Reliabilitaet manualmedizinischer Untersuchungstechniken an der Halswirbelsaeule, Studie zur Qualitaetssicherung in der manuellen Diagnostik, *Z Orthop Ihre Grenzgeb* 138:2, 2000.

61. Smedmark V, Wallin M, Arvidsson I: Interexaminer reliability in assessing passive intervertebral motion of the cervical spine, *Man Ther* 5:97, 2000.

62. Smith AR, Catlin PA, Nyberg RE: Intratester/ intertester reliability of segmental motion testing of cervicothoracic forward bending in a symptomatic population. In Paris SV, editor: *IFOMT Proceedings*, Vail, Colo, June 1-5, 1992, IFOMT.

63. Vincent-Smith B, Gibbons P: Inter-examiner and intra-examiner reliability of the standing flexion test, *Man Ther* 4(2):87, 1999.

64. Carmichael JP: Inter- and intraexaminer reliability of palpation for sacroiliac joint dysfunction, *J Manipulative Physiol Ther* 10:164, 1987.

65. Bronemo L, Van Steveninck J: *A comparison of inter- and intraexaminer reliability of motion palpation of the lower cervical spine (C2-C7) in the oblique-posterior-lateral direction in sitting and supine positions*, Thesis, Bournemouth, UK, 1987, Anglo-European College of Chiropractic.

66. Cooperstein R: The sacral leg check: destructive orthopedic test par excellence, *J Am Chiropr Assoc* 39(8):20, 2002.

67. Bergmann TF, Peterson DH, Lawrence DJ: *Chiropractic technique*, New York, 1993, Churchill Livingstone.

Introduction to Diagnostic Imaging

11

Gary M. Guebert, DC, DACBR,
Terry R. Yochum, DC, DACBR, FACCR

Key Terms

ABDOMINAL AORTIC ANEURYSM	GASTROENTEROLOGIST	PLEURAL EFFUSION
AMERICAN CHIROPRACTIC COLLEGE OF RADIOLOGY	INTRAVENOUS PYELOGRAM	PNEUMOTHORAX
	KILOVOLTS PEAK	POSITRON EMISSION TOMOGRAPHY
	KLIPPEL FEIL SYNDROME	
BONE SCANNING	MAGNETIC RESONANCE IMAGING	PULMONARY CONSOLIDATION
COLONOSCOPY		RADIOGRAPHY
COMPUTED RADIOGRAPHY	MAMMOGRAPHY	RARE EARTH SCREEN
COMPUTED TOMOGRAPHY	METASTASIS	SEPTIC ARTHRITIS
DIPLOMATE OF THE AMERICAN CHIROPRACTIC BOARD OF ROENTGENOLOGY	MICROBUBBLES	SPONDYLOLISTHESIS
	NEPHROLOGIST	SPONDYLOLYSIS
	NIMMO RECEPTOR TONUS	STENOSIS
	NUCLEAR MEDICINE	THROMBOSIS
DOPPLER ULTRASOUND	OSTEOMYELITIS	VIDEOFLUOROSCOPY
FLUOROSCOPY	OSTEOPHYTE	X-RAYS

Diagnostic imaging has been an essential component of chiropractic practice since the early days of the profession. Imaging studies allow the clinician deeper insight into the structural aspects of the body, permitting a degree of specificity in neuromusculoskeletal diagnosis that would otherwise be impossible. Plain-film radiography and other imaging methods allow chiropractors to rule out the presence of dangerous pathologic conditions before proceeding with manual chiropractic procedures and to refer appropriate cases for medical care or comanagement.

All chiropractic colleges provide extensive training in radiology as part of the required curriculum, sufficient to prepare the graduate to own and operate an x-ray machine and to interpret basic radiographic findings. All North American state and provincial licensing laws include radiology within the chiropractor's scope of practice, as do those in many other nations.

Chiropractic practice, with its neuromusculoskeletal focus, requires significant knowledge in skeletal radiology. Recent research by Taylor and colleagues[1] has evaluated students, clinicians, radiology residents, and radiologists from the chiropractic and medical professions in their interpretation of abnormal lumbar spine radiographs. The researchers found no significant difference between the performance of chiropractic radiologists and medical skeletal radiologists or between chiropractic and medical clinicians. Moreover, the chiropractic radiologists, chiropractic radiology residents, and chiropractic students scored significantly higher than the corresponding medical categories (general medical radiologists, medical radiology residents, and medical students, respectively).

This chapter provides an introduction to the history of diagnostic imaging, a brief description of the various imaging technologies in current use, the specific applications of these imaging procedures, the role of imaging in contemporary chiropractic practice, and a look into the future of diagnostic imaging.

HISTORY OF DIAGNOSTIC IMAGING

1895—On November 8, 1895 in Würzburg, Germany, Wilhelm Conrad Roentgen discovers **x-rays** while investigating the properties of cathode ray (Crookes) tubes. Shortly thereafter, Roentgen takes an x-ray of his wife Bertha's hand, an exposure that requires more than 15 minutes.

1898—Thomas A. Edison creates the fluoroscope whereby x-rays are projected on an intensifying screen coated with calcium tungstate as the fluorescent material. Thus human anatomy can be seen in real time. Fluoroscopy was the first widespread application for x-ray technology, allowing visualization of the beating heart, diaphragmatic movement, and intestinal peristalsis. Permanent photographic images were more challenging to obtain because the image was supported on a glass plate; the final image was heavy and subject to breakage. Unfortunately, practitioners were unaware of the whole-body radiation dose delivered to the patient and the physician during such procedures.

Because the deleterious effects of ionizing radiation were unknown at the dawn of the twentieth century, no protection was provided for the patient or physician. Radiation physicians tested the hardness (quality) of the x-ray beam by putting their own hands into the x-ray beam and viewing the resulting image. Within a few short years, some of the adverse biologic effects (skin cancer, thyroid cancer, and cataracts) of radiation exposure became manifest in these physicians who were excessively exposed to this type of radiation on a daily basis.

Fluoroscopy is currently used for contrast studies of the gastrointestinal and genitourinary tracts. The use and interpretation of fluoroscopy in assessing cervical spinal motion is being evaluated.

1901—Roentgen receives the Nobel Prize in physics for the discovery of x-rays.

1910—Palmer School of Chiropractic in Davenport, Iowa, purchases the first x-ray unit in the chiropractic profession.

1913—The Coolidge hot-filament x-ray tube is developed. Belgian glass was in short supply during World War I, thus the Eastman Kodak Company produced a cellulose-based film whereby the emulsion that contains the actual image was coated on one side only.

1917—The Potter Bucky moving grid is introduced, improving contrast on images of large body parts and making larger film sizes (14 × 17 inches) practical. This introduction signals the end of glass plates as film base material.

1922—Arthur Holly Compton describes the scattering of x-rays (Compton effect) for which he later receives the Nobel Prize in 1927.

1929—The rotating anode tube is introduced. Rotating the anode during x-ray production spreads out the heat that is produced and allows for greater radiographic technique (milliampere seconds [mAs]) to be used. By this time, virtually all chiropractic colleges have courses in radiology.

1935—The first standing, full-spine film is taken by New York City chiropractor Warren Sausser using a specially made film, 14 × 36 inches, from the Eastman Kodak Company.

1936—Tomography is introduced whereby reciprocal movement of the x-ray tube and film blur the anatomy above and below the level of interest within the patient's body, allowing the anatomy at the plane of interest to be visualized in greater detail.

1936—The National Council of Chiropractic Roentgenologists (NCCR) is founded. Members were chiropractors in general practice with particular interest in radiography and spinography.

1942—The first automatic x-ray film processor is introduced by Pako.

1946—Purcell and colleagues and Bloch and colleagues publish the principles of nuclear magnetic resonance. The use of magnetic fields for chemical spectroscopy is applied in the analysis of compounds in solution and for determining the structure of biologic macromolecules.[2,3]

1946—National Council of Chiropractic Roentgenologists (NCCR) holds its first meeting at the Palmer House Hotel in Chicago. Speakers include Drs. Leo Wunsch, John Teranel, Fred Baier, Ted Vladeff, and Warren Sausser.[4]

1951—The first nuclear medicine scans of the thyroid gland are produced by Cassen and Curtis.[5]

1956—Eastman Kodak Company introduces the first automatic roller transport film processor.

1958—The American Chiropractic Board of Roentgenology (ACBR) is formed for specialty certification of chiropractic radiologists. The original qualifications to sit for the certifying examination included 200 hours of lecture and maintaining an active chiropractic practice with at least 5-years' use of x-rays. The first three chiropractors to pass the certifying examination were Drs. Joseph Janse, Lester P. Rehberger, and Earl A. Rich. The professional designation for candidates who pass the examination is **Diplomate of the American Chiropractic Board of Roentgenology** (DACBR).

1964—The first annual gathering of chiropractic radiologists takes place at Lincoln Chiropractic College, Indianapolis, Indiana.

1966—Diagnostic ultrasound, which grew out of sonar technology in World War II, is commonly available.

1967—The first resident training program in chiropractic radiology is instituted at the National College of Chiropractic in Lombard, Illinois. Three academic years, encompassing 4400 hours of training, is required before eligibility for certification is possible. Drs. James F. Winterstein and Donald B. Tomkins are the first resident-trained candidates to

become certified as DACBRs after training with chiropractic radiologist Leonard Ritchie.

1968—The American Chiropractic College of Roentgenology (now the American Chiropractic College of Radiology) is formed.

1973—Hounsfield creates the first **computed tomography** (CT) scanner, demonstrating human anatomy in a series of axial "slices." CT begins to replace most plain-film tomography applications.[6]

1973—Raymond Damadian and Paul Lauterbur produce the first nuclear magnetic resonance images (now known as **magnetic resonance imaging** [MRI]), demonstrating the distribution of charged polar protons (primarily hydrogen protons).[7,8]

1974—Rare earth intensifying screens are introduced. **Rare earth screen** phosphors are doubly efficient at converting x-ray photon energy into light energy as compared with non-rare earth compounds such as calcium tungstate. A significant reduction in patient exposure dose is realized from this innovation in x-ray image production.[9]

1980—The first commercial superconducting MRI magnet is introduced by Technicare.

1983—The Eastman Kodak Company develops the first tabular grain film emulsion. Tabular grain films allow for less silver to be used per film, as well as thinner emulsions that contain the actual image. Thinner emulsions result in thinner films, thus reducing the parallax effect and producing more detailed images.

1985—Medium-frequency x-ray generators (6 kHz) are made commercially available, and in 1987, 100-kHz true high-frequency generating systems are developed. These systems are supplied by single-phase electrical power sources but have radiographic power equal to 3-phase generating systems found in hospitals, making this technology affordable for private practices. An added benefit is a significant radiation dose reduction for patients.

1990—Toshiba introduces spiral CT, which allows for a single but continuous exposure of a large body part, such as the chest or abdomen, in a single breath-hold. The total time in the scanner for the patient is reduced, and greater patient throughput is possible.

1992—The U.S. federal government passes the **Mammography** Quality Standards Act (MQSA), significantly improving the quality of mammographic images and reducing patient exposure. MQSA banned the use of single-phase generating systems in the production of mammograms in an effort to further reduce radiation exposure to the breast. Currently, only 3-phase and high-frequency generators are approved for the production of mammograms in the United States.

1998—Multiple rows of detectors (from 4 to 16 rows) and slice acquisition times under 1 second make multislice CT practical for imaging large body cavities such as the chest or abdomen.

CHIROPRACTIC APPLICATIONS FOR DIAGNOSTIC IMAGING

Diagnostic imaging in chiropractic practice includes imaging studies (primarily plain-film x-ray) performed or supervised by the chiropractor and other studies (primarily MRI, CT, and diagnostic ultrasound) performed by chiropractic or medical radiology specialists on referral from the treating chiropractor. At present, most chiropractic general practices have an on-site x-ray machine, but very few have an on-site CT or MRI facility. Therefore patients needing such specialized procedures are referred to larger radiology facilities.

X-Ray

Radiography is the production of photographic images by passing x-rays (a form of electromagnetic energy with a short wavelength) through the body. *X-rays should be taken only when a clinical indication exists that they are needed.* Radiographs may be indicated to rule out contraindications to adjustment/manipulation, such as fracture, dislocation, tumor, or infection, and to evaluate structure and function. This use is sometimes considered a "rule-out" situation in which a single diagnosis is not obvious from the patient's history and physical examination. In a typical chiropractic setting, an older patient might present with localized pain in the neck that radiates into one of the upper extremities. A common cause for this situation might be disk degeneration with or without bone spur **(osteophyte)** formation at the Luschka joint, resulting in intervertebral foraminal **stenosis** (Fig. 11-1). In such a case, a series of neck x-rays should be obtained that would include oblique views showing the intervertebral foramina. If the oblique films demonstrate the foramina to be narrowed by osteophytes, this would confirm a diagnosis of degenerative foraminal stenosis and would be the likely source of the patient's complaint of pain radiating from the neck.

Another patient may present with a productive cough and an elevated temperature. This presentation suggests the potential for pneumonia. Obtaining posteroanterior and lateral chest

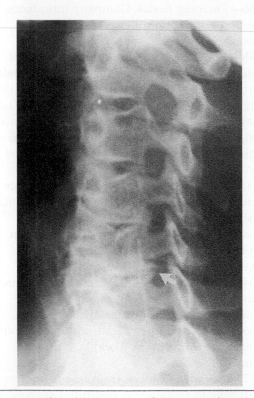

Fig. 11-1 This oblique x-ray of the cervical spine demonstrates degenerative narrowing of the C5-C6 foramen resulting from degenerative hypertrophy of the Luschka joint *(arrow)*. *(From Yochum TR, Rowe LJ: Essentials of skeletal radiology, ed 2, Baltimore, 1996, Williams & Wilkins. Reprinted with permission of Lippincott–Williams & Wilkins.)*

x-rays to see if a **pulmonary consolidation** (fluid accumulation in the airspace of the lung) is present would be most prudent, thus confirming a diagnosis of pneumonia. If consolidation is not evident on the radiographs, then another cause for the symptoms must be sought.

Other clear indications for a chiropractor to order radiographs include concern for the presence of **spondylolisthesis,** congenital or functional short leg, scoliosis, intervertebral fixations, congenital anomalies and variants, and clinical manifestations of vertebral subluxation complex.

Flexion, extension, and lateral bending views of the cervical or lumbar spine may follow static (neutral posture) radiographs, enabling the clinician to evaluate global range of motion, intersegmental biomechanics, and intersegmental stability. Cervical flexion and extension views are commonly obtained. Lateral bending of the cervical spine, lumbar flexion and extension, and lumbar lateral bending views are also obtained.

Fluoroscopy

Fluoroscopy is an x-ray procedure that allows real-time visualization of physiologic motion within the human body. During fluoroscopy, the clinician can watch the progression of a bolus of swallowed barium moving through the esophagus and stomach or peristaltic waves moving iodinated dye down the ureter. Rarely, fluoroscopy is used to watch the cervical spine move in flexion, extension, and lateral bending.

Although the radiation dose associated with traditional fluoroscopy is substantial, it is currently the only practical means to see the dynamics of intestinal and genitourinary function.

Gastrointestinal Fluoroscopy

Upper Gastrointestinal Study

An adult male patient may present with neck pain and difficulty swallowing. Diagnostic considerations for such a presentation include compression of the upper esophagus by large osteophytes on the anterior aspect of the lower cervical vertebrae or possibly a mass arising from the upper esophagus or the surrounding soft tissues. Lateral x-rays of the cervical spine may demonstrate thickening of the soft tissues in front of the C6 and C7 vertebrae, lateral displacement of the tracheal air shadow on the anteroposterior (AP) film, or both. These radiographic findings suggest a tumor of the upper esophagus or adjacent soft tissues.

To further investigate this finding, the chiropractor would be obligated to refer the patient for a barium study that evaluates the upper gastrointestinal (GI) system. For this study, the patient drinks a barium mixture that, when x-rayed, shows the cavity of the esophagus or stomach as white. Displacement of the barium within the esophagus would then confirm the presence of the tumor, and referral to a **gastroenterologist** would be indicated for treatment of the tumor.

Another example would be a case in which, responding to a local television appeal, a 60-year-old man obtains a screening test from the local pharmacy and discovers that occult blood is present in the stool. This man is a chiropractic patient and reports this finding. The chiropractor would then order a confirmatory laboratory test, which also comes back positive. Occult blood in the stool suggests that the bleeding has originated high in the GI system (esophagus or stomach). The most common reason for this bleeding includes gastric ulcer or neoplasm. Referring the patient for an upper GI study to localize the origin of the bleeding would be reasonable and prudent.

If the study shows evidence of a gastric ulcer, the chiropractor may counsel the patient on diet and lifestyle changes to reduce stress while adjusting the spine for any subluxations. However, if the study showed evidence of a tumor of the stomach, the chiropractor would initiate a medical referral for appropriate treatment.

Lower Gastrointestinal Study

Diseases of the lower intestine may express sequelae in the spine. Seronegative enteropathic diseases (certain bowel diseases that do not express a positive rheumatoid factor in the blood) such as Crohn's disease and ulcerative colitis may also cause spinal arthritic disease. These changes include inflammatory bone spurs on the vertebral bodies called syndesmophytes and, in some cases, inflammatory changes affecting the sacroiliac, hip, and shoulder joints.

A chiropractor may first find these distinctive spinal and sacroiliac changes on spinal x-rays and then have to refer the patient for a lower GI study to document any associated intestinal disease.

Genitourinary Fluoroscopy

Kidney disease can be a cause of back pain. To rule out the genitourinary system as the primary cause of back pain, a chiropractor may choose to order fluoroscopy as a specific imaging test to rule out kidney disease or obstruction of the outflow of urine.

Intravenous Pyelogram

Occasionally, on a lumbar spine x-ray, a calcification will be seen lateral to the L2 or L3 vertebra on the AP film, and the calcification superimposes on these same vertebral bodies on the lateral view. The radiographic appearance and anatomic location suggests a kidney stone. To differentiate a kidney stone from a calcified lymph node, referral for an **intravenous pyelogram** (IVP) would be necessary.

To obtain an IVP study, an iodinated dye is injected into the bloodstream, and the dye is then filtered by normally functioning kidneys. If the calcification is shown to displace the dye as it collects in the renal pelvis, the renal stone is confirmed. Once the kidney stone is confirmed, then referral to a **nephrologist** or internist is appropriate.

For another example, a plain-film radiograph of the lumbar spine appears to demonstrate an irregular outline for one of the kidneys. An IVP study would help the chiropractor differentiate a renal mass from superimposed intestinal contents.

Last, in a patient who has multiple block vertebrae, a diagnosis of **Klippel Feil syndrome** would be considered. In addition to the vertebral anomalies, cardiac and genitourinary anomalies may also be present. An IVP study would be appropriate in such a patient to determine if a congenitally malformed *horseshoe* or *cake* kidney is present.

Spinal Motion

A chiropractor may palpate unusual intersegmental motion during motion palpation of the patient's spine. Static radiographs of the cervical spine in the end range of flexion or extension or of the lumbar spine in full left or right lateral flexion do nothing to disclose aberrant coupled motion during the mid-range of motion.

Fluoroscopy of the cervical spine may demonstrate these mid-range abnormalities. The patient is asked to perform a variety of neck motions, including flexion, extension, left and right bending, plus specific motions for the upper cervical spine. Typically, this study requires 2 minutes of beam-on time, is videotaped for later review, and minimizes the patient's radiation exposure, which is considerable compared with plain-film techniques and is always in addition to the plain-film dose.

Videofluoroscopy (VF) of lumbar spine motion is rarely performed because of poor image quality. This loss of image quality is primarily the result of the large amount of scatter radiation that emanates from large body parts when they are x-rayed, resulting in poor contrast among the bones, joints, and soft tissues.

Computed Tomography

CT is an x-ray technique during which the patient usually lies supine on a table and is positioned within the gantry that contains the x-ray tube and radiation detectors. The x-ray tube rotates around the patient, and the detectors record the radiation that is transmitted through the patient. Computers take the information from the detectors and convert it into an image (slice) that is displayed on a computer screen.

Because the information acquired is digital in nature, it can also be manipulated electronically so that images that show bone detail (bone windows) and soft-tissue detail (soft-tissue windows) are acquired. A relatively large

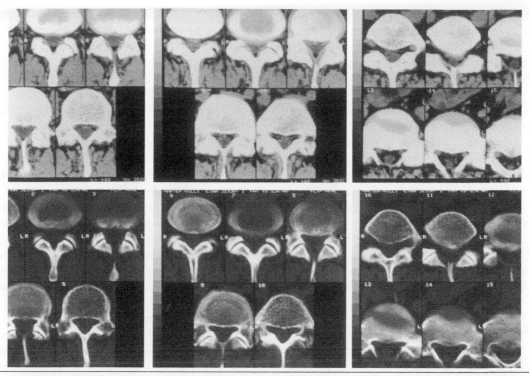

Fig. 11-2 These axial CT images of a lumbar vertebra show how the same information can be digitally altered to show the soft tissues *(top row of images)* or bony anatomy *(bottom row of images)* to the best advantage. *(From Yochum TR, Rowe LJ:* Essentials of skeletal radiology, *ed 2, Baltimore, 1996, Williams & Wilkins. Reprinted with permission of Lippincott–Williams & Wilkins.)*

number of slices through the anatomy of interest is necessary (Fig. 11-2).

Two advantages CT has over plain-film radiography are a three-dimensional anatomic perspective and soft-tissue contrast that is significantly better with CT than it is with plain films.

Bone and Joints

A defect in the pars interarticularis (**spondylolysis**) may not always be evident on plain-film radiographs, particularly when the bony defect is unilateral or when bilateral defects are present without significant anterior slippage of the vertebral body (spondylolisthesis). This false negative finding is primarily caused when the plane of the defect through the pars interarticularis is not oriented parallel to the x-rays as they pass through the defect. Therefore, to confirm the spondylolysis, referral for CT may be required.

Stenosis (narrowing) of the lateral recess and spinal canal stenosis are difficult or impossible to assess with plain-film radiography and are best evaluated by CT.

If a chiropractor has been treating a patient with advanced disk or facet joint degenerative disease, but the patient is slow to respond or does not respond to adjustive/manipulative treatment, a CT examination of the affected region of the spine may disclose lateral recess stenosis or spinal canal stenosis resulting from the bone spurs not revealed on the initial plain-film study. Surgical decompression of the area may be necessary for patients whose symptoms do not respond to chiropractic treatment.

CT can often demonstrate pelvic fractures that are suspected or not evident on plain-film radiography.

Soft Tissues

CT of the chest and mediastinum is useful at localizing a mass found on plain film or to determine if the mass contains calcification. Calcification of pulmonary masses is often a sign of benignancy. CT also is better than plain-film radiographs at finding small **pneumothoraces** (air outside the lung but inside the chest cavity) and **pleural effusions** (fluid outside the lung but inside the chest cavity), as well as intrathoracic aortic aneurysms.

In the abdomen, CT is helpful at finding organ (e.g., liver, kidney) or lymph node metastatic cancer, subphrenic abscess, and diaphragmatic hernias involving the stomach, liver, or intestines. Abdominal aortic aneurysms are well evaluated by CT, particularly if diagnostic ultrasound is unavailable or cannot be performed because of copious intestinal gas (Fig. 11-3).

Last, CT is invaluable in guiding needles into tumors for biopsies and for the placement of catheters to inject contrast materials or to drain abscesses and pleural effusions.

Magnetic Resonance Imaging

MRI is based on the fact that polar protons (particularly hydrogen protons) have a net charge

because of unpaired nuclear elements. Thus these protons behave as tiny bar magnets do in the presence of a strong magnetic field, similar to the way a compass needle points north in the presence of the earth's magnetic field. When a patient is placed in the bore of a superconducting magnet, all of the hydrogen protons inside the patient's body align with the main magnetic field. External radio frequencies are then used to add energy to these protons by pushing them out of alignment with the main magnetic field. When the external radio frequencies are turned off, the hydrogen protons give back the excess energy in the form of radio waves. Antennae that surround the patient receive these radio frequencies emitted by the protons and feed that information to computers that analyze the signal and create an electronic image of that slice of anatomy. The image can then be viewed on a computer screen or printed to film.

Advantages of MRI include the fact no ionizing radiation is utilized as is the case with x-ray and CT, and that any plane within the body can be imaged. Anatomic relationships are better demonstrated than they are using plain-film radiographs. Anatomic detail is exquisite, and fluid (e.g., cerebrospinal fluid, synovial fluid, hydrated disks, urine) can be easily identified and localized.

Soft Tissues

X-rays of the knee do not demonstrate internal derangements such as injuries to the cruciate ligaments or menisci. The integrity of these structures is best evaluated by MRI (Fig. 11-4).

Hematoma, compartment syndrome in the forearm or lower leg, rotator cuff tears or impingement syndrome in the shoulder, joint effusions, tendonitis, and Baker's cyst of the knee are all better demonstrated on MRI images compared with plain-film or CT images. Before the availability of MRI, arthrography (an x-ray study in which contrast is first injected into the joint) was the standard imaging modality for evaluating meniscal tears. The accuracy and noninvasive nature of MRI has led to the replacement of arthrography for most intra- and juxta-articular knee pathologic conditions (Fig. 11-5).

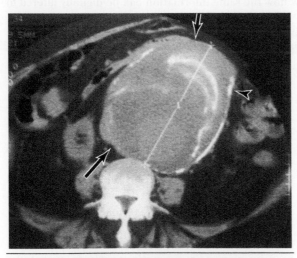

Fig. 11-3 This axial, noncontrast CT image (soft-tissue window) of the mid-abdomen clearly demonstrates a large aortic aneurysm (*arrow*), including the peripheral calcification (*arrowhead*) in the wall of the aneurysm. An electronic cursor has been positioned to measure the diameter of the aneurysm. (*Courtesy of Ralph E. Brewer, DC, Denver, Colorado. From Yochum TR, Rowe LJ: Essentials of skeletal radiology, ed 2, Baltimore, 1996, Williams & Wilkins. Reprinted with permission of Lippincott–Williams & Wilkins.*)

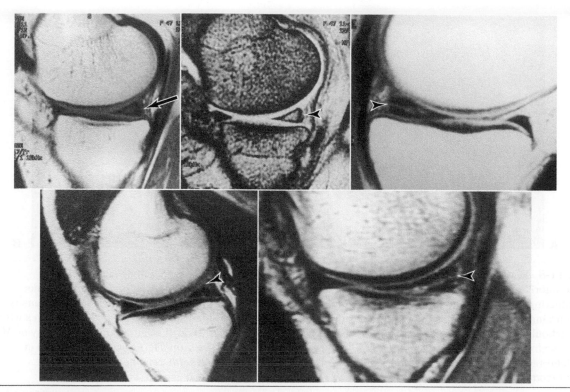

Fig. 11-4 MRI sagittal images, with various pulsing sequences, of different knees demonstrating meniscal tears and degeneration. A normal meniscus is triangular in shape and demonstrates no internal signal (is dark) on MRI *(arrow)*. The bright signal within these menisci proves damage, or a tear, that is unseen on plain-film radiographs *(arrowheads)*. *(From Yochum TR, Rowe LJ:* Essentials of skeletal radiology, *ed 2, Baltimore, 1996, Williams & Wilkins. Reprinted with permission of Lippincott–Williams & Wilkins.)*

Cartilage

Special MRI pulsing sequences can now show the hyaline cartilage that covers the articular end of the bones within a synovial joint. A breakdown, injury, or defect in the articular cartilage, similar to that seen in chondromalacia patella, can now be shown with these MRI sequences.

Bone Bruise

The only method to diagnose the intraosseous edema of a bone bruise accurately is MRI. Patients with this condition will complain of localized pain, with or without localized trauma, but the plain films will be negative. The microfractures of the bony trabeculae and associated bone marrow edema are clearly demonstrated on standard and fat-suppressed MR images.

Marrow Replacement Disorders

MRI will clearly demonstrate the marrow of all bones contained within the field of view. Neoplastic replacement of bone marrow will be easily demonstrated by common MRI techniques. An example might be occult or symptomatic *metastases* to bone. A patient may have or had a primary malignant tumor. Once this condition occurs, the possibility for spread of the tumor **(metastasis)** from the primary site to the bone marrow must be considered and evaluated by MRI (Fig. 11-6).

Diagnostic Ultrasound

Diagnostic ultrasound is an excellent imaging modality for soft-tissue concerns because it is

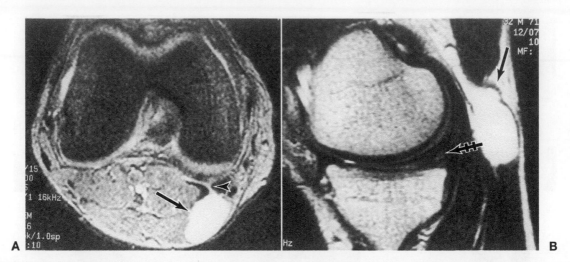

Fig. 11-5 **A,** MRI, axial knee. A large Baker's cyst lies posterior to the femoral condyle *(arrow).* Characteristically, uncomplicated cysts exhibit a very hyperintense signal. The axial images show a tract connecting the cyst to the joint capsule *(arrowhead).* Additionally, a faint, horizontal, high signal–intensity area is coursing through the substance of the posterior horn of the medial meniscus. The area communicates with the articular surfaces *(crossed arrow),* consistent with a grade III tear. **B,** MRI, sagittal knee. *(Courtesy of Alan M. Lesselroth, MD, Mountain Diagnostics, Las Vegas, Nevada. From Yochum TR, Rowe LJ:* Essentials of skeletal radiology, *ed 2, Baltimore, 1996, Williams & Wilkins. Reprinted with permission of Lippincott–Williams & Wilkins.)*

easily and commonly available, does not use ionizing radiation, is price competitive with other imaging technologies, and the images can be viewed in real time. Diagnostic ultrasound is particularly useful at distinguishing solid tumors from fluid-filled cysts. A special form of ultrasound is **Doppler ultrasound,** which allows the color characterization of flowing blood. One shortcoming of diagnostic ultrasound is that it cannot see into or through adult bone. Basically, high-frequency sound waves (from 1 to 20 MHz) are directed into the body region of interest from the transducer. The sound waves are reflected back (echo) from tissue interfaces and collected by the transducer. The time necessary for the sound wave to travel from the transducer and back is a measure of the depth of the tissue plane that reflected the sound waves. A computer takes this information and converts it to a gray scale image that is displayed in virtual real time.

Aortic Aneurysm

Chiropractors need to know if an **abdominal aortic aneurysm** (AAA) is present before treat-

ment. If the patient has an AAA, high-velocity, low-amplitude (HVLA) manipulations of the lumbar spine would be contraindicated, and an urgent medical referral would be in order (Fig. 11-7).

Chiropractors also need to know if an established aneurysm is stable or enlarging over time. A small, nonsurgical aneurysm may eventually enlarge to the point that referral to an internist or vascular surgeon is indicated. One of the best ways to follow an aneurysm to gauge progressive enlargement would be through the use of diagnostic ultrasound.

Chiropractors should also understand that performing or interpreting an ultrasound examination might be technically impossible for evaluating the abdominal aorta if the patient has copious amounts of intestinal gas. Under these circumstances, CT examination would provide a better evaluation of the aortic diameter.

Vertebral and Carotid Arteries

A patient may present to a chiropractor and require adjustment/manipulation of the cervical spine in the management of his or her condition.

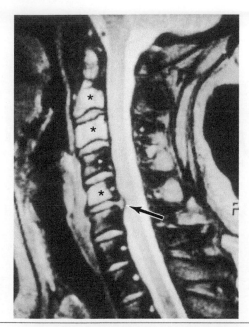

Fig. 11-6 This 48-year-old woman complained of neck and arm pain. Plain films and a bone scan (not shown) were negative. An MRI was performed to rule out a herniated disk. Note the contained disk herniation at C5-C6 *(arrow)*. However, an unexpected finding on this gradient-echo sagittal cervical MRI was the increased signal intensity foci within several cervical vertebrae *(asterisks)*. The marrow infiltrated by the tumor is hyperintense relative to the normally low signal fatty marrow. These findings were proven to be metastatic carcinoma from a primary breast carcinoma. *(Courtesy of James E. Carter, DC, DACBR, Danville, California. From Yochum TR, Rowe LJ: Essentials of skeletal radiology, ed 2, Baltimore, 1996, Williams & Wilkins. Reprinted with permission of Lippincott–Williams & Wilkins.)*

If the patient is also at risk for atherosclerosis, obtaining a Doppler ultrasound may be prudent to evaluate the carotid and vertebral arteries for atheromatous stenosis. The presence of substantial vascular stenosis by fatty or calcified plaques demonstrated by Doppler ultrasound may necessitate the use of a nonforceful chiropractic technique or, in some cases, contraindicate chiropractic adjustment/manipulation of the neck.

Deep Vein Thrombosis

Thrombosis is a condition in which a mass (thrombus) develops within a vein. The danger for the patient is that the thrombus may break

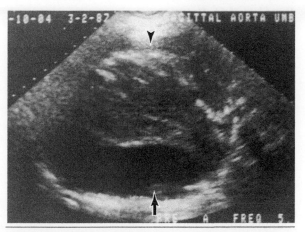

Fig. 11-7 A 76-year-old woman presented with low back pain, at which time plain films were obtained. On discovery of the aortic aneurysm, the patient refused surgery, the aneurysm subsequently ruptured, and the woman died some 10 months later. On this sagittal ultrasound scan of the abdomen, the existing aortic lumen is visible *(arrows)*. The anterior calcified margin that was seen on plain-film radiographs is visible *(arrowhead)*. A large amount of mural thrombus can be identified between the arrows and arrowhead. *(Courtesy of Ralph F. Brewer, DC, Mound, Minnesota. From Yochum TR, Rowe LJ: Essentials of skeletal radiology, ed 2, Baltimore, 1996, Williams & Wilkins. Reprinted with permission of Lippincott–Williams & Wilkins.)*

loose and travel within the blood vessels to a distant site (embolism). The thrombus may then cause an obstruction of blood flow distal to that point (infarction) and result in tissue damage or tissue death.

A patient may present to a chiropractor with leg or calf pain. A method of chiropractic treatment might include the **Nimmo receptor tonus** technique or other soft-tissue technique. However, if the chiropractor was to "strip" the gastrocnemius muscle firmly with the thumbs, he or she might run the risk of dislodging a deep vein thrombus. The situation can be further complicated if the patient is a young female smoker taking oral birth control. This particular patient is at great risk for having deep vein thrombosis because of the smoking history and choice of birth control. Doppler ultrasound may rule out deep vein thrombosis before administering the Nimmo technique or any other soft-tissue technique to the lower leg.

Renal and Gallstones

Most gallstones (85%) and some kidney stones (15%) contain little or no calcium and will not show on plain-film radiographs. Diagnostic ultrasound is effective for diagnosing renal (kidney) stones or gallstones.

Last, a chiropractor may order diagnostic ultrasound for a patient who presents with fracture of the lumbar transverse processes. The concern is that the kidneys or ureters may also have been damaged during the trauma that fractured the transverse processes. Diagnostic ultrasound is used to rule out traumatic injury to the kidneys and ureters.

Nuclear Medicine

Nuclear medicine uses radioactive materials that are usually injected or sometimes inhaled into the body to demonstrate organ-specific pathologic conditions. This type of imaging includes **bone scanning** to demonstrate bone tumors, **osteomyelitis,** and other multicentric diseases, as well as **positron emission tomography** (PET) scanning, which is useful for localizing brain and lung tumors.

Disseminated Metastases

One clear advantage of a bone scan is that the entire body can be inspected for widespread dissemination of skeletal metastases (Fig. 11-8).

Occult Fracture

Plain-film radiography may not always demonstrate all osseous fractures, resulting in a false-negative impression. If a fracture site is not appreciably displaced or the x-ray beam is not directed parallel through the fracture plane, it may be missed on plain-film imaging (Fig. 11-9).

When faced with an apparently negative x-ray, but a patient with symptoms and a history consistent with a bone fracture, a chiropractor would be well advised to refer the patient for a bone scan to rule out an occult fracture (Fig. 11-10).

Infection and Neoplasm

Osteomyelitis (bone infection), **septic arthritis** (joint infection), or tumors may cause a patient to have considerable pain. However, unless these lesions have caused 30% to 50% destruction of

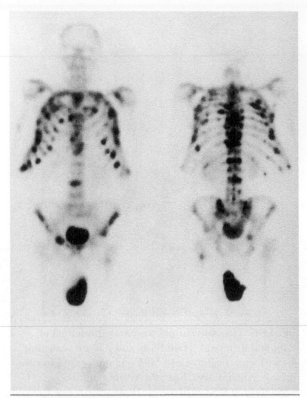

Fig. 11-8 This elderly man had a history of treated small cell carcinoma of the lung and presented with low back pain; bone scan, anterior whole body (*left*), and posterior whole body (*right*). Widespread sites of markedly increased tracer activity are present, consistent with skeletal metastasis. A urine-filled bag from a draining catheter is noted inferior to the pelvis *(arrows)*. *(Courtesy of Timothy Schneider, DC, Racine, Wisconsin. From Yochum TR, Rowe LJ: Essentials of skeletal radiology, ed 2, Baltimore, 1996, Williams & Wilkins. Reprinted with permission of Lippincott–Williams & Wilkins.)*

the bone, the process will not be evident on plain-film x-rays. Bone scans can demonstrate as little as 5% bone destruction and hence can allow for earlier diagnosis and treatment of early infection or neoplasm (Fig. 11-11).

FUTURE HORIZONS

Computed and Digital Radiography

Computed radiography uses a screen inside a conventional x-ray cassette to absorb the x-ray energy transmitted through a patient who is being

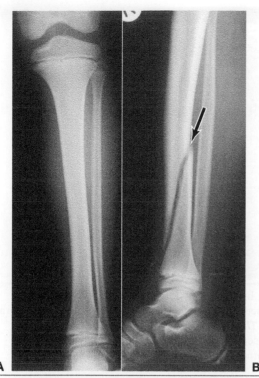

Fig. 11-9 A, On the AP view, no abnormality is evident. **B,** The lateral view clearly shows an oblique fracture line *(arrow)* in the tibia that was not visible on the AP view. *(From Yochum TR, Rowe LJ: Essentials of skeletal radiology, ed 2, Baltimore, 1996, Williams & Wilkins. Reprinted with permission of Lippincott–Williams & Wilkins.)*

x-rayed. This screen is then removed from the cassette and inserted into a laser reader. The stored energy is converted into electrical impulses that are interpreted by computer and converted into an electronic black-and-white image that can be viewed on a computer monitor or printed to film. Radiographic exposure techniques and exposure dose are similar to those used in plain-film radiography.

With digital radiography and the direct digital capture of x-ray transmission through the patient, several improvements over plain-film radiography become evident. Because the contrast of the final image is controlled electronically, the choice of x-ray penetrating power **(kilovolts peak [kVp])** is less important in digital radiography than it is in plain-film radiography. The result is that considerably higher kVp values

can be used, which reduces the patient's exposure dose. Second, because digital radiography involves an electronic image, it can be manipulated electronically to change the brightness, contrast, or both, thus improving the readability of the image. The clinician can also magnify areas of interest on the image and brighten or darken selected portions of the image to improve interpretation. This ability results in the third improvement—virtually no repeat examinations—thereby further reducing patient exposure. Last, an electronic image can be sent to remote locations over telephone lines or other means of electronic communication for interpretation or consultation. With such technology, a chiropractor will also be spared the substantial expense of purchasing and maintaining a film processor or the chemicals to process films, nor does he or she have to clean, maintain, and repair the processor, resulting in a substantial monetary savings over years of use of the digital system. Moreover, electronic images can be stored and retrieved much more efficiently and economically compared with traditional film systems.

Computer-Aided Diagnosis

Another application of computer technology is that mapping software can be used to "read" digital diagnostic images, which appears to improve the accuracy of lesion conspicuity and diagnosis.

Breast Imaging

Evaluation of mammographic films by experienced radiologists routinely finds 85% to 90% of breast cancers. Recent evidence has shown that computer over-read analysis of digital mammographic images, in conjunction with the radiologist's analysis, increases the likelihood that a lesion will be identified and correctly characterized as being benign or malignant. Also in evidence is that the sensitivity of a radiologist using computer-aided diagnosis (CAD) can be improved up to 19%: microcalcifications are yielded with CAD in 100% of cases and masses in up to 80% of cases.[10] If the computer software detects any breast abnormalities on the digital

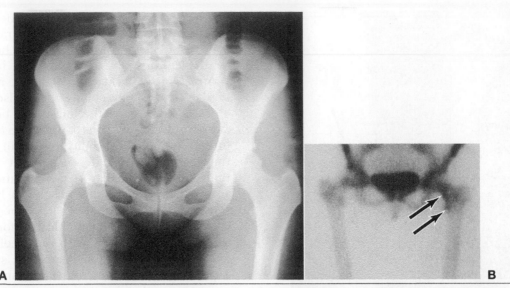

Fig. **11-10** This 31-year-old female runner presented with left hip pain. **A,** AP pelvis. These radiographs are normal. **B,** Bone scan, anterior pelvis. A linear band of increased activity is noted involving the medial femoral neck, consistent with a stress fracture *(arrows)*. *(Courtesy of The Deaconess West Hospital, Department of Radiology, St Louis, Missouri. From Yochum TR, Rowe LJ: Essentials of skeletal radiology, ed 2, Baltimore, 1996, Williams & Wilkins. Reprinted with permission of Lippincott–Williams & Wilkins.)*

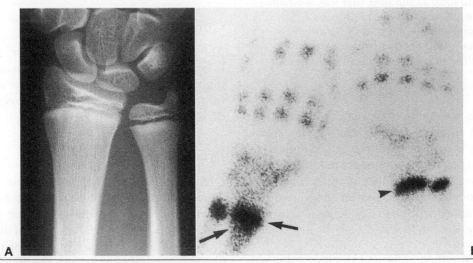

Fig. **11-11** **A,** Despite localized swelling, pain, and a slight fever, the radius shows no radiographic abnormality. **B,** The radioisotope bone scan also obtained at initial presentation shows an increased area of blackness (a "hot spot") in the corresponding symptomatic radius *(arrows)* as compared with the normal side *(arrowhead)*. *(From Yochum TR, Rowe LJ: Essentials of skeletal radiology, ed 2, Baltimore, 1996, Williams & Wilkins. Reprinted with permission of Lippincott–Williams & Wilkins.)*

image, it marks these areas of the image. These abnormalities might be bright spots, suggesting microcalcifications that are highly suggestive of cancer or dense regions with radiating margins (another pattern suggestive of cancer). The radiologist can then go back and review the image to determine whether the marked areas are suspicious and require an additional imaging test or biopsy.

Over time, it is anticipated that not only will the CAD assist in the localization of suspicious findings, but also that CAD software will also make predictions on the likelihood that a mass is cancerous.

Virtual Colonoscopy

Current techniques to visualize the inner surface of the large intestine have been limited to double-contrast lower GI studies, as well as **colonoscopy** using a fiber optic scope inserted rectally. These techniques are time-consuming and difficult for the patient who is being examined. With the advent of spiral CT and computer software, creating a three-dimensional computer representation of the inner surface of the intestine is now possible (Fig. 11-12). The sensitivity and specificity of this technique rivals that of traditional colonoscopy.[11]

PET-CT Fusion

PET uses radioactive substances such as 18F-fluorodeoxyglucose (FDG). FDG is a glucose analog that is radioactive and emits positrons (beta particles) that yield 511 kilo electron volts (keV) of energy. The half-life of FDG is 110 minutes. Anywhere increased glucose metabolism occurs within the body, such as tumor cells, an increased concentration of the FDG (uptake of FDG is proportional to the rate of glycolysis in cells) will be found, allowing differentiation of most malignant from benign tumors.[12]

CT is an x-ray procedure that provides cross-sectional (usually axial) images of human anatomy, as was discussed earlier. The marriage of PET and CT technologies (sometimes MRI images are used instead of CT) allows for precise anatomic localization of specific neoplastic (can-

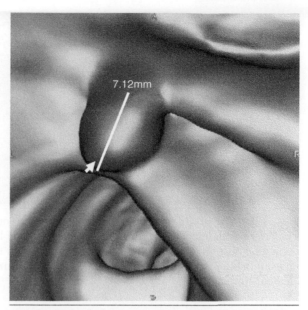

Fig. 11-12 Information from a multislice CT study of the abdomen has been reconstructed by computer to create this virtual colonoscopy image. A 7-mm intraluminal tumor is clearly demonstrated *(arrow)*. *(Courtesy of TeraRecon, Inc.)*

cerous) processes. The time necessary for uptake of the radiopharmaceutical in any tumors that may be present is approximately 60 minutes after injection. Then, in one 30-minute scanning procedure, both CT and PET images are acquired on the same scanning device (known as hybrid systems). The PET and CT images are then anatomically superimposed by computer software, creating a fusion image (Fig. 11-13). Thus anatomically localizing, staging, restaging, planning radiation therapy, and monitoring cancer treatments become much easier. For certain cancers, PET imaging appears to be more sensitive and specific than bone scans at identifying osseous metastases.[13]

If a chiropractor is confronted with a patient with low back pain who also has a history of cancer and now presents with negative x-rays of the spine and a failure to respond to conservative chiropractic treatment, a referral for a PET-CT fusion study may well take place in the near future to determine if the pain represents a recurrence of the primary tumor or metastasis of that tumor to other sites.

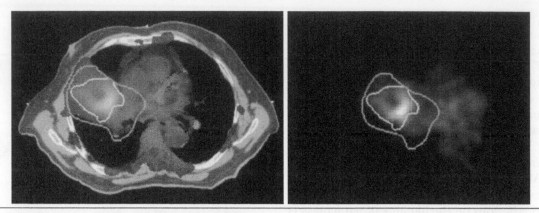

Fig. 11-13 The image on the right demonstrates two outlined areas related to a malignant pulmonary tumor. The larger outlined area represents the area identified by the CT scan, and the inner outlined area represents the actual portion of the lesion that requires radiation treatment. The image on the *left* represents the fused image in which the PET image is combined with the anatomically correlated CT slice. *(Courtesy of Philips Medical Systems.)*

Diagnostic Ultrasound

Musculoskeletal applications for diagnostic ultrasound are gaining acceptance. Evaluating the rotator cuff tendon for tears and of the carpal tunnel to document median nerve swelling are newer uses of this technology.

First available in the early 1980s, **microbubbles** have been used as a vascular contrast agent during Doppler ultrasound to assess myocardial perfusion. The microbubbles of gas enhance ultrasound backscatter so that flowing blood stands out from the surrounding soft tissues. Currently, microbubbles of galactose, coated by a palmitic acid-based agent, are dissolved and agitated in sterile water, creating air-filled microbubbles with a lipid (palmitic acid) coating. During Doppler ultrasound, these microbubbles increase the signal of blood by 10 decibels (dB) to 30 dB. This method is particularly helpful in assessing low-flow or slow-flow situations. Newer developments are leading to vascular enhancers with an active acoustic response and with affinities for specific organs and tissues, heralding the potential for organ or site-specific drug delivery systems.[14] New fluorocarbon-based echocardiographic contrast agents are well suited as echo enhancers because of the difference in acoustic impedance at gas-fluid interfaces.[15] The develop-

ment of microbubble contrast agents for ultrasonic use has also led to second-harmonic imaging, which is the ultrasound equivalent of subtraction angiography (in which bone densities are electronically removed allowing contrast filled blood vessels to be more easily seen) without using radiation. Ultrasound imaging of the vascularity of tumors will become more commonplace with the improvement of microbubble technology.

Enhanced effects of thrombolytic agents such as urokinase and tissue plasminogen activator (TPA) with acoustic energy have been demonstrated. Ultrasound transducer-tipped catheters are being developed for treatment of cardiovascular diseases. Other devices with ultrasound transducers implanted in transdermal drug patches are also being evaluated for possible delivery of insulin through the skin. Echo contrast microbubbles can also be used to carry and release genes to various tissues and lesions. Chemical activation of drugs by ultrasound energy for treatment of cancers is another new field, recently termed *sonodynamic therapy.*[16]

Magnetic Resonance Spectroscopy

Using special pulsing sequences on a conventional MRI scanner, chemical analysis of the tissue in a specified region can be noninvasively assessed, known as *magnetic resonance spectroscopy (MRS)*. Graph results that compare parts per million (PPM) versus concentration or peak height shows the relative amounts of the chemicals contained in the area being tested. The typical chemical peaks found in tissues being analyzed represent, from most to least frequent: lipid, lactate, N-acetyl-aspartate, glutamate-glutamine-γ-aminobutyrate, creatine, choline, myoinositol.

The relative amounts of these chemicals can be strong indicators for disease and often obviate the need for biopsy. For instance, elevated levels of lipid are found in areas of necrosis, and levels of N-acetyl-aspartate are useful indicators of outcome in patients in a coma who have suffered brain injury.[17] Application of MRS in brain imaging has also been shown to reliably predict neoplasms[18] and Alzheimer's disease.[19]

CHIROPRACTIC RADIOLOGY AND THE ROLE OF RADIOLOGY SPECIALISTS

All chiropractors find that, in certain cases, help from a radiology specialist is necessary. This help may be to clarify an uncertain finding, confirm a diagnosis, or perform advanced imaging studies. To meet this need, some chiropractors develop relationships with local medical radiologists, in private practice or in hospitals, who can address issues of pathology.

Additionally, radiology specialists within the chiropractic profession—board certified chiropractic radiologists who are members of the **American Chiropractic College of Radiology** (ACCR)—are also able to address questions of pathology and can provide the additional service of including *clinical comments* in the radiology report that may affect the type of adjustment/manipulation delivered to the patient. For instance, a clinical comment might identify the impropriety of HVLA adjustment/manipulation of the lumbar spine in a patient who has an abdominal aortic aneurysm. A clinical comment may direct the chiropractor toward any additional advanced diagnostic imaging that may be necessary, based on plain-film findings, to either localize a disease process or to make a more specific diagnosis. For example, a patient's lumbar radiographs may show a calcification in the right upper quadrant of the abdomen. Referral for a diagnostic ultrasound of the kidney may confirm if the calcification is a kidney stone, gallstone, hepatic granuloma, or a superimposed calcified lymph node. Chiropractors who choose to send their images out for interpretation not only ensure the highest quality of interpretation and most accurate diagnoses, but also mitigate their liability.[1]

CONCLUSION

The history and development of human diagnostic imaging is rich, and chiropractic has made significant contributions. Clearly, plain-film radiography currently remains the keystone in chiropractic use of diagnostic imaging. However, chiropractors frequently need to avail themselves of the newer imaging modalities such as CT, MRI, and nuclear medicine studies to make informed decisions about their patients' illnesses and to aid in the fundamental decisions as to whether to treat, co-manage, or refer patients for other care. As interdisciplinary relations between chiropractors and medical physicians have evolved and expanded, local practitioners have gained greater access for referring patients to facilities (hospitals and radiology centers) with advanced diagnostic imaging capabilities. Finally, the greatest changes in diagnostic imaging likely to affect chiropractic practice in the near future include affordable digital radiography, as well as the combination of modalities such as PET-CT fusion images to synthesize anatomic and physiologic information. Human diagnostic imaging has yet to provide all the information possible and necessary to assess disease processes fully and should provide many breakthroughs in the twenty-first century in diagnosing and treating various disorders.

Further information on the American Chiropractic College of Radiology is available at http://www.accr.org or www.dacbr.com.

Review *Questions*

1. What were the results of the research by Taylor and colleagues comparing students, clinicians, radiology residents, and radiologists from the chiropractic and medical professions in their interpretation of abnormal lumbar spine radiographs?
2. In what year did Roentgen discover x-rays and Palmer discover chiropractic?
3. List as many circumstances as possible for which plain-film radiographs would be clinically appropriate.
4. Which cervical x-ray view allows the clearest visualization of the intervertebral foramina?
5. What radiographs would be indicated when the clinician suspects pneumonia? What useful information is best revealed by fluoroscopy of the spine?
6. What are two advantages of CT over plain-film radiography?
7. In a case in which damage to the menisci or ligaments of the knee is suspected, what imaging procedure would be recommended?
8. For what clinical situations is diagnostic ultrasound most useful?
9. What imaging modality would be indicated if the chiropractor needed to determine whether a malignancy had metastasized to another area of the body?

Concept *Questions*

1. Should chiropractors take x-rays of all patients? If not, under what circumstances is it appropriate to adjust/manipulate a patient without having performed diagnostic imaging studies?
2. Compare the clinical value of CT and MRI.

REFERENCES

1. Taylor JA et al: Interpretation of abnormal lumbosacral spine radiographs. A test comparing students, clinicians, radiology residents, and radiologists in medicine and chiropractic, *Spine* 20(10):1147, 1995.
2. Purcell EM, Torrey HC, Pound RV: Resonance absorption by nuclear magnetic moments in solids, *Physiol Rev* 69:37, 1946.
3. Bloch R, Hansen WW, Packard M: Nuclear induction, *Physiol Rev* 69:127, 1946.
4. Canterbury R: Radiography and chiropractic spinography. In Peterson D, Wiese G, editors: *Chiropractic: an illustrated history*, St Louis, 1995, Mosby.
5. Cassen B et al: Instrumentation for ^{131}I use in medical studies, *Nucleonics* 9:46, 1951.
6. Hounsfield GN: Computerized transverse axial scanning (tomography): part I. Description of system, *Br J Radiol* 46:1016, 1973.
7. Damadian R et al: Nuclear magnetic resonance as a new tool in cancer research: human tumors by NMR, *Ann NY Acad Sci* 222:1048, 1973.
8. Lauterbur PC: Image formation by induced local interactions: examples employing nuclear magnetic resonance, *Nature* 242:190, 1973.
9. Buchanan RA, Finkelstein SI, Wickersheim KA: X-ray exposure reduction using rare earth oxysulfide intensifying screens, *Radiology* 118:183, 1976.
10. Aichinger U, Schulz-Wendtland R, Bautz W: Value of CAD systems, *Radiologe* 42(4):270, 2002.
11. Rust GF et al: Virtual large intestine imaging with multi-level CT. Pain free coloscopy—that works! *MMW Fortschr Med* 143(45):32, 2001.
12. Delbeke D, Martin WE: Positron emission tomography imaging in oncology, *Radiol Clin North Am* 39(5):883, 2001.
13. Cook GJ et al: Detection of bone metastases in breast cancer by 18FDG PET: differing metabolic activity in osteoblastic and osteolytic lesions, *J Clin Oncol* 16:3375, 1998.
14. Cosgrove D: Echo enhancers and ultrasound imaging, *Eur J Radiol* 26(1):64, 1997.
15. Main ML, Grayburn PA: Clinical applications of transpulmonary contrast echocardiography, *Am Heart J* 137(1):144, 1999.
16. Tachibana K, Tachibana S: The use of ultrasound for drug delivery, *Echocardiography* 18(4):323, 2001.
17. Danielson E, Ross BD: *Magnetic resonance spectroscopy diagnosis of neurological diseases*, New York, 1999, Marcel-Decker.
18. Lin A, Bluml S, Mamelak AN: Efficacy of proton magnetic resonance spectroscopy in clinical decision making for patients with suspected malignant brain tumors, *J Neurooncol* 45(1):69, 1999.
19. Moats RA et al: Abnormal cerebral metabolite concentrations in patients with probable Alzheimer's disease, *Magn Reson Med* 32(1):210, 1994.

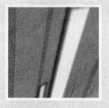

PART FOUR

CHIROPRACTIC CARE

CHAPTER

Chiropractic Manual Procedures

John G. Scaringe, DC, DACBSP, Robert Cooperstein, DC

Key Terms

ADJUSTIVE LOCALIZATION
ADJUSTIVE THRUST
ADJUSTMENT
ANTEROLISTHESIS
CAVITATION
CINERADIOGRAPHY
DYNAMIC THRUST
EPISTERNAL NOTCH
FOSSA
IMPULSE (DYNAMIC) THRUST
INDIFFERENT OR SUPPORT
  HAND
LINE OF DRIVE
LISTING

LONG-LEVER ADJUSTMENT/
  MANIPULATION
MAMMILLARY PROCESS
MANIPULATION
MANUAL PROCEDURES
MASSAGE
MOBILIZATION
MOBILIZATION WITH
  MOVEMENT
MOTOR UNIT
NERVE INTERFERENCE
OSTEOPHYTOSIS
PISIFORM NOTCH
POINT-PRESSURE TECHNIQUES

POSTURALIST
RECOIL THRUST
SEGMENTAL CONTACT
  POINT
SEGMENTALIST
SHORT-LEVER ADJUSTMENT/
  MANIPULATION
SPINOGRAPH
SQUARE STANCE
STAGGERED (FENCER'S)
  STANCE
TISSUE PULL
TRACTION-DISTRACTION
  PROCEDURES

Chiropractic adjustive and manipulative techniques fall within the broad classification of **manual procedures.** As the term indicates, manual procedures encompass all therapeutic procedures performed or administered by hand.[1] Although this form of health care intervention has been traced to numerous ancient civilizations throughout the world,[2] only within the last century has it gained significance in the realm of mainstream health care, primarily via the growth and development of the chiropractic profession.[3-5]

Chiropractic offers a wide variety of technique systems. Many successful chiropractors draw on a variety of techniques, with each chiropractic adjustive procedure made richer through integration with others in a process of cross-fertilization. Although no single technique system can solve all problems, chiropractic technique should be nothing less than systematic.

Approaching patients with a systematic method that is also eclectic is possible.

Manual procedures may be divided into two general categories:
- *Joint adjustment and manipulation,* including spinal and extremity adjustment and manipulation, manual traction-distraction, and the use of mechanical devices to aid adjustment and manipulation
- *Adjunctive manual methods,* including mobilization; manual soft tissue approaches such as point pressure techniques, massage, therapeutic muscle stretching; and visceral techniques (Box 12-1)

A detailed study of all techniques and procedures in these categories is well beyond the scope of this chapter. This section offers the reader an overview of the more commonly used methods employed in the practice of chiropractic.

Box **12-1**   CLASSIFICATION OF MANUAL
METHODS

**JOINT ADJUSTMENT AND MANIPULATION
PROCEDURES**

Adjustment
Manipulation
Manual traction or distraction
Mechanical devices to aid adjustment

ADJUNCTIVE MANUAL PROCEDURES

Mobilization
Point pressure techniques
Massage
Therapeutic muscle stretching or relaxation
Visceral techniques

JOINT ADJUSTMENT AND MANIPULATION PROCEDURES

Joint manipulation procedures are techniques designed to introduce motion into a joint. These procedures may involve the application of a dynamic thrust, as in many adjustive procedures, or they may be of a nonthrusting nature, as in mobilization and traction-distraction procedures.[1,3,6] In either case, the procedure is specifically intended to affect some element of the neuromusculoskeletal system and, in doing so, to produce beneficial results for the patient via the action on the tissues involved. Although the precise mechanism of action is not fully understood, various authors believe it to be the result of improved intra-articular relationship (alignment), restoration of proper joint range of motion, improved nerve function, and reduction in tissue irritation and dysfunction.[1,3,7-11]

Careful distinctions, often based on interpretations of varying perspectives or philosophies in chiropractic, have been drawn between the terms **manipulation** and **adjustment**. Much has been written on the subject, with the distinguishing characteristic being that a chiropractic adjustment uses a specific short-lever osseous contact point (such as a transverse or spinous process) to correct a segmental misalignment or joint dysfunction, whereas a manipulation, commonly performed outside the scope of traditional chiropractic, uses longer leverage to increase

range of motion, usually with less specificity. Some chiropractors would add that an adjustment corrects **nerve interference** or in some other way exerts a normalizing effect on the nervous system, whereas manipulation is intended to affect only musculoskeletal structures by mechanisms such as increasing joint range of motion. An important point to note is that some chiropractors within the profession use the terms *adjustment* and *manipulation* as synonyms. However, using the terms interchangeably usually describes the procedure in the context of a short-lever, specific contact manual procedure that uses controlled force, leverage, direction, amplitude, and velocity directed at specific joint or anatomic regions.

In this chapter, the terms *adjustment* and *manipulation* are interpreted more operationally than they are philosophically. The term manipulation refers to a high-velocity, low-amplitude (HVLA) thrust, sometimes simply described as a **dynamic thrust,** that moves a joint into the paraphysiologic joint space (see Fig. 10-4 in Chapter 10), beyond what is accessible through active and passive movements. The term adjustment refers to procedures designed to effect improvement in the neurologic component of vertebral subluxation, or joint dysfunction. Therefore the terms adjustment and manipulation are not mutually exclusive. An adjustment may use a manipulative (i.e., thrusting) approach, although it need not. An adjustment may use a different approach instead, such as having the patient lie on padded wedges or delivering a force using a percussive device. Similarly, a manipulation may be intended to adjust the spine (reduce nerve interference) but does not have to be delivered with this intent in mind. In this chapter, the context therefore defines whether the term manipulation or adjustment is more appropriate.

The terms *chiropractic adjustment* or *chiropractic manipulation* include a wide variety of manual and mechanical procedures applied with the intent of correcting a clinically identified adjustive/manipulative lesion (e.g., subluxation, muscle dysfunction, motion dysfunction).[3] The adjustment is characterized by the application of a specific dynamic thrust using controlled force, leverage, direction, amplitude, and velocity directed to a joint of the axial or extremity skeleton, after the involved joint has been tensioned to the end of its physiologic limits. The clinician must control the speed, amplitude, and direction of the thrust precisely[1] to ensure the effectiveness of the procedure and minimize patient discomfort.

The adjustive or manipulative procedure forms the foundation of chiropractic case management and constitutes the most common procedure associated with the practice of chiropractic.[1,3] Simply stated, the procedure is characteristic of the profession and represents application of the chiropractic art. As such, the student, as well as the practitioner of chiropractic, must devote significant time and energy to developing and maintaining the necessary cognitive and psychomotor skills.

Adjustive Procedures Decision Making

Once a clinical impression is determined, the chiropractor must decide if manual procedures are indicated. The decision to apply this intervention must be balanced against the existence or absence of pain and the extent of the functional limitations. If no contraindications for the adjustment/manipulation are present, the chiropractor may choose from a wide variety and styles of procedures. Factors influencing the selection of manipulative procedures include[4]:

1. Age of the patient
2. Acuteness or chronicity of the problem
3. General physical condition of the patient
4. Clinician's size and technical abilities
5. Effectiveness of the previous therapy, present therapy, or both

Other factors to consider are knowledge of the local anatomy, including the geometric planes of the articulations, the nature of the condition and presence of co-morbidities, and the mechanical characteristics of the adjustive/manipulative procedure. These factors will determine whether to use a long- or short-lever procedure, the positioning of the patient, specific contact points, the magnitude and vector of the force, and the type of thrust. Box 12-2 lists the factors governing the selection of adjustive methods.

Box **12-2**   FACTORS GOVERNING THE SELECTION OF AND SPECIFIC APPLICATION OF ADJUSTIVE METHODS

ANATOMIC LOCATION OF JOINT DISORDER OR DYSFUNCTION

Morphology of tissues: size, strength, and mobility of structures. Some areas necessitate more power (mass and leverage).

PATIENT'S AGE AND PHYSICAL CONDITION

Ability to assume specific positions
Degree of pretension (force, mass, leverage, and depth of thrust) the patient can withstand
Stress to adjacent spinal or extremity joints and soft tissues

PATIENT'S SIZE AND FLEXIBILITY

Large or inflexible patient: needs increased mechanical advantage in the development of pretension and thrust

Table selection: height, articulating versus nonarticulating, release or drop pieces, mechanized
Method: leverage and type of thrust (e.g., push versus pull)
Flexible patient
Focus force by preloading the joint: removal of articular slack, use of nonneutral patient positions
Selection of method: shorter lever methods

PRESENCE OF MITIGATING DISORDERS OR DEFECTS

Preexisting congenital or developmental defects
Preexisting degenerative defects
Coexisting disease states
Adjacent motion segment instability (focused force minimizes stress to adjacent joints)

Continued

Box **12-2**   Factors Governing the Selection of and Specific Application of Adjustive Methods—cont'd

DOCTOR'S TECHNICAL ABILITIES AND PREFERENCES	Amplitude (depth)
	Mass
	Point of delivery
PATIENT'S TREATMENT PREFERENCES	Pause-nonpause
Cannot compromise safety and effectiveness	Short lever preferred to long lever
	Issue of specificity
	Patient of manageable size
SPECIFIC MECHANICAL AND PHYSICAL ATTRIBUTES OF ADJUSTIVE METHODS	Flexible patient
	Patients with clinical motion segment instability
Adjustive localization and pretension	Long lever preferred to short lever
Patient position	Spinal regions where additional leverage is desired
Doctor position	Patient size and flexibility demand additional leverage and power
Contact points	
Leverage	
Adjustive thrust	
Leverage	
Velocity	

From Peterson DH, Bergmann TF: *Chiropractic technique: principles and procedures*, ed 2, St Louis, 2002, Mosby.

Achieving Adjustive Specificity

As stated earlier, a wide variety of manual procedures are available from which to choose. As properly applied adjustment or manipulation is usually specific, induces joint separation, and is free of pain. The procedure should not produce joint compression, injury, or distractive forces at adjacent, undesired segmental levels. Achieving adjustive specificity depends on the procedures leading to **adjustive localization** and the actual delivery of the adjustive thrust. According to Peterson and Bergmann[1] "adjustive localization refers to the preadjustive procedures designed to localize adjustive forces and joint distraction." Adjustive localization depends on proper patient positioning, doctor positioning, and adjustive contact points. Once appropriate preadjustive tension is developed, the application of a specific, controlled force can be applied. This force, when accompanied with a specific vector (line of drive), is known as the **adjustive thrust**. Together, adjustive localization and the adjustive thrust will improve adjustive specificity and minimize the effects of unwanted distractive forces to adjacent joints (Box 12-3).

Box **12-3**   Achieving Adjustive Specificity

ADJUSTIVE LOCALIZATION AND PREADJUSTIVE TENSION

Patient position
Doctor position
Doctor's contact point
Doctor's indifferent (supporting) hand
Segmental contact point
Tissue pull

ADJUSTIVE THRUST

Line of drive (vector)
Type of thrust

Adjustive Localization and Preadjustive Tension

Patient Position

The patient may be placed in several positions before and during the adjustment/manipulation. Each posture offers different advantages and disadvantages for both the clinician and the patient. Proper patient positioning is crucial when developing preadjustive tension and achieving adjustive specificity. Standard patient postures include prone, supine, standing, sitting, knee-chest, and side lying.

Prone: The patient lies face down on his or her abdomen with the table headpiece positioned below the horizontal plane, allowing slight flexion of the cervical and upper thoracic spine. The table's footrest is positioned above the ankle region allowing the feet to be in a neutral position. The feet may be slightly elevated to decrease the tension of the hamstrings. Another effective option in the prone position is to place the patient on the table and release the breakaway abdominal suspension table-piece. This position creates suspension of the abdomen or extension of the spine. Functionally, the position results in separation of the anterior vertebral bodies, which decreases the resistance to the specific dynamic posterior-to-anterior thrust.

Supine: The patient lies on his or her back. The table headpiece is slightly raised to support the patient's head.

Standing: The patient is erect with his or her feet shoulder-width apart allowing for appropriate balance. This position is commonly used for assessment (postural analysis, sacroiliac dynamic [motion] palpation) and upper extremity adjustment/manipulation procedures.

Sitting: The sitting posture is commonly used during cervical and upper extremity adjustive/manipulative procedures. Thoracic and lumbopelvic procedures can also be performed in the sitting position.

Knee-chest: The patient is placed in a kneeling position with his or her chest, neck, and head supported on a special table (Fig. 12-1).

This position may be used when adjusting the thoracic and lumbar spines. The knee-chest position, similar to the prone position with the breakaway abdominal suspension piece released, does not restrict lower thoracic and lumbar extension, thus decreasing resistance to the posterior-to-anterior thrust. Therefore the clinician should exercise care regarding the depth of the posterior-to-anterior thrust.

Side lying (side posture): The patient is lying on his or her side with the table headpiece elevated to support the head and neck. The lower shoulder is placed slightly anterior so that the patient's upper torso is resting on the scapula and not on the shoulder itself. The lower arm is placed across the patient's chest with the hand resting on the anterior deltoid of the upper shoulder. The upper leg is flexed at the hip and knee, and the foot is placed in the popliteal **fossa** of the lower leg (Fig. 12-2).

Many mechanical devices and sophisticated tables have been designed to enhance the comfort and positioning of the patient and assist the clinician in the delivery of the adjustment. These devices and aids are briefly discussed later.

Doctor Position

The doctor position may refer to the position of the doctor in reference to the patient or to the type of stance or body posture the doctor is maintaining during a specific adjustive/manipulative procedure. The following list describes the doctor's position in reference to the patient:

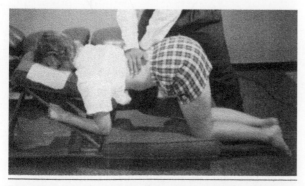

Fig. **12-1** An adjustment of the thoracolumbar junction with the patient positioned on a knee-chest table.

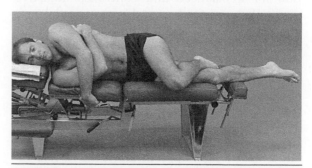

Fig. **12-2** Side-posture position. (*From Peterson DH, Bergmann TF*: Chiropractic technique: principles and procedures, *ed 2, St Louis, 2002, Mosby.*)

- *Cephalad*: The doctor is facing toward the head of the patient.
- *Caudad*: The doctor is facing toward the feet of the patient.
- *Ipsilateral*: The doctor is standing on the same side as the segmental contact point. For example, while making a hypothenar contact on the left transverse process of T6, the doctor may stand on the ipsilateral side, or left side, of the patient.
- *Contralateral*: The doctor is standing on the side of the patient opposite the segmental contact point.

In addition to these positions, the doctor may position himself or herself in a **square stance** or a **staggered (fencer's) stance.** In a *square* stance, the doctor's feet are approximately shoulder width apart and aligned in the coronal plane. The knees and hips are slightly flexed to allow the doctor to be comfortably positioned over the patient while maintaining an erect, neutral spine. When accommodating a lower table height, the doctor should avoid bending at the waist, and instead widen his or her stance, bending at the hips and knees while maintaining a neutral spine. In a staggered or fencer's stance, the doctor positions one foot forward and one foot back. The knees are bent, and the doctor's spine is maintained in a neutral position. As with the square stance, the doctor's hip and knees should bend while accommodating a lower table. This stance allows the doctor to transfer his or her weight from the back foot to the front foot during the adjustive/manipulative thrust.

Doctors' positioning and stance is the foundation for a balanced and controlled adjustive/manipulative procedure and is an essential component for achieving comfort for both the doctor and the patient. Positioning and stance is the foundation for a balanced and controlled adjustive/manipulative procedure. During the patient and doctor setup, the clinician should attempt to place his or her center of gravity over or near the *segmental contact point* (see later discussion). By controlling the center of gravity and using one's body weight appropriately, the doctor can increase the efficiency (by saving energy) of the adjustment/manipulation and reduce unwanted stresses to the doctor's upper extremity.

Performing manual procedures can be physically demanding. Occupational risks for the doctor of chiropractic are significant when performing numerous procedures all day long, day after day, and year after year. By being aware of sound body mechanics, established with appropriate doctor positioning, the chiropractor can decrease the risk of common postural and repetitive disorders.

Doctor's Contact Point

Approximately 12 areas on the hand (Fig. 12-3) can be used to specifically contact the patient.[1,12-14] The doctor's contact point is an attempt to localize the adjustive force to a specific area on the patient (i.e., the transverse process, spinous process, or lamina). However, an overly prominent or *bony* contact point (e.g.,

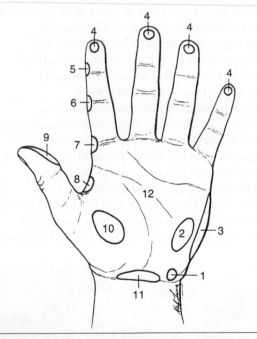

Fig. 12-3 Contact points of the hand: *(1)* pisiform; *(2)* hypothenar; *(3)* metacarpal or knife-edge; *(4)* digital; *(5)* distal interphalangeal (DIP); *(6)* proximal interphalangeal (PIP); *(7)* metacarpophalangeal or index; *(8)* web; *(9)* thumb; *(10)* thenar; *(11)* carpal; and *(12)* palmar. *(From Peterson DH, Bergmann TF:* Chiropractic technique: principles and procedures, *ed 2, St Louis, 2002, Mosby.)*

pisiform) can sometimes be uncomfortable or painful for the patient. The clinician must attempt to be firm but comfortable with the various hand contact positions.

Many adjustive/manipulative procedures can be executed using several different contact points. The selection of which specific area of the hand a clinician uses is often a result of personal preference rather than one contact point being more efficient or *specific* than another.

Doctor's Indifferent (Support) Hand

The hand that is used to stabilize the patient, support adjacent joint structures, or reinforce the contact hand during an adjustive/manipulative procedure is known as the **indifferent or support hand**. The indifferent hand is also used to assist the contact hand during the adjustive/manipulative thrust. For example, when adjusting/manipulating lateral to medial glide of the ulna on the distal humerus at the elbow, both hands deliver a low-amplitude, dynamic thrust in opposite directions. At other times, the indifferent hand may support the patient's head while positioning the patient's neck for a cervical procedure aimed at reducing a rotation dysfunction. When performing lumbopelvic side-posture procedures, the indifferent hand is used to contact the patient's upper torso in a manner that helps stabilize the patient throughout the procedure.

Segmental Contact Point

Segmental contact points are anatomic structures, commonly referred as bony landmarks, located on the patient. Examples of common bony (osseous) landmarks used as segmental contact points are listed in Table 10-1. The clinician uses these structures as focal points for the adjustive force. That is, although many of these points are under deep layers of soft tissue, the doctor contacts over or near these osseous points in an attempt to generate forces to the specific *segmental contact points*. How close the *doctor's contact point* is to the *segmental contact point* defines the difference between short- and long-lever adjustive procedures. Peterson and Bergmann[1] have the

following to say about short- and long-lever procedures:

Adjustive contacts established at or near the level of the dysfunctional joint are referred as *short-lever* (*direct*) adjustments. Adjustive contacts established at some distance from the level of the dysfunctional joint are referred to as *long-lever* (*indirect*) adjustments . . .

Additional information about short- and long-lever procedures will be described later in this chapter.

Tissue Pull

Establishing a firm contact over the segmental contact point is extremely important. Possible slipping away from the intended target point when applying the adjustive/manipulative thrust may dissipate the force and decrease the specificity of the procedure.[1,13] One precaution to avoid slipping or unnecessary movement involves the use of **tissue pull**. Tissue pull is established by applying traction to the superficial soft tissues over the segmental contact point. The indifferent hand is commonly used for this purpose. Typically, one finger of the indifferent hand tractions the soft tissue overlying the segmental contact point in the direction of the adjustive thrust (line of drive). While maintaining the traction, the finger of the indifferent hand is withdrawn and simultaneously replaced by the doctor's contact point of the thrusting hand, allowing a secure and specific contact between the doctor and the patient.

Adjustive Thrust

Line of Drive (Vector)

The **line of drive** (vector) indicates the direction of the adjustive thrust. Along with the plane of the articulation, the line of drive determines the movement of the articular segment. Appropriate adjustive/manipulative vectors are necessary to induce joint distraction at desired joint levels. Vectors aimed in unsuitable directions may induce joint compression, **cavitation,** or both at undesired levels. (Cavitation is the formation of vapor and gas bubbles within fluid through the local reduction of pressure. HVLA adjustments and manipulations are theorized to produce a cavity within a joint, eliciting a characteristic cracking sound.) The line of drive is commonly described in anatomic terms. For example, a clinician may induce a line of drive from posterior to anterior and inferior to superior while contacting the right transverse process of T7. The following common anatomic terms are used to describe specific line of drives:

Posterior to anterior	P-A
Anterior to posterior	A-P
Inferior to superior	I-S
Superior to inferior	S-I
Medial to lateral	M-L
Lateral to medial	L-M

Anatomic descriptors are used in one plane of movement, as with P-A, or they can be used in combination, as with P-A and I-S. Notably, however, a single adjustive thrust may not prove sufficient to restore mobility to more than one direction of restriction. Several thrusting procedures, all with different vectors, may be necessary to normalize a single spinal motion unit or peripheral joint complex.

Type of Thrust

Dynamic adjustive thrusts can be divided into two physical forms: *recoil thrusts* and *impulse (dynamic) thrusts*. **Recoil thrusts** are HVLA ballistic thrusts that are immediately followed by a passive recoil. The thrust is initiated by simultaneously contracting the extensor muscles of the arms (triceps and anconeus) and pectorals. The force of the thrust should be applied equally with both arms, with the doctor positioned such that a straight line can be drawn from the doctor's **episternal notch** to the segmental contact point. Immediately following the thrust is a rapid recoil of the doctor's arms created by the relaxation and a rebound effect of the extensor muscles of the arms. The recoil thrust is commonly used with the joints in the neutral position, with little to no preadjustive tension (Fig. 12-4, *A*).

Preadjustive tension in a recoil adjustment is accomplished by exerting P-A pressure in the plane of the intervertebral disk or the vertebral body, maximizing the separation of the anterior bodies (i.e., increasing spinal extension) immediately before the dynamic recoil thrust is delivered. The depth and force of this adjustment is modulated through the degree of flexion in both arms at the time the thrust is delivered.

Impulse (dynamic) thrusts are HVLA procedures without the dramatic recoil following the thrust. Generating force with the doctor's arms, body, or both can change the adjustive velocity. When less force is desired, as with cervical and some extremity joints, the thrust is generated

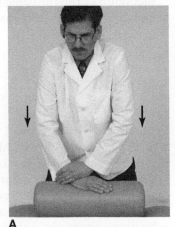
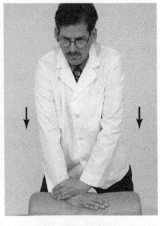

A

Fig. **12-4 A,** Illustration of recoil thrust. The body is held in stationary position, and the thrust is generated by rapid acceleration at the elbows. The thrust is very shallow, with a quick termination, followed by an elastic recoil (the recoil phase is not illustrated here) as full elbow extension is reached.

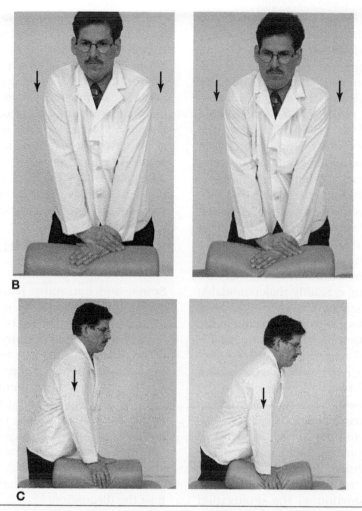

Fig. 12-4 cont'd B, Illustration of shoulder-drop thrust. The body is held in a stationary position, and the thrust is generated through a quick depression (elongation) at the doctor's shoulder. The doctor maintains a light contact after terminating the thrust to dampen reverberations generated by the shoulder thrust. C, Illustration of body-drop thrust. The thrust is generated by accelerating the doctor's body weight through the adjustive contact. Transfer of body weight is generated by transferring weight from the doctor's heels toward the front of his feet. This transfer is usually accomplished by inducing slight ankle dorsiflexion, knee flexion, and flexion of the trunk. Body-drop thrusts are often combined with shoulder-drop thrusts to produce a more rapid and rigid thrust and kinetic chain. *(From Peterson DH, Bergmann TF: Chiropractic technique: principles and procedures, ed 2, St Louis, 2002, Mosby.)*

with the arms only. When more force is desired, as with larger patients and using side-posture procedures, the doctor can transition additional weight from his or her trunk and lower extremity to the contact point. Impulse thrusts are commonly delivered when the target joint is near or at the elastic barrier and the joint is at tension. Shoulder drop and body drop thrusts

are two examples of impulse thrusts (see Fig. 12-4, *A* and *B*).

CHIROPRACTIC SEGMENTALISM AND STRUCTURALISM

Throughout most of its history, starting with the Palmers, chiropractic has emphasized *segmental subluxations*, that is, spinal problems attributed to two adjacent vertebra and the related soft tissues. This emphasis has been generalized by all chiropractors to also include the atlantooccipital, lumbosacral, and sacroiliac joints, and by many chiropractors to also include the extremity joints. On the other hand, a *structuralist* or **posturalist** tendency has existed as well, probably starting with the work of Carver, which emphasized spinal regional considerations, and beyond that, the relation of the various spinal regions to one another.

The **segmentalist** chiropractor asserts that subluxations occur at specific motor units consisting of two bones, be they vertebrae, the skull, any of the pelvic bones, or combinations thereof. As a general rule, the segment above is characterized with respect to the one below, whether solely for the purpose of creating a readily understandable clinic record or to indicate the specific contact point for the adjustment. From the segmentalist perspective, subluxation in the specific motor unit results in postural distortions, such as scoliosis in the frontal plane, and loss or exaggeration of the two kyphotic and two lordotic curves in the sagittal plane. These postural distortions are seen as compensatory consequences of specific segmental subluxations and not as the problems in and of themselves. Gonstead technique is a classic example of the segmentalist approach.

The *structuralist* or *posturalist* chiropractor sees postural distortion as the subluxation in and of itself and proposes a language of listings that describes the linear and angular relationship of entire regions of the axial skeleton. A given **motor unit** (composed of two vertebrae and contiguous soft tissues) may exhibit more signs and symptoms of dysfunction than another, but this is seen by the posturalist to be the consequence rather than the cause of the primary postural distortion. For example, the apex of a lateral curvature in the frontal plane may present with more pain, and show more **osteophytosis** (degeneration) on x-ray, than the other segments that comprise the curvature. Nonetheless, the curvature, not its apex, is considered the subluxation. The posturalist claims that the spine subluxates as groupings of adjacent vertebrae and is to be adjusted accordingly, with relatively nonspecific contacts. Pettibon's Spinal Biomechanics

and Harrison's Chiropractic Biophysics are classic examples of posturalist approaches.

An essential point to note is that a *third way* exists, an eclectic approach to chiropractic technique in which clinicians need not choose between segmentalist and structuralist thinking, endorsing one and rejecting the other. More likely, individual patients are better understood as suffering from either segmental or regional complaints and that a segmental problem is very much affected by the local environment in which it occurs, just as the local spinal environment is partially governed by segmental problems.

SPINAL AND EXTREMITY LISTINGS

Spinal and extremity listings describe abnormal joint positions or movements. In common parlance, a **listing** is a direction of tilt, a leaning to one side. Chiropractors have been using this term since the profession's beginning to describe the direction in which a vertebra has misaligned. A segment can be misaligned only with respect to some other reference point: the segment above or below, the floor, or perhaps the central ray of the x-ray tube. Chiropractors have not been able to agree on a standard listings system.

The following factors have interacted to confuse the discussion:

- A common reference point for listings is lacking.
- Many different methods can be used for obtaining listings, including x-ray, motion palpation, static palpation, muscle palpation, reflex methods employing leg checks, and kinesiologic challenges.
- Some practitioners use the vertebral body, and others use the vertebral spinous process, as the reference point for their listings system.

Certain rules of nomenclature have been adopted to facilitate discussion of biomechanical dysrelationships. For example, if one supposes that a segment can be seen on a **spinograph** to reside anteriorward in relationship to the segment below, should one describe this situation in terms of an anteriority of the superior segment or a posteriority of the inferior segment? Established among medical physicians, as well as chiropractors, is that this condition should be termed an **anterolisthesis** (slipping forward or anterior misalignment) of the segment above. Unfortunately, this convention is seen by some clinicians to contain mechanical significance, with the inference that the superior segment has subluxated and should be contacted directly in any corrective thrust.

The terminologic convention should not imply that the underlying biomechanical fault resides in the one segment rather than the other, because the subluxation actually occurs in the joint between the two. Furthermore, no *a priori* reason exists to suppose that when a clinician attempts to reduce the subluxation by applying a thrust, the force that is applied moves a segment with respect to the one below any more than with respect to the segment above.

Cineradiography (a fluoroscopic technique in which the image is recorded on motion picture film) has demonstrated that a manipulative thrust introduces a damped disturbance into the spine that extends to several motor units both above and below the point of contact, although it directly affects the immediately adjacent articulations (the most). Listing L4 with respect to L5 is one thing, but it is quite another to suppose that a contact on L4 affects only the joint between the two (as opposed to L3-L4), whether this be a matter of introducing motion or realigning the osseous structures.

Listing Systems

Common listing methods reference either the spinous process or the vertebral body when describing a malposition (static listing) or restricted motion direction (dynamic listing). Fig. 12-5 compares static listing systems for Medicare (vertebral body reference), Palmer Gonstead (spinous process reference), and National (vertebral body reference). Dynamic listings are also included, and spinal movements are described in kinesiologic terms with refer-

ence to the direction of limited or restricted movements. Spinal malpositions or restrictions compare the upper vertebra in reference to the lower vertebra. Extremity listings are commonly described statically with reference to anatomic malpositions (i.e., lateral tibia, anterior talus). The more contemporary dynamic view is described in kinesiologic (i.e., flexion, rotation) and accessory motion (i.e., anterior, lateral) terms.

SHORT-LEVER AND LONG-LEVER PROCEDURES

Adjustive procedures may be further classified according to the type of lever system employed in delivery of the dynamic thrust and the specificity associated with it. The two types commonly used are the specific *short-lever adjustment* (Fig. 12-6, *A*) and the *long-lever adjustment* (see Fig. 12-6, *B*). Although both types of adjustment involve administering a controlled HVLA thrust, they vary in the method of doctor-patient contact relative to the specificity of the target area.

The **short-lever adjustment/manipulation** (Fig. 12-7; see also Fig. 12-6, *A*) incorporates a doctor contact directly on or over some part of the soft tissue and osseous structures directly associated with the adjustive/manipulative lesion. Stabilizing the patient can be achieved with contacts in the immediate vicinity or at some distance away from the lesion.[1,3] Once contact and stabilization are established, the clinician tensions the joint to the end of its normal physiologic range (*locks* the joint) and delivers a controlled thrust, taking the joint into its paraphysiologic range. This movement into the paraphysiologic joint space is believed to initiate cavitation, resulting in the production of the audible "pop" or "click" associated with the adjustment. However, absence of this sound does not indicate failure to achieve an effective adjustment. The short-lever method is one of the most specific joint manual procedures available, allowing the experienced practitioner to affect individual target joints when skillfully applied.

By contrast, the **long-lever adjustment/manipulation** (see Fig. 12-6, *B*) method involves a doctor contact that may lie some distance from the

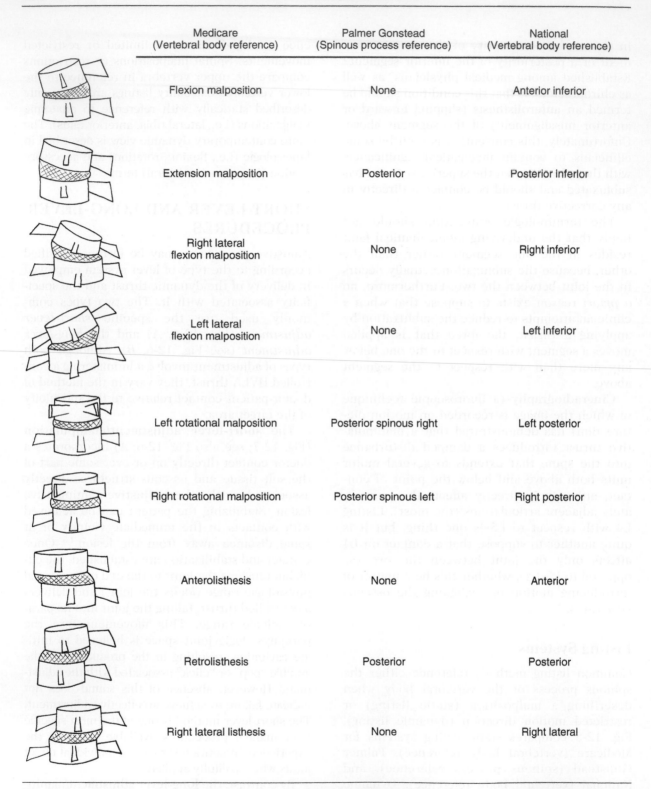

	Medicare (Vertebral body reference)	Palmer Gonstead (Spinous process reference)	National (Vertebral body reference)
	Flexion malposition	None	Anterior inferior
	Extension malposition	Posterior	Posterior inferior
	Right lateral flexion malposition	None	Right inferior
	Left lateral flexion malposition	None	Left inferior
	Left rotational malposition	Posterior spinous right	Left posterior
	Right rotational malposition	Posterior spinous left	Right posterior
	Anterolisthesis	None	Anterior
	Retrolisthesis	Posterior	Posterior
	Right lateral listhesis	None	Right lateral

Fig. 12-5 Comparative chart of listing systems. *(Modified from Peterson DH, Bergmann TF:* Chiropractic technique: principles and procedures, *ed 2, St Louis, 2002, Mosby.)*

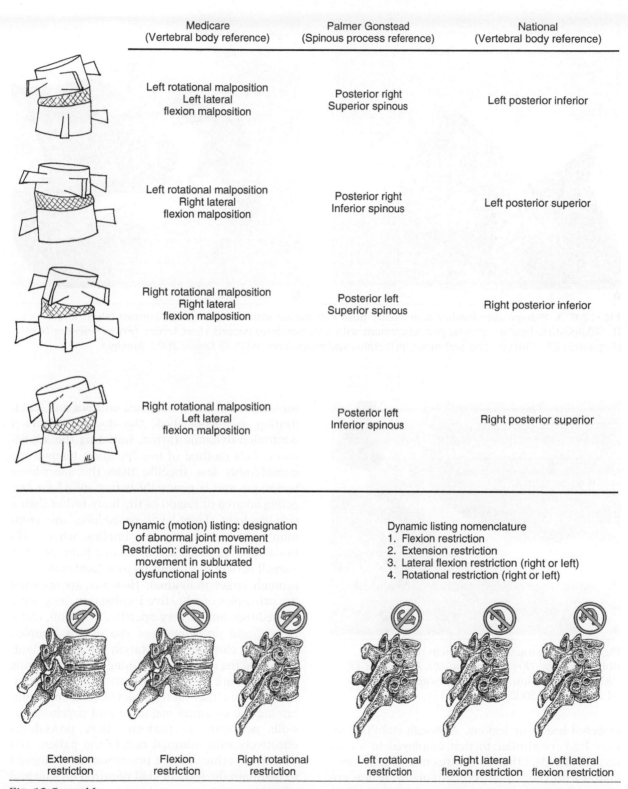

Medicare (Vertebral body reference)	Palmer Gonstead (Spinous process reference)	National (Vertebral body reference)
Left rotational malposition Left lateral flexion malposition	Posterior right Superior spinous	Left posterior inferior
Left rotational malposition Right lateral flexion malposition	Posterior right Inferior spinous	Left posterior superior
Right rotational malposition Right lateral flexion malposition	Posterior left Superior spinous	Right posterior inferior
Right rotational malposition Left lateral flexion malposition	Posterior left Inferior spinous	Right posterior superior

Dynamic (motion) listing: designation of abnormal joint movement
Restriction: direction of limited movement in subluxated dysfunctional joints

Dynamic listing nomenclature
1. Flexion restriction
2. Extension restriction
3. Lateral flexion restriction (right or left)
4. Rotational restriction (right or left)

Extension restriction   Flexion restriction   Right rotational restriction   Left rotational restriction   Right lateral flexion restriction   Left lateral flexion restriction

Fig. 12-5 cont'd

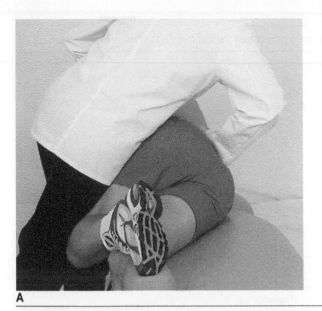 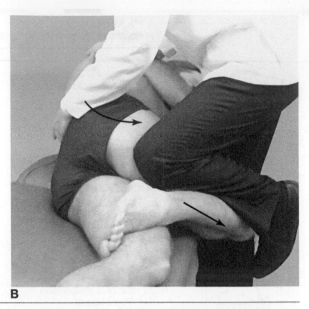

Fig. **12-6 A,** Side-posture lumbar mammillary push adjustment with a thigh-to-thigh contact (short lever). **B,** Side-posture lumbar spinous pull adjustment with a shin-to-knee contact (long lever). *(From Peterson DH, Bergmann TF:* Chiropractic technique: principles and procedures, *ed 2, St Louis, 2002, Mosby.)*

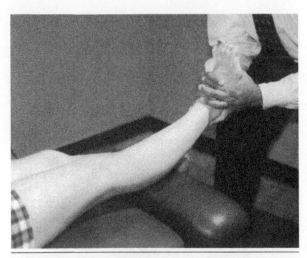

Fig. **12-7** A distraction adjustment of the right tibiotalar joint. *(From Peterson DH, Bergmann TF:* Chiropractic technique: principles and procedures, *ed 2, St Louis, 2002, Mosby.)*

targeted lesion or lesions. Although stabilization may be very similar to that employed in short-lever methods, other structures not directly associated with the adjustive/manipulative lesion are interposed between the target area and the doc-

tor contact.[1,3] Similarly, once contact and stabilization are established, the doctor delivers a controlled dynamic thrust, initiating the adjustment. This method of manipulation tends to be considerably less specific than the short-lever technique and is generally better suited for targeting an area or region of the body rather than a specific joint. Long-lever procedures are commonly used, as their name implies, when additional leverage is needed to affect a joint, as when a small person is attempting to adjust/manipulate a much larger individual. However, by applying the principles of adjustive localization, long-lever procedures can be very specific. The skill, experience, and proficiency of the doctor, coupled with the clinical presentation of the patient, should be the major determining factors dictating the procedure of preference in any given situation.[15] With either method, developing and maintaining the essential cognitive and psychomotor skills necessary to perform these procedures effectively with minimal risk to the patient and doctor are critical. Each practitioner is obligated to maintain the level of skill required for safe and effective practice.

ADJUSTIVE/MANIPULATIVE PROCEDURES

The following procedures represent a variety of patient positions (seated, supine, prone, and side posture), doctor positions (staggered or square stance), doctor's contact points (hypothenar, index finger, thumb), segmental contact points (spinous process, transverse process, femoral condyles), and types of thrusting action (push, pull, toggle).

Cervical Adjustive Procedures

Supine Ipsilateral A-P Rotation Thumb Pull

This procedure is used to induce A-P rotation and ipsilateral joint gapping at the articulation below the segmental contact (Fig. 12-8). The procedure can be used from C2 to C7. The patient is supine and the clinician stands at the head of the table slightly to the side opposite the contact point. The clinician's hands cradle the patient's occiput and cervical spine. The clinician contacts the anterolateral articular pillar of the superior vertebra with a thumb contact. The patient's head is laterally flexed away and rotated toward the adjustive contact. At tension, the impulse is directed through the side of the thumb contact in a posterior direction. Notably, the adjustive impulse is *not* originated with the support hand in a P-A direction.

Supine Contralateral P-A Rotation Index Push

Similar to the ipsilateral procedure described previously, the contralateral P-A index push can be used from C2 to C7 (Fig. 12-9). The patient is supine and the clinician stands at the head of the treatment table at the side of the adjustive contact. The posterolateral articular pillar of the superior vertebra is contacted with the lateral aspect of the clinician's index finger. The clinician's stabilizing hand cradles the patient's occiput and cervical spine on the opposite side. The patient's head is laterally flexed toward and rotated away from the adjustive contact. At tension, the impulse is directed P-A with a slight I-S line of drive with the adjustive contact hand.

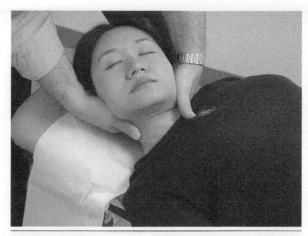

Fig. 12-8 Supine ipsilateral A-P rotation thumb pull adjustment.

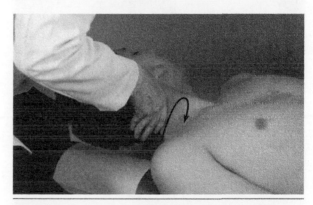

Fig. 12-9 Supine contralateral P-A rotation index push. *(From Peterson DH, Bergmann TF: Chiropractic technique: principles and procedures, ed 2, St Louis, 2002, Mosby.)*

Seated Contralateral P-A Rotation Digit Pull

This procedure is used to induce P-A rotation from C2 to C7 (Fig. 12-10). The patient is seated and the clinician stands facing the patient on the opposite side of the segmental contact. The clinician's hands cradle the patient's occiput and cervical spine while using the palmar surface of the middle finger to contact the patient's articular pillar of the superior vertebra. The patient's head is laterally flexed toward and rotated away from the adjustive contact. At tension, a P-A impulse along the plane of the facets is created by pulling with the contact hand.

Prone Contralateral P-A Rotation Index Pillar Push

The patient lies prone with the headpiece slightly lowered to induce some cervical flexion (Fig. 12-11). The clinician stands on the opposite side of the adjustive contact, facing cephalically. The lateral aspect of the metacarpophalangeal joint of the clinician's index finger contacts the

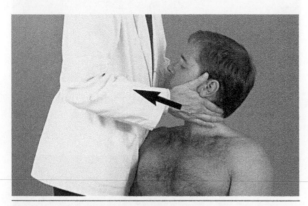

Fig. **12-10** Seated contralateral P-A rotation digit pillar pull. *(From Peterson DH, Bergmann TF: Chiropractic technique: principles and procedures, ed 2, St Louis, 2002, Mosby.)*

posterior articular pillar of the superior vertebra. The thumb-web of the clinician's opposite hand contacts the patient's contralateral occiput and the rest of the stabilizing hand gently supports the patient's cheek and side of the face. The patient's head is laterally flexed toward and rotated away from the adjustive contact. At tension, a P-A and slightly superior impulse along the plane of the facets is created with the contact hand.

Prone P-A Pisiform Spinous Thrust

This procedure is used from C2 to C5 (Fig. 12-12). The patient lies prone with the headpiece in the neutral position with the abdominal piece suspended. The patient's head is turned toward the side of spinous laterality to bring the spinous back toward the midline neutral position. The clinician, standing on the side opposite the spinous listing or deviation, backs up to the patient and pivots in a cephalic direction in a modified fencer's stance. The lateral fifth metacarpal distal to the pisiform, knife-edge, contacts the spinous process. This superior contact hand (the doctor's hand closest to the head of the table) is arched

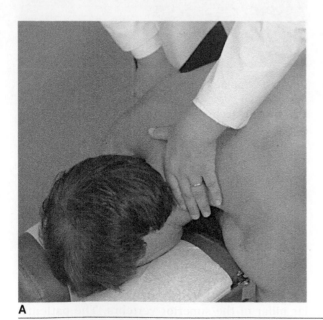

A

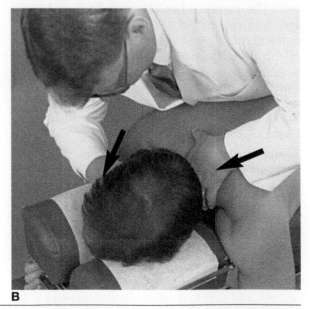

B

Fig. **12-11** Prone contralateral P-A rotation index pillar push. **A,** Index contact established over the posterior aspect of the left C5 articular process. **B,** Procedure shown to left laterally flex and right rotate the left C5-C6 articulation. *(From Peterson DH, Bergmann TF: Chiropractic technique: principles and procedures, ed 2, St Louis, 2002, Mosby.)*

(the wrist extended and the metacarpophalangeal joints flexed), and the indifferent hand grasps the wrist. Both arms are slightly flexed. The clinician is flexed at the hips to the extent that it brings the episternal notch and the line of drive to 90 degrees to the slope of the spine. At tension, the clinician executes a P-A thrust in the plane of the vertebral body or disk through an instantaneous and simultaneous contraction of the extensors of both arms and followed by immediate arm muscle relaxation and a passive recoil release.

Thoracic Adjustive Procedures

Prone Bilateral Thenar Transverse Push for Extension

This procedure is used to induce extension from T4 to T12 (Fig. 12-13). The patient is prone and the clinician stands in a staggered stance on either side of the patient, facing cephalically. The clinician contacts the transverse processes of the superior vertebra with a bilateral thenar contact. At tension, the impulse is directed through the contact points in a P-A direction.

Supine Opposite-Side Contact for Flexion

This procedure is used to induce flexion from T3 to T12 (Fig. 12-14). The patient is supine with the arms crossed and hands grasping shoulders. The clinician stands in a staggered stance on either side of the patient, facing cephalically, and reaches around the patient with a clenched

fist contact. The clinician contacts the transverse processes of the superior vertebra with the thenar on one transverse process and the flexed index finger on the opposite transverse process

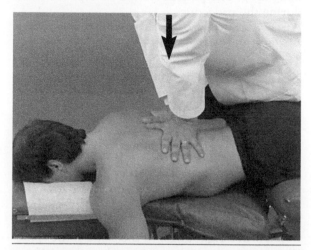

Fig. 12-13 Prone bilateral thenar transverse push for extension. *(From Peterson DH, Bergmann TF: Chiropractic technique: principles and procedures, ed 2, St Louis, 2002, Mosby.)*

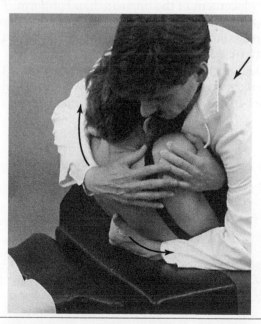

Fig. 12-14 Supine opposite-side contact for flexion. *(From Peterson DH, Bergmann TF: Chiropractic technique: principles and procedures, ed 2, St Louis, 2002, Mosby.)*

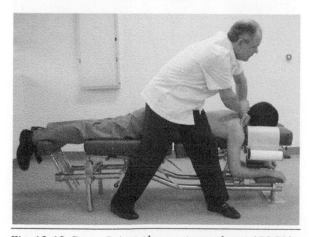

Fig. 12-12 Prone P-A pisiform spinous thrust (C2-PL).

of the same vertebra. The clinician's support arm cradles the patient's neck and upper back. At tension, the impulse is directed through the contact points in a P-A and I-S direction using a body drop. The patient should be kept in flexion during the procedure.

Prone P-A Thoracic-Lumbar Spinous Thrust

This procedure is used from T2 to L3 (Fig. 12-15). The patient lies prone with the headpiece in the neutral position and the abdominal piece suspended. The patient's head is turned toward the side of spinous laterality to bring the spinous back toward the midline neutral position. The clinician, standing on the ipsilateral side of spinous listing or deviation, faces the patient with feet at least shoulder-width apart. One foot is at the level of the subluxation and the other moved in the opposite direction until the episternal notch is at a right angle to the slope of the spine. The superior hand forms an arch as the **pisiform notch** (intercarpal space just distal to the pisiform) straddles the spinous process. The fingers are straight and spread to anchor to the patient's back, and the thumb is raised to create a fossa for placement of the opposite hand pisiform. The opposite hand grasps the wrist and the shoulders, arms, and hands rest in the plane of the patient's spine. P-A pressure is exerted to enhance the extension of the spine and bring the joint to tension. At tension, a P-A thrust is delivered in the plane of the vertebral body or the

disk using contraction of the extensors of both arms simultaneously.

The lateral fifth metacarpal distal to the pisiform, or *knife-edge* hand contact point, contacts the spinous process. This superior contact hand is arched (the wrist extended and the metacarpophalangeal joints flexed), and the indifferent hand grasps the wrist. Both arms are slightly flexed. The clinician is flexed at the hips to the extent that it brings the episternal notch and the line of drive to 90 degrees to the slope of the spine. At tension, the clinician executes a P-A thrust in the plane of the vertebral body or disk through an instantaneous and simultaneous contraction of the extensors of both arms and followed by immediate arm muscle relaxation and a passive recoil release.

Lumbopelvic Adjustive Procedures

Prone Unilateral Hypothenar Mammillary Push for Rotation

This procedure is used to induce rotation from L1 to L5 (Fig. 12-16). The patient is prone and the clinician stands in a staggered or square stance on the side of the adjustive contact. The clinician contacts the patient's **mammillary process** with his or her hypothenar or pisiform with the fingers running parallel to the patient's

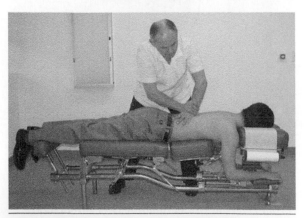

Fig. **12-15** Prone P-A thoracic-lumbar spinous thrust.

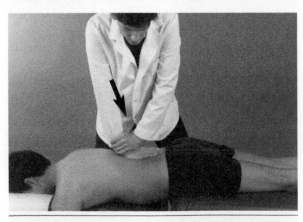

Fig. **12-16** Prone unilateral hypothenar mammillary push for rotation. (*From Peterson DH, Bergmann TF*: Chiropractic technique: principles and procedures, *ed 2, St Louis, 2002, Mosby.*)

spine. The clinician's opposite hand reinforces the contact hand by grasping the wrist. At tension, the impulse is directed through the contact point in a P-A direction using a body drop.

Side-Posture Short-Lever Hypothenar Mammillary Push for Rotation

This procedure is used to induce rotation from L1 to L5 (Fig. 12-17). The patient lies in a side-posture position and the clinician stands in a staggered stance at approximately 45 degrees to the patient. The clinician's thigh contacts the patient's thigh, which helps stabilizes the patient's pelvis (Fig. 12-18). The clinician contacts the patient's mammillary process with his or her hypothenar or pisiform with the fingers

running parallel to the patient's spine. The clinician's opposite hand reinforces the patient's shoulder and overlapping hand. At tension, the impulse is directed through the body and contact point in a P-A direction using a body drop.

Side-Posture Long-Lever Digit-Contact Spinous Pull

This procedure is used to induce rotation from L1 to L5 (Fig. 12-19). The patient lies in a side-posture position and the clinician stands in a squared stance facing the patient. The clinician's knee or distal aspects of the leg contacts the patient's knee (Fig. 12-20). The clinician contacts the patient's spinous process with his or her fingertips of the inferior hand with the fore-

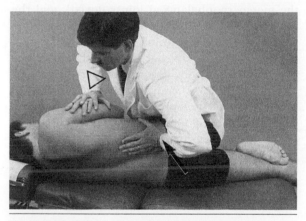

Fig. 12-17 Side-posture short-lever hypothenar mammillary push for rotation. *(From Peterson DH, Bergmann TF:* Chiropractic technique: principles and procedures, *ed 2, St Louis, 2002, Mosby.)*

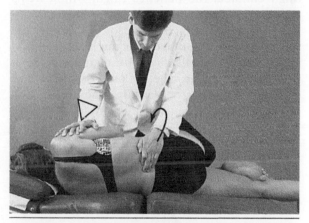

Fig. 12-19 Side-posture long-lever digit-contact spinous pull. *(From Peterson DH, Bergmann TF:* Chiropractic technique: principles and procedures, *ed 2, St Louis, 2002, Mosby.)*

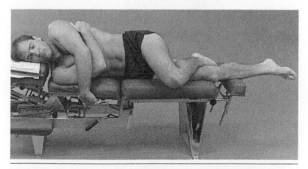

Fig. 12-18 Side-posture short-lever leg position. *(From Peterson DH, Bergmann TF:* Chiropractic technique: principles and procedures, *ed 2, St Louis, 2002, Mosby.)*

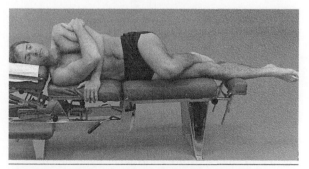

Fig. 12-20 Side-posture long-lever leg position. *(From Peterson DH, Bergmann TF:* Chiropractic technique: principles and procedures, *ed 2, St Louis, 2002, Mosby.)*

arm resting on the patient's posterolateral buttock and hip. The clinician's opposite hand reinforces the patient's shoulder and overlapping hand. Rotating the patient's pelvis with the clinician's leg and forearm develops tension. A M-L pulling impulse is directed through the finger contacts while simultaneously rotating the patient's pelvis by extending the knee.

Side-Posture Short-Lever Hypothenar-Ischium Push for Sacroiliac Flexion

This procedure is used to induce sacroiliac flexion (Fig. 12-21). The patient lies in a side-posture position with the involved side up and the clinician stands in a staggered stance at approximately 45 degrees to the patient. The clinician's thigh contacts the patient's thigh, which helps stabilizes the patient's pelvis. The clinician contacts the patient's medio-inferior ischium with a soft hypothenar contact with the fingers spread and pointed cephalically. The clinician's opposite hand reinforces the patient's shoulder and overlapping hand. At tension, the impulse is directed through the body and contact point in a P-A direction on the ischium using a body drop.

Prone Contralateral Posterior-Inferior Ilium-Hypothenar Thrust

The patient lies prone with the headpiece in the neutral position (Fig. 12-22). The clinician stands on the side opposite the posterior ilium, facing toward the table. In the toggle recoil hand positioning, the doctor's superior shoulder (the shoulder closest to the head of the table) is dropped slightly to achieve a S-I and the P-A line of drive (direction of thrust). The doctor's inferior foot (the foot closest to the foot of the table) is positioned on the floor, in line with the patient's posterior-superior iliac spine. The doctor's feet are placed at least shoulder width apart. The superior hand hypothenar, knife-edge, contacts the posterolateral crest of the ilium. This contact hand is arched (the wrist extended and the metacarpophalangeal joints flexed), and the indifferent hand grasps the wrist. Both arms are slightly flexed. The clinician is flexed forward at the hips to the extent that it brings the episternal notch, the shoulders, elbows, and wrists into the plane of the ilium. The line of drive is 90 degrees to the slope of the spine in a cephalic direction (or approximately a 45-degree angle to the table or floor). At tension, the clinician executes a combined P-A and inferior thrust through instantaneous and simultaneous contraction of the extensors of both arms and followed by

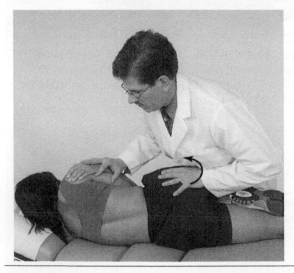

Fig. **12-21** Side-posture short-lever hypothenar-ischium push for sacroiliac flexion. *(From Peterson DH, Bergmann TF:* Chiropractic technique: principles and procedures, *ed 2, St Louis, 2002, Mosby.)*

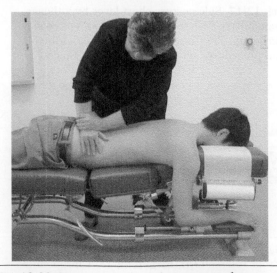

Fig. **12-22** Prone contralateral posterior-inferior ilium-hypothenar thrust (right ilium posterior).

immediate arm muscle relaxation and the passive recoil release.

Upper and Lower Extremity Adjustive Procedures

Posterior Glide with Lateral Distraction of the Humeral Head on the Glenoid

If the greater tuberosity of the humerus does not simultaneously depress and rotate in a gliding motion during shoulder abduction, subacromial impingement may occur (Fig. 12-23). Posterior glenohumeral capsule tightness is also a cause of subacromial impingement syndrome by forcing the humeral head in an anterior and superior direction toward the subacromial space. The following procedure may be indicated in cases in which shortened posterior glenohumeral structures are causing subacromial impingement syndrome.

The patient is supine with the shoulder and elbow flexed to 90 degrees, with the hand resting on his or her chest. The clinician sits with knees perpendicular to the patient on the involved side. Both hands grasp the proximal aspect of the humerus and the patient's elbow is supported by examiner's shoulder. At tension, the clinician pulls the humerus toward his or her chest in a quick (lateral and posterior) scooping motion.

L-M Glide of the Ulna on the Humerus

The patient is either standing or sitting with the elbow slightly flexed, the forearm supinated (palm toward ceiling), and the shoulder flexed comfortably (Fig. 12-24). The clinician stands on the lateral side of the patient's arm and contacts the lateral aspect of the patient's proximal forearm (below the joint line) with his or her outside hand with a thumb web contact. The clinician's opposite (inside) hand supports the patient's distal humerus. With the patient's elbow slightly flexed (just out of terminal extension), the examiner applies a slight valgus stress to the lateral side of the elbow, bringing the joint to tension. At tension, the clinician thrusts L-M with the contact hand and M-L with the indifferent hand, creating a shearing motion between the ulna and the humerus (thrusting into excessive valgus stress is avoided).

Prone Hypothenar–Greater Trochanter P-A Glide

This procedure is used to induce P-A glide of the proximal femur at the hip joint (Fig. 12-25). A loss of P-A glide may decrease active and passive hip extension and external rotation. The patient lies prone and the clinician stands on the same or opposite side of the involved hip. One hand should be placed under the patient's distal femur; the other contacts the posterior aspect of the trochanter. The joint is brought to tension by extending the hip by lifting the knee off the

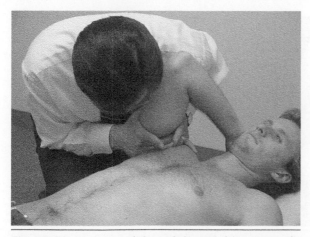

Fig. **12-23** Posterior glide with lateral distraction of the humeral head on the glenoid.

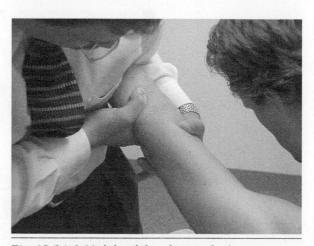

Fig. **12-24** L-M glide of the ulna on the humerus.

table. The clinician should be careful not to over-extend the hip and create too much lumbar lordosis. Once at tension, a P-A thrust with the contact hand on the trochanter can be delivered. A drop piece can also be used.

Side-Posture P-A Glide (Figure-4 Position)

This procedure is used to induce P-A glide of the proximal femur at the hip joint (Fig. 12-26). A loss of P-A glide may decrease active and passive hip extension and external rotation. The patient is placed in the side-lying position with the affected leg up in the figure-4 position. The clinician reaches through the legs with one hand

and contacts the posterior aspect of the trochanter while the other hand reinforces the contact hand. The hip is brought to tension by using the examiner's shoulder as a fulcrum against the patient's distal thigh while pulling the proximal femur toward his or her chest. At tension, an impulse is delivered in a P-A direction.

Long-Axis Distraction of the Tibiotalar (Ankle) Joint

The patient is supine with knee flexed to 90 degrees and the hip flexed at 90 degrees, slightly abducted and externally rotated (Fig. 12-27). The clinician sits on the involved side with his or

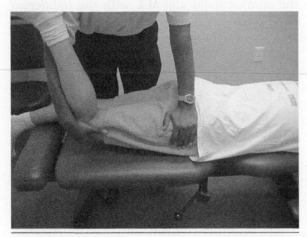

Fig. 12-25 Prone hypothenar greater trochanter P-A glide.

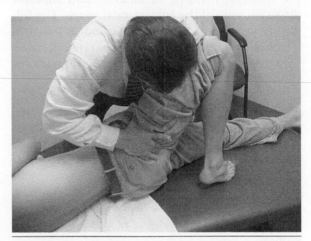

Fig. 12-26 Side-posture P-A glide of the hip (figure-4 position).

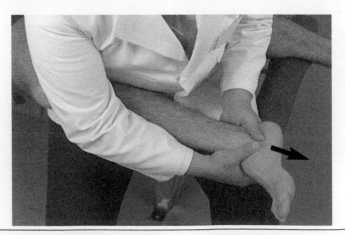

Fig. 12-27 Long-axis distraction of the tibiotalar (ankle) joint. *(From Peterson DH, Bergmann TF: Chiropractic technique: principles and procedures, ed 2, St Louis, 2002, Mosby.)*

her low back against the patient's posterior thigh, facing caudally. The clinician cradles the ankle with both hands, with the lateral hand contacting the dorsal surface of the foot at the talus. The clinician's indifferent (medial) thumb web contacts the posterior aspect of the ankle joint just above the insertion of the Achilles tendon. The foot should be *everted* to lock the subtalar joint. At tension, the clinician applies a distractive thrust by pushing the hands away from his or her body while producing counter pressure against the patient's upper leg.

Traction-Distraction Procedures

Traction-distraction procedures, which include flexion-distraction and extension-distraction methods, are manual procedures designed to produce a pulling or distractive force at the target tissues and joints. As with other manual procedures, traction-distraction procedures range from the very specific, targeting one joint, to the very general, targeting a region of the body. In either situation, the primary reason for applying the distractive force is to reduce joint compression, stretch tight painful tissues, and reduce intracapsular and intradiskal pressure, as clinically indicated.[1,16] Traction-distraction techniques include purely manual procedures and others that incorporate highly sophisticated mechanical tables specifically designed to assist in precisely administering the appropriate force at a very specific target joint or area (Fig. 12-28).

Again, this method may be very effective as a primary or sole therapy or may be enhanced by the inclusion of adjustive/manipulative and other procedures.

Mechanical Devices to Aid Manual Procedures

Since the founding of the chiropractic profession, and with the evolution of approximately 100 named technique systems[17] (Box 12-4), many mechanical devices and aids have been developed to assist in the effective delivery of the chiropractic adjustment. These devices range from sophisticated adjusting tables, incorporating features such as spring or hydraulically operated drop pieces, to much simpler devices such as pelvic wedges, blocks, Dutchman's roll, and thoracic-pelvic boards (Fig. 12-29). All of these devices are designed to enhance the positioning of the patient or the doctor (Figs. 12-30 and 12-31) or to afford the doctor some mechanically assisted advantage in delivery of the dynamic thrust.

Tables that incorporate features such as cervical, thoracic, lumbar, or pelvic drop pieces amplify the effect of the thrust and thereby allow less exertion or force by the adjuster. Devices such as cervical chairs, knee-chest benches (see Fig. 12-1), and wedges, to mention a few, are designed to position the patient effectively so as to afford the doctor a biomechanical advantage in delivering a particular adjustment/manipulation.

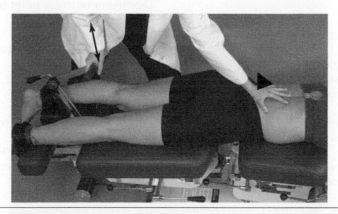

Fig. **12-28** Cox-flexion distraction. *(From Peterson DH, Bergmann TF:* Chiropractic technique: principles and procedures, *ed 2, St Louis, 2002, Mosby.)*

Box **12-4**   NAMED CHIROPRACTIC TECHNIQUES

Access seminars
Activator technique
Alternative chiropractic adjustments
Applied chiropractic distortion analysis
Applied spinal biomechanical engineering
Applied kinesiology
Aquarian age health
Arnholz muscle adjusting
Atlas orthogonality technique
Atlas specific
Bandy seminars
Bio kinesiology
BioEnergetic synchronization technique (BEST)
Bioenergetics
Biomagnetic technique
Blair upper cervical technique
Bloodless surgery
Body integration
Buxton technical course of painless chiropractic
Chiroenergetics
Chiro plus kinesiology
Chirometry
Chiropractic concept
Chiropractic manipulative reflex technique
   (CMRT)
Chiropractic neurobiomechanical analysis
Chiropractic spinal biophysics
CHOK-E system
Clinical kinesiology
Collins method of painless adjusting
Concept therapy
Cranial technique
Craniopathy
Directional nonforce technique (DNFT)
Distraction technique
Diversified technique
Endonasal technique
Extremity technique
Focalizer spinal recoil stimulus reflex effector
   technique
Freeman chiropractic procedure
Fundamental chiropractic
Global energetic matrix
Gonstead technique
Herring cervical technique
Holographic diagnosis and treatment
Howard system
Keck method of analysis
King tetrahedron concept
Lemond brainstem technique
Logan basic technique

Master energy dynamics
Mawhinney scoliosis technique
McTimody technique
Mears technique
Meric recoil technique (full spine specific)
Micromanipulation
Motion palpation
Muscle palpation
Muscle response testing
Musculoskeletal synchronization and
   stabilization technique
Nerve signal interference
Network chiropractic
Neuroemotional technique (NET)
Neuro-organizational technique
Neurolymphactic reflex technique
Neurovascular reflex technique
Olesky 21st century technique
Ortman technique
Pettibon spinal biomechanical technique
Pierce-Stillwagon technique
Polarity technique
Posture imbalance patterns
Perianal postural reflex technique
Pure chiropractic technique
Reaver's 5th cervical key
Receptor tonus technique
Riddler reflex technique
Sacro-occipital technique (SOT)
Soft tissue orthopedics
Somatosynthesis
Spears painless system
Specific majors
Spinal stress (stressology)
Spinal touch technique
Spondylotherapy
Thompson terminal point technique
Tiezen technique
Toftness technique
Top notch visceral techniques
Tortipelvis/torticollis
Total body modification
Touch for health
Truscott technique
Ungerank specific low force chiropractic
   technique
Upper cervical technique (HIO)
Van Fox combination technique
Variable force technique
Zindler reflex technique

Adapted from Bergmann TF: Various forms of chiropractic technique, *Chiropr Tech* 5:53, 1993 with permission.

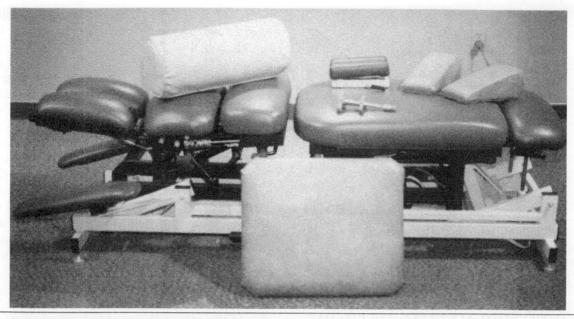

Fig. 12-29 A Chattanooga hydraulic chiropractic table with adjustable cervical, thoracic, lumbar, and pelvic drop sections. On the table, from *left to right*, a Dutchman's (thoracic) roll, a portable toggle-recoil board *(rear)*, an activator instrument *(front)*, and a set of pelvic wedges. Resting on the floor, a thoracic-pelvic board.

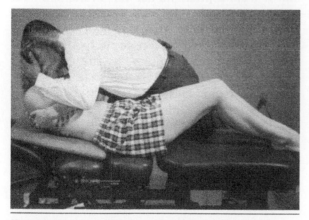

Fig. 12-30 A supine thoracic adjustment using a thoracic-pelvic board to assist the procedure.

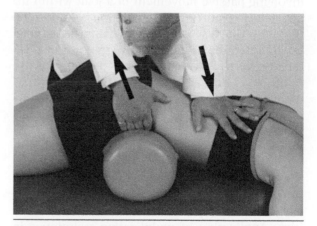

Fig. 12-31 A Dutchman's roll is used to mobilize the lumbar spine. *(From Peterson DH, Bergmann TF: Chiropractic technique: principles and procedures, ed 2, St Louis, 2002, Mosby.)*

The Activator Instrument—a hand-held, spring-loaded percussion device (Fig. 12-32)—is unique in that it is a precision device specifically designed to administer an impulse of a very controlled and uniform speed and amplitude. The Activator Instrument, with vectoring directed by the doctor, imparts the forces necessary for administering the adjustment/manipulation.

As is true in the effective application of all chiropractic manual adjustive procedures, safe and effective use of any equipment depends on the knowledge and skill of the user and the appropriateness of application in clinical situations.

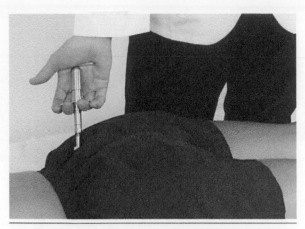

Fig. **12-32** Prone sacroiliac adjustment using an Activator Instrument. *(From Peterson DH, Bergmann TF:* Chiropractic technique: principles and procedures, *ed 2, St Louis, 2002, Mosby.)*

ADJUNCTIVE MANUAL METHODS

Mobilization

Mobilization is a form of joint manipulation involving passive movement of a joint within its physiologic passive range of motion.[1,3] Important to note is the absence of the dynamic thrust that is characteristic of the adjustive procedures. The target joint thus never enters its paraphysiologic range. As with HVLA adjustive procedures, mobilization may involve a specific articulation or a broader region of the body. In either situation, the primary goal of the procedure is to increase the range and quality of motion of the target joints. As with other manual procedures, the effectiveness and safe application of mobilization procedures depend on the development of the necessary psychomotor and cognitive abilities. Application of mobilization techniques is effective only when performed with the level of skill that can produce positive therapeutic results, while minimizing risk of further injury to the patient.

Mobilization procedures may be an effective form of patient care in and of themselves, or they can be used as a prelude to the administration of adjustive/manipulative procedures. In fact, a large number of commonly used mobilization techniques, both for axial and for the extremity skeletal structures, are identical in both doctor and patient positioning to adjustive/manipulative procedures for the same joint, lacking only the dynamic (HVLA) thrust into the paraphysiologic joint space characteristic of the adjustment. As always, the practitioner must judge the type and extent of treatment required in each clinical situation.

A wide variety of mobilization procedures are in common use. Many of these procedures have common features; others are rather unique. Interestingly, some authors have stated that many of the mobilization techniques differ more on the basis of the philosophy and training of the practitioner rather than on the validity of any specific theory.[18] Additionally, a fair amount of overlap may be seen between the various schools of thought.

Maitland Method

One of the more influential individuals to teach mobilization techniques is Geoffrey Maitland, an Australian physical therapist. Maitland's concepts have been widely taught around the world, but his conceptual model for evaluation and treatment is also known as the Australian approach.[19] Maitland advocates treating all joints in a passive manner and uses the patient's presenting signs and symptoms as the foundation for treatment. Maitland states that no set or invariable techniques exist, and the clinician must never do it "this way." Instead, Maitland insists that the technique must be constantly modified until the objective is achieved. Simply stated, the treatment technique will change as the patient's signs and symptoms change.[20] Maitland stresses the importance of continuous analytical assessment, which he calls the keystone of treatment.[21]

After a comprehensive history and complete physical evaluation of the patient is performed, the patient is placed into one of the following five categories[20]:

- Group 1: The main criterion is pain, which limits motion.
- Group 2: The main criterion is loss of movement, with pain being of little significance.
- Group 3a and 3b: Pain and joint stiffness occur simultaneously, and the increase in

pain intensity is proportional to the increase in strength of resistance (a = pain dominant; b = stiffness dominant).

- Group 4: Periodic pain and transient pain are present.

These groupings are used to help in determining the treatment technique. An important point to note is that the patient is not locked into any one group. In fact, patients move from one group to the next during a course of treatment. As patents move from one group to another, treatment procedures must be altered accordingly.[20]

According to Maitland, the goal of mobilization is to restore normal function to a joint and the surrounding tissue. The techniques use oscillatory mobilizations when treating joint dysfunction. For the most part, Maitland's treatments are directed at the joint's inherent resistance.[19] An important contribution to using mobilization procedures is the following grades of mobilization[19,21]:

- Grade I: A small-amplitude movement performed only at the beginning of the active end range
- Grade II: A large-amplitude movement performed through the freely mobile range but not through any part of the restricted range
- Grade III: A large-amplitude movement performed up to, but not exceeding, the passive end range
- Grade IV: A small-amplitude movement applied well into resistance
- Grade V: Equivalent to a manipulation in which a low-amplitude, high-velocity force is performed at end range in an attempt to exceed elastic barrier to movement

Maitland's grades of mobilization are compared with those of Kaltenborn in Fig. 12-33.

Clinically, painful joints are treated with accessory movements of grades I and II, whereas stiff and painless joints are treated with techniques of grades III and IV. Most peripheral mobilization is used within or up to the pathologic limit of a joint, and only rarely does it reach the anatomic limit.[22] (See Chapter 10 for more on accessory movements and anatomic limits.)

After each treatment, the patient is asked to perform the movement that produced the pain and dysfunction. This movement is used as an outcome for the effectiveness of the chosen tech-

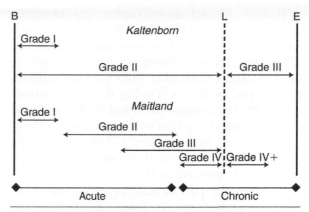

Fig. 12-33 Comparison of Kaltenborn's and Maitland's grades of mobilization. *B,* Beginning of range (joint surfaces approximated; *L,* limitation of range due to dysfunction; *E,* end of normal anatomical range. *(Modified from Scaringe JG, Kawaoka C: Mobilization techniques. In Haldeman S, editor:* Principles and practice of chiropractic, *ed 3, Appleton-Lange [in press].)*

nique and is referred to as the asterisk (*) sign. Maitland began using the asterisk sign; he would mark an asterisk next to the patient's limited functional activity in the treatment notes. A constant reassessment of functional status is preformed throughout the course of treatment and allows the clinician to change or progress the treatment as needed.[20]

Kaltenborn Method

Freddy Kaltenborn, a Norwegian osteopath and physical therapist, founded and greatly influenced the Nordic system of manual therapy, which is an integration and systematic review of physical therapy, medicine, and physical education. Kaltenborn's evaluation process was based not only on the biomechanics of joint motion, but was also influenced, in part, by his osteopathic roots and the concepts of somatic dysfunction. Kaltenborn labeled the examination as *present episode,* a process that involves inspection, palpation, functional examination, neurologic tests, and other examinations as needed.[23] Spinal disorders are divided into lesions with or without neurologic findings. Lesions with neurologic signs are usually treated with traction, and lesions without neurologic signs are treated based on the findings of hypomobility or hypermobility of the joint.[24,25]

Before manual mobilization, the clinician must determine (1) whether the problem is primarily in the joint or in associated soft tissues, (2) if joint hypomobility or hypermobility is present, and (3) whether joint pain and inflammation predominates. During the examination, accessory movements are used to determine if the pathologic joint is of a biomechanical nature, and providing that a treatable lesion is present with a suitable working diagnosis, a gentle trial treatment is performed.[23]

An essential part of Kaltenborn's joint mobilization procedures is long-axis distraction. Traction and gliding movements are divided into three grades or stages. These grades are determined by the amount of *slack* remaining in the joint capsule and surrounding soft tissues. Grade-1 traction nullifies pressures within the joint without separation of the joint surface. This type of traction can be applied with many mobilization movements to prevent trauma to the joint, or it may be used alone for pain relief. Grade-1 traction is used with grade-2 and grade-3 gliding procedures. Grade-2 traction takes up allowable soft tissue laxity in the joint, causes the joint surfaces to separate, and relieves pain. Grade-2 movements do not produce appreciable stretch on the joint capsule. Grade-3 traction is the most aggressive of the three grades, with distraction applied to the point that the soft tissues around the joint are stretched.[22,24]

A summary of Kaltenborn's three grades of movement are as follows[25] (see Fig. 12-33):

- Grade 1: Small-amplitude movement is made at beginning of the range to loosen joint, used for pain modulation and symptom control and as an adjunct to all gliding procedures.
- Grade 2: Larger amplitude is used at end range that takes up slack to tighten joint, used for pain modulation and symptom control and for mobilization of minor joint restrictions.
- Grade 3: Greater force is applied after slack is taken up to stretch tissue crossing the joint, used for both manipulation and mobilization.

For optimal results, appropriate sequencing of treatment technique is important when using multiple treatment techniques in one session (e.g., soft tissue massage, stretching before mobilization treatment for relaxation, strengthening or coordination exercises after treatment to maintain gains achieved through treatment). According to Kaltenborn[25] and many doctors of chiropractic, it is important to inform, instruct, and train patients on exercises and to educate them to improve function, compensate for injuries, and prevent reinjury. Kaltenborn also educates patients on relevant ergonomics and self-care techniques.

Mulligan Method

In 1980, Brian Mulligan, a physiotherapist from New Zealand, developed a technique he termed **mobilization with movement** (MWM).[26,27] This type of technique is articular in nature and is thought to produce both a biomechanical and neurologic effect. Unlike other mobilization procedures, Mulligan performed his techniques on a patient while they were moving, either actively or passively, or while they were performing a resisted muscle contraction. The technique is performed in symptom-free ranges, a factor that probably increases their safety.[28]

In addition to his mobilization with movement techniques that were used in the peripheral joints, Mulligan also developed a series of gliding techniques for the spine. The physiotherapist called these techniques natural apophyseal glides (NAGs) and sustained natural apophyseal glides (SNAGs). NAGs are accessory movements that involve gliding a spinal facet on an adjacent spinal facet while the patient remains passive. SNAGs are NAGs performed while the patient is actively moving through a painful or restricted range of motion. MWM is used to denote SNAGs that are used in peripheral joints.

Mulligan's concepts are outlined as follows[26,28]:

1. The techniques are all performed within a pain-free range. Some palpable or pressure pain is acceptable but not to the point of the initial pain. The symptoms of pain, weakness, stiffness, or any combination must be eliminated, otherwise different types of therapies should be considered. A minimal amount of force is used in the

glide; however, the force can be increased if the treatment is for stiffness rather than pain. Over-pressure may be applied but only if it is painless. In the presence of a highly irritable joint, under-treating is preferable in the early stages of care.

2. The accessory treatment force, as applied in NAGs and SNAGs, follows the facet planes of the spinal joints; therefore the direction of force will change at different vertebral levels. In MWM, the shape of the articular surfaces, forces around the joint, and the type of joint dictates the direction of treatment force. Treatment force is tested in various directions until the most effective one is discovered. Once discovered, the force is usually applied in one direction and is sustained until the patient is able to move the painful or restricted joint freely.

3. Pain and restricted joint motion are caused by a positional fault or by tracking problems. These conditions may develop as a result of subtle biomechanical changes after injury or stresses from normal activities of daily living. For such subtle biomechanical changes to develop in a normal joint, an alteration in one or all of the following needs to occur: the joint surface shape, cartilage thickness, fiber orientation of ligaments and capsule, and direction of forces in muscles and tendons. These structures allow controlled movements while minimizing compressive forces produced by locomotion. These normal movements are kept in balance by the proprioceptive feedback system.

In addition to Maitland, Kaltenborn, and Mulligan, several other individuals have had a significant influence on the development of manual therapeutics. Some of the more recognizable contributors from the medical profession include James Cyriax and John Mennel. Although not typically considered in reference to mobilization procedures, physiotherapist Robin McKenzie and chiropractor James Cox have also developed procedures that use repetitive joint movements, both as evaluation and treatment methods.

Oscillatory Mobilization Procedures

Cervical Seated Spinous Contact for Posteroanterior Glide

This procedure is used to improve P-A glide of the cervical facets (Fig. 12-34). The clinician stands on the left side of the patient in such a position that the patient's left shoulder is stabilized with the clinician's lower trunk (see Fig. 12-34). The clinician should cradle the patient's head with his or her left hand so that the forearm is comfortably resting across the patient's right temporomandibular area. The patient should not move. The clinician should then attempt to "mold around" the patient and support the patient's head against the clinician's abdomen or chest.

The middle phalanx of the clinician's left little finger hooks around the spinous process (SP) of the superior vertebra (the SP of C5 is hooked to mobilize the C5-C6 joint). The thenar of the opposite hand (right) covers one half of the little finger, and an anterosuperior force toward the patient's eyeball (along the facet plane) is applied with the thenar contact. From 6 to 10 oscillations should be applied. This procedure can also be used unilaterally over the facet joint. An improved contact on the SP can be achieved by flexing the patient's cervical spine to the level of involvement.

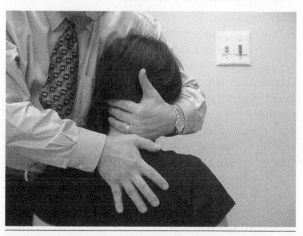

Fig. 12-34 Cervical seated spinous contact for posteroanterior glide mobilization.

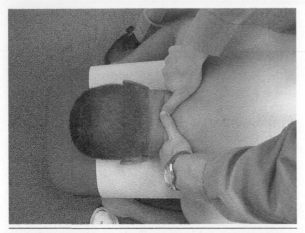

Fig. 12-35 Cervical prone double-thumb spinous process contact posteroanterior glide mobilization.

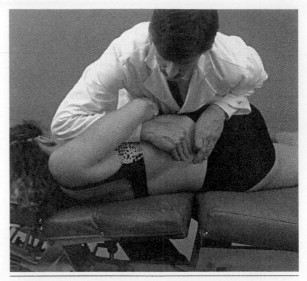

Fig. 12-36 Lumbar side-posture intersegmental (push-pull) rotation mobilization. *(From Peterson DH, Bergmann TF:* Chiropractic technique: principles and procedures, *ed 2, St Louis, 2002, Mosby.)*

Cervical Prone Double-Thumb SP Contact Posteroanterior Glide

An alternative to the previous procedure may be performed while the patient lies prone with the head resting in the neutral position and the chin slightly tucked in (Fig. 12-35). The clinician contacts the involved spinous process with a reinforced thumb (double-thumb) contact. Force is transmitted through the clinician's thumbs in a P-A direction by movement of the trunk and arms. Oscillations should be gentle and rhythmic in the desired grades.

Lumbar Side-Posture Intersegmental (Push-Pull) Rotation Mobilization

This procedure is used to increase intersegmental rotation in the lumbar spine (Fig. 12-36). With the patient in the side-lying position, the clinician places his or her index finger on the interspinous ligament at the affected levels. With the opposite hand, the superior leg is gently flexed while palpating for tension at the interspinous ligament and gapping of the spinous processes. At this position, the leg is fixed, and the superior foot is tucked behind the popliteal fossa of the inferior leg. While palpating the interspinous ligament of the affected levels, the patient's upper body is gently rotated by pulling on the inferior arm (the arm resting on the table) until the palpating finger feels movement of the superior SP. The clinician fixes the patient's upper body by resting his

or her forearm against the patient's upper chest near the axilla while placing the opposite forearm over the patient's ischium. The clinician's thumb of the superior hand is placed on the lateral side of the superior SP and presses downward toward the floor. The index finger of the inferior hand hooks the inferior SP and pulls it upward. At tension, the segments are rotated gently with short amplitude oscillatory movements.

Mobilization with Movement Procedures

Cervical SNAGs

SNAGs are concurrent joint-gliding and active-movement techniques performed with the patient in the weight-bearing (seated) position. When possible, overpressure at the end range of motion should be performed. SNAGS are not an oscillatory-mobilization procedure and can be performed throughout the cervical and upper thoracic spine (thoracic and lumbar SNAGS will be described later) and are applied along the treatment planes of the levels involved. This technique is used to increase motion, decrease the pain associated with it, or both. SNAGS should not be painful.

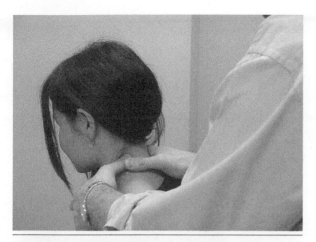

Fig. 12-37 Sustained natural apophyseal glides (SNAG) for cervical rotation (articular pillar contact).

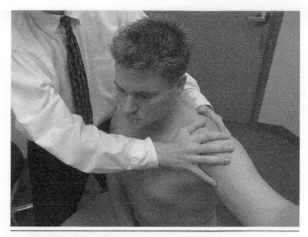

Fig. 12-38 Glenohumeral mobilization with movement (MWM).

Cervical Rotation SNAGS

The patient is seated with the clinician standing behind (Fig. 12-37). The medial border of the distal phalanx is used to contact the articular pillar of the involved (painful) side. The clinician's other thumb is placed over the contact thumb and generates the force needed to glide the facet. The thumbnail should be placed at a 45-degree angle sloping up toward the patient's eye (along the treatment plane of the facets). The clinician's other fingers should rest gently on each side of the neck or upper thorax. While the appropriate glide is being maintained, the patient slowly rotates his or her head in the restricted painful direction. Having the patient push on the side of his or her face with a hand provides over-pressure at the end range of motion. Over-pressure should be used if the patient can achieve full pain-free rotation. The movement is repeated several times, and then the patient's range of motion without applying SNAGS is reassessed.

In a patient presenting with right-sided neck pain when rotating to the right, the involved painful facet on the right is contacted while the patient rotates to the right. If this procedure does not relieve the pain, another level is attempted. If this action is not successful, the line of drive should be slightly changed, or the force of contact is altered. If this action is unsuccessful, the clinician contacts and glides the facet on the left (opposite) side while the patient rotates to the right.

Cervical Lateral Flexion SNAGS

This technique is used to increase lateral flexion in the cervical spine and is performed the same way as that for rotation, except the patient performs active lateral flexion. The clinician can apply an SP or articular pillar contact. The clinician must remember to maintain the glide along the treatment plane and have the patient apply over-pressure for a few seconds.

Glenohumeral Joint MWM

Indications for MWM of the shoulder include painful arc or painful and restricted flexion or abduction (Fig. 12-38). The clinician stands on the opposite side of the involved glenohumeral joint and contacts the head of the humerus with his or her thenar eminence. Because of the orientation of the glenoid and scapula, the best action is to contact the coracoid process and slide off onto the anterior humeral head (too much pressure over the sensitive coracoid should be avoided). The other hand stabilizes the scapula. The patient is asked to abduct or flex his or her arm while applying posterolateral pressure on the humerus. Progressions include wall push-ups, weighted or resisted shoulder presses, and wall techniques for flexion and extension.

Manual Soft Tissue Procedures

Soft tissue procedures (for further details, see Chapter 13) are manual therapies that apply forces to the nonosseous tissues of the body to improve function, reduce pain, or improve health. These procedures generally involve the application of a pressure, stretching, or distractive force to the involved tissues, with the desired effect of increasing circulation, reducing inflammation and edema, and reducing muscle spasm.[1] As with the previously mentioned mobilization procedures, it is not uncommon in the chiropractic practice for soft tissue procedures to be applied in preparation for a dynamic HVLA adjustment/manipulation. Soft tissue procedures are believed to both facilitate and enhance the effects of the adjustment. Included under this heading are point-pressure techniques, massage techniques, therapeutic muscle-stretching techniques, and visceral procedures.[1,3]

Point-Pressure Techniques

Point-pressure techniques of soft tissue care, as the term suggests, involve the application of digital pressure to specific target tissue areas. The applied pressure may be of a steady, sustained nature, or it may be increased progressively, depending on the judgment of the practitioner and the response of the patient. In addition, the practitioner may apply vibratory patterns, movement patterns, or both to enhance the stimulation and therefore the therapeutic effect of the treatment.[1,3] This form of manipulation is commonly associated with techniques such as acupressure, Nimmo receptor tonus technique, Shiatsu, and Chapman-Bennett procedures.

Massage Techniques

Massage techniques involve the manual application of forces to the body to stimulate the soft tissues. The intended goal, as with most soft tissue procedures, is to increase blood flow, reduce inflammation and edema, and relax taut musculature. Included under this heading are procedures such as cross-friction massage (Fig. 12-39) and stripping methods (e.g., Graston technique, Active Release Technique [ART]), which are

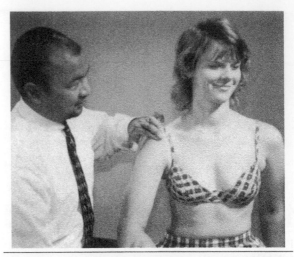

Fig. 12-39 Cross-friction massage technique applied over the right supraspinatus tendon.

particularly helpful in minimizing and reducing adhesions in myofascial and tendinous tissues.

Although a large number of individual massage methods have been developed, many of these incorporate combinations or variations of basic massage techniques. The following list,[14] although not comprehensive, offers an overview of some of the methods not uncommon in chiropractic practice:

- Cupping. A quick tapping of the skin with palms cupped
- Effleurage. A light stroking procedure
- Pétrissage. Manipulation of large folds of skin and tissue
- Pincement. Manipulation of small folds of skin
- Pressure technique. The application of full hand pressure, incorporating a simultaneous kneading component
- Roulement. The manipulation of large folds of skin with a progressive wavelike movement along the target tissue
- Tapotement. A quick tapping of the skin with the medial aspect of loosely held hands

The therapeutic effect of massage treatment, as with all other manual methods, depends on the skill of the practitioner, the clinical picture that

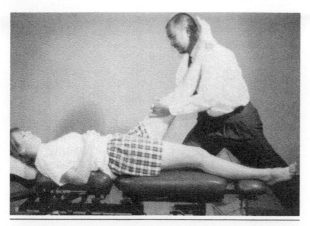

Fig. 12-40 Postcontraction stretch (PCS) applied to the left hamstring muscle group.

the patient presents, and the individual patient response to the particular type of procedure.

Therapeutic Muscle Stretching and Relaxation Techniques

Therapeutic muscle stretching and relaxation procedures include all techniques intended to produce the previously mentioned soft tissue effects through the stretching (lengthening) of muscles and their related fascia.[1,29] Commonly employed methods include the *postcontraction stretch (PCS)*, *postisometric relaxation (PIR)*, and *reciprocal inhibition (RI)* techniques. As the name might suggest, PCS (Fig. 12-40) involves the active contraction of the target muscles against resistance, followed by an aggressive passive stretch administered by the clinician. This technique is especially useful in treating chronic myofascial conditions.

PIR methods incorporate a more gentle active muscle contraction or resistance, followed by a gentle stretch of the involved musculature. PIR can be more useful in the handling of some acute and subacute problems.

Finally, RI uses active contraction of the antagonistic muscle groups to facilitate an inhibitory response in the targeted muscle or muscles followed by a gentle stretch of the tissues. This method can be of significance in treating acute and painful injuries.[30] The type, duration, and frequency of treatment using the noted procedures must be determined based on the clinical picture presented and on the skill and confidence of the practitioner.

Visceral Techniques

Visceral manipulation refers to all manual methods designed to improve or foster the mobility or motility (or both) of the internal organs of the body. This effect is achieved by applying very specific and very gentle forces or pressures over key areas of the body. The forces are intended either to manipulate the tissues in a particular direction or to stimulate the organ tissue or those tissues that may have a direct effect on the organ.[1]

Rehabilitation Procedures

With each patient, the doctor must decide if the goal of care is mostly for short-term crisis intervention, mostly for the purpose of alleviating the patient's pain (over 90% of chiropractic patients list pain as their primary complaint), mostly for long-term maintenance, wellness, preventative, or rehabilitative (these terms overlap) care, or some combination of these. Rehabilitation procedures are largely used for chronic patients, who account for the bulk of spine-related health care costs in the United States. These procedures are not adjustive per se, but they serve as a useful adjunct to adjustive procedures. (See Chapter 14 for a thorough discussion of rehabilitation.)

CONCLUSION

Although the HVLA thrust adjustment remains the backbone of the profession, the art of chiropractic is not limited to this singular method of intervention. The clinical interventions, procedures, and equipment available to the contemporary chiropractor provide a wide array of choices for application in treating a variety of neuromusculoskeletal conditions. Each method can provide substantial value to the needy patient in and of itself. In combination, these modalities provide a repertoire that is well suited to the patient who desires an alternative or integrated approach to health care.

Review *Questions*

1. What are the two basic categories of manual procedures described in this chapter, and what procedures are included in each?
2. What factors must be considered in selecting an adjustive method?
3. Briefly contrast the short-lever and long-lever methods of adjustment and manipulation.
4. How do the segmentalist and posturalist perspectives differ?
5. Name two or more forms of chiropractic adjustment that do not involve a dynamic thrust.
6. What is tissue pull, and how does it aid in the delivery of an adjustment or manipulation?
7. How do recoil thrusts differ from impulse thrusts?
8. According to cineradiography studies, can an adjustment or manipulation be localized to one segmental level?
9. List and describe some of the mechanical devices that can be employed to assist in the effective delivery of chiropractic manual procedures.
10. How does mobilization differ from manipulation and adjustment?

Concept *Questions*

1. Is it possible at this time to reach an evidence-based conclusion as to which chiropractic techniques are more effective than others and for which conditions? What sort of evidence would be needed to determine this accurately?
2. How should a doctor of chiropractic determine which technique or techniques to use in a particular case?

REFERENCES

1. Peterson DH, Bergmann TF: *Chiropractic technique: principles and procedures*, ed 2, St Louis, 2002, Mosby.
2. Willis J: Forerunners of the chiropractic adjustment. In Redwood D, Cleveland CS III, editors: *Fundamentals of chiropractic*, St Louis, 2003, Mosby.
3. Haldeman S et al: Spinal manipulative therapy. In Frymoyer JW, editor: *The adult spine: principles and practice*, ed 3, Baltimore, Lippincott, Williams & Wilkins (in press).
4. Greenman PE: *Principles of manual medicine*, ed 2, Baltimore, 1996, Williams & Wilkins.
5. Cherkin DC, MacCornack FA: Patient evaluations of low back pain from family physicians and chiropractors, *West J Med* 150:351, 1989.
6. Scaringe JG, Kawaoka C: Mobilization techniques. In Haldeman S, editor: *Principles and practice of chiropractic*, ed 3, New York, Appleton-Lange (in press).
7. Haldeman S: Neurologic effects of adjustments, *J Manipulative Physiol Ther* 23(2):112, 2000.
8. Bolton PS: Reflex effects of vertebral subluxations: the peripheral nervous system. An update, *J Manipulative Physiol Ther* 23(2):101, 2000.
9. Budgell BS: Reflex effects of subluxation: the autonomic nervous system, *J Manipulative Physiol Ther* 23(2):104, 2000.
10. Giles LG: Mechanisms of neurovascular compression within the spinal and intervertebral canals, *J Manipulative Physiol Ther* 2(2):107, 2000.
11. Zusman M: Spinal manipulative therapy: review of some proposed mechanisms, and a new hypothesis, *Aust J Physiother* 32:89, 1986.
12. Byfield D: *Chiropractic manipulative skills*, Oxford, 1996, Butterworth-Heinemann.
13. Schafer RC, Faye LJ: *Motion palpation and chiropractic technique: principles of dynamic chiropractic*, Huntington Beach, Calif, 1989, The Motion Palpation Institute.
14. States AZ: Introduction. In Kirk CR, Lawrence DJ, Lalvo NL, editors: *States manual of spinal, pelvic and extravertebral techniques*, ed 2, Baltimore, 1985, Waverly Press.
15. Terrett AG: *Current concepts in vertebral complications following spinal manipulation*, ed 2, West Des Moines, Iowa, 2001, NCMIC Group.
16. Cox JM: *Low back pain: mechanism, diagnosis, and treatment*, ed 5, Baltimore, 1990, Williams & Wilkins.
17. Bergmann TF: Various forms of chiropractic technique, *Chiropr Tech* 5:53, 1993.
18. Saunders HD: *Evaluation, treatment and prevention of musculoskeletal disorders*, Minneapolis, 1985, Viking Press.
19. Farrell JP, Jensen GM: Manual therapy: a critical assessment of role in the profession of physical therapy, *Phys Ther* 72(12):843, 1992.
20. Maitland GD: *Peripheral manipulation*, ed 3, London, 1991, Butterworth-Heinemann.
21. Maitland GD: *Vertebral manipulation*, ed 5, London, 1990, Butterworth-Heinemann.
22. Cookson JC, Kent BE: Orthopedic manual therapy—an overview. Part I: the extremities, *Phys Ther* 59(2):136, 1979.
23. Kaltenborn FM: *Manual mobilization of the extremity joints: basic examination and treatment techniques*, ed 4, Oslo, Norway, 1989, Olaf Norlis Bokhandel.

24. Kaltenborn FM: Orthopedic manual therapy for physical therapists Nordic system: OMT, Kaltenborn-Evjenth concept, *J Manual Manipulative Ther* 1(2):47, 1993.

25. Kaltenborn FM: *The spine: basic evaluation and mobilization techniques*, ed 2, Oslo, Norway, 1993, Olaf Norlis Bokhandel.

26. Mulligan BR: *Manual therapy "NAGS," "SNAGS," "MWM," etc.*, ed 4, Wellington, New Zealand, 1999, Plane View Services.

27. Mulligan BR: Mobilization with movement (MWMs), *J Man Manipulative Ther* 1(4):154, 1993.

29. Cantu RI, Grodin AJ: *Myofascial manipulation: theory and clinical application*, Gaithersburg, Md, 1992, Aspen.

30. Leibenson C: *Rehabilitation of the spine: a practitioner's manual*, Philadelphia, 1996, Williams & Wilkins.

Manual Soft Tissue Procedures

Warren Hammer, DC, DABCO

Key Terms

ACTIVE RELEASE
  TECHNIQUES
COUNTERSTRAIN
DECOAPTATION
GRASTON INSTRUMENTS
INTEGRATIVE FASCIAL
  RELEASE

MUSCLE ENERGY
  TECHNIQUE
MYOFASCIAL RELEASE
  TECHNIQUE
PERIARTICULAR
POSTISOMETRIC
  RELAXATION

POSTFACILITATION
  STRETCH
SOFT TISSUE
SHERRINGTON'S LAW OF
  RECIPROCAL INNERVATION
TRANSVERSE FRICTION
  MASSAGE

A patient has a Grade II traumatic cervical sprain as a result of a rear-end automobile accident. The patient's chief complaint is severe pain located at the anterior cervical area. How should this case be approached from a manual point of view? A professional piano player reports pain and paresthesia in the first three and one-half fingers of his right hand. Surgery for carpal tunnel syndrome has failed to relieve his symptoms. What manual methods are appropriate in this case? Another patient complains of chronic lumbar pain, and examination reveals a chronically shortened iliopsoas muscle. What is the manual approach for treating the shortened iliopsoas muscle? Still another patient has consulted several orthopedists and chiropractors with chronic midscapular pain. He has a forward head and shoulder posture. Spinal adjustments have relieved the problem but offered no sustained solution. What alternative manual approach could be the primary treatment for this condition?

All these conditions will benefit from spinal adjustments, but in each case, **soft tissue** therapies can either completely resolve the condition or (in the acute first case) provide symptomatic relief until a spinal adjustment is feasible.

RATIONALE FOR MANUAL SOFT TISSUE PROCEDURES

Differentiating Spinal from Peripheral Causes for Pain

The first responsibility of doctors of chiropractic dealing with the total locomotor system is to find the source of the pain. The location of the source, along with its acuteness or chronicity, generally determines the type of treatment. In evaluating spinal subluxations related to musculoskeletal pain, the following question must always be asked: How much of the pain is directly related to the articular component of the subluxation? In many cases of peripheral soft tissue pain, the primary cause is in fact peripheral, in the local soft tissue itself, not in the spine. Thus although the lumbar spine and sacroiliac joint may be indirectly related to an Achilles tendinosis or a trochanteric bursitis, the majority of the treatment in these cases must be directed to the involved soft tissue.

From a soft tissue point of view, the problem may be located in various areas, including the muscle belly, musculotendinous portion, body of the tendon, insertion point of the tendon, bursa, ligament, or fascia. The soft tissue may be under tension because of a spinal source of pain; a postural, structural, or functional aberration; a viscerosomatic problem; or a problem located at the local soft tissue level. Chiropractors pay particular attention to the vertebral subluxation complex (VSC), with special emphasis on joint kinesiopathology, usually hypomobility.[1] If a primary reason for a subluxation is restriction within paraspinal or outlying muscles (i.e., the myofascial component of VSC) or connective tissue (i.e., the histopathologic component of VSC) because of microtraumatic or macrotraumatic injury, sedentary living, or altered motor patterns that have created muscular imbalances, then spinal adjustments alone may not fully address the condition.

In addition to influencing vertebral joint mechanics, spinal adjustments also directly affect soft tissues. Facet movement externally elicited by an adjustment affects the joint capsules and surrounding **periarticular** connective tissue including muscles, ligaments, and fascia. A joint is a space built for motion, and connective tissue structures surrounding that space are soft tissues affected by movement. The human spine, which is composed of vertebral bodies, disks, and supporting ligaments, lacks the ability to move on its own; it depends on the dynamic muscular system as its prime mover. Although spinal adjustments affect surrounding muscles, ligaments, and fascia, treatment of these soft tissue structures similarly affects spinal joint mechanics. It is important that chiropractors not limit their focus to only one side of this equation.

Evaluating and Treating the Whole System

Those seeking to develop expertise in treating functional conditions of the musculoskeletal system must evaluate and treat the whole system. The brain is a sensory and motor organ that delivers orders based on the sensory information it receives. Any persistent or chronic peripheral dysfunction (i.e., shortened muscle or fascia, trigger points, hyperpronation) will elicit a compensatory response from the central nervous system, which may result in an altered movement pattern. A typical example of such alteration is abnormal hip extension caused by a weak gluteus maximus. The weakened gluteus maximus could be caused by its antagonist, a shortened iliopsoas, based on **Sherrington's law of reciprocal innervation** (contraction of muscles is accompanied by the simultaneous inhibition of their antagonists), or a sacroiliac fixation could have caused the weakened muscle. Abnormal hip extension could create a change in gait (weakened hip extension), resulting in compensatory lumbar lordosis and hypermobility at the L4 and L5 vertebral segments.

Many altered patterns of movement remain in place even after the original painful lesion has disappeared[2,3] and are significant factors in subluxations that fail to respond to chiropractic adjustments or refixate after adjustment. Treatment of peripheral lesions not related to the spine, as well as treatment and prevention of spinal joint dysfunctions (subluxations), require evaluation and treatment of extraarticular soft tissue.

Distinguishing the Results from the Rationale

Clinicians using soft tissue methods usually report results through case studies because controlled studies are often difficult and sometimes impossible to perform. The rationales that clinicians use to explain their results are not necessarily valid, and researchers will eventually prove or disprove these theoretical explanations. For example, in 1984, Cyriax[4] described the effects of his method of frictional massage as increasing circulation and breaking down scar tissue. However, it was eventually demonstrated through microscopy that friction massage increased fibroblastic proliferation, which is essential for synthesizing and maintaining collagen, fibronectin, proteoglycans, and other proteins of the connective tissue matrix for tissue repair.[5] Judgment regarding technique rationales must be withheld until scientific documentation confirms the reason a method works. What is most important is that the technique creates consistently positive results.

VARIETIES OF SOFT TISSUE TECHNIQUES

Literally hundreds of soft tissue techniques exist, among them friction massage, **Active Release Techniques** (ARTs), postisometric relaxation, postfacilitation stretch, counterstrain, myofascial release, and muscle energy technique. This chapter surveys a variety of common soft tissue methods. It will not make the practitioner an expert in these techniques; rather, it provides a clear rationale for soft tissue work and a basis for further education in these methods. All soft tissue techniques require hands-on supervision and practice.

Soft tissue techniques require the use of the hands as a sensor to evaluate the status of soft tissue. The practitioner learns to feel for end ranges of motion, barriers, and looseness, as well as types of tissue organization often characterized as "lumpy," "leathery," "stringy," "doughy," "boggy," "nodular," "mobile," "taut," and "springy." Through manual palpation, the skilled practitioner discerns change in the tension of tissues, which helps determine the type of soft tissue treatment best suited to the patient's needs and to monitor progress and patient response to treatment.

Certain soft tissue techniques are most effective in acute conditions, whereas others are effective in both acute and chronic conditions. The larger the number of effective soft tissue techniques in the practitioner's repertoire, the better the overall quality of care.

Effect of Mechanical Load on Soft Tissue

Mechanical load on soft tissues, such as compression and tensile loading (Chapter 6), has been experimentally evaluated. Research has demonstrated that the form and function of musculoskeletal soft tissues are influenced by mechanical loading.[5] Loading methods such as transverse friction massage, deep massage, and the use of Graston instruments, can now be explained on a cellular level. Davidson and colleagues[5] have produced a remarkable study on the effect of soft tissue mobilization on the rat tendon. By way of light and electron microscopy, the effects of augmented soft tissue mobilization (i.e., Graston technique or friction massage) on injured rat Achilles tendon causes an absolute increase in fibroblast proliferation. Gehlsen and colleagues[7] have demonstrated that the proliferative response is directly dependent on the magnitude of the applied pressure.

Kolega[8] has found that stretching tissues with mobile clusters of epithelial fibroblasts causes the microfilaments within the cells to align along the long axis of that tension, thus offering a structural mechanism for fibroblast realignment with longitudinal mechanical stress. As a result, loading the tissue (in this case by stretching) alters the structure of the cytoskeleton (i.e., the microfilaments that make up the structure of the cell). This allows the fibroblasts produced by mechanical load (e.g., stretching, friction massage), which eventually become new collagen, to form with normal longitudinal lines of stress rather than with an abnormal cross-linking pattern. Excessive cross-linking of collagen is responsible for restrictive inelastic tissue, resulting in the potential for soft tissue abnormalities and eventual pain. Many studies[8] have shown that "cells in muscle, tendon, ligament, skin, and cartilage generally respond to 'windows' of increased loading by increasing matrix synthesis, increasing metabolic activity, and increasing cellular replication rates, and modifying their production of matrix components."

A piezoelectric phenomenon is another important effect of mechanical load on soft tissue.[9] Massage, especially deep massage, causes deformation of collagen, which generates electrical signals. Piezoelectricity (i.e., pressure electricity) is the result of mechanical energy turning into electric energy. The effect is activation of the healing processes by the creation of electrical commands into the extracellular matrix, which affects extracellular events such as the proper alignment of collagen bundles in tendons, fascia, ligaments, and arteries.[10] Piezoelectric energy is currently used in medicine to accelerate fracture healing and callus formation.

TRANSVERSE FRICTION MASSAGE

Transverse friction massage (TFM) is localized pressure usually administered on a ligament or on the components of muscle (e.g., belly, musculotendinous portion, body of the tendon, insertion). It has recently been described for use on chronically painful bursae.[11] This technique is extremely valuable in the treatment of tendinosis, ligamentous sprains, muscular lesions, and chronic bursitis. It is useful in both acute and chronic conditions, depending on the condition and area involved. Light friction may be used on a recent partial tear and in recent ligamentous sprains, but caution is required because cells in the process of repair are in an immature state. The application of stronger friction, respecting the patient's tolerance, is useful in the chronic stage.

Cyriax,[4] a medical physician, has proposed that the pressure and movement concentrated in a small local area by TFM can create greater therapeutic movement than strenuous exercise or manipulation. He states that TFM creates traumatic hyperemia (increase in blood) and movement that breaks down connective tissue (CT) adhesions. Recent studies on the effect of loading on cells has shown increased matrix synthesis, increased metabolic activity, increased cell replication rates (i.e., fibroblastic proliferation), and remodeling of matrix.[11] The digital stimulation of TFM acts on the local mechanoreceptors and may create temporary anesthesia, allowing for increased levels of pressure. After 10 to 20 minutes of TFM, if the massage is terminated while anesthesia is still present, functional isometric muscle testing of the involved area will demonstrate decreased pain, providing positive feedback to both doctor and patient.[12]

The exact placement of the practitioner's finger is extremely important. Cyriax emphasizes a functional evaluation of the area stressing particular tissues, thus allowing the practitioner to apply friction to the precisely correct location. He notes that the most painful area is not necessarily the source of the pain and that painful isometric muscle testing often reveals a pain source that is not the most tender area.

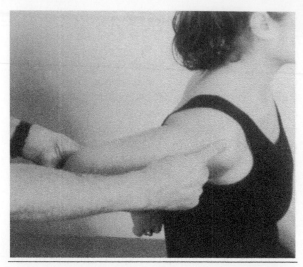

Fig. **13-1** Optimal position for palpating and treating supraspinatus tendon insertion.

The practitioner's finger and the patient's skin should move as if they are attached. Otherwise, the skin will be frictioned, and bruising will occur. Knowledge of surface anatomy is necessary to ascertain that the exact location is being treated. Recent cadaver studies have demonstrated new approaches to palpation for some rotator cuff muscle and tendon areas.[13]

The new optimal position for palpating the supraspinatus insertion for maximum exposure has the patient sitting, with arm behind back, in maximal adduction, with medial rotation, and up to 30 to 40 degrees of hyperextension, depending on patient tolerance (Fig. 13-1). The maximal exposure for palpating and treating the insertion of the teres minor and infraspinatus has the patient sitting with shoulder in flexion to 90 degrees, combined with 10 degrees of shoulder adduction and 20 degrees of shoulder lateral rotation (Fig. 13-2).

Cyriax,[4] who used injectable steroids for many conditions, nevertheless considered certain anatomic areas curable only by deep friction. These include the following:
- Belly of the subclavius
- Musculotendinous junction of the supraspinatus
- Long head and lower musculotendinous junction of the biceps

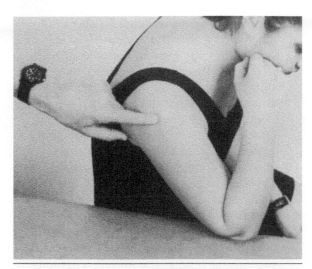

Fig. **13-2** Optimal position for palpating and treating insertion of infraspinatus and teres minor *(just below infraspinatus)*.

- Belly of the brachialis
- Belly of the supinator
- Ligaments about the carpal lunate bone
- Adductors of the thumb
- Interosseous belly at the hand
- Interosseous tendon at the finger
- Intercostal muscles
- Oblique muscles of the abdomen
- Lower musculotendinous junction of the iliopsoas (Fig. 13-3)
- Quadriceps expansion at the patella
- Coronary ligament of the knee
- Lower musculotendinous junction of the biceps femoris
- Musculotendinous junction of the anterior and posterior tibial and peroneal
- Posterior tibiotalar ligament
- Anterior fascia of the ankle joint
- Interosseous belly at the foot

ACTIVE RELEASE TECHNIQUES

Developed by chiropractor P. Michael Leahy, ART is a patented method used for the examination, diagnosis, and treatment of repetitive stress disorders such as carpal tunnel syndrome and epicondylosis (i.e., tennis elbow).[14-17] Leahy states that acute injury or repetitive injury of a constant pressure or tension may lead to a cumu-

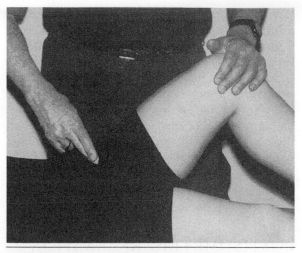

Fig. **13-3** Position for friction massage of lower musculotendinous junction of iliopsoas.

lative injury cycle, which may result in a state of adhesion and fibrosis.[14] Unless connective tissue is free of adhesions, a *traction neurodesis* may occur, resulting in peripheral nerve entrapment. A traction neurodesis represents fibrosis (formation of fibrous tissue) around the nerve, resulting in the nerve being stretched instead of performing its normal gliding function. Peripheral nerves must be able to glide during movement. For example, the brachial plexus moves 15.3 mm during shoulder abduction or adduction, and median nerve excursion proximal to the elbow is 7.3 mm during full elbow flexion and extension.[14] Any restriction to this motion will affect transmission of impulses through the peripheral nerve. Peripheral nerve entrapment is far more common than spinal nerve root entrapment.

As with all other soft tissue techniques, ARTs require a hands-on learning experience. Through palpation, the practitioner must evaluate tissue texture, tension, movement, and function, along the lines of the PARTS (*P*ain/tenderness; *A*symmetry; *R*ange-of-motion abnormality; *T*issue tone, texture, and temperature abnormality; and *S*pecial tests) paradigm described in Chapter 10. According to Leahy, it is possible to determine the duration of a condition through skilled palpation.[14] For example, in the inflammatory phase (i.e., 24 to 72 hours after injury), a movable, fluidlike swelling with associated signs of inflammation may be palpated. After 2 days to 2 weeks, a "stringy, guitar string" feeling will be elicited. A lumpy feeling will be palpated after 2 weeks to 4 months, and finally after 3 months a leathery feeling will be present.

ART is an appropriate treatment for the failed carpal tunnel surgery discussed at the beginning of this chapter. It is an excellent procedure for treating entrapment of the median nerve as it passes through or under the pronator teres muscle. Often percussion of the pronator teres at its midbelly elicits a positive Tinel's sign, referring paresthesia (abnormal sensation such as burning or prickling) to the median nerve distribution in the hand.

POSTISOMETRIC RELAXATION

Lewit uses **postisometric relaxation** (PIR) to relax tense muscles, comparing this method with the Travell spray-and-stretch technique.[2] For muscle tension caused by spinal fixation or viscerosomatic reflexes, this technique will not be effective. The patient with acute whiplash and muscle spasm offers the classic case for the appropriate use of PIR, with treatment directed to the upper trapezius.

The technique is as follows (Fig. 13-4):

1. The practitioner lengthens the muscle until the slack is taken up at the point where slight resistance is encountered without creating pain.
2. The patient is then asked to contract the muscle isometrically with minimal force (this should cause little or no pain) and to inhale and look with the eyes to the side of contraction. The patient should contract the muscle for 10 seconds. Gaymans[18] has shown that inhalation has a facilitating effect on muscles and exhalation an inhibiting effect; moving the eyes toward the side of muscle activity facilitates the contracting muscle, whereas looking away from the side of contraction inhibits the contracting side.
3. The patient is then told to "let go," to relax, exhale, and look in the opposite direction. The practitioner allows the muscle to lengthen by spontaneous decontraction. Relaxation can last 10 to 20 seconds, as long as the muscle lengthens, at which point a new barrier is reached. The procedure can be repeated three to five times. If the patient has difficulty relaxing, the isometric contraction phase can be increased up to 30 seconds.

An example of appropriate use of PIR for the lower extremity would be a patient who is in acute pain and who is forward flexed as a result of iliopsoas spasm assumes a modified Thomas position (Fig. 13-5, *A*, under postfacilitation stretch); a flexed right hip is observed because of spasm of the right iliopsoas. The patient executes the same procedure as performed for the upper trapezius, but in this case the eyes look up during inspiration. The doctor exerts minimal pressure on the knee, feeling the psoas contract (Fig. 13-6, *A*). During inspiration phase, the patient

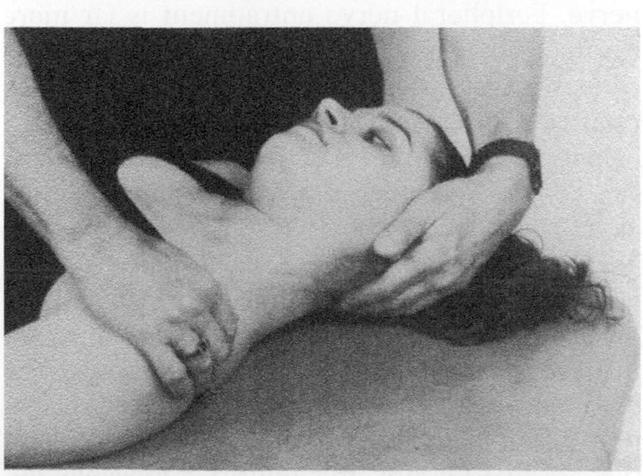

Fig. **13-4** Patient lets go, exhales, and looks in opposite direction as practitioner allows muscle to lengthen by spontaneous decontraction.

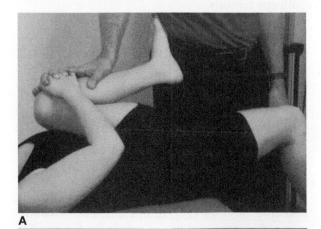

A

Fig. **13-5 A,** Modified Thomas' test indicating a tight right iliopsoas. Note slight flexion of right hip.

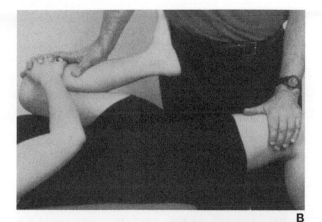

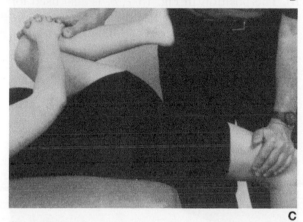

Fig. 13-5 cont'd B, Patient isometrically resists doctor's pressure for 7 seconds. C, Patient lets go, and doctor stretches iliopsoas for 12 seconds.

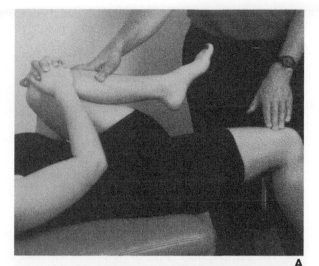

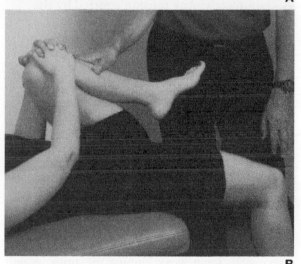

Fig. 13-6 A, Postisometric relaxation (PIR) for iliopsoas. B, Relaxation phase of PIR for iliopsoas.

may minimally contract isometrically as long as pain is not elicited. Fig. 13-6, B, shows the patient "letting go" with expiration and eyes downward for 10 to 20 seconds or until relaxation occurs.

Unlike the Travell spray-and-stretch method, an attempt is make to avoid the stretch reflex in this case. Lewit believes that this method should eliminate trigger points and pain points where the tendon is attached to the periosteum.[2] Methods that relax muscles usually improve joint range of motion.

POSTFACILITATION STRETCH

Postfacilitation stretch (PFS) is primarily used to stretch chronically shortened muscles. Popularized

by Janda, a medical physician, this technique restores muscle balance. Certain muscles, principally postural slow-twitch muscles such as the iliopsoas, tensor fascia lata, piriformis, and erector spinae, tend to tighten; other phasic muscles including the serratus anterior and the gluteus maximus, medius, and minimus tend to become weak and inhibited.[19] With as few as six PFS treatments over 6 weeks, tight muscles will normalize. Janda describes typical "muscle imbalance patterns," which perpetuate many spinal problems. Often a tight muscle is the cause of a weak, inhibited antagonistic muscle, and after using PFS the inhibited muscle spontaneously strengthens.

The iliopsoas, which can be evaluated with the modified Thomas' test (see Fig. 13-5, *A*), is considered tight if the extended femur does not easily reach 5 to 15 degrees extension below the table. The PFS technique for the iliopsoas is as follows:

1. The shortened psoas is placed in the midposition. The patient isometrically resists for 7 seconds (see Fig. 13-5, *B*) and then lets go (see Fig. 13-5, *C*) while the practitioner stretches the muscle for 12 seconds.
2. The patient may have to be taught to relax completely. Any tension exerted by the patient after they let go will inhibit the relaxation phase, which is necessary for this stretching procedure.
3. The practitioner must wait 20 seconds before attempting to restretch. Three to five passes may be applied. The procedure should not be continued if pain ensues. As range of motion increases, isometric contraction is started at the new range.
4. The patient should then perform active movement of the muscle in its new range of motion.

One reason that some low back problems never completely resolve is that a tight iliopsoas may be responsible for a weak gluteus maximus, which creates an abnormal pattern of hip extension.

Normal hip extension begins with contraction of the ipsilateral gluteus maximus and hamstrings, followed immediately by contraction of the contralateral lumbar muscles. This sequential muscular contraction creates a lever that crosses the lumbosacral area to stabilize the lower spine and pelvis during hip extension.

When the gluteus maximus is weak, the hamstrings work harder, creating abnormal sequences of motion. Contraction of the ipsilateral lumbar muscles instead of the contralateral lumbar muscles can occur, as can contraction of the ipsilateral thoracic muscles or even the trapezius muscles, as the body attempts to accomplish extension. Abnormal hip extension may result in

an increased lumbar lordosis and hypermobility of the lower lumbar spinal segments.

Treatment of the tight iliopsoas by PFS or ARTs may allow the inhibited weak gluteus maximus to regain its strength spontaneously. Fig. 13-7, *A*, and 13-7, *B*, demonstrate PFS for the left upper trapezius. Fig. 13-7, *A*, shows the patient's neck in maximum flexion, contralateral side bending, and ipsilateral rotation. The patient isometrically pushes her left shoulder cephalad against the doctor's resistance for 7 seconds. The patient is told to let go and to allow the doctor to push the shoulder caudal for 12 seconds (Fig. 13-7, *B*). The position in Fig. 13-7, *B*, is also used for screening to determine the end feel for tightness. This end feel is compared with the opposite side.

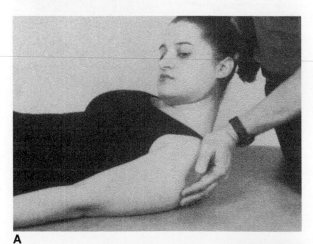

A

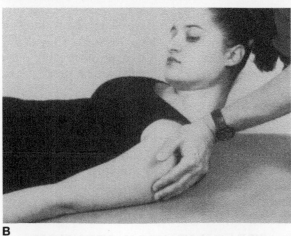

B

Fig. **13-7** **A,** Postfacilitation stretch (PFS) for left upper trapezius. **B,** PFS for left upper trapezius.

The exact mechanism for proprioceptive neuromuscular facilitation techniques such as PFS is still under examination.[20,21]

STRAIN AND COUNTERSTRAIN

In *Jones' Strain and Counterstrain*,[22] osteopathic physician Lawrence H. Jones relates the discovery of this technique. A patient was unable to stand erect or sleep because of continuous pain and failed to respond to 2 months of treatment by two chiropractors and 2 additional months of manipulative osteopathic therapy by Dr. Jones himself. Dr. Jones finally spent 20 minutes attempting different positions that relieved the patient until he "achieved a position of surprising amount of comfort" (p. 1). When the patient stood he was "overjoyed." His posture was erect, and the pain substantially decreased. No manipulation was performed. In subsequent years, Jones found almost 200 small zones of tense, tender, edematous muscle and fascial tissue about a centimeter in diameter all over the body, along with specific associated positions that relieved the local tender points.

Counterstrain is a system of evaluation and treatment of joint pain based on the idea that joint pain is the result of a strain of the proprioceptive and neuromuscular reflexes, which cause muscular imbalance and joint dysfunction. Uses for the technique have been described for supraspinatus tendinitis,[23] forward and backward torsions of the sacrum,[24] and acute ankle sprains,[25] as well as for a variety of conditions in the hospital population.[26]

Irwin Korr's Theory of Proprioception

The work of physiologist Irwin Korr,[27] the premier osteopathic researcher of the twentieth century, offers a model to explain counterstrain. A good illustration is a cervical trauma in which the head extends posterior and the anterior cervical muscles are stretched while the posterior cervical muscles are maximally shortened. Spindle activity is reduced to almost zero in the passively shortened posterior muscles, reflecting the lack of stimulation of primary afferent (Ia) fibers. After receiving no feedback from the muscle spindle, the central nervous system (CNS) then activates the gamma system (high gamma gain), which reactivates the spindle. Gamma motor neuron cells originate in the ventral horn, pass through the ventral root, stimulating the intrafusal fibers, which stimulates further afferent spindle firing. Normally, controlling the contraction of the intrafusal fibers through gamma stimulation allows the CNS to set and reset the muscle length and tone, as well as the sensitivity of muscle spindles to stretch.[28] However, the high gamma gain does not return to normal, and it continues to provide inaccurate information to the CNS regarding muscle length. The posterior muscle in its shortened position therefore reports that it is being stretched.

Korr states that the muscle resists returning to its resting length because of the increased spindle discharge. The sustained contraction prevents the spinal segment from returning to its original resting position. Eventually, segmental facilitation occurs, which can last for years. Counterstrain points may overlap with trigger points or acupuncture points, but they tend to be more segmental.[28]

General Counterstrain Technique

1. The tender point is located.
2. The muscle or joint is moved into a position of comfort until a pain level estimated at 10 is reduced to 2. This position shortens the muscle containing the dysfunctional proprioceptors and allows the primary endings to "shut off" the abnormal elevated activity. As the gamma system shuts off, the annulospiral endings reduce the output to the alphas and the muscle relaxes. The patient will feel the tender points shut off.
3. The position of comfort is held for no less than 90 seconds, which is the minimum time required to allow the gamma system to return to normal.
4. Returning to the neutral position occurs very slowly to ensure that the sensitive proprioceptors are not reactivated.

As an example of counterstrain technique for anterior neck pain, a tender point at the anterior

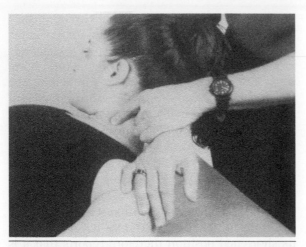

Fig. 13-8 Counterstrain position for treatment of anterior cervical tender point.

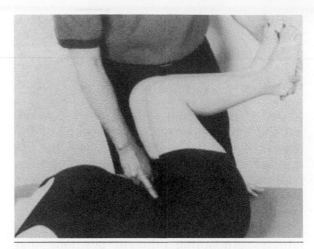

Fig. 13-9 Counterstrain position for painful psoas point.

surface of the tip of the left transverse process of C5 is considered. Such tenderness may be due to involvement of the scalenus anticus and longus colli. In Fig. 13-8 the patient's neck is flexed (position of comfort for this point) while the doctor presses the sensitive point with up to 2 pounds of pressure. For this particular point, the neck is brought into increasing flexion while the doctor palpates for diminution of the tender point. Positioning the neck into flexion shortens the muscle, which reduces the tenderness. Jones has found that with tenderness in this particular location, adding contralateral rotation and possibly lateral bending away from the pain will further diminish the pain. The point is held for 90 seconds, and the neck is then slowly returned to its neutral position. For most of the tender points found in this technique, the area is first brought into its most shortened position, although occasionally the area (muscle or joint) is brought into a lengthened position to decrease the tenderness.

In treating the anterior cervical points, the most painful point is treated first. This technique is very beneficial in acute cervical problems with anterior cervical pain with active or passive cervical extension. The painful point usually reduces in two visits, with a 50% reduction in pain typically noted after the first visit.

For counterstrain treatment of a painful psoas point, the previous procedure is followed (Fig.

13-9). The iliopsoas muscle is treated similarly to the anterior cervical muscles; in both situations the points are on the anterior portion of the body and therefore treated in flexion. For rare cases, an anterior point is treated in extension or a posterior point is treated in a flexed position.

MYOFASCIAL RELEASE TECHNIQUE

Myofascial release technique is a method of evaluating and treating abnormally cross-linked, restrictive (though not necessarily painful) fascia. Barnes[29] estimates that 90% of patients treated with musculoskeletal problems have myofascial dysfunction. He asserts that this physiologic system has been widely ignored, resulting in poor or temporary results from many treatments.

The fascia is a three-dimensional web of connective tissue that spreads throughout the body without interruption. Fascial restriction can cause abnormal pressure on nerves, muscles, blood vessels, osseous structures, and visceral organs.[29] An obvious fascial restriction occurs in "compartment syndrome," in which an increase in lower extremity blood pressure prevents a runner from continuing. Blood vessels are supported and surrounded by fascia, which, upon shortening, restricts the blood supply to the muscles. Pain that is the result of ischemia and increased blood pressure prevents the runner from continuing. This condition is often treated by a surgical fasciotomy. Compartment syndrome even occurs in the lumbar paraspinal areas, where restrictive thoracolumbar fascia that surrounds the erector spinae muscles affects the circulation of the back muscles, resulting in a painful lower back.[30]

Barnes finds that chronic poor posture, inflammation, or trauma most commonly cause restrictions. Pelvic torsion, forward head and shoulders, lumbar lordosis, and spinal fixations are among the structural aberrations directly related to restricted fascia. Fascia from patients with low back pain who are evaluated by light-and-electron microscopy have been found to display "a primary ischemic pathoanatomy in the fascia that may be of relevance to back pain syndromes"[31].

Greenman[32] states that a wide variety of myofascial release techniques are in use. He describes a technique taught by Ward, an osteopath, in which the practitioner evaluates the fascia by applying compression and transverse shear in opposite directions, sensing for tension or laxity in both superficial and deep fascial levels. Contact is applied against the barrier, and the practitioner follows the "inherent tissue motion," during which time the patient performs enhancing motions using the eyes or breathing for physiologic summation.[3] Physiologic summation refers to the facilitative use of the eyes or breathing on the muscular system as discussed earlier in this chapter under "Postisometric relaxation."[2]

Lewit[2] simply takes up the slack (engages the barrier) and with minimal change in pressure waits until release occurs, which generally takes between a few seconds and one-half minute. He then follows the release.

Barnes[29] maintains that some myofascial techniques only affect the elastic and muscular components rather than the collagenous viscous portion of the ground substance embedded in the interstitial spaces of the fascial system. He states that the connective tissue ground substance loses some of its fluid content and undergoes colloidal solidification, thereby restricting both local and distal areas. Manual intervention provides a mechanical, electromagnetic, and thermal force that can change the consistency of the colloid to a more liquid gelatinous arrangement.

Theoretic Foundations of Myofascial Release

Practitioners who use myofascial methods often obtain results distant from the location of their contact. In 1931, Columbia University anatomist B.B. Gallaudet dissected 34 adult cadavers to determine the relationship of the fascial planes of the body. He concluded that the "planes of fascia in one region of the body are directly continuous with the same planes in all other regions"[33] (Preface). Barker[34] used 41 embalmed cadavers to show the relationship of the superficial and deep thoracolumbar fasciae. She demonstrated direct connections between the fasciae that extend from the occiput and neck to the lower back, upper and lower limbs, trunk, abdomen, pelvis, and biceps femoris, demonstrating as well that mechanical forces were transmitted among these areas. Willard[35] showed that the interspinous and supraspinous ligaments can act as force transducers, translating the tension originating from the fasciae of the extremities and torso into the lumbar vertebral column to the facet joint capsules. Thus restricted fasciae in the extremities can be responsible for restricted movement of the spine. This provides a sound rationale for evaluating soft tissue distant from the spine as part of addressing spinal problems.

The tensegrity model of biomechanics (see Chapter 4) reveals even more of the effects of treating the abnormal tensions of the body by soft tissue methods. Tensegrity, a concept originated by pioneering designer and inventor Buckminster Fuller and architect Kenneth Snellsen, is defined as a system that stabilizes itself mechanically because of the way tensional and compressive forces are distributed and balanced within the structure. Continuous tension and discontinuous compression[36,37] exist within the body; the connective tissue is under constant tension, whereas the bones may be considered the compression elements. Increased tension in any part of the body results in increased tension in individual structural elements throughout the body.[4] Restricted areas in this tension system therefore can affect the balance of any part of the system.

Barnes Myofascial Release Technique

1. The practitioner first palpates the skin for deeper restrictions and determines the direction of the barrier.
2. Contact is made against the barrier with one hand while the other hand provides a counter pressure.
3. The practitioner waits 1 to 2 minutes until the barrier releases and follows the direction of release.

Barnes emphasizes that waiting for the release is essential since early motion is due to the elastic rather than the viscous component of the fascia.

Fig. 13-10 depicts a release on the side of an anterior ilium as a result of a restriction of fascia on the anterior thigh. Fig. 13-11 depicts a position for fascial release in the area of the psoas. The thigh is shifted through its range of motion to palpate for fascial restrictions.

A cross-handed position on the pectoral areas of the chest is an excellent method of freeing fascia responsible for causing forward shoulders. Forward shoulders and head are often responsible for chronic upper thoracic pain as a result of pressure on the posterior upper thoracic spine. Releasing the anterior chest fascia will often allow the shoulders to shift posteriorly, taking the strain off the posterior thoracic spine.

INTEGRATIVE FASCIAL RELEASE

Hammer's **Integrative Fascial Release**[38] integrates several myofascial methods.[29,32,39,40] The practitioner tests muscles (fasciae) for shortening, palpates the body surface for tissue restrictive barriers, and posturally evaluates for potential shortened tissues. Treatment involves choosing the most restricted tissue and contacting the area in the direction of the barrier. The fascial restriction can be in any plane, because in many areas of the body the fascia is multidirectional. Often the barrier releases over the bellies of several muscles. After contacting the barrier the practitioner waits for the barrier to release. To enhance the release, the patient is told to inhale and hold the breath for 5 or 10 seconds. The patient may have to inhale several times until the release occurs. As the release occurs (whether during inhalation or exhalation), the practitioner follows the release, exerting a stretch on the tissue by moving the local area or a related extremity in a direction, if possible, that linearly increases the tension (stretch) in the line of the barrier. Releasing fascial barriers is proposed to

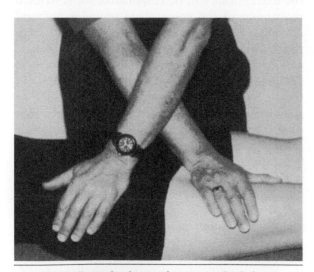

Fig. 13-10 Fascial release of anterior thigh fascia. Doctor's left hand is pressing cephalad against anterior superior iliac spine (ASIS) while right hand is pressing against barrier.

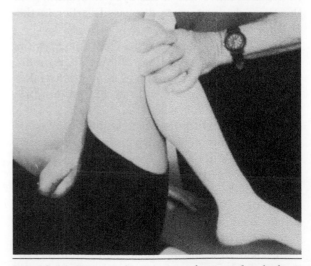

Fig. 13-11 Position for releasing fascia at level of psoas.

restore balance to the muscular system, remove nerve entrapments, aid circulation, and play a proprioceptive role.

MUSCLE ENERGY TECHNIQUE

Developed by osteopath, Fred L. Mitchell, **muscle energy technique** involves voluntary contraction of the patient's muscles in a precisely controlled direction at varying levels of intensity against a distinctly executed counterforce applied by the practitioner.[32] According to Greenman,[32] this technique can be used to mobilize a restricted articulation. Other uses are to lengthen shortened, contracted, or spastic muscles, to strengthen physiologically weakened muscle groups, and to reduce localized edema caused by congestion by using muscles to pump the lymphatic and venous systems.

The muscle energy method used for the cervical spine is based on the theory of reciprocal innervation. A short hypertonic muscle prevents normal motion in the opposite direction and also inhibits its antagonistic muscle. After isometrically contracting the hypertonic muscle, the hypertonic muscle can be stretched to a new resting length. At the same time the weakened antagonist develops increased tone, thereby balancing the area. Muscle energy treatment takes into consideration coupled motions of the cervical spine for C1-7 side bending and rotation to occur to the same side. Therefore both side bending and rotation are treated. These coupled motions are evaluated in both flexion and extension. If the segment is fixed in flexion or extension or both, treatment would also include the additional coupled motion of flexion or extension or both.

For example, palpation in both flexion and extension is first performed to determine restricted lateral motion. If in the flexed position, lateral motion is restricted because of localized hypertonicity at C5 pushing from right to left; the assumption is that C5 is restricted in flexion, right lateral bending, and right rotation (coupled motions).

1. The articular pillar of C6 is contacted to enable C5 to move upon it.
2. The patient's head is flexed forward as far as the C5-6 interspace.

3. Next, move the neck into the barrier of right rotation and right side bending. From this position the three-coupled motions are treated with muscle energy.
4. The patient rotates isometrically left against resistance for 3 to 5 seconds, three to five times (Fig. 13-12).
5. The patient then moves the head laterally left against resistance for 3 to 5 seconds, three to five times.
6. Finally, the patient isometrically resists into extension for 3 to 5 seconds, three to five times.

After each of these movements, the practitioner may observe enhanced mobility, with barriers becoming progressively less restrictive (Fig. 13-13).

If C5 were fixed in extension, right lateral bending, and right rotation, something would prevent the right facet from closing. The same procedure would be used, except that isometric resistance by the patient toward flexion would be used because of the restriction found in cervical extension.

Although chiropractic adjustments can in many cases accomplish all of the previously discussed results, in certain circumstances, high-velocity, low-amplitude thrusts are inadvisable. Such

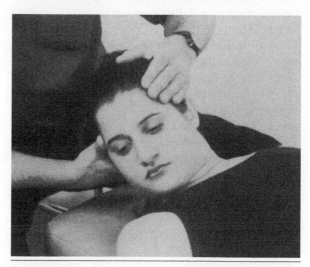

Fig. **13-12** Patient's head is rotated rightward to barrier. She is then asked to resist against rotation to her left.

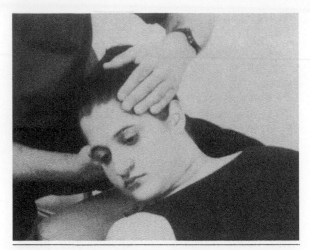

Fig. **13-13** Patient has increased range of rotation to a new barrier and is resisting against rotation to her left.

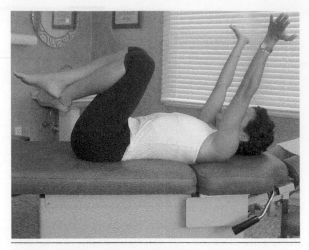

Fig. **13-14** Decoaptation, C5-C6.

circumstances include various acute pain situations, severe osteoporosis, and bony abnormalities. In these cases, muscle energy technique and other soft tissue methods offer a valuable addition to the chiropractor's repertoire.

LONGITUDINAL STRETCHING WITH OSTEOARTICULAR DECOAPTATION

Guy Voyer has developed stretching positions that are effective as a daily exercise for intervertebral disk problems.[41] He states that depending on the position of the body, particular disk levels will be affected. This method represents a **decoaptation** (from *coapt*, to approximate or draw together), which is an increased separation or traction occurring at a local level by stretching all the connected fasciae related to that particular area. The results of this 1-minute per day stretch are disk and zygopophyseal separation, disk imbibition (absorption of liquid), increased venous return, and normalization of muscle tone. The patient must be taught to develop an awareness of the specific position for C5-C6 decoaptation (Fig. 13-14).

1. Coccyx is lifted by pressing the sacral base to ground.
2. Arms are lifted sagittally overhead about 135 degrees; shoulder blades are lifted off the ground.
3. Elbows are extended, wrists are dorsiflexed, and hands are externally rotated.
4. Chin is tucked to chest, and head is lifted approximately 2 inches off ground.
5. Action: Sacral base is pressed down, heels of hands are pushed out with *extreme* effort, and top of head is pushed cephalad, also with *extreme* effort.
6. Position is held for 1 minute. It may take several visits for patient to learn exact position and to hold position at first for a full minute.

The positioning for L4-L5 (Fig. 13-15):

1. Patient sits straight, feet are hip-width apart, and knees are flexed 90 degrees.
2. Ankles are everted and dorsiflexed.
3. Patient should push abdomen out, attempting to flatten lumbar curve.
4. Arms should be extended, externally rotated with wrists dorsiflexed.
5. Chin is tucked to chest, and head is lifted cephalad.
6. Extreme effort is used to push head and hands toward ceiling. Position is held for 1 minute. It may take several visits for patient to learn exact position and to hold the position for a full minute.

GRASTON TECHNIQUE

David Graston and Andre Hall are nonpractitioner inventors who suffered with chronic knee

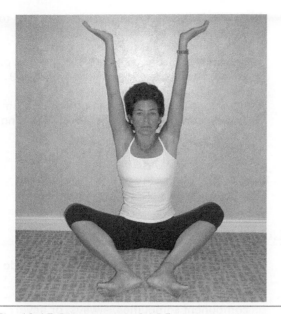

Fig. 13-15 Decoaptation, L4-L5.

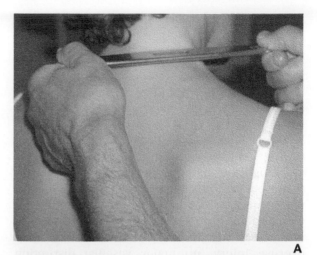

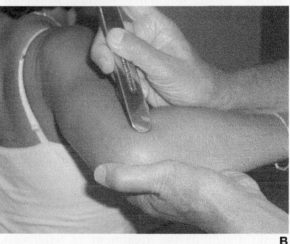

Fig. 13-16 A, The use of a Graston instrument for paracervical myofascial release. B, The use of a Graston instrument for lateral epicondylosis.

problems, one of which remained after surgery. They benefited from Cyriax's friction massage technique and attempted to treat themselves. Graston fabricated metal instruments to give his hands relief from the strain of the massage, and eventually he designed instruments to fit the contours of the human body (Fig. 13-16). Positive outcome studies have been reported for numerous soft tissue conditions[42] treated with these instruments. The fat pads of human fingers compress tissues, whereas instruments with a narrower edge have the ability to separate the fibers, allowing the practitioner to increase the sensitivity of palpation for chronic deep collagen cross-links. One of the main theories for the efficacy of this method is the accepted theory of friction massage (i.e., to elicit a controlled microtrauma to the affected soft tissue, stimulating a local inflammatory response leading to normal remodeling and repair). The **Graston instruments** help the practitioner penetrate and remove fibrotic tissue that is not amenable to the human hand (Fig. 13-17). As with friction massage and all fascial release methods, combining a targeted stretching and strengthening exercise program with the technique is important.[43]

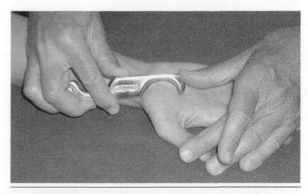

Fig. 13-17 The use of a Graston instrument for carpal tunnel syndrome.

TENDINITIS AND TENDINOSIS

Recent research has led to reconsideration of the term *tendinitis* (also spelled *tendonitis*). This widely used term is now considered a misnomer because biopsies of the rotator cuff, Achilles tendon, elbow tendon, and patellar tendon have failed to exhibit cells with acute inflammation.[44,45] Most injuries observed in a chiropractic clinical setting deal with chronic overuse conditions resulting from microtraumatic injuries, rather than from macrotraumatic injuries. A true inflammatory process occurs more readily in a macrotraumatic injury because vascular disruption initiates an inflammatory cascade. In a chronic overuse injury, no major vascular disruption exists and the pathologic result is therefore a degenerative process consisting of hypertrophy and hyperplasia of fibroblasts, increasingly disorganized collagen production, and vascular hyperplasia sometimes referred to as angiofibroblastic degeneration.[46] This type of histopathology is referred to as *tendinosis*.

Although nonsteroidal antiinflammatory drugs (NSAIDs) are commonly prescribed for tendinitis or tendinosis, the lack of inflammation calls their use into question. Soft tissue methods such as deep friction massage and Graston technique, which can initiate a new inflammatory cascade within the degenerated tendinosis, represent a breakthrough in the treatment of tendinosis. Inflammation is a necessary component of healing, and the final stage of inflammation, known as the remodeling phase, represents the formation of new collagen along the normal lines of stress.

Review *Questions*

1. What are the two causes of a weakened gluteus maximus? Describe.
2. What is the effect of manual soft tissue techniques on connective tissue cells?
3. In what situations is light rather than strong friction massage appropriate?
4. What is the benefit of creating soft tissue anesthesia by manual methods?
5. What is the ideal position for transverse friction of the supraspinatus muscle?

6. Why is it necessary for peripheral nerves to have freedom of motion?
7. In palpating soft tissue, how would the practitioner distinguish between a lesion of 2 weeks compared with a lesion of over 3 months?
8. How does Lewit's PIR technique differ from Travell spray-and-stretch method regarding the muscle stretch?
9. What is Irwin Korr's theory relating to counterstrain? Describe.
10. Why is the muscle put into a shortened position in the counterstrain technique?

Concept *Questions*

1. Based on your chiropractic perspective, do you believe that the spinal (osseous) component supersedes the soft tissue component sometimes, always, or never? Explain.
2. What percentage of patients requires a soft tissue evaluation? Explain.
3. How do soft tissue procedures interface with the operational model of subluxation complex?

REFERENCES

1. Seaman D: Subluxation: causes and effects, *Dyn Chiropr* 14(3):12, 1996.
2. Lewit K: *Manipulative therapy in rehabilitation of the locomotor system*, ed 2, Boston, 1991, Butterworth-Heinemann.
3. Janda V: Muscles and motor control in low back pain: assessment and management. In Twomey LT, Taylor J: *Physical therapy and the low back*, New York, 1987, Churchill Livingstone.
4. Cyriax J: *Textbook of orthopaedic medicine*, vol 2, ed 11, London, 1984, Baillere Tindall.
5. Davidson CJ et al: Rat tendon morphologic and functional changes resulting from soft tissue mobilization, *Med Sci Sports Exerc* 29(3):313, 1997.
6. Frank CB, Hart DA: Cellular response to loading. In Leadbetter WB, Buckwalter JA, Gordon SL: *Sports-induced inflammation*, Park Ridge, Ill, 1989, American Academy of Orthopedic Surgery.
7. Gehlsen GM, Ganion LR, Helfst R: *Effects of pressure variations on tendon healing. Research binder*, Muncie, Ind, 1998, Performance Dynamics.
8. Kolega J: Effects of mechanical tension on protrusive activity and microfilament and intermediate filament organization in an epidermal epithelium moving in culture, *J Cell Biol* 102:1400-1411, 1986.

9. Turchaninov R: Research and massage therapy: part 2, *Massage & Bodywork* 48-56, Dec/Jan 2001.

10. Basset CAL: Biophysical principles affecting bone structure. In Bourne GH: *The biochemistry and physiology of bone*, vol 3, New York, 1971, Academic Press.

11. Hammer WI: The use of transverse friction massage in the management of chronic bursitis of the hip or shoulder, *J Manipulative Physiol Ther* 16:107, 1993.

12. Hammer WI: Friction Massage. In Hammer WI: *Functional soft tissue examination and treatment by manual methods: the extremities*, Gaithersburg, Md, 1991, Aspen Publishers.

13. Mattingly GE, Mackarey PJ: Optimal methods for shoulder tendon palpation: a cadaver study, *Phys Ther* 76:236, 1996.

14. Leahy PM: Active release techniques. In Hammer WI: *Functional soft tissue examination and treatment by manual methods*, ed 2, Gaithersburg, Md, 1996, Aspen Publishers.

15. Leahy PM, Mock LE: Myofascial release technique and mechanical compromise of peripheral nerves of the upper extremity, *J Sports Chiropr Rehabil* 6:139, 1992.

16. Leahy PM, Mock LE: Altered biomechanics of the shoulder and the subscapularis, *J Sports Chiropr Rehabil* 5:62, 1991.

17. Leahy PM, Mock LE: Synoviochondrometaplasia of the shoulder: a case report, *J Sports Chiropr Rehabil* 6:5, 1992.

18. Gaymans F: Die Bedeutung der Atemtypen fur Mobilisation der Wirbelsaule, *Manuell Medizin* 18:96, 1980.

19. Jull GA, Janda V: Muscles and motor control in low back pain. In Twomey LT, Taylor JR, editors, *Physical therapy of the low back*, New York, 1987, Churchill Livingstone.

20. Moore MA, Kukulka CG: Depression of Hoffmann reflexes following voluntary contraction and implications for proprioceptive neuromuscular facilitation therapy, *Phys Ther* 71:321, 1991.

21. Guissard N, Duchateau J, Hainaut K: Muscle stretching and motoneuron excitability, *Eur J Appl Physiol* 58:47, 1988.

22. Jones LH, Kusunose R, Goering E: *Jones' strain-counterstrain*, Boise, Ind, 1995, Jones Strain-Counterstrain.

23. Jacobson EC et al: Shoulder pain and repetition strain injury to the supraspinatus muscle: etiology and manipulative treatment, *J Am Osteopath Assoc* 89(8):1037, 1989.

24. Cislo S, Ramires MA, Schwartz HR: Low back pain: treatment of forward and backward torsions using counterstrain technique, *J Am Osteopath Assoc* 1(3):255, 1909.

25. Jones LH: Foot treatment without hand trauma, *J Am Osteopath Assoc* 72(1):481, 1973.

26. Schwartz H:. The use of counterstrain in an acutely ill in-hospital population, *J Am Osteopath Assoc* 86(7):433, 1986.

27. Korr I: Proprioceptors and somatic dysfunction, *J Am Osteopath Assoc* 74(3):638, 1975

28. Kusunose RS: Strain and counterstrain. In Basmajian JV, Nyberg R: *Rational manual therapies*, Baltimore, Md, 1993, Williams & Wilkins.

29. Barnes JF: *Myofascial release: a comprehensive evaluatory and treatment approach*, Paoli, Penn, 1990, MFR Seminars.

30. Kitajima I et al: Acute paraspinal muscle compartment syndrome treated with surgical decompression, *Am J Sports Med* 30(2):283, 2002.

31. Bednar DA, Orr FW, Simon GT: Observations on the pathomorphology of the thoracolumbar fascia in chronic mechanical back pain, *Spine* 20(10):1161, 1995.

32. Greenman PE: *Principles of manual medicine*, ed 2, Baltimore, 1996, Williams & Wilkins.

33. Gallaudet BB: *A description of the planes of fascia of the human body*, New York, 1931, Columbia University Press.

34. Barker PJ: Attachments of the posterior layer of lumbar fascia, *Spine* 24(17):1757, 1999.

35. Willard FH: The muscular, ligamentous, and neural structure of the low back and its relation to back pain. In Vleeming A et al: *Movement stability and low back pain*, New York, 1997, Churchill Livingstone.

36. Ingber DE: The architecture of life, *Sci Am* 278(1):48, 1998.

37. Levin SM: *Continuous tension, discontinuous compression: a model for biomechanical support of the body*, http://www.biotensegrity.com/tension.html, February 26, 2003.

38. Hammer WI: Genitofemoral entrapment using integrative fascial release (IFR), *Chiropr Tech* 10(4):169-176, 1998.

39. Leahy MP: *Active Release Techniques: soft tissue management system for the upper extremity*. Colorado Springs, Colo, 1994, Active Release Techniques.

40. Lewit KI: Soft tissue relaxation techniques in myofascial pain. In Hammer WI: *Functional soft tissue examination and treatment by manual methods: the extremities*, ed 2, Gaithersburg, Md, 1998, Aspen Publishers.

41. Voyer G: *Longitudinal stretching with osteoarticular decoaptations manual*, Somatotherapy Interactive Seminars. Jane@somatotherapy.com.

42. TherapyCare Resources: *TherapyCare resources clinical outcomes (as of 12-98)*, poster presentation, Seattle, Wash, 1999, APTA Combined Sections Meeting.

43. Carey T: *Graston technique manual*, Indianapolis, Ind, 2001, TherapyCare Resources.

44. Astrom M, Rausing A: Chronic Achilles tendinopathy: a survey of surgical and histopathologic findings, *Clin Orthop* 316:151, 1995.

45. Uhthoff HK, Sano H: Pathology of failure of the rotator cuff tendon, *Orthop Clin North Am* 28(1):31, 1997.

46. Budoff JE, Nirschl RP, Guidi EJ: Debridement of partial-thickness tears of the rotator cuff without acromioplasty, *J Bone Joint Surg* 80(5):733, 1998.

14

Reactivation and Rehabilitation

Craig Liebenson, DC, Clayton Skaggs, DC

Key Terms

ACTIVE CARE	DISTRESS	PHASIC
ACTIVE MODALITIES	ENDPLATE	PRIMARY PREVENTION
ACTIVITY INTOLERANCES	ENKEPHALINERGIC	QUOTA
AGONIST	FEAR-AVOIDANCE BEHAVIOR	RECONDITIONING
ANTAGONIST	FUNCTIONAL RANGE	RED FLAG
BIOMEDICAL	GRADED ACTIVITY	SECONDARY PREVENTION
BIOPSYCHOSOCIAL	GROOVING	SEGMENTAL SPINAL
CENTRALIZATION	HABITUATION	STABILIZATION EXERCISES
COCHRANE COLLABORATION	HYPERTONUS	SENSITIZATION
COGNITIVE-BEHAVIORAL	ISOTONIC EXERCISES	SYNERGIST
APPROACH	JOINT BLOCKAGE	SYNERGIST SUBSTITUTION
DECONDITIONING	NONSPECIFIC BACK PAIN	TONIC
DISK BULGE	OPERANT-CONDITIONING	TRENDELENBURG SIGN
DISK EXTRUSION	PASSIVE MODALITIES	WINDLASS MECHANISM

Chiropractic has always emphasized manual treatment of the locomotor (neuromusculoskeletal) system—particularly the spinal column—in its approach to health care. The emphasis on the spinal column is based on the tenet that the nervous system controls healing and that normalization of the function of the vertebral column joints will have a positive effect on health of the entire organism.

Because of chiropractors' success in managing lower back pain (LBP), the profession has gained increased legitimacy for treating a variety of spinal disorders (e.g., headache, whiplash syndrome, sciatica). Chiropractors with expertise in sports and orthopedics have also gained credibility for their skill in managing musculoskeletal problems involving the extremities. Chiropractic management of somatovisceral disorders affecting the cardiovascular (e.g., high blood pressure), respiratory (e.g., asthma), digestive (e.g., ulcers), and other systems of the body has

not attained this degree of credibility. As a result, the vast majority of patient visits to chiropractors are for musculoskeletal problems, with LBP ranking as the number one reason for a patient to visit a doctor of chiropractic.[1]

LBP has a generally positive natural history but can be a very complex disorder. LBP is estimated to be at least a $30-billion problem in the United States.[2] The traditional view of back problems was that they represent primarily acute, self-limiting conditions that resolve within 4 to 6 weeks.[3] However, recent epidemiologic studies contradict this rather optimistic picture. Back problems are now recognized as chronic ailments that are characterized with frequent acute spikes.[4] Although back pain is rarely disabling,[5] the minority of cases that involve disability account for a disproportionate percentage of the overall health care costs.[6]

A great deal of evidence now exists regarding appropriate treatment for many spinal disorders, and international guidelines have flourished since 1986.[7-10] Waddell has stated that the most cost-effective approach to managing this problem is to pursue secondary prevention efforts more aggressively on *subacute patients before chronic disability is fully established*.[11] (**Primary prevention** is the prevention of a disorder before it has begun; **secondary prevention** efforts seek to keep a subacute disorder from becoming chronic.)

In particular, the major patient management errors have involved the traditional emphasis on a **biomedical** rather than a **biopsychosocial** approach. The biomedical approach has too often included *labeling* patients as damaged (arthritis) or injured (ruptured disk), overprescribing bed rest, recommending early imaging, and selecting surgical candidates inappropriately.[12] In contrast, the biopsychosocial model emphasizes early *reassurance* (unambiguous explanation that the patient's back pain is not the result of serious disease processes and has an overall good prognosis) and *reactivation* (advice that recovery is accelerated by gradual resumption of activities) along with spinal adjustment/manipulation and exercise.[11,13,14]

The biomedical approach leads to the cascade effect in the clinical management of patients with back pain. The downward spiral begins when high-tech imaging replaces a thorough history and examination. Medicalization of back pain results from an underestimation of the iatrogenic (harmful) effects of overly aggressive diagnosis (imaging) and treatment (surgery).[15] In addition, the psychologic consequences of *labeling* patients with pain resulting from coincidental structural pathologies are commonly ignored.[12]

When a patient feels persistent pain, this reinforces negative attitudes about the relationship of activity and pain as the patient takes on the "sick" role.[16] The result is activity avoidance and further deconditioning of the involved portions of the musculoskeletal system. Unfortunately, **reconditioning** time is longer than deconditioning time.[17] Therefore reactivating patients as early as possible is important. Numerous studies have shown that gradually resuming activities is both safe and effective for acute, subacute, and chronic back pain.[7-9,18-20]

Chiropractors are ideally suited to play a leading role in managing neuromusculoskeletal disorders. LBP is an excellent proving ground for the profession. However, if chiropractors are to benchmark themselves as experts, then they must gain greater knowledge and skill in the area of rehabilitation and exercise. Generally referred to as **active care**, this approach encourages patients to participate actively in the resolution of their conditions rather than waiting for clinicians to "fix" them. The ancient role of the physician as helper or teacher must accompany the contemporary medical emphasis that defines the doctor's role in terms of curing or fixing.

SCIENTIFIC PRINCIPLES
Diagnosing Back Pain: Current Evidence and Deficiencies

Appropriate management of any condition depends on accurate diagnosis of the patient. Treatment should be guided by classification of patients into discrete groups that have unique characteristics amenable to specific interventions. Unfortunately, most consensus guidelines suggest that less than 20% of patients with back pain can be given a clear structural diagnosis of their condition.[7] Fortunately, new evidence indicates the promising role of determining the patient's *functional diagnosis*,[21] which consists of identifying the relevant physical performance deficits (e.g., strength, endurance, mobility, balance, coordination).

Meta-analysis of the scientific literature on diagnosis of back pain reveals various labels being used without appreciable evidence of validity.[22] International consensus guidelines agree that back pain can be classified in three groups: (1) those with **red flags,** such as tumor, infection, fracture, and serious medical diseases (less that 2%); (2) those with nerve root compression (less than 10%); and (3) **nonspecific back pain** (85% to 90%). Most research on the effectiveness of different interventions has assumed that the *nonspecific* back pain is a homogenous group.[22] However, to categorize most back pain in this generic fashion may cause researchers and practitioners to lose sight of potentially significant distinctions in this broad category. LaBoeuf-Yde explains that specific interventions, which may be beneficial for a certain subgroup, may not have demonstrable clinical effectiveness if given to a heterogeneous population.[23] Thus many hopeful methods will be erroneously assumed to be ineffective. Future research should therefore strive to determine if the *nonspecific* classification actually represents a homogeneous or heterogeneous population.

Erhard and Delitto have shown that subclassification of the *nonspecific* group is possible with reliable tests.[24] Treatment that is then matched to the appropriate subclassification has been shown to be superior to unmatched treatments.[24] Furthermore, a treatment that is driven by subclassification has been shown to be superior to the *generic* treatment recommended by the Agency for Health Care Policy and Research (AHCPR) for the broad *nonspecific* category.[25] Researchers at Washington University have similarly validated a subclassification scheme based on functional evaluation of movement patterns.[26,27]

Although ordering advanced imaging tests to find the *cause* of pain is tempting, structural pathologic conditions are quite common and usually coincidental. ***Disk bulges,** facet joint degeneration,* **endplate** *changes, and mild spondylolisthesis all correlate more with age than they will with symptoms.* Exceptions include **disk extrusions,** moderate or severe canal stenosis, and nerve root compression.[28]

Although recent literature points out past errors, unanswered questions remain. The fundamental problem in dealing with back pain continues to be identifying which patients will respond best to which interventions. For instance, which patients respond best to adjustment/manipulation, to reassuring counsel, to exercise, to medication, and to various combinations? General guidelines adhering to a biopsychosocial model have emerged and suggest a new path.

Psychosocial and Performance Factors

The inherent difficulty in diagnosing LBP has led to great frustration for both patients and clinicians. Given that most back problems are not the result of structural pathologic abnormalities (arthritis, herniated disk) or serious disease (tumor, infection, fracture), and because the majority of patients benefit from prompt reassurance and early reactivation advice, a primary goal of care should be to reassure patients about the benign nature of their pain and the safety and value of resuming normal activities. Thus prevention of deconditioning—both physical and psychologic—is a fundamental goal of the modern management of spinal disorders.

Deconditioning is the diminished ability to perform tasks involved in a person's usual activities of daily living. The AHCPR LBP guidelines explain that the main goal for treatment of back pain has shifted from treatment of pain to treatment of activity intolerances related to pain.[7] Although a variety of measurements of deconditioning are available, as yet, no "holy grail" has been found (Box 14-1).

A patient's self-report of **activity intolerances** is a valuable tool in measuring clinical outcomes and even in goal setting. These self-reports are typically questionnaires and, despite being subjective, are excellent outcomes tools because they are highly reliable and responsive.[29] However, the validity of these reports as prescriptive tools is doubtful because they do not correlate well with actual measurements of functional performance ability.[30]

Simmonds and colleagues have shown how general functional ability can be measured with simple, reliable, inexpensive, and time-efficient tests.[30,31] Tests such as functional reach, loaded reach, timed up and go, distance walked, and so forth are valuable tools for identifying functional limitations and establishing realistic goals.[32]

Clinicians typically make the improvement of specific functions such as range of motion a central goal of care. However, *because impairments correlate poorly with pain or disability, they are better used as a means to an end.*[33-36] Mannion

Box **14-1** Measurements of Deconditioning

- General functional ability or disability
- Self-report of activity intolerances (e.g., Oswestry form)
- Tests of walking, standing, reaching
- Specific functional deficits or impairments
- Tests of strength, range of motion

From *ICDH-2: International classification of functioning and disability*, beta-2 draft, full version, Geneva, 1999, World Health Organization.

suggests that one half of self-reported disability before treatment and more than one half of it after therapy is unaccounted for by structural, psychologic, voluntary performance, or electromyographic (EMG) fatigue findings. Therefore Mannion believes that new aspects of physical function relating to motor control are worthy of future investigation.[37] These aspects include those involved in nonvoluntary, reflex control of movement, such as position sense, delayed reaction times, and balance tests.[38-43] McGill has identified that *motor control errors* can occur as a result of prolonged or repetitive strain or poor aerobic fitness.[44,45]

Pain Behavior

Patients' expectations, motivations, and behaviors influence their performance.[46-49] Patient performance can therefore be limited by psychologic and physical factors. Patients who equate hurt with harm develop **fear-avoidance behavior,** which promotes deconditioning.[50] Pain behavior can also include maneuvers during which the patient repeatedly checks to see if the pain is still present.[51] This behavior can lead to **habituation, sensitization,** or both.[52] Maras also suggests that personality characteristics associated with increased muscle tension can negatively influence biomechanical performance.[53]

A recent study measuring psychologic characteristics related to pain showed improvement using three different active care approaches.[37] No psychologic intervention took place, thus it appears that exercise and activity modification have both psychologic and physical effects. Growing evidence and guidelines suggest that educating patients on the nature and science of back pain is of utmost importance for their recovery.[8,54] Self-help books are available that support the active-care approach and guide the patient through the restorative process.[55,56]

Ciccione and Just found that pain expectancies were important not only in chronic patients, but also in acute patients.[57] Thus fear-avoidance beliefs such as pain expectancies begin in acute pain and precede other psychosocial problems that develop as acute pain becomes chronic. In Box 14-2, Vlaeyen and colleagues summarize the impact of fear-avoidance

behavior on both general and specific functional abilities.[50]

Does Evidence of Effectiveness Exist for Active Care in Acute and Chronic Patients?

Acute and Subacute Phase (up to 12 Weeks)

Information and advice emphasizing the value of fitness and the safety of resuming activities achieved superior outcomes to advice that reinforced rest, activity restrictions, and the notion that the spine was injured or damaged (e.g., arthritis, herniated disk).[18] Reassuring workers and encouraging resumption of ordinary activities was superior to medication, bed rest, or mobilization exercises.[20] Early behavior modification through exercise reduced disability 1 year later.[58] An eightfold reduction in the risk of becoming chronic was achieved from information designed to reduce fear and anxiety and provide self-care advice.[59] Little and colleagues recently demonstrated that educational advice that encourages early exercise (not just advice to stay active) or endorsement by a physician of a self-management booklet has been shown to increase patient satisfaction and function while reducing pain.[19]

COCHRANE COLLABORATION META-ANALYSIS QUESTIONED

A Cochrane Collaboration systematic analysis on acute LBP concluded that ..." there is strong evidence (Level 1) that exercise therapy is not more effective for acute LBP than other active treatments with which it has been compared."[60] Faas and colleagues conducted one notable study that influenced these conclusions, which reported that in the treatment of uncomplicated, acute LBP patients, exercise was no better than usual care from a general practitioner.[61] However, the exercise approach was not individualized to the patients, and a relatively small sample of only three studies were used by the Cochrane Collaboration to reach level-1 conclusions.[62]

The **Cochrane Collaboration** is an international organization formed for the purpose of preparing systematic reviews of the effects of health care interventions.

Box **14-2**   THE IMPACT OF FEAR-AVOIDANCE BEHAVIOR

PROBLEM:

a. Pain catastrophizing (fearing the worst) is a precursor of pain-related fear.

b. Fearful patients tend to be more hypervigilant (being acutely aware of possible signals of threat).

c. Psychophysical reactivity is present in individuals with fear-avoidance behavior if activities are perceived as harmful, even if they are not actually harmful.

d. *Guarded movements* such as altered flexion-relaxation ratio are correlated with fear-avoidance beliefs, *not* actual pain.

e. Anxious patients predict pain earlier during performance of physical tasks such as range-of-motion or straight leg raise tests.

f. Fear and anxiety lead to the tendency to avoid the perceived threat.

g. Pain-related fear leads not only to poor physical performance, but also to restrictions in activities of daily living.

h. Avoidance behavior is highly resistant to treatment because the individual rarely comes into contact with the actual (nonharmful) consequences of the feared situation.

SOLUTION:

a. A cognitive-behavioral approach addresses the individual's inaccurate predictions about the relationship between specific activities and pain.

b. Education of patients with pain-related fear should emphasize that the fear can be self-managed after repeated desensitization from *graded exposures* to the feared stimuli.

c. Pain expectancies are corrected with repeated performance of the movements or exercises on subsequent days.

d. After multiple exposures, overpredictions of pain intensity change to match actual pain experience.

From Vlaeyen JWS, Linton S. Fear-avoidance and its consequences in chronic musculoskeletal pain. A state of the art, *Pain* 85:317, 2000.

In most studies of exercise evaluated with meta-analysis techniques, the same exercise type is given randomly to a heterogeneous group of patients with nonspecific LBP. Nonetheless, in clinical practice, most exercise approaches are taught with great emphasis on individualizing the type of exercise to the functional or mechanical attributes of the individual.[24,63] In fact, when a comparison was made between individuals performing exercises that were matched to them versus those that were unmatched, the matched group significantly outperformed the unmatched exercise group.[24] Additionally, a recent paper by the same group describes a study comparing the general exercise recommendations of the AHCPR guidelines to matched treatment based on their subclassification scheme.[25] *Their conclusion was that specific treatments matched to appropriate patients are superior to a general approach recommended by recent guidelines.*

Hides and colleagues have demonstrated that **segmental spinal stabilization exercises** (SSSE) can prevent multifidus muscle atrophy in subject with acute LBP.[43] SSSE are training maneuvers designed to enhance coordination and endurance of the local, deep muscles that are responsible for segmental control of the spine. Although symptomatic and functional recovery as assessed by Oswestry occurs independent of this intervention, those not receiving the exercises continued to have multifidus muscle atrophy. More recently, Hides and colleagues have demonstrated that such exercises have a secondary preventive effect by reducing recurrences.[42]

As with patients experiencing LBP, similar early activation has been found to be effective for neck pain following a whiplash injury.[64-66]

Because the natural history of low back syndromes reveals that most acute patients recover satisfactorily with minimal intervention, theories suggest that the subacute phase is the ideal time for both active and aggressive treatment.[11,59,67] Hagen and colleagues reported on a recent study using light activity, education about the benign nature of pain, and encouragement to stay active.[68] At 1-year follow-up, a significantly greater number of patients in the experimental group returned to work than those who received more traditional management. Lindstrom and colleagues showed that a graded activity program reduced disability more than traditional medical intervention.[69] **Graded activity** uses exercise to reach a **quota** (set amount) rather than being guided by pain (e.g., less on bad days and more on good days).

Chronic Phase—Reactivation and Exercise (after 12 Weeks)

According to the Cochrane Collaboration, evidence strongly supports activation (advice to gradually resume activities) and exercise for chronic patients.[60] One excellent study involving long-term follow-up is that of Indahl and colleagues.[14] This program provided education designed to reduce fear. Patients were informed that light activity would not injure the disk, but instead, speed recovery. The rate of returning to work was double that seen in the control group.[70] O'Sullivan and colleagues showed that specific *spine stabilization exercises* achieved superior outcomes to **isotonic exercises** (involving movement against resistance) in chronic patients with spondylolysthesis.[70] Manniche and colleagues demonstrated that an isotonic regime emphasizing endurance training was successful in improving outcomes.[71] A significant number of exercise regimes using a **cognitive-behavioral approach** (a structured, goal-oriented method emphasizing functional analysis and skills training) has demonstrated their effectiveness in a variety of settings.[72-77] Quota-based exercises not guided by pain were used in these studies. Interestingly, several studies have shown that exercises without a cognitive-behavioral component are less successful.[78]

What is the Evidence for Passive Modalities?

Many of the most popular adjunctive treatments for acute LBP lack evidence of effectiveness. The recent Danish guidelines state, "One of the greatest errors in the treatment of LBP in this century has been the unquestioned usage of passive treatments, often-times initiated when spontaneous recovery has already begun."[8] **Passive modalities** rely completely, or

in large part, on intervention by the doctor, in contrast to **active modalities** (such as exercise) in which the patient's effort constitutes the primary intervention. Passive modalities such as electrical muscle stimulation, ultrasound, diathermy, and traction were recommended only as optional. Although such passive modalities may engender higher levels of patient satisfaction, they have not been demonstrated to improve outcomes related to recovery.[3] Thus similar to routinely taking x-rays, patients may like passive modalities. However, because passive treatment does not improve outcomes, better patient education about appropriate management techniques for acute LBP is needed.[2,4,5]

UNDERSTANDING SPINE STABILITY

How Does Injury Occur?

Injury occurs when applied loads exceed tissue tolerance. The spinal column devoid of its musculature has been found to buckle at a load of only 90 newtons (approximately 20 lb) at L5.[79] However, during routine activities, loads 20 times greater are encountered on a routine basis. Panjabi writes, "This large load-carrying capacity is achieved by the participation of well-coordinated muscles surrounding the spinal column."[80] Not surprisingly, the motor control system functions well when under a load. Muscles stabilize joints by stiffening in a manner similar to the rigging on a ship. However, when load is at a minimum, such as when the body is relaxed or a task is trivial, the motor control system may be *caught off guard,* and injuries are often precipitated.[21]

Agonist-Antagonist Muscle Imbalance

Agonist-antagonist muscle co-activation is a central aspect of joint stability. Dysfunction of **agonist** (the muscle acting as prime mover) and **antagonist** (the muscle opposing the prime mover) will compromise joint stability. Early research on the elbow and knee showed that antagonist muscle co-activation is important for helping ligaments in maintaining joint stability.[81]

A well-known fact is that certain muscles such as those in the knee, lumbar spine, or cervical spine respond to inflammation or injury by becoming inhibited or developing atrophy.[82-84] Also commonly accepted is that other muscles such as the upper trapezius, sternocleidomastoid (SCM), and lumbar erector spinae respond to injury or overload by tensing or becoming overactive.[85-87]

Lund and colleagues theorized that when pain is present, a decreased activation of muscles occurs during movements in which they act as agonists, and increased activation occurs during movements in which they are antagonists.[88] In a wide variety of studies involving such diverse locomotor tasks as gait, trunk bending, mastication, head raising, reaching, and carrying activities, agonist inhibition, synergist substitution, and antagonist overactivity have repeatedly been demonstrated.[86,89-92] (**Synergist** muscles complement the activity of the prime mover.) For instance, Jull has shown that when chronic neck pain develops after whiplash, during cervicocranial flexion maneuvers, the deep neck flexors are inhibited, and the sternocleidomastoid muscles are overactivated.[86]

Spine Stabilizers

Specific muscles have been shown to stabilize the low back in various situations: (1) the rotators and intertraversarii have been shown to resist twisting movements; (2) the pars thoracis component of both the iliocostalis lumborum and longissimus thoracis can produce the greatest amount of extensor moment with a minimum of compressive penalty to the spine; and (3) the multifidus creates extensor torque but only at individual joints.[93] Anteriorly, the oblique abdominal muscles are involved in twisting, side bending, and stabilizing when the spine is being axially compressed.[94-96] Surprisingly, the one muscle that is highly active during tasks involving flexion, extension, and lateral bending is the quadratus lumborum.[96] This muscle's architecture is ideally suited to be a stabilizer because it attaches each transverse process to the more rigid pelvis and rib cage, thereby facilitating a bilateral buttressing effect for the vertebrae.[93]

Interestingly, strength (not coordination and endurance) between agonist and synergist muscles plays a pivotal role in resisting injury. Two muscles that have been studied extensively are the multifidus and transverse abdominus. The multifidus has been shown to be atrophied in patients with acute LBP.[83] This atrophy was ipsilateral to the pain and at the same segmental level as palpable joint dysfunction. Recovery from acute pain did not automatically result in restoration of the normal girth of the muscle. However, spinal stabilization exercises did successfully rebuild the muscle's size.[43] Recent research demonstrates that individuals who successfully restore normal multifidus girth have fewer recurrences of LBP at both 1- and 2-year follow-up.[42]

EMG studies have shown that the transverse abdominus was recruited before any other abdominal muscle when the trunk was subjected to sudden destabilizing forces.[97] In a study that examined abdominal activity during upper limb movements, the transverse abdominus was the only muscle active before initiation of arm motions.[98] The same result was found to be true during lower limb movements.[97]

Rood first proposed that muscles can be grouped into broad categories on the basis of their functional characteristics.[99] Certain muscles were hypothesized to function as stabilizers and others as mobilizers. In recent decades Janda[100,101] and Sahrmann[102] promoted the concept that muscle imbalance is a key dysfunction in altering movement patterns and influencing joint stability and pain. Janda suggested that certain muscles had a tendency to become overactive, and others tended to become inhibited. The author had observed that individuals with neurologic diseases such as cerebral palsy have predictable spasticity in certain muscles (e.g., short thigh adductors) and, in conditions such as polio predictable paralysis, occurs in other muscles (e.g., abdominal wall). Janda also noted that these same tendencies were seen in individuals without neurologic disease who were either highly sedentary or were training their muscles inappropriately.

Muscle imbalance has a neurodevelopmental basis. The neonatal fetal position is maintained by **tonic contraction** (sustained, low-level muscle activity) of trunk and extremity flexors and extremity adductors and internal rotators. *Reciprocal inhibition (Sherrington's law)*, which is present in early infancy, inhibits the antagonists of the **tonic** muscle chains, thus maintaining muscle imbalance. As the infant develops, the reciprocal inhibition becomes dampened, thus allowing the **phasic** muscle system (brief, forceful muscle activity) to activate (failing in cerebral palsy). As the *reflex-bound* infant begins to develop his or her postural control system, *tonic* activity of muscles that maintain the fetal posture is superceded by agonist-antagonist co-activation of muscles necessary for movement control and production of the upright posture. Thus extensors, abductors, and external rotators co-activate with their fetal partners to stabilize joints in *centrated postures* and allow neurodevelopment of posture.

Bergmark summarized the scientific evidence that muscles can be divided into two broad categories based on their function, one functioning to produce movement and the other to control movement.[103] Superficial muscles are responsible for producing voluntary movement or torque production, and deep muscles are responsible for maintaining joint stability. The deep *(intrin-sic)* muscles are responsible for joint stability on an involuntary or subcortical basis, and movement production is largely a voluntary act. The following charts show the different divisions of muscles according to their dysfunctional tendencies (Box 14-3).

CLINICAL APPLICATION

The traditional orthopedic approach to managing musculoskeletal problems focuses on treating the site of injury or pain. Orthopedics originated as a way to deal with acute, traumatic injuries in modern factories, emphasizing rest and treatment of symptoms. This approach was grounded in the Renaissance ideas of Descartes, which states that most pain occurs as a result of injury. Therefore if an activity causes pain, the activity should be avoided. From this philosophy came the adages "hurt equals harm" and "let pain be your guide." This viewpoint forms the basis of the traditional biomedical approach to pain, which includes symptomatic treatment, rest, activity avoidance, and surgery.

With today's epidemic of chronic, disabling pain, this traditional biomedical model is inadequate. In the 1960s Melzack and Wall[104]

Box **14-3** MUSCLE SYSTEM CLASSIFICATIONS

GLOBAL—SUPERFICIAL MUSCLES: TYPICALLY BECOME OVERACTIVE OR SHORTENED

Gastro-soleus
Adductors
Hamstrings
Tensor fascia lata
Hip flexors
Piriformis
Quadratus lumborum (lateral)
Rectus abdominus
External obliques
Lateral and thoracolumbar erector spinae
Upper trapezius
Levator scapulae
Pectorals
Subscapularis
Suboccipitals
SCM

Lateral pterygoids
Masseters

LOCAL—DEEP MUSCLES: TYPICALLY BECOME INHIBITED OR LENGTHENED

Quadratus plantae
Peronei
Vastus medialis
Gluteals
Transverse abdominus
Internal oblique
Multifidus
Quadratus lumborum (medial)
Medial and lower erector spinae
Lower and middle trapezius
Serratus anterior
Deep neck flexors
Digastricus

From Bergmark A: Stability of the lumbar spine. A study in mechanical engineering, *Acta Orthopedica Scandinavica* 230:20, 1989.

formulated the revolutionary *gate control theory of pain,* which demonstrates how pain is modulated in the dorsal horn of the spinal cord by both ascending facilitatory and descending inhibitory pathways, which are **enkephalinergic** (i.e., part of the body's internal opiate system of pain modulation). When the descending pain inhibitory pathway is dampened, pain can be perpetuated beyond the normal course of tissue healing. This circumstance can occur from addiction to pain relievers, as well as from depression and inactivity. The biopsychosocial model focuses on reducing disability and activity intolerances caused by pain. The emphasis is on increasing the patient's functional capabilities and psychosocial coping abilities. This approach involves persistent reassurance that the patient is not damaged, coupled with the recommendation that gradual reactivation will not only restore activity tolerance, but also accelerate recovery. Patients are advised that "hurt does not necessarily equal harm."

Action Steps

This reactivation approach consists of four fundamental action steps (Box 14-4). First, a detailed history is taken of the patient's activity intolerances associated with their pain. Second, a thorough examination is conducted of the functional pathologic conditions related to their activity intolerances. Third, treatment (advice, adjustment/manipulation, and exercise) is directed to restoring function to the *key link,* which is believed to be responsible for biomechanical overload of the pain-generating tissue. Fourth, audit (assessment) of the results takes place.

Restoring function depends on expanding the patient's **functional range** (FR). The FR consists of the patient's activity intolerances, mechanical

sensitivities, and relevant functional pathologic conditions. Making this functional diagnosis is an essential starting point in patient care; it also facilitates regular audit of meaningful outcomes of care because each component is easily reevaluated.

The FR is limited by the patient's aggravating movements and positions and chief motor control deficits. According to Dennis Morgan, a pioneer in spinal stabilization training, "the functional position is the most stable and asymptomatic position of the spine for the task at hand."[105] Thus, before exercise can be prescribed, a thorough history and examination of the patient's mechanical sensitivities should be carried out.[106,107]

History of Activity Intolerances

The history should identify the activity intolerances that are present. Initial inquiries regard basic functions, such as sitting, standing, walking, and bending activities. Such activity intolerances, once identified, automatically become excellent *patient-centered* goals of care. This identification helps the patient focus on the (dys)function instead of the pain.

Sitting or forward-bending sensitivities strongly suggest a disk problem and that self-treatment would be biased toward extension. Some patients may have a weight-bearing sensitivity, but they may be relatively pain-free in non–weight-bearing positions. Such patients may tolerate and thus benefit from recumbent exercise.[106]

CLINICAL UTILITY OF THE HISTORY OF ACTIVITY INTOLERANCES

- Restoring those functions becomes the main *goal* or *end point of care.*
- When greeting patient on follow-up visits *always* ask if activity intolerances are same or different (e.g., sitting, standing, walking intolerances).
- *Challenge: Can you uncover from the patient's history what specific activity intolerances are present?*

Box **14-4** FUNCTIONAL REACTIVATION ACTION STEPS

1. History of any activity intolerances
2. Assessment of relevant functional condition
3. Treatment of dysfunctional kinetic chain
4. Audit of the results

Assessment of Relevant Functional Pathologic Conditions

Once the patient's activity intolerances are identified, the next step is to find the functional pathologic abnormality responsible for them. For instance, if the patient has a walking intolerance, the feet or sacroiliac regions may have relevant dysfunction that is responsible for pain with walking.

The object is to focus on the source of biomechanical overload that can cause or perpetuate symptoms in the pain-generating or injured tissue.[108] In particular, locating the specific functional anomaly or dysfunctional kinetic chain that has led to the patient's mechanical sensitivity is crucial.[108]

Mechanical Sensitivity

Initial examination of the patient should identify the movements and positions that are painful or painless. McKenzie has provided one of the best guides to exercise prescription in his description of the **centralization** phenomenon. According to McKenzie's assessment method, the positions or repetitive movements that increase, decrease, or centralize symptoms should be identified.[107] The movements and positions found to aggravate symptoms are used as an audit before and after testing to assess the patient's progress. In contrast, the pain-centralizing or pain-relieving positions and movement ranges are used for self-treatment.

Myofascial Pain

If eliciting a patient's characteristic pain is difficult with orthopedic or range-of-motion tests, then a myofascial examination can be valuable. If active trigger points that reproduce the patient's characteristic pain can be found, then a sure-fire treatment guide is at hand, especially as a recheck of patient response and status before and after treatment.

Identifying Key Functional Abnormalities Responsible for Pain or Activity Intolerances

The cause of 90% of spine pain is unknown. Therefore most medical guidelines recommend using the unsatisfactory label *nonspecific* back pain.[7,8,10] Even though most back pain is called *nonspecific,* assuming that this pain is psychogenic or that no cause or mechanism of injury exists would be a mistake. In fact, new research is pointing toward *motor control deficits* as the most promising candidates for playing an etiopathologic (causative) role in spinal disorders.*

The relevant functional conditions are those related to the pain generator or injured tissue, primarily because these are the source of biomechanical overload that eventually leads to repetitive strain of the painful tissue.[108] An example of this idea would be a patient presenting with neck pain in which the functional aspect responsible for the pain may be the head-forward posture and poor motor control of cervicocranial flexion. Another example is a patient presenting with knee pain in which the key functional condition may be a kinetic chain dysfunction whereby subtalar hyperpronation causes internal tibial rotation during gait or squatting. Thus muscle (kinesiopathologic) or joint dysfunction may be responsible for the repetitive strain of a vulnerable part of the locomotor system.

CLINICAL UTILITY OF THE EXAMINATION OF MECHANICAL SENSITIVITIES

- As a baseline outcome for rechecks of patient status before and after treatment
- To determine the starting point of care (e.g., if flexion peripheralizes symptoms and extension centralizes them, extension movements are indicated)

PRACTICE-BASED PROBLEM

Patients often present with numerous functional abnormalities relating to poor motor control. Therefore how can the *key link* or relevant dysfunctional chain be identified?

*References 37, 39, 40, 109, 110.

CLINICAL UTILITY OF IDENTIFYING THE KEY FUNCTIONAL CONDITION

- As a tool to increase the patients FR:
  a. Identify and treat the key manipulable lesion (e.g., hypomobile joint).
  b. Identify and treat the key kinesiopathologic condition (i.e., altered movement pattern).
- *Problem:* Functional assessment often produces a high percentage of false positives. Therefore the functional condition must be linked to the pain generator biomechanically (source of overload) or neurophysiologically (dysfunctional kinetic chain).

Note: The hypothesis must be empirically proven by retesting the FR after treatment.

CLINICAL CHALLENGE

Can the movement dysfunction (kinesiopathologic condition) that is responsible for the patient's symptoms or activity intolerances be found?

TESTS OF FUNCTIONAL ABNORMALITIES OF THE MOTOR SYSTEM

A broad array of tests of the locomotor system are available (Box 14-5).

Lower Quarter (Legs and Trunk)

Dorsiflexion Mobility of the First Metatarsal-Phalangeal (MTP) Joints[110a]

Test: The patient is supine. The metatarsal bone is stabilized, and the first phalangeal bone is mobilized into dorsiflexion. Sixty-degree flexion is normal.

Clinical relevance: Decreased dorsiflexion of the first MTP joint limits the push-off phase at terminal stance because of slackening of the plantar fascia and inability to activate the windlass mechanism. The **windlass mechanism** occurs when the plantar fascia is tensed during the late stance phase of gait. This action aids resupination of the

---

Box 14-5   FUNCTIONAL TESTS

LOWER QUARTER
Mobility of first metatarsal-phalangeal joint
Transverse arch reflex stability test of Vele
Hyperpronation of the longitudinal arch during gait
Hip extension mobility
Hip abduction coordination
Hip extension coordination
Single-leg balance
Squat (two leg)
One-leg squat

LUMBOPELVIC
Active straight leg raising
Trunk curl-up
Side bridge
Sorensen
Prone abdominal hollowing

THORAX
Arm elevation
Respiration

CERVICAL
C0-C1 flexion

OROFACIAL
Mouth opening

UPPER QUARTER
Scapulohumeral rhythm
Push-up

---

foot and thus helps promote a smooth early propulsive phase of the gait cycle.

Vele's Reflex Foot Stability Test (Lower Extremity Stability)[111]

Test: The patient stands with feet shoulder-width apart. The patient is requested to lean forward from his or her ankles without bending from the knees or spine (similar to a ski jumper). The clinician notes if delayed *reflex* gripping of the toes occurs. Asymmetry is noted.

Clinical relevance: Disturbed reflex stability of the *intrinsic foot* flexors, located on the sole of the foot.

Hyperpronation of the Longitudinal Arch of the Foot[110a]

Test: The patient is asked to walk a few steps. The clinician observes the medial longitudinal arch for excessive pronation during the stance phase.

Clinical relevance: Excessive pronation can lead to other faults in the kinetic chain resulting from medial bowing of the Achilles tendon, tibial torsion, and anterior pelvic tilt.

Hip Extension Mobility (Modified Thomas Test)[110b,110c]

Test: The patient is positioned with his or her pelvis at the foot of the examination bench. One knee is held close to the chest to flatten the lumbar lordosis. The other leg is allowed to extend passively. Hip and knee extension mobility are noted.

Clinical relevance: Decreased hip extension mobility (less than 10 degrees) significantly alters the normal biomechanics of the toe-off or propulsive phase of gait. Decreased hip extension mobility can also lead to secondary hypermobility or repetitive overstrain of the lumbosacral spine in extension causing facet irritation.

Hip Abduction after Janda (Lower Extremity and Lumbo-Pelvic Coordination) (Fig. 14-1)[113,115]

Test: While in a side-lying position, the patient slowly raises the top leg straight up to the ceiling.

Pass-Fail (PF) criteria:
- Failure if initiation occurs (with)
- Cephalad shift of the pelvis (overactive quadratus lumborum)
- Pelvic rotation
- Thigh flexion (overactive tensor fascia latae)

Clinical relevance: Poor function of the gluteus medius can increase ankle, knee, hip, or lumbopelvic instability in the transverse and frontal planes.

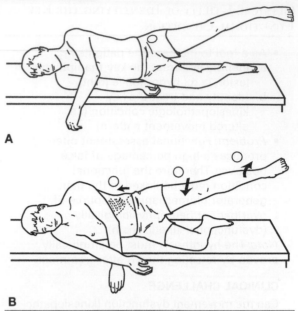

Fig. 14-1 Hip abduction. **A,** Normal—hip abduction to 45 degrees. **B,** Abnormal—if hip flexion, external rotation, "hiking," or pelvic rotation takes place during movement. *(Reprinted with permission from Liebenson CS: Manual resistance techniques in rehabilitation. In Chaitow L, editor:* Muscle energy techniques, *ed 2, Edinburgh, Churchill Livingstone, 2001.)*

Hip Extension after Janda (Lower Extremity and Lumbo-Pelvic Coordination) (Fig. 14-2)[110b,110d]

Test:
- Patient is in a prone position.
- One leg is raised straight up to the ceiling.

PF criteria:
- Failure if initiation occurs (with)
- Anterior pelvic tilt
- Lumbar rotation (or hyperextension)
- Delayed gluteus maximus contraction
- Muscular contraction above T8
- Knee flexion

Clinical relevance: Altered hip extension typically leads to overstress of the lumbar facet joints during extension and can lead to hamstring strain resulting from substitution for the gluteus maximus.

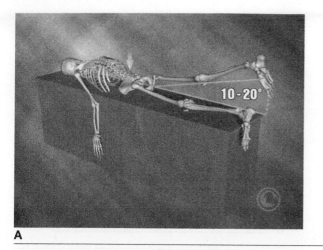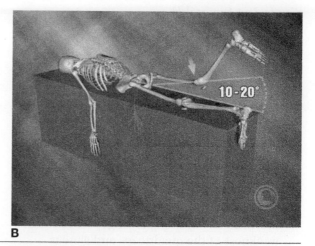

Fig. 14-2 Hip extension. **A,** With lumbar hyperextension. **B,** With overactivity of the hamstrings. *(Reprinted with permission from Liebenson CS, Chapman S: Lumbar spine: making a rehabilitation prescription, Baltimore, 1998, Williams & Wilkins.)*

One-Leg Standing Balance Test[110e,110f]

Test:
- The patient stands on one leg, with the opposite leg flexed at the hip and knee.
- The subject should be instructed to fix his or her gaze at a point on the wall directly in front of the patient.
- The patient should practice with eyes open two times for up to 10 seconds.
- The patient should then attempt to balance as long as possible on one leg with eyes closed for up to 30 seconds.
- The best score with eyes closed for each leg is recorded.
- If the subject lasts 30 seconds on the first eyes-closed attempt, he or she should make a second attempt.
- The exercise may be repeated two times for each leg to account for learning.

Quantification: Each test is timed until the subject:
- Reaches out
- Hops
- Puts foot down
- Touches the foot to weight-bearing leg

Observation: The length of time the patient stands on one leg with eyes open (maximum of 30 seconds) and then repeated with eyes closed (maximum of 30 seconds) is recorded. Both legs are tested.

Normative data:

Age (in Years)	Eyes Open (in Seconds)	Eyes Closed (in Seconds)
20-59	29-30	21.0-28.8 (average 25)
60-69	22.5 average	10
70-79	14.2	4.3

Clinical relevance: Poor balance is associated with ankle and knee instability and can predispose older adults to falls.

Dynamic Squat Test[110g]

Test: The patient stands with feet shoulder-width apart. Arms are outstretched. Patient is instructed to perform repetitive squats to a depth at which the thighs are horizontal. Repetitions are performed until fatigue, knee pain, or back pain stops; until the test is over; or until 50 repetitions are achieved.

Clinical relevance: Poor squat endurance is associated with stoop-lifting strategies replacing squat-lifting strategies.

Single-Leg Squats[110h]

Test:
- The patient stands on one foot with eyes open.
- The patient squats as deeply as possible without losing balance.

PF criteria:
- Depth of squat
- Trendelenburg sign
- Tibial torsion
- Subtalar hyperpronation or supination
- Hip or trunk flexion

Clinical relevance: Asymmetry of depth indicates any of the following: poor balance, weakness of the quadriceps and gluteus maximus, or knee instability. The **Trendelenburg sign** indicates weakness of the lateral hip stabilizers, in particular the gluteus medius. Hip flexion indicates weakness of the hip extensors. Tibial torsion is a sign of knee instability and can be secondary to either hyperpronation in the subtalar region or gluteus medius insufficiency. Hyperpronation is a sign of subtalar instability. Excessive trunk flexion indicates weakness or inhibition of the hip extensors.

Lumbopelvic

Active Straight Leg Raising (ASLR) Test[110i]

Test: The patient is supine and is asked to raise one leg up slowly until it is elevated to a height of 20 cm. Low back or sacroiliac pain, lumbopelvic torsion, or both are noted. Resistance may be added just above the ankle. Pain, lumbopelvic torsion, and strength (0-5 to 5-5 scale) may be recorded.

Clinical relevance: A positive ASLR and resisted SLR have been shown to be associated with postpartum sacroiliac pain, as well as poor pelvic floor and diaphragm function.

Trunk Curl-Up after Janda (Lower Extremity and Lumbo-Pelvic Coordination) (Fig. 14-3)[110b,110d]

Test:
- Patient is supine with knees flexed

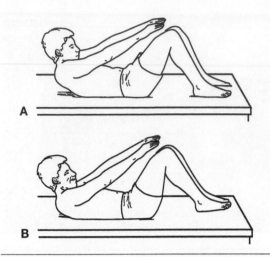

Fig. 14-3 Trunk curl-up. **A,** Normal—trunk curl until scapulae are off the table without the feet rising up or low back arching. **B,** Abnormal—feet rising up before scapulae do. *(Reprinted with permission from Liebenson CS: Manual resistance techniques in rehabilitation. In Chaitow L, editor: Muscle energy techniques, ed 2, Edinburgh, Churchill Livingstone, 2001.)*

- Trunk is slowly raised until shoulder blades are off the table while reaching fingers toward knees.

PF Criteria: Failure if:
- Anterior pelvic tilt is present.
- Feet rise up off the table before shoulder blades.

Clinical relevance: Failure to raise the trunk without the feet lifting up is a sign of an overactive psoas. If the trunk is lifted in lordosis, weakness of the abdominal wall is suggested.

Horizontal Side Bridge (Fig. 14-4)[122]

Test:
- The subject lies on one side supported by his or her pelvis, lower extremity, and forearm (elbow bent with hand facing forward).
- The top leg is in front of the lower leg with both feet on the floor.
- The upper arm is placed across the chest with the hand touching the anterior lower shoulder.

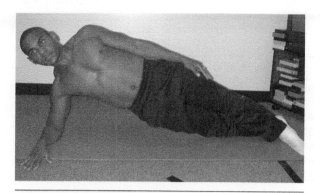

Fig. 14-4 Horizontal side bridge.

- The pelvis is raised off the table as high as possible and held in a line with a long axis of the body supporting the weight between the feet and elbow.
- Subject statically maintains this elevated position.

Termination criteria:

- Subject is unable to lift his or her body up from the floor.
- Subjects thigh touches the floor.
- Subject drops his or her pelvis or thigh part way and cannot raise it up to the start position again.
- Significant LBP causes the test to be stopped.

Quantification: Comparative data is presented here for young, healthy adults for the trunk extensor endurance test of Sorensen, a modified static sit-up (isometric partial curl-up), and the horizontal side bridge. A predictable relationship exists among anterior (abdominal sit-up), posterior (extensor-Sorensen), and lateral trunk (side bridge) muscle static endurance. The extensors are strongest, followed by the abdominal muscles, and finally the side bridge muscles. Table 14-1 gives the mean times for healthy, young men and women and the ratios of the abdominal and side bridge endurance compared against the extensor endurance. *Clinical relevance:* Side bridge endurance deficits correlate with back pain.

Trunk Extensor Endurance (Sorensen Test)[110g,110j,122]

Test:

- Patient is prone with the inguinal region at end of a table. Arms are at the sides, ankles are fixed, and the patient is holding a horizontal position.
- Patient maintains in the horizontal position as long as possible.
- The duration that the position can be held is observed (maximum of 240 seconds).

Quantification:

Prone Abdominal Drawing in Test (Table 14-2)[110k]

Clinical relevance: This test measures the function of the transverse abdominus muscle. Poor activation of this muscle is associated with low back disorders.

Thorax

T4 Active Extension (Thoracic Mobility)[110l,110m]

Test:

- Patient is standing with his or her back against a wall and feet slightly forward.

Table **14-1** TRUNK EXTENSION, TRUNK FLEXION, AND SIDE BRIDGE (YOUNG, HEALTHY ADULTS)[122]

Task	Men			Women			All		
	Mean (in Seconds)	SD	Ratio	Mean	SD	Ratio	Mean	SD	Ratio
Extensor	146	51	1.0	189	60	1.0	177	60	1.0
Flexor	144	76	0.99	149	99	0.79	147	90	0.86
Side bridge, right	94	34	0.64	72	31	0.38	81	34	0.47
Side bridge, left	97	35	0.66	77	35	0.40	85	36	0.5

SD, Standard deviation.

Table **14-2** TRUNK EXTENSOR ENDURANCE[122]

	Men (n = 242)						Women (n = 233)					
	Blue Collar		White Collar		All		Blue Collar		White Collar		All	
Age	Mean	SD	X	SD	X	SD	X	SD	X	SD	X	SD
35-39	87	38	113	47	97	43	91	61	95	48	93	55
40-44	83	51	129	57	101	57	89	57	67	51	80	55
45-49	81	45	131	64	99	58	90	55	122	73	102	64
50-54	73	47	121	56	89	55	62	55	99	78	69	60
35-54	82	45	123	55	97	53	82	58	94	62	87	59

SD, Standard deviation; *X*, average.

- Patient is instructed to raise both arms fully overhead.

PF criteria: Failure if:
- Lumbopelvic junction hyperextends.
- Arms do not become vertical (reach wall).
- Thoracic kyphosis remains.

Clinical relevance:
- Decreased active arm flexion mobility results in fixed thoracic kyphosis or reduced glenohumeral mobility.
- Compensatory lumbopelvic hyperlordosis occurs during arm elevation tasks.

Respiration (Abdomen and Anterior Chest Wall Coordination)[110n,111]

Test:
- The seated patient is observed during natural breathing for any visible elevation of the shoulder girdle (or girdles) or scalene muscle activity. Breathing should normally occur in a horizontal plane, not a vertical plane.
- The supine patient is observed for a predominance of chest breathing over abdominal breathing. Normally, abdominal breathing predominates. Clinically, an advanced sign of respiratory dysfunction is present when the abdomen moves in during inhalation (normally it moves out) and out during exhalation. This condition is termed *paradoxical respiration.*

Clinical relevance: Faulty respiration is associated with excessive activity in the shoulder girdle elevators and scalene muscles. This condition can be a key perpetuating factor of cervicothoracic and upper quarter repetitive strain disorders.

Cervical

Cervicocranial Flexion Test of Jull[110o]

Test:
- An inflatable cushion (e.g., Stabilizer, Chattanooga South Pacific) is placed under the neck to support it without pushing it up.
- The cushion is inflated to 20 mm Hg.
- The patient is instructed to breathe in and out and, on exhalation, signal an increase in pressure to 22 mm Hg by nodding his or her head without cervical retraction (chin tucking).
- The patient is instructed to hold this pressure steady while breathing normally.
- If successful, the patient is instructed to perform chin nod movements to increase the pressure by 2 mm Hg increments up to a maximum of 30 mm Hg.
- Five-second holds are performed at each level.
- When the greatest level of resistance that the patient can control is found, then the patient is tested for his or her ability to maintain the pressure for 10 seconds for 10 repetitions.

Quantification:
- The ability to target and hold the position steady (based on the pressure recording) is measured while observing activity in the superficial neck flexor muscles (e.g., SCM muscles, anterior scalene muscles).

Failure results if any of the following occurs:

a. Patient is unable to reach target pressure.
b. Patient is unable to hold target pressure steady for 10 seconds.
c. Superficial muscle substitution is observed.
d. Breath holding occurs.
e. Patient cannot perform 10 repetitions.

Being able to perform 10 repetitions at 28 mm Hg is considered normal.

Clinical relevance: Using this method, Jull studied 12 subjects with whiplash-associated disorder (WAD) and 85 volunteers who were asymptomatic. In the asymptomatic subjects, 22 mm Hg holds yielded the least superficial mm strength, and the 30 mm Hg target was highest. The WAD group had significantly greater superficial mm activity versus the norm group (least at 22, greatest at 30 mm Hg, similar).

Orofacial

Mouth Opening (Orofacial Coordination)[110p]

Test: The patient is asked to open his or her mouth, and the clinician notes if any protrusion of the chin occurs. Any protrusion is considered abnormal.

Clinical relevance:

- Dysfunctional mouth opening signifies muscle imbalance with overactive mouth closers (e.g., masseters, lateral pterygoids) and inhibited mouth openers (digastricus).
- An abnormality can result in temporomandibular joint and cervicocranial overstrain.

Upper Quarter

Arm Abduction—Scapulothoracic Rhythm (Upper Extremity Coordination) (Fig. 14-5)[110b,110,110n]

Test:

- The patient is seated.
- The bent arm is slowly raised out to the side.

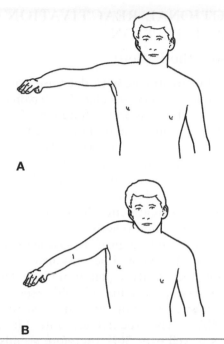

A

B

Fig. 14-5 Arm abduction—scapulothoracic rhythm. **A,** Normal—elevation of the arm without shoulder shrugging before 60 degrees arm abduction. **B,** Abnormal—shoulder shrugging before 60 degrees arm abduction. *(Reprinted with permission from Liebenson CS: Manual resistance techniques in rehabilitation. In Chaitow L editor: Muscle energy techniques, ed 2, Edinburgh, Churchill Livingstone, 2001.)*

PF criteria: Failure occurs if shoulder shrugs before arm is raised 60 degrees.

Clinical relevance: Poor scapulohumeral rhythm coordination is related to head or neck disorders (e.g., headache, whiplash) and shoulder disorders (e.g., impingement).

Push-Up[110b,110n,110q]

Test: The patient performs a push-up on either his or her toes or knees. While lifting the body up from the floor, scapular position is noted. Shrugging, full retraction, and "winging" would all be considered signs of dysfunction. Asymmetry should be noted.

Clinical relevance: Poor scapulothoracic coordination is related to shoulder disorders (e.g., impingement, anterior instability).

FUNCTIONAL REACTIVATION OR REHABILITATION

Advising the Patient

The goal of treatment is to decrease symptoms and **distress** (anxiety associated with pain or fear of pain) and to improve function. Typically, some degree of functional improvement is noted before any decrease in pain. Therefore the patient's expectation of immediate pain relief must be tempered. Additionally, the patient should be informed that soreness after treatment is *not* a sign of treatment failure, because sensitive tissues are often reactive.

Patients should be given reassuring reactivation advice; they should be informed that "hurt does not necessarily equal harm." In fact, in chronic cases, patients should expect that "rusty" tissues will hurt at first when they are remobilized. The recurrence rate for acute patients is well over 50%, therefore promising a cure would be a mistake. Chronic patients are particularly vulnerable to unrealistic expectations. Therefore these patients should be told that a relapse is expected. Hopefully, the relapses will be less severe, but the goal is to teach them how to manage these recurrences better. *Control rather than cure is the operational end point in chronic pain management.*

Advice begins with *reassurance* to dispel the myth that hurt equals harm. Promotion of gradual resumption of activities is recommended to prevent deconditioning and improve nourishment to the painful tissues. This phase is followed with specific activity modification advice regarding how to reduce inappropriate biomechanical loading of vulnerable tissues. This phase consists of advice regarding workstation ergonomics; sleep posture and pillows; bending, lifting, and carrying; and pushing and pulling.

Karel Lewit [112] teaches that the first treatment is for the patient to avoid what harms him. To allow recovery from injury, loads known to precipitate injury must be avoided. By removing exposure to harmful load, the healing and adaptation process can fulfill its objective of increasing the failure tolerance of the tissues. However, if all load is removed, deconditioning involving

How Can Knowledge of Mechanism of Injury Influence Management?

> McGill states that "evidence from tissue-specific injury generally supports the notion of a neutral spine (neutral lordosis) when performing loading tasks to minimize the risk of low back injury.... Avoiding spine end-range of motion, during activity, can reduce the risk of several types of injury." [119a]
>
> For example, lifting should occur without end-range flexion of the spine. The patient should learn to hinge from the hips while maintaining the lumbar lordosis during squatting or forward bending.

disuse atrophy will occur, and instability will be created as an iatrogenic consequence of overly conservative treatment.

What Type of Load Is Safe?

Epidemiologic evidence in athletes such as gymnasts and Australian cricket bowlers demonstrates that vertebral posterior arch damage leading to spondylolisthesis is not simply the result of shear forces, but is also correlated with repetitive full-range activities. [112] Disk injury was shown to be related to three factors: (1) full end-range flexion in younger spines (caused by higher discal water content), [113-115] (2) repetitive joint end-range flexion loading motion in excess of 20,000 to 30,000 cycles, [116,117] and (3) epidemiologic association between disk herniation and sedentary sitting occupations. [118]

When Is the Ideal Time to Load the Spine?

Knowledge of when injury is most likely to occur can also influence what people do. Evidence suggests that the low back is particularly vulnerable in the early morning or after periods of prolonged sitting. Reilly and colleagues showed that 54% of the loss of disk height (water content) occurs in the first 30 minutes after arising. [137] Disk-bending stresses are increased significantly in the morning. [138] After even a brief period of sitting or stooping in end range, protective joint stiffness is compromised. Even after 30 minutes of rest, residual joint laxity persists.[139] Therefore avoidance of high-risk activities early in the morning or after sitting or stooping in full flexion is crucial to injury or reinjury prevention.

Behavioral Principles

Ciccione and Just showed that, in susceptible individuals, discordance exists between pain expectancies and pain intensity with activities.[57] However, this difference is unknown to the patient. To decrease fear-avoidance behavior, the patient should be gradually and incrementally exposed to perceived painful activities. The clinician should teach patients that their expectation is *not* accurate. In particular, reducing anxiety and pain expectations associated with the specific movements that generate the greatest fear in the patient should become a key goal of care.[140] As part of this process, **operant-conditioning therapy** (behavioral therapy involving repeated exposures to activities inaccurately perceived to be harmful) involves *graded exposures* to progressively greater durations, intensities, and frequencies of exercises. This type of therapy is often referred to as exercise administered and progressed *by quota* with preestablished goals.[58,69,72]

Patient education should focus on the fact that normal activities (e.g., walking, swimming, biking) can be resumed safely and informing the patient about simple activity modifications to reduce biomechanical strain (e.g., hip hinge, cat scratch, abdominal bracing). The patient should be advised: (1) to stay as active as possible, (2) to gradually increase his or her physical activity, (3) that increasing activity is safe so as long as pain is not radiating to the periphery, and (4) that the hurt he or she experiences does not necessarily equal harm but is just a sign that stiff areas are being mobilized. Indahl has described a few general tenets of the behavioral approach that are provided in Box 14-6.[14]

A problem-solving approach can be used through teaching patients how to (a) take an active role, (b) reduce modifiable risk factors (e.g., using ergonomics), and (c) avoid impulsively seeking relief that is mainly symptomatic[141] (Box 14-7).

Role of Adjustment/Manipulation

Randomized, controlled trials indicate that adjustment/manipulation is one of the most effective initial treatments for either acute or chronic musculoskeletal problems, especially LBP. (See Chapter 23 for an extensive discussion of this research.) However, the reason why adjustment/manipulation works so well is unclear. One possible reason is that the source of a kinetic chain dysfunction may be found in a dysfunctional tissue, such as a hypomobile joint, fascial restriction, inhibited muscle, or old scar.

Adjustment/manipulation or manual therapy acts as a catalyst to recovery. The tissue that is interfering with function in the kinetic chain, which is related to the pain generator or activity

---

Box **14-6** SPECIFIC REACTIVATION ADVICE

Patients were informed or assured that:
a. Pain or anticipation of pain can increase muscle activation and tension and thus increase pain.
b. Light activity would not further injure the disk or other structures causing pain.
c. Light activity would enhance the repair process.
d. Flare-ups of pain are normal occurrences and do not signify further damage.
e. Emotions such as worry or anxiety increase muscle tension and pain; therefore trying to relax and remain active when pain flare-ups occur is best

From Indahl A et al: Five-year follow-up study of a controlled clinical trial using light mobilization and an informative approach to low back pain, *Spine* 23:2625, 1998.

Box **14-7** PROBLEM-SOLVING PROCESS

1. Identifying and selecting a problem
2. Analyzing problem
3. Generating potential solutions
4. Selecting and planning solution
5. Implementing solution
6. Evaluating solution

From Shaw WS et al: Working with low back pain: problem-solving orientation and function, *Pain* 93:129, 2001.

intolerance, should receive joint or soft tissue adjustment or manipulation.

If this intervention is successful, the clinician should seek the self-treatment that reproduces the effects of the adjustment/manipulation. For example, if a patient with LBP has a "key link" in the foot, then manipulation of the relevant **joint blockage** (hypomobility) will expand his or her FR. This procedure should then be followed up with self-treatment advice to train a relevant motor control dysfunction, such as the longitudinal and transverse arches of foot.

Exercise

Exercise serves a variety of purposes in restoring function. First, exercise may overlap with adjustment/manipulation as a catalyst to recovery. Second, exercise may help stabilize the dysfunctional kinetic chain by **grooving** (reeducating and reprogramming) appropriate movement patterns, such as in agonist-antagonist co-activation or sensory-motor training. Third, exercise may help prevent recurrences by reconditioning functional patterns (i.e., functional training), which mimic the actual challenges that the individual confronts at home and work or during sports activities.

What Exercises Are Safe?

Safe exercises for patients with acute and subacute LBP should have favorable biomechanical load profiles. Properly functioning muscles controlled by the central nervous system enable stability to be maintained. McGill recommends that, for subacute exercise training, a safe limit is approximately 3000 newtons (N).[144] Box 14-8 lists several exercises with both safe and unsafe load profiles.

CLINICAL CHALLENGE

Which exercises will reeducate the movement patterns responsible for biomechanical overload in the patient's home, occupational, or sports activities?

Box 14-8   LUMBAR SPINE LOAD PROFILES FOR COMMON EXERCISES AND ACTIVITIES

SPINAL LOAD PROFILES

- Without muscles the spine buckles at 90 N[80,127a]
- However, routine daily activities involve 2000 N[80]
- According to McGill, recommended subacute exercise training = < 3000 N.[127]
- National Institute for Occupational Safety and Health (NIOSH) limit for repetitive tasks = 3300 N.
- NIOSH work demand limit = 6400 N.[117,125]
- 7000 N (1568 lb) begins to cause damage in very weak spines.[127b]
- Tolerance of average healthy young male spine approaches 12,000-15,000 N (2688-3660 lb).[127b]
- Competitive weight lifters manage loads in excess of 20,000 N (4480 lb).[127c]

EXERCISES

- Quadruped single-leg raise = 2000-2300 N (one side of lumbar extensors at 20% of maximum).[119]
- Opposite arm and leg raise = 3000 N (one side thoracic extensors approximately 30%-40% max + opposite side lumbar extensors at 20% of maximum (McGill book).[119]
- Side bridge on ankles = 2600 N.[119]
- Curl-up = 2000 N.[119]
- Sit-ups bent knee = 3300 N (730 lb)[119,127d]
- Sit-ups straight knee = 3500 N.[119]
- Roman chair exercise = > 4000 N (890 lb) (McGill).[119]
- Prone superman = up to 6000 N (over 1300 lb) (McGill).[119]

PRACTICE-BASED PROBLEM

"How does a clinician progress a patient's functional program, and when is enough really enough?"

How to Progress the Patient

Many exercises are touted as training stability or *core* muscles. However, unless agonist, antagonist, and synergist muscles are trained as a functional unit rather than in isolation, or with one dominating, then *core* training is not occurring. An example of such poor stability is when a joint's *neutral range* is compromised during a task as a result of muscle imbalance, such as excessive synergist substitution or inadequate agonist-antagonist co-activation. **Synergist substitution**—which is often termed *global muscle overactivity*—occurs when superficial muscles compensate for inhibited deep, segmental (local) muscles. According to Richardson and colleagues, "In approaching treatment, the clinician must answer two basic questions: (1) does the patient present with unwanted global muscle activity, and (2) if so, which muscles are problematic? These questions must be answered in order to institute best-practice therapeutic exercise."[128]

An example of global muscle **hypertonus** (excessive contraction) is when thoracolumbar hypertonus occurs during an activity such as standing. An example of a common "trick" movement synergy resulting from this overactivity is leg raising into extension that occurs with an anterior pelvic tilt (rather than *neutral* spine positioning) (Fig. 14-2, *A*). Another example is when hip abduction occurs with excessive hip flexion or hip hiking (Trendelenburg sign) resulting from excessive substitution of the tensor fascia lata or quadratus lumborum for the gluteus medius (Fig. 14-1, *A*).

Besides using exercises with acceptable load profiles and maintaining core stability, several traditional exercise science principles should be followed so results can be maximized. These principles relate to training with the appropriate intensity, frequency, and duration. Motor control or stability training requires an emphasis on endurance rather than on strength.[110,119,128] For this reason, the *intensity* of training should be submaximal. As an example, a typical prescription would involve 8 to 10 repetitions of slow movements with prolonged hold times (5 to 6 seconds/repetition). A *frequency* of twice a day with a *duration* of up to 3 months is often required to remediate chronic spinal pain.[71]

In motor learning, the adage asserting that "practice does not make perfect; it makes permanent" applies. The manner by which patients acquire the skill of core stability during functional activities generally follows certain established stages of motor learning (Box 14-9). These stages may be unnoticed by the patient, but the astute clinician guides the patient effortlessly through these stages with the help of encouraging and facilitory cues, contacts, resistance, commands, and so forth.

Functional stability training is goal oriented. Initially, stability patterns that avoid global muscle substitution are reeducated. Isolated or nonfunctional positions, such as recumbent positions, may be used as stepping stones to *groove* these movement patterns. However, as soon as possible, core stability must be trained in exercises mimicking the demands the patient faces in home, occupational, and recreational activities. One key way in which stability patterns are learned is by adding unstable surfaces such as balance boards and gymnastic balls. This addition provides enhanced proprioceptive stimulation, which facilitates motor learning. Box 14-10 shows a progressive model of how to stay on track toward functional goals. The earlier that actual functional activities are trained in the program, the better. However, at each step, core stability must be demonstrated.

Box **14-9**   STAGES OF MOTOR LEARNING

1. Cognitive-kinesthetic awareness
2. Associative
3. Autonomous (involuntary control)

From Shumway-Cook A, Woollacott M: Motor control-theory and practical applications, Baltimore, 1995, Lippincott-Williams & Wilkins.

Clinical note: Training begins in the patients FR. The goal is to expand the FR to include the patient's home, occupational, and sports activities.

PRACTICE-BASED PROBLEM: HOW TO PROGRESS THE PATIENT TOWARD FUNCTIONAL GOALS AND EXERCISES

Part of the art of prescribing exercises is determining how long to stay with exercises that require the patient to hypervigilantly (voluntarily) control posture versus having the patient practice simple, functional movements that he or she automatically (involuntarily) performs with good core control. As Karel Lewit concludes, "remedial exercise is always time consuming, and time should not be wasted.... We should not attempt to teach patients ideal locomotor patterns, but only correct the fault that is causing the trouble."[111]

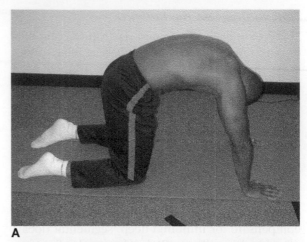

A

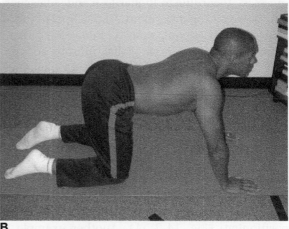

B

Fig. 14-6 **A,** Cat; **B,** Camel.

Level-One Training: Functional Range Exercises

In level-one training, postural control is the focus, which requires an emphasis on cognitive-kinesthetic awareness (KA). Most patients have poor kinesthetic awareness of how to produce or control motion in their problem area. The patient learns to "discover" how to move and centrate an important region such as the lumbopelvic, scapulothoracic, or cervicocranial area. Patients acquire the skill to perform the movement and then to limit it to a pain-less or *pain-centralizing* FR. Examples include the following:

Lumbopelvic control: cat-camel (Fig. 14-6), abdominal hollowing (AH) (Fig. 14-7), and bracing

Scapulothoracic: shoulder rolls or Brügger exercise (Fig. 14-8)

Cervicocranial: flexion (nodding of the head as if saying "yes")

Respiration: diaphragmatic (Fig. 14-9)

Once patients learn to move and position their spines in fundamental ways, then a progression to more complex exercises and functional activities can occur. Two aspects to the decision are always presented as to whether a patient is ready to progress. The first is concerned with motor control (MC) and the second with mechanical sensitivity (MS). The earlier that actual functional activities are trained in the program, the better. However, it is necessary at each step that (a) MS is not increased and (b) that MC is reeducated. MC involves functional centration or *neutral posture* of key joints, normal respiration (i.e., no breath holding), and avoiding global muscle substitution.

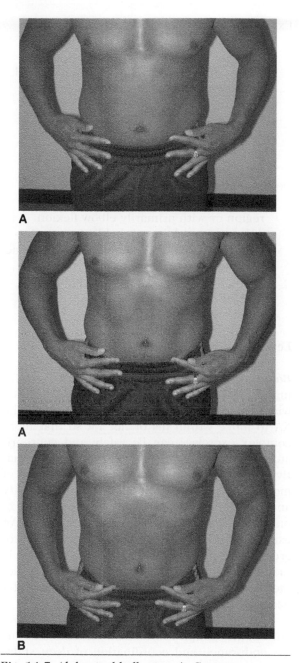

Fig. **14-7** Abdominal hollowing. **A,** Correct.
B, Incorrect.

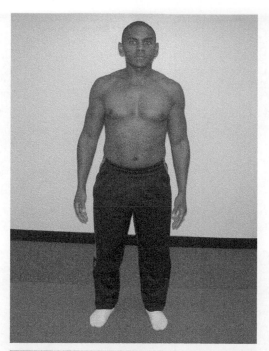

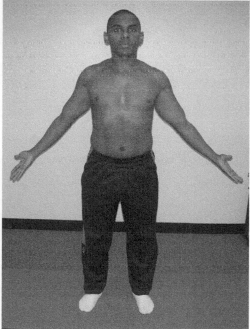

Fig. **14-8** The Brügger relief position.

When to Move On?

- MC: Is KA present to the following extent?
- Can full range of motion of the involved joints be actively produced?
- Can a *neutral* centrated position be found and held?

- Can global muscle overactivity be avoided?
- Is normal respiration maintained?
- MS: Are symptoms increasing or peripheralizing with the training?

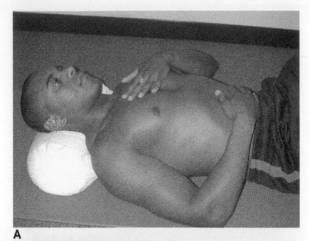

A

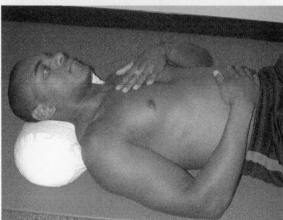

B

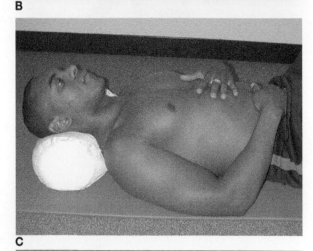

C

Fig. 14-9 Breathing exercises. A, Incorrect.
B, Correct. C, Ideal.

Examples:
Move on if:
- Cat-camel occurs with full spine flexion-extension and *neutral* positioning control.
- AH occurs with the abdomen below the navel moving inwards (see Fig. 14-7, *A*).
- Inhalation occurs with horizontal movement forward of the abdomen and laterally of the lower rib cage (see Fig. 14-9, *B* and *C*).

Do not move on if:
- Cat-camel occurs only in the thoracic region or with primarily elbow flexion.
- AH occurs with breath holding, posterior-pelvic tilt, or thoracolumbar erector spinae hypertonus (see Fig. 14-7, *B*).
- Inhalation occurs with the abdomen moving inwards or vertical rib elevation predominating (see Fig. 14-9, *A*).

Level-Two Training: Stability Exercises

Basic stability (beginner). In level-two training, stability is the focus. Stability is entered when the patient has sufficiently developed the KA to move within his or her FR so that more complex exercises can be safely and appropriately performed using a key region. Such associative motor learning involves a grooving of movement patterns, which enhances stability and coordination. Repetitions are performed to build endurance into these movements. An example of this concept is when a movement progresses from simple, unresisted concentric motions (e.g., cat-camel) to one requiring isometric core stabilization during peripheral mobilization (e.g., quadruped single-leg reach).

This level of training incorporates postural control into simple low-load movements that target endurance and coordination of *deep* stabilization muscles. For instance:
- *The Big Three*
  - Quadruped leg reach (extensors) (Fig. 14-10)
  - Horizontal side bridge (lateral muscles) (Fig. 14-11)
  - Trunk curl-up (flexors)
- C0-C1 flexion versus resistance (e.g., with the feedback cuff or against gravity)

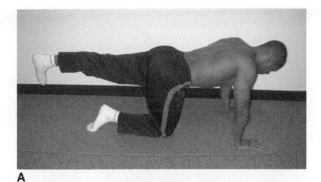

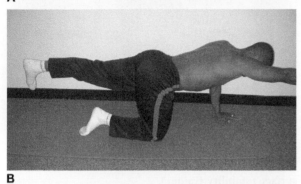

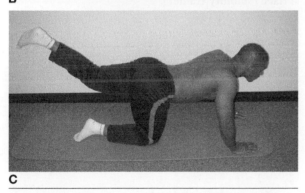

Fig. **14-10** Quadruped single leg reach. **A,** Correct. **B,** Advanced. **C,** Incorrect.

When to Move On?

- MC: When KA is "automatizing" so that associative training occurs with good motor control (i.e., core stability)
- MS: When symptoms are reducing or centralizing

Examples:

Move on if:

- Quadruped leg reach occurs with *neutral* spine control.

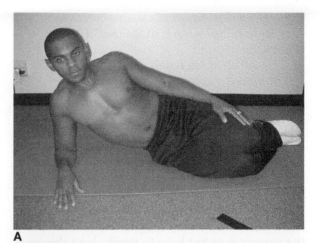

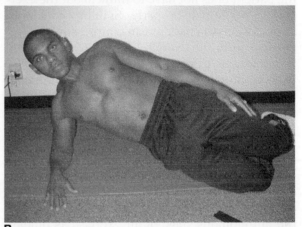

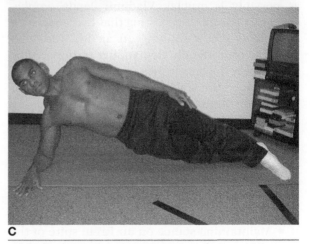

Fig. **14-11** Horizontal side bridge. **A,** Start position. **B,** End position. **C,** Advanced.

- C0-C1 flexion occurs with a nodding motion against cuff at 28 mm Hg.

Do not move on if:
- Quadruped leg reach occurs with lumbosacral hyperextension or thoracolumbar hypertonus.
- C0-C1 flexion occurs with cervical retraction, SCM overactivity, or breath holding.

Sensory-motor (advanced). A progression from beginner to advanced stability training occurs when *autonomous* control of core stability is challenged. This stability is accomplished when the patient does not have to think about the exercise to perform it properly. Stability is demonstrated when the patient can control lumbopelvic posture during an exercise in spite of unexpected perturbations from a labile surface (e.g., stability pad, mini-trampoline) or from the clinician (quick, gentle pushes). In this way, training for the unexpected nature of real-life situations involving sudden movements and jostles is accomplished.

Gymnastic balls, rocker boards (RBs), or even reducing the base of support during a quadruped exercise from 4 to 3 to 2 points of support. Because many patients lack the motivation to concentrate during exercise training, reaching the autonomous stage of an exercise as quickly as possibly is crucial. Vladimir Janda emphasized this point by suggesting that exercises such as sensory-motor training on an RB were preferred over cortically demanding training, such as complex floor exercises, because it automatically trained the stability system without requiring much voluntary control.[101]

Examples of sensory-motor stability training include:
- Single-leg stance on a stability pad (Fig. 14-12)
- Curl-ups on a gymnastic ball (Fig. 14-13)
- Using the RB in double-stance in the sagittal plane (see Fig. 14-13)
- Maintaining stance on an RB in spite of the clinician giving unexpected perturbations

When to move on?
- MC: When KA is automatizing so that autonomous training occurs with good motor control (i.e., core stability)

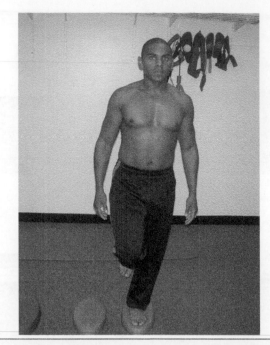

Fig. 14-12 Single-leg stance balance on an unstable surface (stability trainer).

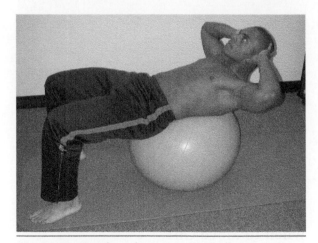

Fig. 14-13 Trunk curl-up on a gym ball.

- MS: When symptoms are reducing or centralizing

Examples:

Move on if:
- Curl-up on a gymnastic ball occurs with flexion in the thoracic spine only.
- Single-leg stance on a stability pad with eyes closed can be done for 10 seconds.

Do not move on if:

- Curl-up on a gymnastic ball with cervical or lumbar flexion-extension occurs.
- Single-leg stance on a stability pad with eyes open and hyperpronation, tibial torsion, or Trendelenburg sign occurs.

Level-Three Training: Functional Training

The third level of training involves functional activities that mimic the patient's daily living, occupational, or recreational demands.[129-132] The most functional movement that the patient can perform well is determined. This movement is used as the starting point for the patient's functional training. This concept is termed "attacking success." [129]

Unless functional training occurs, no guarantee can be made that other training will actually stabilize an individual's vulnerable joints during "real world" challenges. Examples of functional training include squats, lunges, pushing, pulling, catching, carrying, and so forth.

A patient's FR should be identified for each functional training exercise. For instance, to train for lifting activities, squatting should be analyzed and practiced. If *squatting* is found to occur with poor control of the lumbar lordosis, then it can be modified by having the patient perform the movement with a gym ball supporting his or her lumbar spine in lordosis or with the patient facing the wall and keeping his or her arms stretched overhead (Fig. 14-14).

Functional stability during activities such as walking, climbing stairs, or kneeling can be reeducated with an exercise such as the *lunge* (Fig. 14-15). A typical dysfunction or faulty movement pattern with forward lunging is excessive hip and trunk flexion.

A simple exercise that is usually within the patient's FR is to perform a forward lunge while raising the arms overhead. This movement will usually reeducate *neutral* lumbopelvic posture automatically.

If the forward lunge occurs with subtalar hyperpronation, an excellent way to "attack success" is to attempt an angle lunge with an arm reach (Fig. 14-16). This movement will typically "drive" the foot into supination automatically! Whatever is the

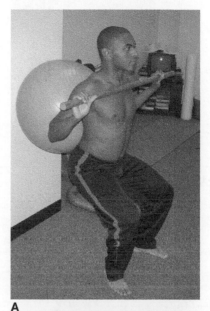

A

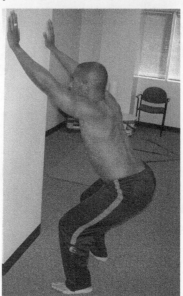

B

Fig. **14-14** Squats. A, With ball. B, Facing wall.

Continued

PRACTICE-BASED PROBLEM

How can training be made as functional as possible so as to stabilize the patient in his or her home, sport, and occupational activities?

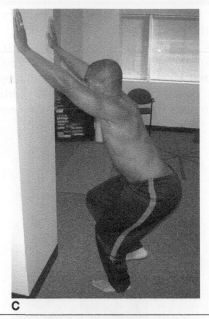

C

Fig. **14-14** cont'd C, Advanced single leg.

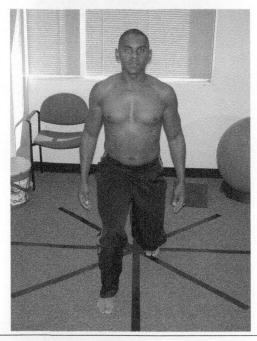

Fig. **14-15** Forward lunge.

most challenging functional activity the patient can perform with appropriate stability should be the one selected for exercise. Lunging on an unstable surface such as a Stability Trainer is a perfect example of such a progression (Fig. 14-17).

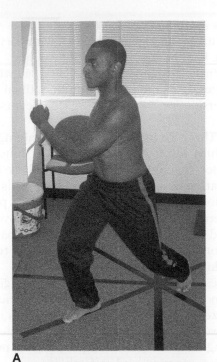

A

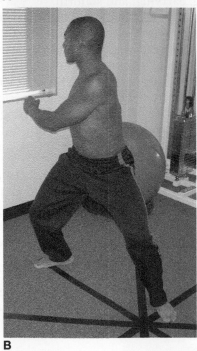

B

Fig. **14-16** Angle lunges with arm reaches. **A,** Angle lunge with arm reach. **B,** Back lunge with trunk twist and arm reach.

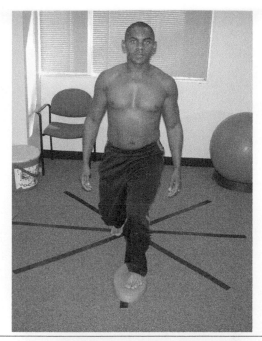

Fig. **14-17** Lunge on an unstable surface (stability trainer).

Balancing is a component of walking, reaching, and any activity or sport requiring a weight transfer from one leg to the other (e.g., golf, tennis). Testing of single-leg stance balance ability that produces a Trendelenburg sign indicates gluteus medius insufficiency. A simple way to reeducate functional stability in the frontal plane is to perform a single-leg stance position with the involved hip in the Trendelenburg position. The patient then reaches across the body with the opposite arm to automatically correct the pelvic obliquity and facilitate the gluteus medius (Fig. 14-18). This movement can also be applied to the single-leg squat (Fig. 14-19).

Common movements such as pushing and pulling require the patient to make simple multiplanar *weight transfers*. Pushing is part of functional activities such as a tennis forehand, boxing punch, or pushing a shopping cart or vacuum cleaner. Pulling is part of functional activities such as a tennis backhand, throwing a Frisbee, or lifting a grocery bag out of a car or a baby out of a crib. Pushing and pulling can be trained with simple pulley or tubing exercises (Figs. 14-20 and 14-21).

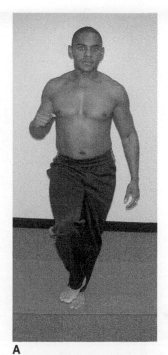

A

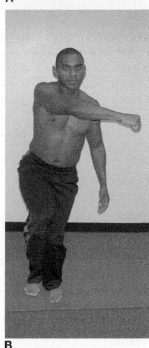

B

Fig. **14-18** Single-leg stance with arm reach. **A,** Start position. **B,** End position.

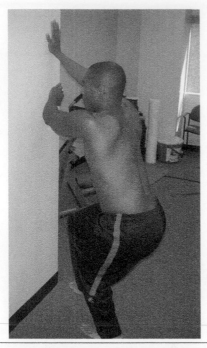

Fig. **14-19** Single-leg squat with arm reach.

Although functional training is listed here as the third and final level of training, a patient may actually begin with functional exercises. The key is to find the most functional movement that is within the patient's FR. Reactivation progressions should continue until patients' FR includes their home, sports, and occupational demands.
Examples include:
a. Balancing:
 One-leg stance
 RBs
 Wobble boards
 Balance sandals
 Stability pads
 Adding perturbations from the clinician to each of the above leg stance leg reaches
 One-leg stance arm reaches
 One-leg stance trunk twists
b. Squats:
 Two-leg squats:
  With ball against back
  Facing wall with arms overhead
  Standing free
  With weights
  On an unstable surface (i.e. rocker board, stability pads)

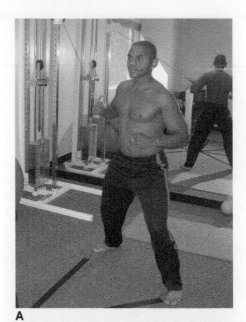

A

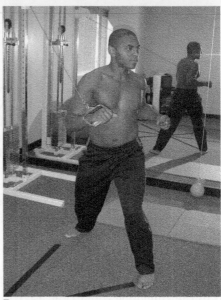

B

Fig. **14-20** Pushing. **A,** Punch—beginning position. **B,** Punch—end position.

Continued

 One-leg squats:
  With the ball against the back
  Facing the wall with arms overhead
  Standing free
c. Lunges:
 Forward lunges
 Angle lunges

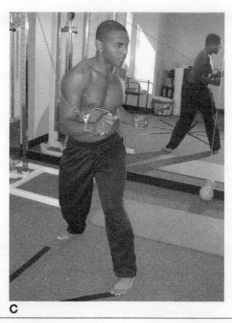

Fig. **14-20 cont'd C,** Punch with trunk twist.

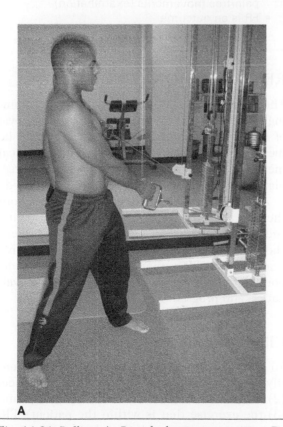

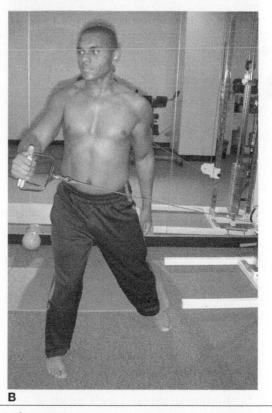

Fig. **14-21** Pulling. **A,** Sword—beginning position. **B,** Sword—end position.

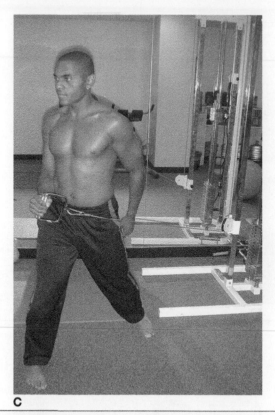

C

Fig. **14-21** cont'd C, Sword with trunk twist.

Side lunges
Back lunges
Add:
    Arm reaches
    Trunk twists
    Hand weights
d. Step-ups:
    Front
    Side
    Back
e. Weight Transfers:
    Double-to-single stance on stability trainer
      pads
    Quadruped single-leg reach
    Single-leg bridges
    Pushing, reaching, punches, or trunk twists
      with cables or tubing
    Pulling, sword (lawn mower or
      tennis backhand), and seatbelt
      (proprioceptive neuromuscular
      facilitation diagonals) with cables or
      tubing

THE ART, SCIENCE, AND CRAFT OF THE CLINICAL METHOD

- Evaluation → Hypothesis → Treatment → Audit (reevaluate for improvement after treatment)
- Patient's FR (history and examination)
- Treatments are prescribed that are safe for the patient's condition and have empirically been found to increase the FR.
- The FR is always reassessed after treatment

THE FR MUST BE FOUND FOR *all* PATIENTS

- Improvement in FR is a goal of treatment. This goal focuses the doctor and patient on function!
- FR is an empirical guide to treatment. Treatment should decrease activity intolerances (history) and increase the pain-free movements (examination).
- FR is an outcome.

REEVALUATION (AUDIT)

The process of functional reactivation and training should be goal oriented toward the removal of activity intolerances. These goals should be measurable via reliable, valid, and practical means.[133,134] Finally, patient status should be regularly reevaluated and goals adjusted as needed.

A patient's functional diagnosis includes both the MS and relevant functional abnormality, such as aberrant MC. Successful treatment should improve MC and reduce MS. Functional evaluation enables an audit process to be incorporated into patient care through regular reevaluation and program modification as needed.

Clinical Examples

To prescribe reactivation properly requires identifying (1) the patient's activity intolerance, (2) the patient's key functional abnormality, and (3) the exercise that is within the patient's FR. Patients are progressed if they demonstrate good

MC and diminishing MS. MC is demonstrated if *neutral* joint control is present and global muscle overactivity is absent. MS is demonstrated if the patient can exercise without an increase or peripheralization of symptoms.

Patient with LBP

History and activity intolerance: Patient with LBP presents with chronic symptoms that become worse with weekend golf.

Examination and functional condition: Poor MC is found involving global muscle overactivity and thoracolumbar hypertonus during observation of:
- Standing postural analysis
- Janda's prone leg extension test
- Hodges' quadruped leg reach exercise

Treatment Plan:

Advice: Warm-up needed; training also needed during week for weekend sport.

Manipulation: Psoas release, thoracolumbar junction adjustment/manipulation.

FR exercise: MC treatment of the patient's lumbopelvic region involves deep stabilizer training with quadruped leg reach within the FR.

Progression: This exercise is progressed to quadruped opposite arm and leg reach and finally to functional training involving squat-lunge, balance, and push-pull training.

Patient with Neck Pain

History and activity intolerance: A patient with neck pain presents with chronic symptoms that become worse with prolonged sitting work in front of the computer.

Examination and functional condition: Poor MC is found involving head forward posture with SCM overactivity during observation of:
- Standing or seated postural analysis
- Jull's cervicocranial flexion test[86]

Treatment plan:

Advice: Micro-breaks during day when sitting; ergonomic workstation advice

Manipulation: C0-C1 and T4-8 adjustment/manipulation; inhibition of upper quarter flexion muscle chain

FR exercise: MC treatment of the patient's cervicothoracic region involves deep stabilizer training, such as cervicocranial flexion training or facilitation of upper quarter deep stabilization chain (e.g., Brügger exercise).

Progression: Cervicocranial flexion is progressed from the recumbent position to upright sitting and standing positions. Ergonomic advice regarding the workstation is customized. Brügger's exercise is progressed to functional movements involving pushing and pulling such as with punches, trunk twists, sword, and seatbelt maneuvers.

CONCLUSION

Two key questions must be answered before prescribing an exercise program for a patient with spinal pain:

What exercises can the individual patient best tolerate?

What is the most relevant dysfunction that is responsible for specific activity intolerances?

This approach provides a simple filter that can be used to aid in the selection of the appropriate treatment.

Review *Questions*

1. What are some signs that a patient has assumed a "sick role" in response to back pain?
2. What is the essential difference between active and passive methods of care?
3. How do the biomedical and biopsychosocial models of health care differ?
4. What are the possible negative consequences of viewing people with nonspecific back pain as a homogenous group?
5. True or false? Disk bulges, facet joint degeneration, endplate changes, and mild spondylolisthesis all correlate more with age than they do with symptoms.
6. How can deconditioning be prevented? How can reassuring patients about their back pain help prevent deconditioning?

7. For what clinical purposes might a chiropractor use self-reports of activity intolerance?

8. How can McKenzie's centralization phenomenon be applied in formulating an exercise program for a patient?

9. How do acute and chronic cases differ in terms of setting realistic goals for chiropractic management?

10. At what time of day is the lower back most susceptible to injury?

Concept *Questions*

1. Aside from the physical diagnostic characteristics of a patient's back or neck pain, what other factors should be considered in determining how best to aid recovery? A biopsychosocial perspective should be applied in formulating the answer.

2. What is the appropriate role for passive modalities, such as electronic muscle stimulation, that bring higher levels of patient satisfaction but have not been demonstrated to improve outcomes related to recovery?

REFERENCES

1. Cherkin DC et al: A comparison of physical therapy, chiropractic manipulation and provision of an educational booklet for the treatment of patients with low back pain, *N Engl J Med* 339:1021, 1998.
2. Frymoyer JW: Predicting disability from low back pain, *Clin Orth* 279:107, 1992.
3. Hadler NM: Regional back pain, *N Engl J Med* 315:1090, 1986.
4. Croft PR et al: Outcome of low back pain in general practice: a prospective study, *BMJ* 316:1356, 1998.
5. Carey TS et al: Beyond the prognosis, *Spine* 25:115, 2000.
6. Hashemi L et al: Length of disability and cost of worker's compensation low back pain claims, *J Occup Environ Med* 40:261, 1998.
7. Bigos et al: Agency for Health Care Policy and Research (AHCPR): *Acute low-back problems in adults,* Clinical Practice Guideline number 14, Washington, DC, 1994, US Government Printing.
8. Manniche C et al: Danish Health Technology Assessment (DIHTA): *Low back pain: frequency management and prevention from an HAD perspective* 1:1, 1999.
9. Waddell G et al: Royal College of General Practitioners (RCGP): *Clinical guidelines for the management of acute low back pain,* London, 1999, Royal College of General Practitioners (also available at www.rcgp.org.uk).
10. Spitzer WO et al: Scientific approach to the assessment and management of activity-related spinal disorders: a monograph for clinicians. Report of the Quebec Task Force on Spinal Disorders, *Spine* 12(suppl 7):S1, 1998.
11. Waddell G: *The back pain revolution,* Edinburgh, 1998, Churchill Livingstone.
12. Bogduk N: What's in a name? The labeling of back pain, *Med J Aust* 173:400, 2000.
13. Liebenson CS, editor: *Rehabilitation of the spine: a practitioner's manual,* Baltimore, 1996, Lippincott-Williams & Wilkins.
14. Indahl A et al: Five-year follow-up study of a controlled clinical trial using light mobilization and an informative approach to low back pain, *Spine* 23:2625, 1998.
15. Mold JW, Stein HF: The cascade effect in the clinical care of patients, *N Engl J Med* 314:512, 1986.
16. Main CJ, Watson PJ: Psychological aspects of pain, *Man Ther* 4:203, 1999.
17. Booth FW: Physiologic and biochemical effects of immobilization on muscle, *Clin Orthop* 219:15, 1987.
18. Burton K, Waddell G: Information and advice to patients with back pain can have a positive effect, *Spine* 24:2484, 1999.
19. Little P et al: Should we give detailed advice and information booklets to patients with back pain? A randomized controlled factorial trial of a self-management booklet and doctor advice to take exercise for back pain, *Spine* 26:2065, 2001.
20. Malmivaara A et al: The treatment of acute low back pain—bed rest, exercises, or ordinary activity? *N Engl J Med* 332:351, 1995.
21. McGill SM: *Low back disorders: evidence-based prevention and rehabilitation,* Champaign, Ill, 2002, Human Kinetics.
22. Van Tulder WE et al: Disseminating and implementing the results of back pain research in primary care, *Spine* 27:E121, 2002.
23. Laboeuf-Yde C, Manniche C: Low back pain: time to get off the treadmill, *J Manipulative Physiol Ther* 24:63, 2001.
24. Erhard RE, Delitto A: Relative effectiveness of an extension program and a combined program of manipulation and flexion and extension exercises in patients with acute low back syndrome, *Phys Ther* 74:1093, 1994.
25. Fritz JM et al: The role of fear-avoidance beliefs in acute low back pain: relationships with current and future disability and work status, *Pain* 94:7, 2001.
26. Van Dillen LR et al: The effect of active limb movements on symptoms in patients with low back pain, *J Orthop Sports Phys Ther* 31(8):402, 2001.

27. Maluf KS et al: Use of a classification system to guide non-surgical treatment of a patient with chronic low back pain, *Phys Ther* 80(11):1097, 2001.

28. Jarvik JG et al: The longitudinal assessment of imaging and disability of the back (LAIDBack) study, *Spine* 26:1158, 2001.

28a. *ICDH-2: international classification of functioning and disability*, beta-2 draft, full version, Geneva, 1999, World Health Organization.

29. Bombardier C: Outcome assessments in the evaluation of treatment of spinal disorders: summary and general recommendations, Spine 25:3100, 2000.

30. Simmonds MJ et al: Psychometric characteristics and clinical usefulness of physical performance tests in patients with low back pain, Spine 23(22):2412, 1998.

31. Novy DM et al: Physical performance: differences in men and women with and without low back pain, Arch Phys Med Rehab 80:195, 1999.

32. Simmonds MJ, Lee CE: Physical performance tests: an expanded model of assessment and outcome. In Liebenson C: editor, Rehabilitation of the spine: a practitioner's manual, ed 2, Baltimore, 2003 (scheduled publication), Lippincott–Williams & Wilkins.

33. Klein AB et al: Comparison of spinal mobility and isometric trunk extensor forces with electromyographic spectral analysis in identifying low back pain, Phys Ther 71(6):445, 1991.

34. Nattrass CL et al: Lumbar spine range of motion as a measure of physical and functional impairment: an investigation of validity, Clin Rehab 13(3):211, 1999.

35. Newton M et al: Trunk strength testing with iso-machines. Part 2: experimental evaluation of the Cybex II Back Testing System in normal subjects and patients with chronic low back pain, Spine 18(7):812, 1993.

36. Waddell G et al: Objective clinical evaluation of physical impairment in chronic low back pain, Spine 17:617, 1992.

37. Mannion AF et al: Active therapy for chronic low back pain. Part 3: factors influencing self-rated disability and its change following therapy, Spine 26:920, 2001.

38. Cholewicki J et al: Effects of external loads on lumbar spine stability, J Biomech 33:1377, 2000.

39. Radebold A et al: Muscle response pattern to sudden trunk loading in healthy individuals and in patients with chronic low back pain, Spine 25:947, 2000.

40. Radebold A et al: Impaired postural control of the lumbar spine is associated with delayed muscle response times in patients with chronic idiopathic low back pain, Spine 26:724, 2001.

41. Wilder DG et al: Muscular response to sudden load. A tool to evaluate fatigue and rehabilitation, Spine 21:2628, 1998.

42. Hides JA, Jull GA, Richardson CA: Long-term effects of specific stabilizing exercises for first-episode low back pain, Spine 26:e243, 2001.

43. Hides JA, Richardson CA, Jull GA: Multifidus muscle recovery is not automatic after resolution of acute, first-episode of low back pain, Spine 21(23):2763, 1996a.

44. Cholewicki J, McGill SM: Mechanical stability of the in vivo lumbar spine: implication for injury and chronic low back pain, Clin Biomech 11(1):1, 1996.

45. McGill SM, Sharratt MT, Seguin JP: Loads on the spinal tissues during simultaneous lifting and ventilatory challenge, Ergonomics 38(9):1772, 1995.

46. Al-Obaidi SM et al: The role of anticipation and fear of pain in the persistence of avoidance behavior in patients with chronic low back pain, Spine 25(9):1126, 2000.

47. Council JR et al: Expectancies and functional impairment in chronic low back pain, Pain 33:323, 1988.

48. Lackner JM, Carosella AM, Feuerstein M: Pain expectancies, pain, and functional self-efficacy expectancies as determinants of disability in patients with chronic low back disorders, J Consult Clin Psych 64:212, 1996.

49. Geissner M, Haig A, Theisen M: Activity avoidance and function in persons with chronic back pain, J Occup Rehab 10(3):215, 2000.

50. Vlaeyen JWS, Linton S: Fear-avoidance and its consequences in chronic musculoskeletal pain. A state of the art, Pain 85:317, 2000.

51. Teasall RW: The denial of chronic pain, J Pain Res Manage 2:89, 1997.

52. Teasall RW, Shapiro AP: Whiplash injuries: an update, J Pain Res Manage 3:81, 1998.

53. Maras WS et al: The influence of psychological stress, gender and personality on mechanical loading of lumbar spine, Spine 25:3045, 2000.

54. Koes BW et al: Clinical guidelines for the management of low back pain in primary care: an international comparison, Spine 26:2504, 2001.

55. Siegal RD et al: Back sense, New York, 2001, Broadway Books.

56. Waddell G et al: The back book, ed 2, Norwich, UK, 2002, The Stationary Office.

57. Ciccione DS, Just N: Pain expectancy and work disability in patients with acute and chronic pain: a test of the fear avoidance hypothesis, J Pain 2:181, 2001.

58. Fordyce WE et al: Pain measurement and pain behavior, Pain 18:53, 1984.

59. Linton SJ, Hellsing AL, Bergström G: Exercise for workers with musculoskeletal pain: does enhancing compliance decrease pain? J Occup Rehab 6:177, 1996.

60. Van Tulder MW et al: Exercise therapy for low back pain. A systematic review within the framework of the Cochrane Collaboration Back Review Group, Spine 25(21):2784, 2000.

61. Faas A et al: A randomized, placebo-controlled trial of exercise therapy in patients with acute low back pain, Spine 18:1388, 1993.

62. Manniche C, Jordan A: Letter to the editor, Spine 26:840, 2001.
63. Stankovic R, Johnell O: Conservative treatment of acute low-back pain. A prospective randomized trial. McKenzie method of treatment versus patient education in "mini back school," Spine 15:120, 1990.
64. Borchgrevink GE et al: Acute treatment of whiplash neck sprain injuries, Spine 23:25, 1998.
65. McKinney LA: Early mobilisation and outcome in acute sprains of the neck, BMJ 299:1006, 1989.
66. Rosenfeld M, Gunnarsson R, Borenstein P: Early intervention in whiplash-associated disorders: a comparison of two treatment protocols, Spine 25(14):1782, 2000.
67. Frank J et al: Preventing disability from work-related low-back pain. New evidence gives new hope—if we can just get all the players onside, CMAJ 158:1625, 1998.
68. Hagen EM, Eriksen HR, Ursin H: Does early intervention with a light mobilization program reduce long-term sick leave for low back pain? Spine 25:1973, 2000.
69. Lindstrom A et al: Activation of subacute low back patients, Phys Ther 4:279, 1992.
70. O'Sullivan P, Twomey L, Allison G: Evaluation of specific stabilizing exercise in the treatment of chronic low back pain with radiologic diagnosis of spondylolysis or spondylolisthesis, Spine 24:2959, 1997.
71. Manniche C et al: Intensive dynamic back exercises for chronic low back pain, Pain 47:53, 1991.
72. Frost H et al: Randomized controlled trial for evaluation of fitness programme for patients with chronic low back pain, BMJ 310:151, 1995.
73. Frost H et al: A fitness programme for patients with chronic low back pain: two-year follow-up of a randomised controlled trial, Pain 75:273, 1998.
74. Frost H, Lamb SE, Shackleton CH: A functional restoration programme for chronic low back pain: a prospective outcome study, Physiotherapy 86(6):285, 2000.
75. Klaber Moffet J et al: A randomized trial of exercise for primary care back pain patients: clinical outcomes, costs and preferences, BMJ 319:279, 1999.
76. Larsson UB et al: Rehabilitation of long-term sick-listed patient in Sweden through techniques of sports medicine, J Back Musculoskel Med 15:67, 2000.
77. Skouen JS et al: Relative cost-effectiveness of extensive and light multidisciplinary treatment programs versus treatment as usual for patients with chronic low back pain on long-term sick leave, Spine 27:901, 2002.
78. Waling K et al: Effects of training on female trapezius myalgia, Spine 27:789, 2002.
79. Gardner-Morse MG, Stokes IAF: The effects of abdominal muscle coactivation on lumbar spine stability, Spine 23:86, 1998.
80. Panjabi MM: The stabilizing system of the spine. Part 1: function, dysfunction, adaptation, and enhancement, J Spinal Disorders 5:383, 1992.
81. Baratta R et al: Muscular coactivation. The role of antagonist musculature in maintaining knee stability, Am J Sports Med 16:113, 1988.
82. Spencer JD, Hayes KC, Alexander IJ: Knee joint effusion and quadriceps reflex inhibition in man, Spine 26:994, 2001.
83. Hides JA et al: Evidence of lumbar multifidus muscle wasting ipsilateral to symptoms in patients with acute/subacute low back pain, Spine 19(2):165, 1994.
84. Hallgren R, Greenman P, Rechtien J: Atrophy of suboccipital muscles in patients with chronic pain: a pilot study, J Am Osteopath Assoc 94:1032, 1994.
85. Nederhand MJ et al: Cervical muscle dysfunction in the chronic whiplash associated disorder Grade II (WAD-II), Spine 15:1938, 2000.
86. Jull GA: Deep cervical flexor muscle dysfunction in whiplash, J Musculoskeletal Pain 8:143, 2000.
87. Shumway-Cook A, Woollacott M: Motor control—theory and practical applications, Baltimore, 1995, Lippincott–Williams & Wilkins.
88. Lund JP et al: The pain-adaptation model: a discussion of the relationship between chronic musculoskeletal pain and motor activity, Can J Physiol Pharmacol 69:683, 1991.
89. Arendt-Nielsen L et al: The influence of low back pain on muscle activity and coordination during gait, Pain 64:231, 1995.
90. Graven-Nielsen T, Svensson P, Arendt-Nielsen L: Effects of experimental muscle pain on muscle activity and co-ordination during static and dynamic motor function, Electroencephalogr Clin Neurophysiol 105:156, 1997.
91. Svensson P, Houe L, Arendt-Nielsen L: Bilateral experimental muscle pain changes electromyographic activity of human jaw-closing muscles during mastication, Exp Brain Res 116:182, 1997.
92. Edgerton VR et al: Theoretical basis for patterning EMG amplitudes to assess muscle dysfunction, Med Sci Sports Exerc 28:744, 1996.
93. McGill SM: Clinical biomechanics of the thoracolumbar spine. In Zeevi Dvir, editor: Clinical biomechanics, Philadelphia, 2000, Churchill Livingstone.
94. McGill SM: A myoelectrically based dynamic 3-D model to predict loads on lumbar spine tissues during lateral bending, J Biomech 25(4):395, 1992.
95. McGill SM: Electromyographic activity of the abdominal and low back musculature during generation of isometric and dynamic axial trunk torque: implications for lumbar mechanics, J Orthop Res 9:91, 1991.
96. McGill SM, Juker D, Kropf P: Quantitative intramuscular myoelectric activity of the quadratus lumborum during a wide variety of tasks, Clin Biomech 11(3):170, 1996.

97. Hodges PW, Richardson CA: Contraction of the abdominal muscles associated with movement of the lower limb, Phys Ther 77:132, 1997b.

98. Hodges PW, Richardson CA: Feedforward contraction of transversus abdominus is not influenced by the direction of arm movement, Exp Brain Res 114:362, 1997a.

99. Goff B: The application of recent advances in neurophysiology to Miss M. Rood's concept of neuromuscular facilitation, Physiotherapy 58:409, 1972.

100. Janda V: Muscles, central nervous motor regulation and back problems. In Korr IM, editor: The neurobiologic mechanisms in manipulative therapy, New York, 1978, Plenium Press.

101. Janda V: On the concept of postural muscles and posture in man, Aus J Physioth 29:83, 1983.

102. Sahrmann S: Diagnosis and treatment of movement impairment syndromes, St Louis, 2001, Mosby.

103. Bergmark A: Stability of the lumbar spine. A study in mechanical engineering, Acta Orthopedica Scandinavica 230:20, 1989.

104. Melzack R, Wall PD: Pain mechanisms: a new theory, Science 150:978, 1965.

105. Morgan D: Concepts in functional training and postural stabilization for the low-back-injured, Top Acute Care Trauma Rehab 2(4):8, 1988.

106. Vollowitz E: Furniture prescription for the conservative management of low-back pain, Top Acute Care Trauma Rehab 2(4):18, 1988.

107. McKenzie RA: Mechanical diagnosis and therapy for low back pain. In Twomey LT, Taylor JR, editors: Physical therapy of low back pain, Edinburgh, 1987, Churchill Livingstone.

108. Kibler WB, Herring SA, Press JM: Functional rehabilitation of sports and musculoskeletal injuries, Gaithersburg, Md, 1998, Aspen Publishers.

109. McGill SM: Low back stability: from formal description to issues for performance and rehabilitation, Exerc Sport Sci Rev 29(1):26, 2001.

110. McGill SM: Spine Instability. In Liebenson C, editor: Rehabilitation of the spine: a practitioner's manual, ed 2, Baltimore, 2003 (scheduled publication), Lippincott–Williams & Wilkins.

110a. Michaud TC: Foot orthoses and other forms of conservative foot care, Baltimore, 1993, Williams & Wilkins.

110b. Janda V: Evaluation of muscle imbalance. In Liebenson C, editor: Rehabilitation of the spine: a practitioner's manual, Baltimore, 1996, Williams & Wilkins.

110c. Liebenson C, Murphy D: Rehabilitation of the spine post-isometric relaxation techniques for the lumbar spine and lower quarter [videotape], Baltimore, 1998, Williams & Wilkins.

110d. Liebenson C, Chapman S: Rehabilitation of the spine: functional evaluation of the lumbar spine [videotape], Baltimore, 1998, Williams & Wilkins.

110e. Bohannon RW: Decrease in timed balance test scores with aging, Phys Ther 64:1067, 1984.

110f. Byl NN, Sinnot PL: Variations in balance and body sway, Spine; 16:325, 1991.

110g. Alaranta H et al: Non-dynametric truck performance tests: reliability and normative data, Scand J Rehab Med 26:211, 1994.

110h. Gray G: Total body functional profile, Adrian Mich, 2001, Wynn Marketing.

110i. Mens JMA: The active straight leg raising test and mobility of the pelvic joints, Eur Spine J 8:468, 1999.

110j. Biering-Sorenson F: Physical measurements as risk indicators for low back trouble over a one-year period, Spine 9:45, 1984.

110k. Richardson CA et al: Therapeutic exercise for spinal segmental stabilisation in low back pain: scientific basis and clinical approach, Edinburgh, 1999, Churchill Livingstone.

110l. Kolar P: Seminar at Anglo European College of Chiropractic, March 1999.

110m. Norris CM: Back stability, London, 2000, Human Kinetics.

110n. Liebenson C, DeFranca C, Lefebvre R: Rehabilitation of the spine: functional evaluation of the cervical spine [videotape], Baltimore, 1998, Williams & Wilkins.

110o. Jull G: Further clinical clarification of the muscle dysfunction in cervical headache, Cephalgia 19:179, 1999.

110p. Skaggs C, Liebenson CS: Orofacial pain, Top Clin Chiropr 7(2):43, 2000.

110q. Murphy D: Conservative management of cervical spine syndromes, New York, 2000, McGraw-Hill.

111. Lewit K: Manipulative therapy in rehabilitation of the motor system, ed 3, London, 1999, Butterworth-Heinemann.

112. Hardcastle P, Annear P, Foster D: Spinal abnormalities in young fast bowlers, J Bone Joint Surg 74B(3):421, 1992.

113. Adams P, Muir H: Qualitative changes with age of proteoglycans of human lumbar discs, Ann Rheum Dis 35:289, 1976.

114. Adams MA, Hutton WC: Prolapsed intervertebral disc: a hyperflexion injury, Spine 7:184, 1982.

115. Adams MA, Hutton WC: Gradual disc prolapse, Spine 10:524, 1985.

116. King AI: Injury to the thoraco-lumbar spine and pelvis. In Nahum AM, Melvin JW, editors: Accidental injury, biomechanics and presentation, New York, 1993, Springer-Verlag.

117. Gordon SJ et al: Mechanism of disc rupture—a preliminary report, Spine 16:450, 1991.

118. Videman T, Nurminen M, Troup JDG: Lumbar spinal pathology in cadaveric material in relation to history of back pain, occupation and physical loading, Spine 15(8):728, 1990.

119. McGill SM: Low back exercises: evidence for improving exercise regimens, Phys Ther 78(7):754, 1998.

119a. McGill SM: Low back exercises: prescription for the healthy back and when recovering from injury. In: American College of Sports Medicine: ASCM's resource manual for guidelines for exercise testing and prescription, ed 3, Philadelphia, 1993, Lippincott, Williams & Wilkins.

120. Reilly T, Tynell A, Troup JDG: Circadian variation in the human stature, Chronobiol Int 1:121, 1984.

121. Adams MA, Dolan P, Hutton WC: Diurnal variations in the stresses on the lumbar spine, Spine 12(2):130, 1987.

122. McGill SM, Childs A, Liebenson C: Endurance times for stabilization exercises: clinical targets for testing and training from a normal database, Arch Phys Med Rehab 80:941, 1999.

123. Van den Hout JHC et al: The effects of failure feedback and pain-related fear on pain report, pain tolerance, and pain avoidance in chronic low back pain patients, Pain 92:247, 2001.

124. Shaw WS et al: Working with low back pain: problem-solving orientation and function, Pain 93:129, 2001.

125. Stokes IAF et al: Decrease in trunk muscular response to perturbation with preactivation of lumbar spinal musculature, Spine 25:1957, 2000.

126. McGill, personal correspondence.

127. McGill SM: The biomechanics of low back injury: implications on current practice in industry and the clinic, J Biomech 30(5):465, 1997.

127a. Crisco JJ III, Panjabi MM: Postural biomechanical stability and gross muscular architecture in the spine. In Winters JM, Woo SL-Y, editors: Multiple muscle systems, New York, 1990, Springer-Verlag.

127b. Adams MA, Dolan P: Recent advances in lumbar spine mechanics and their clinical significance, Clin Biomech 10:3, 1995.

127c. Cholewick J, McGill SM, Norman RW: Lumbar spine loads during lifting extremely heavy weights, Med Sci Sports Exer 23(10):1179, 1991.

127d. Axler C, McGill SM: Low back loads over a variety of abdominal exercises: searching for the safest abdominal challenge, Med Sci Sports Exerc 29(6):804, 1997.

128. Richardson C et al: Therapeutic exercise for spinal stabilization in lower back pain, Edinburgh, 2000, Churchill Livingstone.

129. Gray G, Rehabilitation Institute of Chicago: Functional Approach to Musculoskeletal System II Seminar, October 2001. For further information: wynnmarketing.com.

130. Risberg MA et al: Design and implementation of a neuromuscular training program following anterior cruciate ligament reconstruction, J Orthop Sports Phys Ther 31:620, 2001.

131. Rutherford OM: Muscular coordination and strength training, implications for injury rehabilitation, Sports Med 5:196, 1988.

132. Liebenson CS: Advice for the clinician and patient: functional exercises, J Bodywork Movement Ther 6(2):108, 2002.

133. Fairbank JCT et al: The Oswestry low back pain index, Physiotherapy 66:271, 1980.

134. Vernon HT, Mior S: The neck disability index: a study of reliability and validity, J Manipulative Physiol Ther 14:409, 1991.

CHAPTER

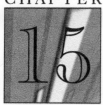

15

Pediatrics

Joel Alcantara, DC, Claudia A. Anrig, DC,
Gregory Plaugher, DC

Key Terms

ADAPTABILITY
ADOLESCENT IDIOPATHIC
 SCOLIOSIS
DEFORMATION
DISRUPTION
ENURESIS

LEGG-CALVÈ-PERTHES
 DISEASE
MALFORMATION
MALLEABILITY
MORPHOGENESIS

PHYSIOLOGIC
 HYPERMOBILITY
PSEUDOSUBLUXATION
SCOLIOSIS
SKIN TEMPERATURE
 DIFFERENTIALS

At a time when adult use of complementary and alternative medicine (CAM) continues to increase,[1,2] with chiropractic the most widely used nonallopathic professional service,[3] one would expect commensurate use in children. Moreover, with increasing concerns about the safety, effectiveness, and long-term outcomes of several types of pediatric medical interventions,[4] particularly those involving the use of psychotropic medications, many parents are seeking alternative approaches for the care of their children,[5] often without telling their medical pediatricians.[6] In one study on the use of CAM therapies for children, the most common types were self-care methods such as herbs, prayer healing, high-dose vitamin therapy and other nutritional supplements, and folk and home remedies, along with two professionally administered interventions: massage therapy and chiropractic.[7] In a cross-sectional survey study by Lee and colleagues[8] on chiropractic care of pediatric patients, an estimated 420,000 pediatric visits took place in the Boston metropolitan area alone in 1998, representing a health care expenditure of approximately $14 million.

In this introductory chapter, the biomechanical features unique to the pediatric spine are reviewed, which provide the rationale and foundation for the discussion on pediatric adjusting, the hallmark of pediatric chiropractic care.[9,10] A series of case presentations follows, along with an examination of current research.

BIOMECHANICAL CONSIDERATIONS

The pediatric spine has unique biomechanical features that distinguish it from the adult spine, particularly with regard to its greater flexibility of both soft and hard tissues. These factors are incorporated into the process of detecting and correcting spinal subluxations in the pediatric patient. Inattention to these differences may lead to misdiagnosis and *iatrogenesis* (i.e., causation of an adverse condition as the result of a health intervention). For example, normal physiologic ligamentous laxity of the pediatric spine may result in a false impression of subluxation of C2 on C3. Attempt at correction through the application of a high-velocity, low-amplitude (HVLA) thrust would be inappropriate for this **pseudosubluxation**. On the other hand, true instability of C2 on C3 may be misdiagnosed if the chiropractor is not aware of the limits of physiologic ligamentous laxity in his or her patients. Both situations may have serious consequences.

Growth

Central to the uniqueness of pediatric spinal bio-mechanics[11] is the capacity for active growth and remodeling. The development of the neuromusculoskeletal system is multifactorial, with ongoing dynamic interactions at the molecular and cellular levels, as well as increasingly complex processes of control over developing tissues, organs, and systems. Embryogenic development is characterized by **morphogenesis** (formation and growth of bodily structures) involving programmed development of the embryonic cells of the endoderm, mesoderm, and ectoderm. Abnormal progression of the previously listed processes (i.e., malformation, deformation, disruption) may lead to structural defects, particularly in the spine and spinal cord.[12] Understanding the spine's growth process and potential alterations in this process is an essential aspect of pediatric chiropractic.

Malformation, Disruption, and Deformation

Malformation results from dysfunctional embryogenesis of a specific anatomic structure. Once a malformation is anatomically established, the asymmetry may continue, resulting in adverse spinal development throughout the fetal and postnatal periods. The malformation will affect three-dimensional development and growth of the individual, contributing to dysfunction.

Disruption results from the destruction of a normally formed structure. The cause may involve altered growth patterns resulting from trauma, infection, tumors, or metabolic alterations. This condition involves the limbs more frequently than the spine during the fetal stage.

Deformation results from altered structure (and hence function) of normally developed structures during the fetal period, the postnatal period, or both. The nature of the deformity is contingent on the extrinsic and intrinsic properties of the structure, as well as the forces involved. For example, deformations may develop whenever normal movements, whether prenatal or postnatal, are constrained.

CHIROPRACTIC APPLICATIONS

How do the biomechanical features of growth and the potential abnormalities involved (i.e., deformation, malformation, disruption) become important considerations for the doctor of chiropractic? An example is the common use of leg length measurements, sometimes used by chiropractors as an indicator of lumbosacral subluxation. Because children can have asymmetrical growth in the long bones of the legs, interpreting leg length inequalities should always be augmented by other procedures. Similarly, using orthotics in young children should also be approached with caution.

A fetus may undergo physical alteration if constrained for a sufficient period. For the developing fetus, several factors are associated with uterine constraint. These factors include intrauterine (i.e., multiple fetuses) and extrauterine (i.e., increased abdominal and pelvic muscle tone) factors, as well as aberrant fetal position (i.e., malposition, malpresentation). The range of deformities and their health consequences (short- and long-term) may not yet be fully appreciated, particularly for adverse fetal presentation. Larry Webster (1937-1997), a pioneer in chiropractic pediatrics, advanced a technique for altering adverse fetal presentation.[13] The Webster technique is described by Forrester and Anrig[14] and taught in the postgraduate program of the International Chiropractic Pediatric Association (ICPA).

Adaptability

The ability of the pediatric spine to adapt to stresses is much greater than that of the adult spine. This **adaptability** can be attributed to the tissue plasticity and growth potential of the pediatric spine, which permit children to maintain a high level of functionality despite considerable structural dysfunction. Chiropractors experienced in detecting and correcting subluxation in the pediatric patient are sensitive to minor structural alterations in the developing child by virtue of their hands-on approach.

Some health practitioners unfamiliar with chiropractic procedures have expressed concern about the application of dynamic thrust adjustments to the pediatric spine. However, the adaptability of the pediatric spine allows it to absorb the dynamic force of modified HVLA adjustments safely.

Malleability

In addition to the active process of *adaptability*, the pediatric musculoskeletal system has **malleability;** that is, it may be deformed with the application of external forces. In the past, some cultures have applied this principle in destructive ways that have caused aberrant structure in children, such as binding the feet of Chinese baby girls to limit growth and molding the skulls of young Chinook Indians with leather splints. In general, forces applied inappropriately will have detrimental effects.

Hypermobility

The physiologic range of motion of the pediatric spine is much greater than that of the adult as a result of differences in the ability of soft tissue structures to act as restraints, as well as differences in facet joint orientation. An appreciation of hypermobility in the pediatric spine will assist the pediatric chiropractor in his or her clinical assessment procedures and will lead to appropriate modifications in adjusting procedures. An example is the pseudosubluxation of C2 on C3 mentioned previously. Unlike hypermobility in adult spinal joints, this normal **physiologic hypermobility** in the child will not result in pathologic changes when subjected to normal or appropriately delivered forces.

Changing Spinal Contours

The sagittal spinal curvature of the pediatric spine begins as a C-shaped arc. The lordotic cervical and lumbar curvatures form gradually with spinal development. These secondary curves have considerable biomechanical relevance, because the transitional regions are sites where stress concentrates and are therefore more susceptible to developing vertebral subluxations. During periods of rapid growth, such as the typical adolescent growth spurt, the spine may be susceptible to both rotational and coronal plane deformities, potentially resulting in subluxations or **scoliosis**.

Changing Applied Forces

The forces to which the spine is subjected are important in the initiation, perpetuation, and exacerbation of the vertebral subluxation complex. The day-to-day forces applied to the pediatric spine change during the process of growth and development. For example, the infant is subjected to lesser biomechanical forces because of the relative inactivity during the period before the child is able to stand upright, walk, and run. As the child develops, these forces increase as play becomes more vigorous, subjecting the musculoskeletal system to repetitive stresses. Sports injuries are a common cause of trauma for the growing child.[15]

The infant's head is relatively large compared with the body mass. As a result, the pediatric patient's cervical spine experiences relatively larger forces during acceleration or deceleration compared with the adult patient. In situations involving vigorous shaking of a baby during play, or in cases of abuse, the pediatric patient is vulnerable to injury. The types of injuries sustained in patients undergoing whiplash are well documented.[16] Controversy exists as to the extent of injuries sustained from low-versus high-impact collisions. For the pediatric patient, forces involving even relatively low impact collisions can have significant consequences, due, in part, to the lack of stabilization of the cervical spine in the immature neuromusculoskeletal system. Although myelination of the central nervous system is completed during the first 2 years of a child's life, development of balance and coordination continues well into adulthood. As a result, the child's musculoskeletal system has an increased risk of injury and consequent predisposition to structural abnormalities.

SCOLIOSIS

Adolescent idiopathic scoliosis (AIS) is an important consideration for the pediatric chiropractor.

Scoliosis can be found in any area of the spine but is most common in the thoracic region. AIS is a three-dimensional entity, with spinal curvatures commonly including deviation not only laterally, but also in the anterior-posterior dimension and obliquely. When such curvatures are present, inequality of paraspinal muscle tension on the right and left sides is inevitable. This condition may represent an application of Wolff's Law, which states that bone is shaped by the forces or lack of force placed on it.

When scoliosis develops in the adolescent spine, the resultant biomechanical stresses can cause permanent wedging of the vertebral bodies. Once significant deformation occurs, the curvature cannot be reversed by nonsurgical means. Aside from the pain and structural imbalances that patients with scoliosis can endure, it must also be understood that the most severe cases of scoliosis can involve mechanical pressure on the heart and lungs.

Nottingham Theory

Research has not determined the cause of AIS, but genetic predisposition may play a role in some cases (Figs. 15-1 and 15-2). One concept in the pathogenesis of AIS is the *dinner plate-flagpole* theory as proposed by the Nottingham group.[17] Briefly, the concept involves developmental disturbance in the central nervous system, which causes asymmetry of trunk muscle function as a result of asymmetrical central pattern generators in the spinal cord. During normal two-legged walking, rotation-inducing forces arise in the pelvis (the dinner plate) with counter-rotational forces in the upper trunk as a result of muscle action. The central pattern generators in the spinal cord control spinal rotators attached to ribs. Failure of control leads to failure of rotational control of the spine. A biomechanical breakdown ensues, resulting in the three-dimensional spinal deformity of scoliosis.

Subsequently, the biomechanical features of the pediatric spine as previously discussed (e.g., growth, malleability, etc.), together with gravity, add to the neuromuscular asymmetry to exaggerate spinal curve progression. This concept suggests a rationale for care through motor control

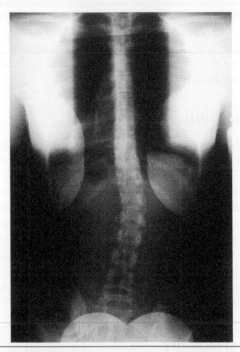

Fig. **15-1** Sixteen-year-old adolescent with scoliosis.

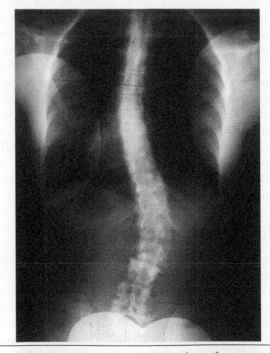

Fig. **15-2** Forty-seven-year-old mother of patient depicted in Fig. 15-1 with scoliosis. The degenerative changes at the apex of the curvature are noted.

function by balancing the healthy trunk dynamically through activating nerve afferents of trunk muscles, tendons, and joints. This proprioceptive mechanism may involve *rewiring* during the process of learning. Other potential neurologic causes of central pattern asymmetry initiating AIS may arise in the spinal cord or higher centers. Pediatric chiropractic care is consistent with this theory. Recent research has demonstrated that spinal adjustments activate mechanoreceptors,[18] as well as affect brain function.[19]

PALPATION AND ADJUSTMENT OF THE PEDIATRIC PATIENT

As with all patients, chiropractic pediatric care begins with a thorough history and examination. Discussing all the salient features of such an undertaking is beyond the scope of this chapter; the reader is therefore referred to the relevant chapters[13,20] in Plaugher's *Textbook of Clinical Chiropractic: A Specific Biomechanical Approach* and Anrig and Plaugher's *Pediatric Chiropractic* for a more complete discussion. This introductory chapter will address the palpation and adjustment of the pediatric patient.

Palpation

Static and motion palpation are core procedures in examining the chiropractic patient, pediatric or adult. Static palpation involves detecting edema or bogginess in musculature, as well as anatomic sites of tenderness. Tenderness is often present in regions of hypermobility as a result of a compensation for segments or regions of hypomobility. Motion palpation involves two types: end-play motion palpation and intersegmental range of motion. Both types warrant further investigation because the reliability of palpation has demonstrated mixed results.[21,22] (See Chapter 10 for a detailed discussion of palpation research.) Posteriority, as detected on flexion-extension motion palpation of the spine from C2 to S2, is the most common listing (specific description of abnormal joint position of movement) in the newborn and infant, although lateral flexion dysfunction is generally not a major finding. Spinous rotation is not as common in the

young spine as it is in adults. However, this problem should be suspected in cases of rotational trauma to the spine or when long-term vertebral malposition exists as a result of compensation for a segmental dysfunction elsewhere in the spine.

Adjustment

Adjustment procedures are frequently modified for the adult patient based on factors that include clinical presentation, size, and patient comfort. This practice also holds true for the pediatric patient. The following discussion of pediatric adjusting considers the age and size of the patient, the importance of specificity of contact points, adjusting apparatus, positioning, and thrust characteristics for the pediatric patient.[23]

AGE-RELATED FACTORS

In addition to clinical findings, adjusting procedures for the pediatric patient are guided by the age and size of the patient, particularly regarding the application of force. Older children are adjusted similarly to young adults. In much younger patients, force modification, table positioning, and clinician contact points must be reconsidered to provide effective chiropractic care. The amount of force needed to produce the desired movement or repositioning (or both) of a subluxated segment is generally less in smaller patients.

Young toddlers have special needs as they begin to demonstrate increased muscle control, as well as a will of their own. These factors create additional complexity for the chiropractor, thus rapport must be developed with the young patient so that he or she will follow guidance to relax and remain still before the adjustment. Clinicians should not attempt to overcome these challenges by treating the patient with suboptimal care or specificity or by forcing the patient to submit to procedures against his or her will. Communication and reassurance appear to be the only reasonable way of surmounting these difficulties. Communication may be facilitated in a number of ways. For example, children who have seen their parents being adjusted may be more receptive to participate in the process once their turn arrives. For infants, an explanation of the adjustment process is provided only to the parent.

Because of its smaller dimensions, the pediatric spine requires special care with respect to specificity of segmental contact points. This requirement is necessary to ensure that the appropriate segments are adjusted and to avoid introducing forces into adjacent normal or hypermobile functional spinal units. To achieve the desired level of specificity, clinicians may need to modify their adjusting methods by using smaller digits as contact points. For example, the lack of specificity seen in the double-thenar contacts or the anterior dorsal adjustment makes them unsuitable for the small child's spine.

ADJUSTING OPTIONS FOR THE PEDIATRIC PATIENT

Adjusting the pediatric spine requires the utmost of a chiropractor's psychomotor skills. Modification of adjustive technique is an essential aspect of pediatric care, with these modifications based on the size and age of the patient, as well as the functional segment to be adjusted. Adjustments may be performed prone, seated, or in a lateral recumbent or supine position.

Cervical Spine

The cervical spine, for example, can be adjusted in the prone position with the distal end of the fifth digit on a contact site, such as the C2 spinous process. This type of contact addresses the need for specificity on the small cervical spinous processes and the resulting short-lever adjustment. This type of adjustment will have a line of drive directed primarily from posterior to anterior and inferior to superior, with an arcing movement through the plane line of the intervertebral disk (IVD) and facet articulations. If the clinician's hands are small enough and the patient is older, then the pisiform contact can be used on the same segments. If specificity cannot be achieved, then the procedure is contraindicated. Adjustments to the atlas in an infant can be achieved by using a thumb contact. The patient can be seated on the lap of a parent or

assistant. The cervical chair can also be used if the child is large enough. The anterosuperior occiput can be adjusted in the supine position. An adjustment for an anterosuperior condyle subluxation (in hyperextension) may use a small-sized condyle block to support the posterior ring of the atlas and the inferior cervical segments. The thrust is made from anterior to posterior with the contact at the glabella of the frontal bone to achieve flexion of the C0-C1 functional spinal unit.

Thoracic Spine

Adjustments to the thoracic pediatric spine can be performed in the prone position. For the newborn, the patient can be positioned on the parent's lap. For the juvenile and adolescent patient, a variety of adjusting tables, including the hi-lo, pelvic bench, or knee-chest table, may also be used to achieve specific adjustments. The knee-chest table can be modified to the small child's dimensions. By using a double-thumb contact, specificity is combined with the ability to generate sufficient force to move the segment. Similar patient positioning can be achieved on the hi-lo table with a slackening of the tension of the abdominal section. However, the smaller child usually does not adapt well to the adult lengths of the head, abdominal, and pelvic sections. The pelvic bench usually has a breathing or nose vent at one end and is acceptable for prone adjustments, especially those of the upper thoracic–lower cervical region.

Lumbar Spine, Ilium, and Sacrum

The lumbar spine, ilium, and sacrum can be adjusted with the patient placed in the prone or side posture position. The choice of patient positioning depends on several factors. However, patient comfort is most important, especially in the patient with an acute injury. The doctor's contact point should be appropriate to the size of the patient. For example, finger contact points are preferred over broad thenar contacts to achieve specificity. As in all adjustments to the low back, excessive rotation should be avoided over several spinal segments, and the preload (taking the articulation to tension) should be to a specific segment rather than multisegmental. Contraindications to adjusting may include the inability of the doctor to prevent rotation in the thoracic spine, excessive body-drop, or multiple contact points. Notably, in certain diseases of childhood, such as **Legg-Calvè-Perthes disease** or slipped femoral capital epiphysis, the involved hip should be placed side down or the correction performed in the prone position.

Thrust Characteristics

With HVLA adjustments, significant effects and alterations can be achieved based on the malleability and adaptability of the pediatric spine. Given the physiologic hypermobility of the pediatric spine, a greater amount of preload is necessary to bring the segment to tension. Moreover, greater displacement into the paraphysiologic space occurs with a minimal amount of effort and force needed to achieve end range. Only in rare circumstances should the thrust be made as the patient resists the force. A vertebral segment should be adjusted with the minimum necessary force, taking into account prior adjusting experience, biomechanics, and anatomy (i.e., facet joint orientation, disk angles). The doctor uses palpation to determine the patient's tolerance and adjustment requirements. For example, two patients may have similar morphologic characteristics but require differing preloading, set-up time, relaxation, and degree of force to accomplish the adjustment successfully. A thorough clinical evaluation and clinical experience will assist in achieving a successful adjustment.

For the adult patient, a set-hold procedure is the norm and is well tolerated. Therefore followthrough is important in achieving a successful outcome. Cavitations may be very small or nonexistent in the very young pediatric patient and should not be considered a necessary component of a successful adjustment, although cavitation will often occur even with the controlled force appropriate for pediatric patients. The focus in the thrust should be the extent of motion in the vertebral segment. Such feedback provides information about the health of the articulation and considerations for future adjustments.

CASE MANAGEMENT

Case 1: Headaches, Dizziness, Sinusitis, Allergies, Asthma

BreeAnn (age 9 years) was presented by her mother for chiropractic evaluation and care for complaints associated with the cervical spine. History revealed "popping and grinding" in the neck for the previous 6 months, headaches at least once a week, and positional dizziness for the previous few weeks. Since the age of 7, she had also experienced sinusitis, allergies, and asthma. Prescription medication included 17 g Albuterol inhaler (two puffs every 4 hours), 34 ml Astelin 137MCG (one spray twice daily), 20 g Azmacort 100MCII inhaler (two puffs twice daily), and Singular Tab (one tablet at bedtime).

Cervical and lumbar orthopedic examinations were negative. Lumbar range of motion (ROM) was within normal limits. However, the patient's active and passive ROM in the cervical spine was abnormal such that on extension and left rotation, "popping sounds" were heard by both examiner and patient. A decreased ROM was observed in right rotation and in left and right lateral flexion. Static palpation of the paraspinal musculature revealed taut and tender muscle fibers at C5 through C7 and T3 through T8 bilaterally and tenderness to palpation at the spinous process of L5 and over the left ala of the sacrum. Motion palpation demonstrated reduction of joint play at C6, T5, T8, and L5, and at the left sacrum. Abnormal instrumentation findings (i.e., **skin temperature differentials**) were found at the C6, T5, T8, and L5 vertebral levels.

Based on the history and examination findings, a full-spine radiographic examination was undertaken. The lateral view showed a loss of cervical curvature (Fig. 15-3) and an increased lumbar curvature, and the anteroposterior film view revealed a left sacral rotation and mild thoracic deviation from the midline between T3 and T10 (Fig. 15-4).

Based on these examination findings, the following subluxations were detected: C6 P-inf, T5 PRS, T8 PRI-t, sacrum P-L5, and L5 PR-m. (See Chapter 12 for further detail on adjusting procedures.) Adjustments to sites of vertebral sublux-

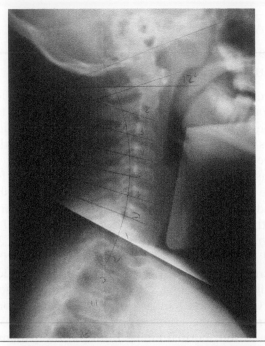

Fig. 15-3 Lateral cervical radiograph demonstrating a reduction in the cervical lordosis.

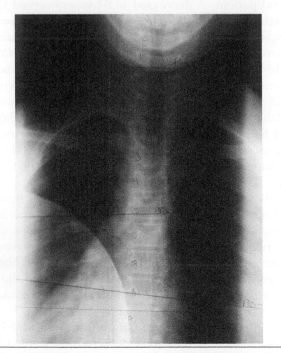

Fig. 15-4 Anteroposterior radiograph shows lateral flexion misalignments of midthoracic spine.

ations were performed at the levels of C6, T6, and the sacrum as follows:

C6 P-inf:

Patient position: Seated on the parent

Doctor's position: Standing behind the patient

Contact site: Inferior aspect of the spinous process

Supportive assistance: Parent stabilizing the chest and back of the patient

Pattern of thrust: Posterior to anterior and inferior to superior with an arcing movement through the plane of the intervertebral disk and facet articulations

Possible contraindications to consider in similar cases:

1. The newborn or infant is unable to be stabilized in the seated position.

2. The doctor is unable to prevent excessive lateral flexion, extension, or rotation during the thrust.

T5 PRS:

Procedure: Pelvic table, pisiform set-up

Patient position: Prone on the pelvic or slot table

Doctor's position: Standing inferior to the contact line, to the side of spinous laterality

Contact site: Right inferior aspect of the spinous process (Tissue pull occurs with the stabilization hand from inferior to superior and lateral to medial.)

Pattern of thrust: Posterior to anterior, lateral to medial with an inferiorward arcing motion toward the end of the thrust

Sacrum P-L5: Standing to either side, the doctor will contact the lateral aspect of the sacral ala (Fig. 15-5). Careful consideration must be taken not to contact the posterior superior iliac spine (PSIS) or the sacral tubercle. While bilaterally raising and lowering the legs, the doctor moves the joint posterior to anterior and slightly medial to lateral. If a rotated sacral tubercle exists, the joint will generally present with both restriction and slight edema. Although rare, it has been noted by this author (CAA) that severe sacral tubercle rotation can inhibit the infant's crawling development.

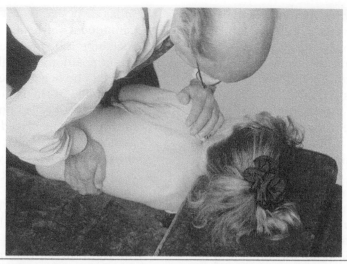

Fig. 15-5 Rotated sacrum adjustment in side posture position.

Patient position: Preadolescent or adolescent is placed involved side up in the side posture position on the pelvic bench

Doctor's position: Side posture position for the pelvic bench, with the doctor straddling the superior bent leg

Contact site: Left sacral ala (Tissue pull is performed by the stabilization hand from inferior to superior and medial to lateral.)

Pattern of thrust: Posterior to anterior and slightly medial to lateral (To improve the line of correction, the doctor leans over the patient to lower the elbow to the level of the plane of the sacroiliac joint.)

At the fourth visit, observations included a notable decrease of grinding and popping in the cervical spine and, according to BreeAnn and her mother, a decrease in her asthma symptoms. At the seventh visit, BreeAnn's mother informed the chiropractor that her daughter was "50% off her medications." A reexamination of the patient at her ninth visit (6 weeks since starting care) revealed the patient's cervical ROM had improved. According to BreeAnn and her mother, the following had changed: neck popping and grinding were "90% improved," the patient had no headaches for the past 5 weeks, no positional

dizziness since the second week of care, sinus problems and allergies were "50% improved," asthma was "70% improved," and no colds. Additionally, the patient's mother noted a dramatic change in her child's ability to play. Fourteen visits later, the patient's asthma symptoms were "90% improved." BreeAnn's mother informed the medical physician treating her sinus, allergy, and asthma of the improvement in her child's condition, resulting in a decrease in all of her medications.

The patient continues to maintain the improvements in her symptoms following chiropractic care. BreeAnn is on wellness care and visits her chiropractor twice a month.

Case 2: Failure to Thrive, Feeding Difficulties, Reflux

Hannah (age 6 months) was brought for a chiropractic consultation for poor feeding, spitting up, failure to thrive, and resistance to feeding. The mother would express her milk and feed Hannah via a bottle to control and encourage her daughter's intake, which was less then 6 oz per day. Her mother was fearful and concerned that her daughter would have to be hospitalized within the next few days given that Hannah's physical condition was rapidly deteriorating.

According to Hannah's mother, Hannah was medically diagnosed with a mild to moderate gastroesophageal reflux. Prescription medication included Zantax (6.2 ml two times a day) since age 3 months and Bethanechol (0.9 ml three times a day) for the previous 2 weeks.

Numerous medical physicians told Hannah's mother that the cause of her daughter's gastroesophageal reflux was unknown. The specialists at the children's hospital "did not know what to do" but suggested that Hannah might grow out of her condition sooner or later.

During the initial chiropractic consultation, it was revealed that during the last trimester of pregnancy, Hannah was in a transverse lie position, that the mother's water was broken in the hospital, and that Hannah had a difficult and rapid delivery. From the time of birth, Hannah would cry from the moment she awoke in the morning until she fell asleep at 4:00 AM the next day. Additionally, from the first day of her birth, Hannah would spit up from her feedings.

Observations during Hannah's feeding revealed that when the bottle was placed in Hannah's mouth, her mother would have to brace her to take in even a few ounces because Hannah would arch back, strain, cry, and then spit up the breast milk. Examination findings revealed hypertonic paraspinal muscles at T4 and T5 and in the left occipital to C2 paraspinal region. Motion palpation detected joint dysfunctions at atlas and T5. Based on the examination as described, a T5 posterior and an atlas (ASL) subluxation were identified.
T5 posterior:
  Technique: Gonstead
  Procedure: Prone hi-lo adjustment
  Contraindications to be screened:
    Hypermobility, instability, destruction or fracture of the neural arch or spinous process, infection of the contact vertebra
  Patient position: Prone on the hi-lo table, with hands resting on the hand plates
  Doctor's position: Either side of the table
  Contact site: Inferior portion of the spinous process
  Tissue pull: With the stabilization hand from inferior to superior
  Pattern of thrust: Posterior to anterior and slightly inferior to superior

ASL atlas:
  Technique: Gonstead
  Procedure: Side posture atlas adjustment
  Patient position: On right side on the pelvic bench (The head piece of the hi-lo or knee-chest table or the lap of the parent may be used. A small rolled up towel or foam pad may need to be placed between the lateral aspect of the patient's cervical spine and the table to reduce any air gap.)
  Contact site: Anterolateral aspect of atlas transverse process
  Supportive assistance: The parent may need to stabilize the chest, lower limbs, or both from activity
  Pattern of thrust: Lateral to medial, inferiorward arc at end of the thrust
  Possible contraindications to consider in similar cases: The newborn or infant is unable to be maintained in a side posture position

After Hannah's first adjustment, her mother reported that her child was calm for several hours. At the third visit, Hannah's mother stated that Hannah had increased her breast milk intake to 8 oz per day. At her fifth visit, Hannah's milk intake increased to 17.5 oz. At the eighth visit, milk intake increased to 21 oz, and at the ninth visit, to 22 oz. At the tenth visit, she was able to eat more solids and was off all medications. The 10 visits were over a 30-day period. Over the following 30 days, Hannah continued to thrive, gain weight, and show increasing calmness. She rarely cried, did not resist the bottle, and the reflux diminished to occasional mild episodes. Hannah was monitored at five visits during this time period.

Case 3: Bedwetting

William (age 7 years) was presented for chiropractic consultation by his mother because of her concern that his bedwetting was beginning to affect his peer relationships. William's bedwetting had been present since he was potty trained, with nocturnal **enuresis** at least three times a week. During the history, William's mother noted that he also experienced headaches, approximately one per week, for the previous several months. No unusual traumas to the head were noted except for "typical" childhood falls.

Orthopedic examination revealed no significant findings. Lumbar ROM was normal. The patient's cervical spine ROM demonstrated a decrease in left rotation and left lateral flexion. Static palpation revealed tenderness over the spinous processes at C5 and T6 and at the right sacroiliac joint. Skin temperature differentials were also present at C5 and T6. Motion palpation revealed joint dysfunction at these sites. Based on the history and physical examination findings, a full-spine plain film radiographic study was undertaken. The lateral radiograph revealed a mild loss of the cervical curve and a mild increase of the lumbosacral curve. The anteroposterior view revealed a spinographic measurement of 7 mm right sacral rotation.

C5 PL:

Technique: Gonstead

Procedure: Prone hi-lo cervical (Fig. 15-6).

Patient position: Prone on the hi-lo table

Doctor's position: Standing on the right side and slightly inferior to the patient

Contact site: Inferior right lateral aspect of the spinous process

Pattern of thrust: Posterior to anterior and inferior to superior with an arcing movement through the plane of the intervertebral disk and facet articulations with a slight rotation

T6 PL:

Technique: Gonstead

Procedure: Cervical chair adjustment

Patient position: Seated in the cervical chair, using the stabilization strap or the parent's hand on the chest of the child

Doctor's position: Standing behind the patient, slightly to the side opposite of spinous rotation

Contact point: Right spinous-lamina junction

Pattern of thrust: Posterior to anterior through the disk plane line, with an inferiorward arcing motion toward the end of the thrust

P-R sacrum:

Technique: Gonstead

Procedure: Side posture sacral finger push adjustment

Patient position: Involved side up in the side posture position on the pelvic bench

Doctor's position: Side posture position for the pelvic bench, straddling the superior bent leg

Contact site: Right second sacral ala, with tissue pull performed by the stabilization hand from inferior to superior and medial to lateral

Pattern of thrust: Posterior to anterior and slightly medial to lateral

William reported at the second visit that he had all dry nights since his visit 5 days previously.

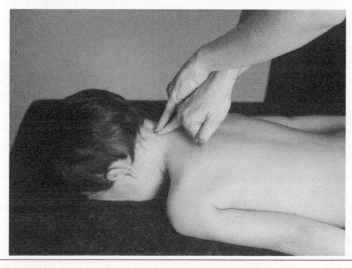

Fig. **15-6** Prone C5 adjustment.

At the third visit, William reported only one wet night over a 4-day period. By the fifth visit, he had an entire dry week. At the fifth visit, the T6 and C5 adjustment were introduced. By the end of a 10-week period involving 14 adjustments, no reports of bedwetting or headaches were reported. William is now seen periodically for wellness care.

PEDIATRIC CHIROPRACTIC RESEARCH

The body of research on chiropractic pediatric care is small but growing. Thus far, the only pediatric conditions for which controlled trials of significant size have been conducted are asthma, infantile colic, and nocturnal enuresis.

An excellent resource addressing chiropractic pediatric research in detail is Anthony Rosner's *Infant and Child Care: An Assessment of Research*,[24] published by the Foundation for Chiropractic Education and Research. In this 2003 monograph, which includes discussion of both medical and chiropractic approaches, the following conditions are covered: otitis media, infantile colic, nocturnal enuresis, asthma, scoliosis, neurologic disorders (e.g., epilepsy, autism, attention deficit-hyperactivity), and headache.

The following is a summary of chiropractic pediatric research published in journals indexed by the National Library of Medicine and listed on MEDLINE. Additional small studies and case studies have been published in other journals. Further reports on chiropractic pediatric care for conditions such as urinary incontinence, gastrointestinal disorders, and tonsillitis are presented in Chapter 25, along with coverage of research on the conditions listed here.

Asthma

In a recent systematic review of the literature for the *Cochrane Collaboration*, Hondras and colleagues[25] found insufficient evidence to support or refute using manual therapy for patients with asthma and also noted that sham-controlled trials (see later discussion) may underestimate the actual benefit of manual therapy.

In 1998, Balon and colleagues[26] conducted a randomized, controlled trial of chiropractic spinal adjustment/manipulation for children with mild or moderate asthma. After a 3-week baseline evaluation period, 91 children who had continuing symptoms of asthma despite conventional medical therapy were randomly assigned to receive either active or simulated chiropractic adjustment/manipulation for 4 months. None of the children had previously received chiropractic care. Small increases (7 to 12 L/minute) were observed in peak expiratory flow in the morning and evening in both treatment groups, with no significant differences between the groups in the degree of change from baseline (morning peak expiratory flow: P = 0.49 at 2 months and P = 0.82 at 4 months).

Symptoms of asthma and use of beta-agonist medication decreased, and the quality of life increased in both groups, with no significant differences between the groups. No significant changes in spirometric measurements or airway responsiveness were observed. The authors concluded that in children with mild or moderate asthma, the addition of chiropractic spinal manipulation to usual medical care provided no benefit, though quality of life scores were more improved in the chiropractic adjustment group.

Of note in the Balon and colleagues' study is the nature of the sham adjustment/manipulation, which consisted of a variety of noncavitating manual maneuvers that may not have been therapeutically inert. (For further discussion of the methodologic controversies in this study, see Chapter 25.)

A 2001 study by Bronfort and colleagues[27] sought to determine whether chiropractic spinal manipulative therapy (SMT) in addition to optimal medical management resulted in clinically important changes in asthma-related outcomes in children. This study also sought to assess the feasibility of conducting a full-scale, randomized clinical trial in terms of recruitment, evaluation, treatment, and ability to deliver a sham SMT procedure. After 3 months of combining chiropractic SMT with optimal medical management for pediatric asthma, the children of the study rated their quality of life substantially higher and their asthma severity substantially lower compared with baseline values. These improvements were maintained at the 1-year follow-up assessment. No important changes were noted in lung function or hyperresponsiveness at any time. The authors cautioned, however, that the observed improvements were unlikely a result of the specific effects of chiropractic SMT alone, but rather other aspects of the clinical encounter.

Colic

Klougart and colleagues[28] published a prospective, uncontrolled study of 316 infants with infantile colic. These investigators demonstrated a satisfactory result of spinal adjustive/manipulative therapy in 94% of the cases. The median age of the infants was 5.7 weeks at the beginning of the treatment. The results were evaluated by analysis of a diary continually kept by the mother and an assessment file based on parent interviews. This assessment was a multicenter study lasting 3 months and involving 73 chiropractors in 50 clinics. The results occurred within 2 weeks and after an average of three treatments.

In 1998, Wiberg and colleagues[29] published a controlled study supporting spinal adjustment/manipulation as a treatment for patients with infantile colic. Patients demonstrated a significant difference between hours of crying per day in two groups of infants, one treated with spinal adjustment/manipulation and the other with dimethicone, a medication used for colic.

In 2001, Olafsdottir and colleagues[30] also investigated the efficacy of chiropractic mobilization in the management of infantile colic. Of 100 infants with typical colicky pain recruited to a randomized, blinded, placebo-controlled, clinical trial, 86 completed the study. Although 32 of 46 infants in the treatment group (69.9%) and 24 of 40 in the control group (60.0%) showed improvement, the study authors concluded that chiropractic spinal manipulation is no more effective than placebo in treating infantile colic. Members of the control group of children were each held by a nurse for 10 minutes.

Nocturnal Enuresis

Several studies have investigated the effectiveness of chiropractic care in patients with noc-

turnal enuresis. Similar to the studies involving asthma and colic, the results are mixed. Leboeuf-Yde and colleagues,[31] in an uncontrolled study involving 171 enuretic children, ages 4 to 15, found no validity in the claim that chiropractic is a treatment of choice for functional nocturnal enuresis. Blomerth,[32] on the other hand, through a case report, asserts that a patient's enuresis resolved with the use of adjustment/manipulation that was not able to be attributed to time or placebo effect. Reed and colleagues,[33] in a controlled clinical trial of 46 nocturnal enuretic children (31 treatment and 15 control group), found that 25% of the treatment group children had 50% or more reduction in the wet night frequency from baseline to post-treatment. None among the control group had such a reduction.

CONCLUSION

Pediatric chiropractic is an established part of the chiropractic college curriculum. With continued interest in postgraduate specialty training, the establishment of professional associations, the creation of textbooks dedicated solely to pediatric chiropractic, and the establishment of the scholarly *Journal of Clinical Chiropractic Pediatrics*, chiropractic pediatrics is on its way to becoming an established specialty. It offers chiropractors the opportunity to provide a needed service to children and parents and is a cornerstone of family practice.

Review *Questions*

1. Under normal circumstances, does the pediatric spine have more or less mobility than the adult spine?
2. What is a pseudosubluxation?
3. What are the differences among malformation, deformation, and disruption?
4. Why is the three-dimensional nature of scoliosis significant?
5. What factors must be considered when determining proper patient positioning for adjusting an infant?
6. What are some modifications in positioning of the chiropractor's hands that

should be considered in adjusting small children?

7. Why should side posture adjustments be avoided in patients with Legg-Calvè-Perthes disease?

8. What was the main conclusion of the Hondras and colleagues' systematic review of the research literature on manual therapy for asthma?

9. How did the conclusions of the Wiberg and Olafsdottir studies on adjustment/manipulation for infantile colic differ from one another?

10. How would you characterize the currently available research data on the effectiveness of adjustment/manipulation for nocturnal enuresis?

Concept *Questions*

1. How would you respond to someone who states that no one under the age of 18 should receive chiropractic care?

2. What modifications of adjusting techniques are required in working with young children?

REFERENCES

1. Kessler RC et al: Long-term trends in the use of complementary and alternative medical therapies in the United States, *Ann Intern Med* 135(4):262, 2001.
2. Eisenberg DM et al: Trends in alternative medicine use in the United States, 1990-1997: results of a follow-up national survey, *JAMA* 280(18):1569, 1998.
3. Smith M, Carber L: Chiropractic health care in health professional shortage areas in the United States, *Am J Public Health* 92:2001, 2002.
4. Bussing R et al: Use of complementary and alternative medicine for symptoms of attention-deficit hyperactivity disorder, *Psychiatr Serv* 53:1096, 2002.
5. Pitetti R et al: Complementary and alternative medicine use in children, *Pediatr Emerg Care* 17:165, 2001.
6. Ottolini MC et al: Complementary and alternative medicine use among children in the Washington, DC, area, *Ambul Pediatr* 1:122, 2001.
7. Sawni-Sikand A, Schubiner H, Thomas RL: Use of complementary/alternative therapies among children in primary care pediatrics, *Ambul Pediatr* 2:99, 2002.
8. Lee AC, Li DH, Kemper KJ: Chiropractic care for children, *Arch Pediatr Adolesc Med* 154:401, 2000.
9. Alcantara J, Plaugher G: Subluxation. In Anrig CA, Plaugher G, editors: *Pediatric chiropractic*, Baltimore, 1995, Williams and Wilkins.
10. Gatterman M: *Foundations of chiropractic: subluxation*, St Louis, 1995, Mosby.
11. Banks GM, Transfeldt EE: Biomechanics. In Weinstein SL, editor: *The pediatric spine*, New York, 1994, Raven Press.
12. Ogden JA et al: Development and maturation of the axial skeleton. In Weinstein SL, editor: *The pediatric spine*, New York, 1994, Raven Press.
13. Anrig C: Chiropractic approaches to pregnancy and pediatric care. In Plaugher G, editor: *Textbook of clinical chiropractic: a specific biomechanical approach*, Baltimore, 1993, Williams & Wilkins.
14. Forrester JA, Anrig CA: The prenatal and perinatal period. In Anrig CA, Plaugher G, editors: *Pediatric chiropractic*, Baltimore, 1998, Williams & Wilkins.
15. Flynn JM, Lou JE, Ganley TJ: Prevention of sports injuries in children, *Curr Opin Pediatr* 14:719, 2002.
16. Boyd R et al: Whiplash associated disorder in children attending the emergency department, *Emerg Med J* 19:311, 2002.
17. Willner S: Adolescent idiopathic scoliosis: etiology. In Weinstein SL, editor: *The pediatric spine*, New York, 1994, Raven Press.
18. Pickar JG, Wheeler JD: Response of muscle proprioceptors to spinal manipulative-like loads in the anesthetized cat, *J Manipulative Physiol Ther* 24:2, 2001.
19. Dishman JD, Ball KA, Burke J: First prize: central motor excitability changes after spinal manipulation: a transcranial magnetic stimulation study, *J Manipulative Physiol Ther* 25:1, 2002.
20. Buerger MA: History and physical assessment. In Anrig CA, Plaugher G, editors: *Pediatric chiropractic*, Baltimore, 1995, Williams & Wilkins.
21. Leboeuf-Yde C et al: Motion palpation findings and self-reported low back pain in a population-based study sample, *J Manipulative Physiol Ther* 25:80, 2002.
22. Panzer DM: The reliability of lumbar motion palpation, *J Manipulative Physiol Ther* 15:518, 1992.
23. Plaugher G, Alcantara J: Adjusting the pediatric spine, *Top Clin Chiropr* 4:59, 1997.
24. Rosner AL: *Infant and child care: an assessment of research*, Norwalk, Iowa, 2003, Foundation for Chiropractic Education and Research.
25. Hondras MA, Linde K, Jones AP: Manual therapy for asthma, *Cochrane Database Syst Rev* (1):CD00100, 2001.
26. Balon J et al: A comparison of active and simulated chiropractic manipulation as adjunctive treatment for childhood asthma, *N Engl J Med* 339:1013, 1998.
27. Bronfort G et al: Chronic pediatric asthma and chiropractic spinal manipulation: a prospective clinical series and randomized clinical pilot study, *J Manipulative Physiol Ther* 24:369, 2001.

28. Klougart N, Nilsson N, Jacobsen J: Infantile colic treated by chiropractors: a prospective study of 316 cases, *J Manipulative Physiol Ther* 12:281, 1989.

29. Wiberg JM, Nordsteen J, Nilsson N: The short-term effect of spinal manipulation in the treatment of infantile colic: a randomized controlled clinical trial with a blinded observer, *J Manipulative Physiol Ther* 22:517, 1999.

30. Olafsdottir E et al: Randomised controlled trial of infantile colic treated with chiropractic spinal manipulation, *Arch Dis Child* 84:138, 2001.

31. Leboeuf-Yde C et al: Chiropractic care of children with nocturnal enuresis: a prospective outcome study, *J Manipulative Physiol Ther* 14:110, 1991.

32. Blomerth PR: Functional nocturnal enuresis, *J Manipulative Physiol Ther* 17:335, 1994.

33. Reed et al: Chiropractic management of primary nocturnal enuresis, *J Manipulative Physiol Ther* 17:596, 1994.

Caring for Aging Patients

Lisa Zaynab Killinger, DC

Key Terms

CEREBROVASCULAR
  ACCIDENT
DERMATOLOGIST
GERIATRICS

MEDITERRANEAN DIET
MORBIDITY
MORTALITY
OSTEOPOROSIS

PAPANICOLAOU (PAP)
  SMEAR
STROKE

Caring for aging patients presents the chiropractor with unique challenges and opportunities. The complex health care needs of older patients demand more of the doctor of chiropractic: sharpness of assessment skills, vigilance for changes in health status, patience, and a gentler touch. Older patients present chiropractors with opportunities to gain insight into the future, insight into a past about which most people have only read, and insight into themselves as chiropractors and human beings.

In working with older patients, chiropractors have the opportunity not only to improve function and relieve pain through the use of chiropractic manual procedures, but also to actively practice health promotion and disease prevention by applying knowledge of health risk factors and encouraging healthy diet and proper exercise.

This chapter summarizes current demographic trends in the aging of the population; discusses risk factors and preventive strategies for heart disease, cancer, **stroke**, and **osteoporosis**; and describes the stages of joint degeneration and their relevance to chiropractic geriatric practice. It begins the discussion of technique options (presented in detail in Chapter 17) for cases in which chiropractic care is needed but certain standard adjustments are contraindicated; and proposes ways to make a chiropractic practice *age-friendly*.

RESPONDING TO SPECIAL NEEDS OF GERIATRIC PATIENTS

Providing health care for an older person forces clinicians to marshal all their abilities and expertise. The clinical presentation of an older patient is often fraught with challenges. An older person may have a complex health history and equally complex physical examination findings, which are further obfuscated by the use of multiple medications, over-the-counter supplements, and folk remedies, all of which may be self-prescribed. The confluence of these factors may challenge the diagnostic skills of even the most skilled practitioner because even a seemingly uncomplicated case of mechanical low back pain may be the result of multiple coexisting factors which might include hypertonic muscles, sprained ligaments, or an undiscovered visceral pathology. Thus, a chiropractor must be vigilant to the possibility that a patient may require co-management, additional consultations, further testing, or referral, even if the clinician determines the patient's chief complaint to be a vertebral subluxation complex amenable to spinal adjustment.

Application of the art of chiropractic for an older person goes far beyond simply 'thrusting less hard.' Chiropractors are fortunate to be able to choose from a long list of technique systems ranging from those focusing on alignment of the uppermost vertebral segments (upper cervical techniques) to those

Continued

primarily emphasizing the stability of the pelvis (Logan Basic). Moreover, the use of high velocity low amplitude (HVLA) thrusting-type adjustments need not be abandoned, as long as normal age-related changes are taken into consideration. Lastly, it must be emphasized that chiropractic care provided to an older person extends beyond the application of adjustments. Evidence-based lifestyle changes and preventive health screenings may also be incorporated to enhance the health status of the older patient. Indeed, such expanded approaches may strengthen the doctor-patient relationship, an area in which chiropractic, as a profession, traditionally excels.

Chiropractic care of an older person is as simple or complex as the older person. It is imperative that chiropractors not erroneously assume that nothing can be offered to a person with chronic pain, structural complications, or a complex health presentation. With so much diversity in the profession, it seems inevitable that one of the myriad approaches will resonate with the special needs of an older patient. The challenge, as with all patients, is to modify care plans to meet the aging patient's special needs, and to set realistic and achievable goals.

Brian Gleberzon, DC
Chiropractic educator and clinician
Toronto, Ontario

RISING AGE WAVE

In the 1990s, approximately one third of the patients in a typical chiropractic practice were over the age of 50, and one half of those were over age 65.[1] On any given day in the United States, 6000 people celebrate their sixty-fifth birthday, and by 2010, nearly 10,000 a day are expected to reach that milestone.[2] If current trends continue, by the year 2030, approximately one in every four Americans will be over the age of 65.[2]

At the top end of the age scale, over 100,000 people in the United States are over the age of 100, and by the year 2050, estimates suggest that one million centenarians will be living in America.[2] The most rapidly growing segment of the population is the over-85 age category,[3] a situation for which no historic precedent exists. With the *graying* of the population, the number of older patients seen in chiropractic practice is rising. People are living longer, living stronger,[4] and seeking alternative health care choices in growing numbers.[5-10]

Caring for an aging population is a major focus in chiropractic today, both in scientific literature and in practice. In recent years, several chiropractic journals have dedicated issues to the topic of aging.[11-16] Articles in a 2002 issue of *Topics in Clinical Chiropractic* highlight key areas of geriatric research and practice, with an interdisciplinary team of authors. This issue is a must-read for chiropractors interested in the care of aging patients. Other authors and journals have published articles on chiropractic geriatric practice, prevention and health promotion for the elderly, and skeletal conditions commonly seen in older people, such as osteoporosis and osteoarthritis.[17-26] **Geriatrics** is an area that will continue to grow as the age wave rolls across society, affecting everything in its path, including the chiropractic profession.

TREATING DISEASE OR PROMOTING HEALTH?

During the last decade, chiropractic, along with complementary and alternative health care in general, has grown in popularity[5,6] to the point at which chiropractic is increasingly viewed as a part of the health care mainstream.[8-10] According to the Council on Chiropractic Education, chiropractors are trained to be primary contact providers. This role includes providing patient education in health promotion and prevention, health screening assessment, and managing common acute and chronic problems.[10] Aging chiropractic patients seek care primarily for musculoskeletal problems,[5-7] but they may also benefit from the approach to care that more patient-centered chiropractors offer. In many cases, these benefits may be in areas not directly related to the symptoms that initially led them to seek chiropractic care.

Patients' health and well being are of primary importance to both the chiropractor and the patient. The chiropractor, whatever his or her philosophic perspective, must engage in activities that will most effectively increase the patient's wellness potential, whether the patient is 20 or 80 years of age. As Daniel David Palmer tellingly noted, "I have never considered anything below my dignity if it is for the good of the patient." To achieve maximum benefits for their patients, doctors of chiropractic, similar to thoughtful health care providers of all professions, can enter into a partnership with each patient to establish a plan for achieving optimal wellness, as well as preventing disease.

Since its inception, chiropractic has sought to improve the quality of life and help patients achieve optimal wellness.[27,28] *Healthy People 2010* (HP 2010) is the prevention agenda for the United States. This document is a statement of national health objectives designed to identify the most significant preventable threats to health and to establish national goals to reduce these threats. With the development and publication of the HP 2010 objectives,[29] the nation's health care paradigm is shifting toward health promotion and prevention (HPP), rather than being strictly concerned with crisis intervention and reaction to chronic, debilitating disease.[29] The HP 2010 document is available online at www.health.gov/healthypeople/. This *wellness* movement is gaining momentum, a trend also reflected in the health promotion–related articles becoming commonplace in chiropractic and other journals and publications.* Chiropractors currently participate in a significant amount of HPP activity, in addition to providing other primary care services.[19-21,33] In fact, chiropractors recommend exercises (one of the HP 2010 objectives)[29] to nearly 70% of their patients.[20,21,29] Chiropractic care, with adjustments and other manual procedures at its core, often includes recommendations about exercise, dietary counseling, and other related health promotion interventions, as appropriate in each patient's case.[20,21] Interestingly, patients under chiropractic care report a decreased use of non-prescription[20,21] and prescription drugs[26] and have fewer medical provider visits than the gen-

eral population.[26] Because prescription drug errors are exceedingly common (one in five older adults is prescribed an inappropriate drug or drug combination) and prescription drug errors are a leading cause of death in older adults,[38] it may be time for the society to explore and use conservative, drug-free health care, such as chiropractic, as a viable choice for health and wellness in the care of the older patient.

In the first major descriptive study on chiropractic maintenance care (MC) for patients over 65, Rupert and colleagues[21] compared patients seen by chiropractors and medical physicians to those seen only by medical physicians (Fig. 16-1). Defining MC as *HPP care* that includes chiropractic adjustments, along with a variety of interventions that may include adjunctive therapies, as well as education on exercise, nutrition, and relaxation, these investigators found that patients undergoing MC (over four visits per year for over 5 years) had annual health care expenditures of $3106 compared with $10,041 for non-MC patients.[21] Although the data do not allow the inference of a direct causal relationship between MC and the decreased health costs, Rupert and colleagues' data do suggest value in conceiving chiropractic practice more broadly than the relief of musculoskeletal symptoms.

TOP HEALTH CONCERNS IN OLDER ADULTS

The statistics on the major causes of **mortality** and **morbidity** in older adults tell a tale of the need for better HPP. As the population ages, these demographic shifts will carry with them increasing

---

My older patients have always been my favorites. They are on time for their appointments. They rarely miss an appointment, but if they *have* to miss, they call to apologize and reschedule. They listen to my advice, they refer new patients, and they inspire me in every way. Older patients truly *need* chiropractic care and are most appreciative of the care they receive.

Paige Thibodeau, DC
Scotts Valley, California

---

*References 20-24, 27, 28, 30-37.

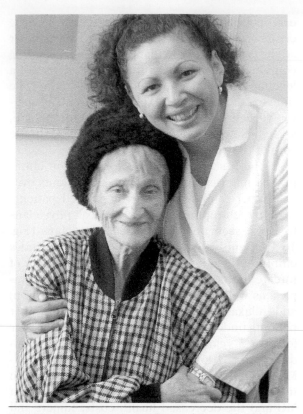

Fig. **16-1** Doctor-patient relationships with older patients can be deeply satisfying.

health costs and an increasing prevalence of the common chronic conditions of the older patient. After all, the elderly population suffers the most disability and has the highest health care costs related to chronic diseases such as arthritis, heart disease, and osteoporosis.[39-41]

The three major illnesses causing death[4,37] for people over the age of 65 in America are:

1. Heart disease
2. Cancer (lung, breast, prostate, colon, and others)
3. Stroke

In many cases, conditions can be prevented or their onset significantly delayed through HPP interventions involving changes in health habits and lifestyle.

Heart Disease

Among people 65 and older, heart disease is the leading cause of both death and hospitalization in the United States. Heart disease is also the second or third leading cause of disability in the geriatric population after arthritis.[4,37]

The risk factors for heart disease[36,37]:

- Family history of heart disease
- High cholesterol
- High blood pressure
- Smoking
- Overweight
- Excessive consumption of saturated fat

The scientific literature strongly supports several dietary recommendations for people with heart disease.[42-48] A variety of diets have been studied in the prevention of heart disease, including the **Mediterranean diet** (higher in fish, fruits, vegetables, omega-3 fatty acids, and fiber; lower in red meats),[42] as well as diets low in sodium[43] and cholesterol[44,45] and high in antioxidants[46,47] and fiber.[44]

Preventive strategies for heart disease[36]:

- Engaging in regular physical activity
- Quitting smoking
- Losing weight, if overweight or obese
- Eating more fruits, vegetables, and whole grains
- Limiting alcohol use
- Using less salt and choosing lower fat foods

Cancer

Cancers are the second leading cause of death among older adults, with millions affected each year in the United States alone.[4] Most common cancers are preventable or are amenable to treatment if identified early.[36] For chiropractors, a worthwhile goal can be to provide regular screenings for various types of cancer (if permitted by state law) or to make sure that patients receive the recommended screenings for various types of cancer (Table 16-1).

Most common and deadly cancers[4,36]:

Skin cancer: The most common form of cancer; preventable and survivable if detected early

Lung cancer: The leading cause of cancer deaths resulting from cancer in geriatrics

Prostate or breast cancer: The second leading cause of cancer deaths in geriatrics

Table **16-1** RECOMMENDED SCREENING SCHEDULE FOR COMMON CANCERS IN OLDER ADULTS

Type of Cancer	Risk Factors	Symptoms	Recommended Screenings
Breast	No children or having first child after age 35, family history of cancer, high-fat diet, alcohol or caffeine intake, oral contraceptives	Lump in breast tissue, change in breast or nipple (e.g., redness, tenderness)	Baseline mammogram at age 40 (every other year after that), monthly breast self-examination, annual breast examination by a physician
Prostate	History of venereal disease or prostate cancer, diet high in animal fat or caffeine, vasectomy, over age 50, African American	Constant pain in low back, pelvis, or thighs; difficult, painful, or interrupted urine flow; frequent or bloody urination	DRE, blood tests, including PSA or PAP
Colon	Family history of colon cancer, low-fiber diet, low calcium intake, high-fat diet, chronic constipation	Persistent diarrhea or constipation, blood in stool, tiredness, loss of weight for no apparent reason, frequent intestinal gas or cramps	Annual fecal occult blood test, sigmoidoscopy every 5 years, colonoscopy every 10 years
Skin	Family history of skin cancer, exposure to the sun or ultraviolet radiation, fair skin, scars from severe sunburns, moles	Change in shape, size, or color of mole; skin lesion that will not heal, especially on the face, hands, ears, or shoulders	Vigilance of all moles and skin lesions, annual dermatologic examination, especially when suspicious lesions are present
Lung	Smoking; exposure to second-hand smoke, asbestos, pesticides, or chemicals; chronic bronchitis; history of TB	Productive persistent cough, bloody sputum, chest pain	Chest x-ray when clinical signs are present

DRE, Annual digital rectal examination; *PSA*, prostate specific antigen; *PAP*, prostate acid phosphatase; *TB*, tuberculosis.

Colon cancer: The third leading cancer incidence in both genders over age 55

Ovarian cancer: The fourth leading cause of cancer deaths in women

Esophagus and stomach cancer: The seventh and ninth leading causes of cancer deaths

Skin Cancer

Chiropractors (DCs) generally see patients more frequently than do allopathic physicians, and they examine areas of the skin not routinely visualized on many medical visits. Thus DCs sometimes have the opportunity to identify skin cancer in its earliest stages, potentially saving lives. Approximately one in four people over age 50 will have at least one incident of skin cancer,

with the face, ears, and neck most susceptible, resulting from cumulative exposure to the sun. As "sun worshippers" age, the incidence of skin cancers may well increase, although this trend may be mitigated by recent public health efforts to increase awareness of the negative effects of overexposure to the sun.

Simple lifestyle changes can prevent the vast majority of skin cancers. Counseling patients of all ages on minimizing exposure to the sun or the ultraviolet radiation of tanning beds is an important primary prevention strategy. DCs should advise patients who work in the sun to wear light-colored, long-sleeved shirts, hats that shade the face, neck, and ears, and sunscreen on any exposed skin. Over one half of all skin cancers can be prevented by practicing these simple preventive measures.[36,37]

DCs must be aware of any suspicious skin lesions, noting the size, location, and shape in the patient's file. On subsequent visits, the lesion should be reevaluated for any changes. Suspicious cases should be referred without delay to a **dermatologist,** with the DC emphasizing to the patient the importance of following through on the referral.

The following pneumonic is a useful, simple tool for early detection of skin cancer in chiropractic practice. Because skin cancers are preventable and treatable if caught early, knowing these signs is crucial[21]:

A — **A**symmetry
B — Irregular **B**orders
C — Variation in **C**olor within the same lesion
D — Growth in **D**iameter greater than 6 mm

Lung Cancer

Lung cancer is the most common type of cancer (and cancer-related death) in both male and female older patients, aside from skin cancer.[36,37] Smoking is, by far, the most significant risk factor for lung cancer. Smoking causes more deaths per year than murder, suicide, and car accidents combined.[4] Because smoking is the habit-lifestyle choice with the most serious negative health consequences and is the key risk factor for lung cancer, heart disease, and stroke, DCs should be motivated as a profession to encourage all patients to quit.

Patients who quit smoking report that the most influential factor in their decision to quit was simply *that their doctor recommended it.*[37] DCs, as members of the largest drug-free health profession, *must* take the time to encourage, request, and implore patients to stop smoking. Because DCs see patients with some regularity, an opportunity is presented to remind patients regularly of the importance of quitting and to support and monitor progress and compliance.

DCs must also recognize the clinical signs that may indicate the presence of lung cancer, including:

• Persistent cough
• Blood in the sputum
• Chest pain
• Shortness of breath
• Painful or labored respiration

Any patient with these symptoms and a history of tobacco use requires a posterior-to-anterior (P-A) chest x-ray film to rule out lung cancer. Even if the DC has taken standard thoracic spine x-rays of the patient, adequate visualization of the lung fields is best accomplished by taking a P-A chest film. In thoracic spine x-rays, to obtain the proper density for the thoracic spine, the air-filled lung fields are often overexposed. This overexposure makes thoracic spine films an inappropriate tool for ruling out significant lung diseases. All questionable radiographs should be referred to a chiropractic radiologist or medical radiologist for further evaluation. With early detection, lung cancer is highly treatable.[36,37] Early detection is also essential to prevent metastasis from the lung to osseous structures, particularly the thoracic spine.

Gender-Related Cancers

The aged population is at the highest risk for gender-related cancers, most of which are quite survivable if detected early. Chiropractic patients should be asked when they had their most recent screening examination for breast or prostate cancer. The recommended screenings are as follows[36,54,55]:

For women over age 50:

• Annual palpatory breast examination by a health professional
• Mammogram every other year
• Monthly breast self-examination
• Annual pelvic examination and **Papanicolaou (Pap) smear**

For men over age 50:

• Annual digital rectal examination
• Annual prostate specific antigen (PSA) blood test

Most patients can easily recall such examinations and will be able to report the month and year of their most recent screening. Patients should also be informed that the scientific literature suggests that a low-fat diet, decreasing obesity and alcohol consumption, and quitting smoking may be protective against gender-related cancers, including prostate and breast cancers.[36,54]

Colon Cancer

Colon cancer, which strikes 1 in every 17 people in the United States, is most common in people over age 50. The scientific evidence is strongly in support of dietary changes for preventing colon cancer.[36,37,55] DCs can participate in preventing colon cancer by recommending[55]:

1. A diet low in fat and high in fiber
2. Restriction of alcohol intake
3. An annual fecal occult blood test

Advising patients on ways to increase fiber in their diet to the recommended intake of 30 grams or more per day is simple.[22,28,55] Some bran breakfast cereals contain one third of the daily recommendation of fiber; beans and seeded berries are close behind. Fruits, vegetables, and whole grain breads or pastas may help prevent colon cancer in chiropractic patients. It all starts with simply bringing up the topic, as well as educating and empowering the patient to choose a lifestyle of prevention rather than risk.

Stroke

Stroke (**cerebrovascular accident**) ranks as the third leading cause of death in older adults, following heart disease and cancer.[4] Every year, over 150,000 people die and many more are disabled as a result of stroke in the United States, with the vast majority over the age of 65.[4,37] Because treatments for stroke are quite limited and costly, *prevention* is of utmost importance. Stroke prevention focuses on the two major causes of stroke: atherosclerosis and hypertension. Numerous studies show that physical activity is associated with lower stroke risks,[4,56-60] thus recommending regular physical activity to patients is important. Diets higher in whole grains, fish, fruits and vegetables, vitamins C and B, potassium, calcium, and magnesium, and foods lower in fat, calories, and meat-based proteins are also recommended to reduce the risk of stroke.[61-63] These dietary recommendations may also have value in preventing other diseases common in older adults (e.g., heart disease, obesity, colon cancer), thus such advice may be useful for most older patients.

Prudent examination of the older patient and attention to the patient's history and stroke risk factors are crucial. Every health care provider must know the risk factors for stroke so that prevention recommendations can be offered and high-risk patients can be identified before chiropractic technique decision-making occurs. Equally important is to know the signs and symptoms of stroke, should one occur.

The risk factors of stroke[36,37]:

- Smoking
- High blood pressure
- Family history of stroke
- Use of oral contraceptives (women)
- Sedentary lifestyle
- High-fat diet
- Atherosclerotic vessels

The signs and symptoms of stroke:

- Unusual visual disturbances
- Difficulty speaking
- Weakness or numbness in face or extremities
- Focal headaches of sudden onset that can last seconds to months
- Dizziness or loss of consciousness

Osteoporosis

Bone health is essential to musculoskeletal well being. Patients should be encouraged to engage in activities and incorporate lifestyle practices that help maintain optimal bone density. The societal impact of osteoporosis is substantial. Currently, approximately $10 billion is spent annually in the United States for diagnosis, treatment, and rehabilitation related to the over 1.3 million fractures sustained in patients with osteoporosis.[64] Osteoporosis is one of the most prevalent conditions in elderly patients, with over 25 million people affected in the United States alone.[64] Osteoporosis is considered a part of *normal aging* for a female patient to lose 1% of bone mass per year after the age of 30, approximately twice the rate of bone loss for men.[65] However, prevention and health promotion can slow or reverse this process in most patients.[66-71]

DCs can and should take an active role in the prevention and early identification of osteoporosis. Osteoporosis risk factors are as follows:

- Preventable risks[22,25,66,67]:
  - Sedentary lifestyle
  - Aversion or avoidance of dairy products and other sources of dietary calcium

- Consumption of caffeinated beverages
- Alcohol consumption
- Consumption of soft drinks ("pop")
- Smoking
- Diet high in meat-based protein
- Nonpreventable risks:
  - Familial history of osteoporosis
  - Fair-skinned and small-framed individuals
  - Asian or European descent
  - Hysterectomy early in adulthood
  - Women

Most osteoporosis risk factors are preventable. When a DC sees a patient who is at high risk for osteoporosis, letting her or him know about their risk factors and recommending ways to increase bone density or at least decrease or stop bone loss is essential. Although the best time to increase bone density is before menopause, it is never too late to slow the rate of bone loss or even to begin to build bone density* through implementing prevention and health-promotion strategies. The real key to preventing osteoporosis is regular physical activity, particularly *axial-loading* exercises, such as walking, running, or stair stepping.[49,66-68]

Numerous controlled clinical trials have measured and compared the bone mineral density of postmenopausal women who completed a program of weight lifting or axial-loading exercise with women who did not participate in such exercise programs. In each study, the women who performed axial-loading exercises actually increased their bone density, as did those engaged in specially tailored weight-lifting programs, even the older, more frail patients.[73-75] The women in the control groups (those who did not exercise) in each of these studies failed to realize any positive changes in bone density. The important evidence-based message for DCs to relay to their patients is that it is *never* too late to get involved in a routine of physical activity to improve bone health. An excellent publication, offering a visual presentation of various exercises appropriate for patients who wish to prevent frailty in their later years, is available free of charge through the National Institute

*References 49, 66, 67, 69, 71, 72.

on Aging.[68] The scientific evidence is also overwhelmingly in support of increasing dietary intake of both calcium and vitamin D as a preventive measure against osteoporosis and related fractures.[69-72] The U.S. National Institutes of Health recommends a daily calcium intake of 1500 mg for people over age 65.[71]

Basics of caring for people at risk for osteoporosis include the following[36,66,67]:

1. Evaluating patients for the presence of clinical risk factors so as to make appropriate prevention and health-promotion recommendations
2. Recommending baseline bone mineral density scan of hip for all patients over age 60
3. Counseling all at-risk patients to exercise, as their health status allows
4. Counseling all patients about the importance of dietary calcium and vitamin D
5. Advising all patients to avoid smoking and excessive alcohol and caffeine intake
6. For all older patients, assessing the risk of falls and providing precautionary measures to improve safety

JOINT DEGENERATION AND PATIENT CARE

Because the vast majority of the patients who seek chiropractic care have a chief complaint of back pain,[5-7] DCs working with older patients require an intimate familiarity with the spinal changes that come with age. McCarthy, in his 2002 article in *Topics in Clinical Chiropractic*, offers an eloquent discussion of the normal aging of the spine, the stages of spinal degeneration, and chiropractic care goals related to these stages.[76] In this article, McCarthy discusses the Kirkaldy-Willis (K-W) model[77] and its relevance to chiropractic practice. (W.H. Kirkaldy-Willis is a renowned Canadian orthopedist at the University of Saskatchewan, where chiropractic is now an essential component of back pain care in the university hospital orthopedics department.) The K-W model of degeneration was designed with an understanding of the role of subluxation or segmental dysfunction in the degenerative process. In this model, three distinct stages are discussed[77]:

- Dysfunction. Trauma or uncoordinated muscle contraction leads to facet subluxation (joint dysfunction), local pain, synovitis, segmental muscle hypertonicity, and muscle splinting, leading to further dysfunction if not addressed.
- Instability. Trauma or long-standing dysfunction leads to laxity of the facet joint capsule and bulging of the annulus, causing abnormal motion at the three-joint complex and increasing instability, often with local and referred pain.
- Stabilization. Chronic, poor biomechanics results in degenerative changes, including destruction of disk and endplates, osteophytic changes, and enlargement of the

facets, resulting in stiffness and decreases in ranges of motion and mobility.[77]

Although an individual older patient may be experiencing any one of these stages of degeneration, the elderly patient is most commonly in the stabilization phase of degeneration. Care plans for patients in the stabilization phase must address loss of mobility. If active intervention does not occur, this loss of mobility may progress to poorer functional status and decreased independence. However, with carefully planned and implemented chiropractic management plans, including stretching and flexibility activities, older patients may experience improvements in function and mobility over time. Table 16-2 summarizes patient care goals and care plans appropriate to the three K-W degenerative stages.

Based on the K-W model, younger patients (or patients with minimal trauma or biomechanical

Table **16-2** CLINICAL IMPLEMENTATION FOR THE KIRKALDY-WILLIS MODEL

Stage of Degeneration	Dysfunction	Instability	Stabilization
Clinical signs	Subluxation: three-joint complex, muscle guarding	Increased ligament laxity, abnormal motion, decreased intrinsic muscle coordination, increased disk degeneration	Decreased motion, loss of function, decreased muscle strength, increased degenerative changes
Chiropractic goals	Remove subluxations, decrease synovitis, return patient to normal activities as soon as possible	Remove stressors and subluxation, stabilize motion, return to normal activities	Maximize motion, maximize function, remove subluxations, return to normal activities
Care plan	Specific adjusting, general	Perform techniques that do not aggravate ligament laxity	Perform techniques that focus on increasing motion to spine and joints
Health and wellness strategies	Assess activities, promote good posture and sleep habits	Encourage smoking cessation, weight loss (if needed), and increase physical activity in sedentary patients	Advise patient to increase flexibility (e.g., yoga) and increase strength and aerobic fitness, maintain hydration
Prevention	Educate patient about proper lifting and physical activities, promote healthy lifestyle choices	Supplementation, osteoporosis checklist, promote healthy lifestyle choices	Home safety checklist, comprehensive geriatric assessment, promote healthy lifestyle choices

Patient Compliance Strategy: *Small Sustainable Changes.*

stress) may need chiropractic care simply to remove a subluxation. Patients who have developed spinal instability (e.g., through trauma or repetitive stress) may require both chiropractic adjustments *and* muscular balancing or strengthening techniques to achieve optimal wellness. In such cases, muscular integrity and altered biomechanics may be addressed through incorporating specifically designed exercise plans,[76] or the DC may prefer co-management with another health care provider, such as a physical therapist or occupational therapist, to design and implement a plan for overall patient rehabilitation and restoring biomechanical stability in the spine. Patients (in the stabilization phase) who have had poorly addressed or chronic biomechanical instability will begin to lose function because of pain or limitations in their ranges of motion. In these patients (usually the older patient), maintaining motion in the spine and joints is essential in delaying or decreasing disability and slowing degenerative processes.[76,77]

Care strategies should be developed only after considering the patient's age, history (including injuries), stage of degeneration, and previous response to chiropractic (and other) care. These considerations should mold the care plan, addressing the needs of *that* patient *at that time*.

AGE-FRIENDLY PRACTICE

As the population grays, the economics of health care in general, and of chiropractic practice in particular, are likely to reflect more of a *patient's market*. Older patients may begin shopping for providers who make the effort to anticipate, understand, and accommodate their needs. Conscious efforts to make a care provider's practice more *age-friendly* are highly recommended. The following checklist (Box 16-1) suggests possible areas for enhancement.

Leading the Healthy Aging Movement in the Community

Actions speak louder than words. DCs can contribute to their communities as advocates for and leaders in *healthy aging* programs. This action takes effort, but given changing demo-graphics, the effort is worthwhile. DCs who take the time to organize activities and events to promote healthy aging soon become recognized as doctors with genuine concern for their older patients. The following is a list of activities a DC might initiate:

1. "The Thousand-Mile Walk": The elder patient base is challenged to walk a thousand miles! Each patient can set a monthly goal appropriate for his or her health status and walk that amount during the month. Patients must keep a diary and are encouraged to walk with a buddy. At the end of each week, patients report their miles to add to the chart in the DC's reception room. (A clever visual of the thousand-mile walk can be created to post in the reception room, and few patients will want to be left behind.) Incentives can be offered for the greatest increase in mileage (according to ability) or for the most miles walked. Some patients may walk a few miles a day, and others may walk a couple of miles a month. The DC can invite the local news station to watch the progress as the older patients walk 1000 miles for health.

2. "Climb Mount Everest": Patients are invited to start at base camp and participate in *wellness* activities that will earn them points that take them higher and higher up a symbolic Mount Everest. Points can be given for any activity that adds to the wellness of the patient: walking, yoga, using seatbelts, eating a low-fat meal, drinking six glasses of water per day, and so forth. A great visual effect may be a large poster of a mountain in the waiting room and watching as the "mountaineers'" game pieces (representing participating older patients) reach the summit. This activity is great for both "flatlanders" and mountaineers alike.

3. Sponsoring a Senior Olympic Team in the community: The DC's office can encourage participation in the Senior Olympics and even offer incentives to patients who represent the "team" in an event that they love. Holding training camps, pre-Olympic

Box **16-1** AGE-FRIENDLY PRACTICE CHECKLIST

STAIRS

1. Are there unnecessary steps?
2. Can a dangerous step be replaced with a ramp?
3. Are all steps clearly marked, with a contrasting color strip on stair itself and a warning sign at eye level saying "Step Up" or "Watch Your Step?"
4. Are *all* steps equipped with a handrail, even single steps?

BATHROOMS

1. Do the bathrooms have a potentially slippery floor?
2. Are paper towels or hand dryers positioned to avoid dripping water on the floor where patients will have to walk?
3. Do the toilets have handrails?
4. Can the doors be opened (or unlocked) if a patient falls or needs assistance in the bathroom?

ADJUSTING ROOMS

1. Do the tables bring the patient to a standing position, and if so, can they be adjusted to bring the patient up more slowly?
2. Can the tables be *stopped* when halfway up to allow time for frailer patients or patients with orthostatic hypotension to accommodate to the upright position?
3. Is there sufficient contrast between the footplate of the table and the carpet?
4. Is the carpet very low pile? Shag or deep pile may cause falls.
5. Is there room on either side of the table for the doctor to stand and support the patient as the table is raised up or as patient gets up from table?

REEXAMINING THE FORMS, THROUGH AGING EYES

1. Do the patient history or intake forms have large print, such as 14-point font bold?
2. Is a set of specific forms available for doing a comprehensive assessment of various aspects of the general health status of aging patients (e.g., Mini-Mental Status examination, Geriatric Depression Scale, Functional Status Index; Nutritional/Oral Health Status forms)?

COMMUNICATING EFFECTIVELY WITH THE OLDEST PATIENTS

1. Can background music be turned off while interviewing or caring for older patients?
2. Can the DC be positioned during a patient interview or history such that the patient can read the DC's lips and hear the voice clearly?
3. Is a prepared resource list available for information on senior services and appropriate referrals based on the needs of the aging patients?
4. Is appropriate health-promotion and disease-prevention information related to the needs or health concerns of older patients available?

GROUNDS AND EXTERIOR

1. Is the office wheelchair accessible?
2. Are the sidewalks in good repair and free of leaves, snow, and loose gravel?
3. Are parking lots well lighted and in good repair?

dinners, or just having patients volunteer to help at the Senior Olympics will work. Senior Olympics is an inspirational event that is held in virtually every major city.

4. Organizing the "Senior Force" in the community: The DC can, starting with his or her patients and their friends, organize a team of volunteers. Incentives can be offered for the most hours of service or the most innovative service to the community.

Volunteering has been shown to improve the health of older people, even when all other factors are constant.

5. Declaring "Bone Health Week": Either independently or in collaboration with a national osteoporosis organization, the DC can sponsor a series of *bone health* events in the office. Activities start with a free osteoporosis risk factor analysis, followed by an osteoporosis prevention

mini-seminar and a series of bone-building activities such a free weight-lifting class, bone building walks, and so forth.

6. Arranging a "Healthy Hearts, Healing Hands" month: The DC can invite a speaker from the American Heart Association to the office and can offer free blood pressure checks one morning a week for a month. The DC's office can be filled with literature on heart health. Additionally, a heart-healthy dinner, a series of heart walks, a heart-smart cooking class by a local chef can be added. The DC can help prevent this number one killer of older men and women!

7. The DC can also plan his or her own event, create a wellness program, and have fun promoting healthy aging.

Health Promotion and the Value of Physical Activity

Providing health-promotion advice to older patients is an essential part of chiropractic practice. Older patients, contrary to the stereotype that they are too set in their ways and unwilling to change, are actually the *most* likely to comply with their doctors' recommendations.[78-81] Older patients are more likely to have experienced a serious health incident, such as a fall, a heart attack, or a brush with death. As a result, older patients are frequently quite motivated to comply with a doctor's recommendations to delay or prevent future health problems. After all, the most valued possession of many aging people is their independence. Wisdom and common sense dictate that if walking will prevent a move to the nursing home, then most older people will be willing to walk on a regular basis. As noted earlier, the scientific literature supports physical activity as a principal key to better health.* A simple and undeniable condition of existence is that life is supported, sustained, and enhanced by staying active, mentally, physically, and spiritually. The DC must play an active role in modeling healthy behaviors and educating patients about the value of activities such as regular physical activity.

The benefits to older patients of staying engaged in life, sharing their skills, and contributing to society are immeasurable. Viewing aging patients in the larger context of their contribution to a world in which wisdom, experience, and the time to share those gifts are valued and appreciated is essential. As society ages, DCs have an excellent opportunity to learn from their older patients while contributing to the enhancement and promotion of health.

*References 49, 56-60, 73, 75.

HPP RESOURCES FOR OLDER PEOPLE AND GERIATRIC CAREGIVERS

Alzheimer's Disease Education and Referral Center
Phone: 800-438-4380
Website: www.alzheimers.org

American Cancer Society
Phone: 800-ACS-2345
Website: www.cancer.org

American Association of Retired Persons
601 E Street, NW
Washington, DC 20049
Website: www.aarp.org

American Heart Association
Phone: 1-800-AHA-USA1

American Society on Aging
Phone: 415-974-9600
Website: www.asaging.org

Arthritis Foundation
Website: www.arthritis.org

Canadian Task Force on Periodic Health Examination
Phone: 519-682-4292, ext. 2327

Elderweb
Website: www.elderweb.com

Alliance for aging Research
Website: www.agingresearch.org

Review *Questions*

1. What are the three major causes of death in Western industrialized nations?
2. What are the key risk factors for heart disease?
3. Which form of cancer is most likely to be detected in a typical chiropractic examination?
4. What dietary advice would be helpful in preventing colon cancer?
5. What are some diagnostic signs indicating possible lung cancer?
6. Is referral to a medical physician always required in cases in which the DC detects the apparent presence of cancer?
7. What are the major risk factors for stroke?
8. What are the major preventable and nonpreventable risk factors for osteoporosis?
9. Describe the K-W model of joint degeneration.
10. What are some of the ways a chiropractic practice can be more age-friendly?

Concept *Questions*

1. Patients under chiropractic care use fewer nonprescription and prescription drugs than the general population. Is this use a result of the benefits of chiropractic care, or does chiropractic attract patients who need or desire fewer pharmaceuticals?
2. In what ways is the graying of the population likely to influence the type of practice the DC has 10 years from now?

REFERENCES

1. Christensen MG et al: *Job analysis of chiropractic 2000: a project report, survey analysis, and summary of the practice of chiropractic within the United States*, Greeley, Colo, 2000, National Board of Chiropractic Examiners.
2. Alliance for Aging Research: *Medical never-never land: ten reasons why America is not ready for the coming age boom*, Washington, DC, 2002, Alliance for Aging Research.
3. Department of Health and Human Services: *A profile of older Americans: administration on aging and the program resources department*, Washington, DC, 1996, American Association of Retired Persons.
4. National Center for Health Statistics: *Health, United States 1998*, Rockville, Md, 1999, Public Health Service.
5. Eisenberg DM et al: Unconventional medicine in the United States: prevalence, costs, and patterns of use, *N Engl J Med* 328:246, 1993.
6. Eisenberg DM et al: Trends in alternative medicine use in the United States, 1990-1997: results of a follow-up national survey, *JAMA* 280:1569, 1998.
7. Hurwitz EL et al: Use of chiropractic services from 1985-1991 in the United States and Canada, *Am J Pub Health* 88:771, 1998.
8. Meeker WC: Public demand and the integration of complementary and alternative medicine in the US health care system, *J Manipulative Physiol Ther* 23(2):123, 2000.
9. Anonymous: The mainstreaming of alternative medicine, *Consumer Reports*, p. 17, May 2000.
10. Gonyea MA: *The role of the doctor of chiropractic in the health care system in comparison with doctors of allopathic medicine and doctors of osteopathic medicine*, Arlington, Va, 1993, Foundation for Chiropractic Education and Research.
11. Morley JE et al: Back to basics: recent advances in geriatrics, *Top Clin Chiropr* 9(2):1, 2002.
12. Thomas DR et al: Nutritional considerations in older people, *Top Clin Chiropr* 9(2):7, 2002.
13. Plezbert J et al: Sensory deficits in elderly patients: progressive disclosure of clinical decision-making in two case studies, *Top Clin Chiropr* 9(2):25, 2002.
14. Nicholson CV: Putting prevention into elder care as if wellness matters most, *Top Clin Chiropr* 9(2):32, 2002.
15. Gleberzon BJ: Combating ageism through student education, *Top Clin Chiropr* 9(2):41, 2002.

16. Downes JW: The master's athlete: defying aging, *Top Clin Chiropr* 9(2):53, 2002.

17. Killinger LZ et al: Development of a model curriculum in chiropractic geriatric education: process and content, *J Neuromusculoskelet Sys* 6(4):146, 1998.

18. Hawk CK et al: Chiropractic training in the care of the geriatric patient: an assessment, *J Neuromusculoskel Sys* 5(1):15, 1997.

19. Hawk CK et al: Chiropractic care for patients aged 55 years and older: report from a practice-based research program, *J Am Geriatr Soc* 48(5):534, 2000.

20. Rupert R et al: A survey of practice patterns and the health promotion and prevention attitudes of US chiropractors: maintenance care: part I, *J Manipulative Physiol Ther* 23(1):1, 2000.

21. Rupert R et al: Maintenance care: health promotion services administered to US chiropractic patients aged 65 and older: part II, *J Manipulative Physiol Ther* 23(1):10, 2000.

22. Killinger LZ: Prevention and health promotion in the older patient. In Gleberzon B, editor: *Chiropractic care of the older patient*, Oxford, UK, 2001, Butterworth Heinemann.

23. Killinger LZ: Trauma in the geriatric patient: a chiropractic perspective with a focus on prevention, *Top Clin Chiropr* 5(3):10, 1998.

24. Killinger LZ: Promoting health and wellness in the older patient: chiropractors and the Healthy People 2010 objectives, *Top Clin Chiropr* 8(4):58, 2001.

25. Gleberzon BG, Killinger LZ: Management considerations for patients with osteoporosis and osteoarthritis: a chiropractic perspective on what's working, *Top Clin Chiropr* 9(1):38, 2002.

26. Coulter ID et al: Chiropractic patients in a comprehensive home-based geriatric assessment, follow up, and health promotion program, *Top Clin Chiropr* 3(2):46, 1996.

27. Hawk CK: Should chiropractic be a wellness profession? *Top Clin Chiropr* 7(1):23, 2000.

28. Hawk CK: Chiropractic and primary care. In: *Advances in chiropractic*, vol 3, 1996, Mosby-Yearbook.

29. US Department of Health and Human Services: *Healthy People 2010: understanding and improving health*, ed 2, Washington, DC, 2000, US Government Printing Office.

30. Fox PJ et al: Effects of a health promotion program on sustaining health behaviors in older adults, *Am J Prev Med* 13:257, 1997.

31. Anderson RT et al: Issues of aging and adherence to health interventions, *Control Clin Trials* 21:171S, 2000.

32. Talarico LD: Preventive gerontology: strategies for optimal aging, *Patient Care*, p. 195, May 1995.

33. Hawk CK et al: A survey of 492 chiropractors on primary care and prevention related issues, *J Manipulative Physiol Ther* 18:57, 1995.

34. Sawyer CE: The role of the chiropractic doctor in health promotion, Proceedings of the 1992 International Conference on Spinal Manipulation, May 15-17, 1992.

35. Kane RL: The public health paradigm. In Hickey T, Speers M, Prohaska T, editors: *Public health and aging*, Baltimore, Md, 1997, John Hopkins University Press.

36. Department of Health and Human Services, Office of Disease Prevention and Health Promotion: *Clinician's handbook on preventive services*, ed 2, Washington, DC, 1998, US Government Printing Office.

37. Hickey T et al: *Public health and aging*, Baltimore, Md, 1997, John Hopkins University Press.

38. Lazarou J, Pomeranz BH, Corey PN: Incidence of adverse drug reactions in hospitalized patients: a meta-analysis of prospective studies, *JAMA* 279(15):1200, 1998.

39. Lubitz J et al: Longevity and Medicare expenditures, *N Engl J Med* 332:999, 1995.

40. Hoffman C et al: Persons with chronic conditions: their prevalence and costs, *JAMA* 276:1473, 1996.

41. Rao JK et al: Use of complementary therapies for arthritis among patients of rheumatologists, *Annals Int Med* 131(6):409, 1999.

42. De Lorgerill M et al: Mediterranean diet, traditional risk factors, and the rate of cardiovascular complication after myocardial infarction: final report of the Lyon diet heart study, *Circulation* 99:779, 1999.

43. Whelton PK et al: Sodium restriction and weight loss in the treatment of hypertension in older persons: a randomized controlled clinical trial of non-pharmacological intervention in the elderly (TONE), *JAMA* 279:839, 1998.

44. Canadian Task Force on the Periodic Health Examination: Lowering the total blood cholesterol level to prevent coronary heart disease. In *The Canadian guide to clinical preventive health care*, Ottawa, 1994, Minister of Supply and Services.

45. US Health and Human Services, National Institutes of Health, National Heart, Lung, and Blood Institute: *Preventing and controlling high blood pressure*, NIH Publication No. 96-3655, Bethesda, Md, 1996, National Institutes of Health.

46. Hercberg S et al: The potential role of antioxidant vitamins in preventing cardiovascular diseases and cancers, *Nutrition* 14:513, 1998.

47. Stephens NG et al: Randomised controlled trial of vitamin E in patients with coronary disease: Cambridge heart antioxidant study (CHAOS), *Lancet* 347:781, 1996.

48. Russell RM et al: Modified food pyramid for people over 70 years of age, *J Nutrition* 129:751, 1999.

49. Jette AM et al: Exercise—it's never too late: the strong for life program, *Am J Pub Health* 89(1):66, 1999.

50. Manello DM: Osteoporosis: assessment and treatment options, *Top Clin Chiropr* 4(3):30, 1997.

51. Miller AL: Cardiovascular disease—toward a unified approach, *Alt Med Rev* 1(3):132, 1996.

52. National Institutes of Health: *Exercise: a guide from the National Institutes on Aging*, Publication No. 99-4258, Bethesda, Md, 1999, National Institutes of Health.

53. Solberg LI et al: A systematic primary care office-based smoking cessation program, *J Fam Pract* 30:647, 1990.

54. Austin S: Recent progress in treatment and secondary prevention of breast cancer with supplements, *Alt Med Rev* 2(1):4, 1997.

55. American Cancer Society: *Colon cancer: what is it, and what you can do to prevent it*, Washington, DC, 1999, American Cancer Society.

56. Lee I et al: Physical activity and stroke incidence: the Harvard alumni health survey, *Stroke* 29(10):2049, 1998.

57. Wannamethee G et al: Physical activity and stroke in British middle aged men, *BMJ* 304:597, 1992.

58. Gillium RF et al: Physical activity and stroke incidence in women and men: NHANES-1, *Am J Epidemiol* 143:860, 1996.

59. Abbott RD et al: Physical activity in older middle-aged men and reduced risk of stroke: the Honolulu heart program, *Am J Epidemiol* 139:881, 1994.

60. Sacco RL et al: Leisure time physical activity and ischemic stroke risk: the northern Manhattan stroke study, *Stroke* 29:380, 1998.

61. Serving K et al: Fish consumption and risk of stroke: the Zutpen study, *Stroke* 25:328, 1994.

62. Ascherio A et al: Intake of potassium, magnesium, calcium, and fiber, and risk of stroke among US men, *Circulation* 98:1198, 1998.

63. Davigus M et al: Dietary vitamin C, B, carotene, and 30 year risk of strokes: results from the western electric study, *Neuroepidemiology* 16:69, 1997.

64. Hawker G: The epidemiology of osteoporosis, *J Rheumatol* 45(23):2S, 1996.

65. Souza T: Normal aging, *Top Clin Chiropr* 3(2):1, 1996.

66. Drugay M: Healthy People 2000. Breaking the silence: a health promotion approach to osteoporosis, *J Gerontol Nurs* 23(6):36, 1997.

67. O'Connor DJ: Understanding osteoporosis and clinical strategies to assess, arrest, and restore bone loss, *Alt Med Rev* 2(1):36, 1997.

68. National Institute on Aging, National Institute of Health: *Exercise: a guide from the National Institute on Aging*, NIH Publication number 99-4258, Bethesda, Md, 1999, National Institutes of Health.

69. Dawson-Hughes B et al: A controlled clinical trial of the effect of calcium supplementation on bone density in post-menopausal women, *N Engl J Med* 323:878, 1990.

70. US National Institute of Health: *NIH consensus development conference on optimal calcium intake*, Bethesda, Md, 1994, National Institutes of Health.

71. Petrovich H et al: Pros and cons of postmenopausal hormone replacement therapy, *Generations* 4:7, 1996.

72. Altkorn D, Vokes T: Treatment of postmenopausal osteoporosis, *JAMA* 285(11):1415, 2001.

73. Kerr D et al: Resistance training over 2 years increases bone mass in calcium depleted post menopausal women, *J Bone Miner Res* 16(1):175, 2001.

74. Snow CM et al: Long term exercise using weighted vests prevents hip bone loss in post menopausal women, *J Gerontol Biol Sci Med Sci* 55(9):M489, 2000.

75. Rikli RE, McManis BG: Effects of exercise on bone mineral content in post menopausal women, *Res Q Exerc Sport* 61(3):243, 1990.

76. McCarthy KA: A chiropractic approach to aging, degeneration, and the subluxation, *Top Clin Chiropr* 8(1):61, 2001.

77. Kirkaldy-Willis WH, Bernard TN: *Managing low back pain*, ed 4, Philadelphia, 1999, Churchill-Livingstone.

78. DiMatteo MR: Adherence. In Feldman MD, Christensen JF, editors: *Behavioral medicine in primary care: a practical guide*, Stamford, Conn, 1997, Appleton and Lange.

79. O'Connell D: Behavior change. In Feldman MD, Christensen JF, editors: *Behavioral medicine in primary care: a practical guide*, Stamford, Conn, 1997, Appleton and Lange.

80. Chao D et al: Exercise adherence among older adult: challenges and strategies, *Control Clin Trials* 21:212S, 2000.

81. Singer C et al: Older patients. In Feldman MD, Christensen JF, editors: *Behavioral medicine in primary care: a practical guide*, Stamford, Conn, 1997, Appleton and Lange.

CHAPTER

17 Adjusting the Aging Patient

Lisa Zaynab Killinger, DC,
Carol Claus, DC

Key Terms

DIVERSIFIED TECHNIQUE
EXPIRATION THRUST
FLEXION DISTRACTION
   TECHNIQUE
FULCRUM

GERIATRIC
GONSTEAD TECHNIQUE
LOGAN BASIC TECHNIQUE
MERIC RECOIL TECHNIQUE
   (FULL SPINE SPECIFIC)

ROTATOR CUFF
SACROOCCIPITAL
   TECHNIQUE
THOMPSON TECHNIQUE

First of all, do no harm.

HIPPOCRATES

Although chiropractic patients of all ages require careful examination and diagnosis before applying adjustive procedures, chiropractors working with older patients must give special consideration to age-related changes of the spine and other structures of the musculoskeletal system. Through the years, chiropractors have developed a broad range of manual techniques to accommodate the needs and preferences of their patients.[1-6] In deciding which technique to use for a particular patient, the doctor of chiropractic should bear in mind that in health care, many questions have more than one correct answer.

This chapter explores chiropractic techniques and their application in the care of older patients, briefly describing the core procedures for each adjustive method along with its potential advantages and limitations. Based on a review of the technique literature, clinical experience, and observation, the authors present a range of options.

Though chiropractic procedures entail less risk to patients than more invasive medical procedures, caution is always appropriate. Thoroughly assessing the overall health status of the older patient, considering issues that affect safety in chiropractic adjusting, and then selecting a course of

care appropriately matched to the patient's clinical picture is important.[6-8] Also important is for the technique choices to take into consideration the patient's stage of degeneration as described in the Kirkaldy-Willis (K-W) model discussed in Chapter 16.[8] Good rules of thumb to avoid patient injury or discomfort include the following:

- Performing a thorough assessment of patient's health status
- Using the least amount of thrust necessary
- Always maintaining cognizance of patient tolerance
- Monitoring patient progress
- If positive outcomes are achieved, continuing with this adjusting strategy
- Continuing to monitor patient progress, noting any negative outcomes
- Adjusting patient care plan to meet patient's needs as health status changes

AVOIDING ADVERSE OUTCOMES

Although injury resulting from spinal adjustive procedures is uncommon, minimizing potential adverse outcomes of the **geriatric** chiropractic adjustment is important. The following are possible adverse outcomes related to chiropractic care of older patients. All results, except transient muscle soreness, are very rare occurrences.

- Muscle soreness or discomfort around adjustment site

- Rib fracture
- Hip fracture, injury, or dislocation of hip prosthesis
- Injury to shoulder and **rotator cuff** injury
- Falls from chiropractic table
- Burns from hot packs or ice
- Stroke[9,10]

Stroke is exceedingly rare. See Chapter 26 for detailed discussion.

COMMUNICATION

> The best risk management tool you have in chiropractic practice is good communication with the patient.
> Director of Claims, National Chiropractic Mutual Insurance Company

As with all patient interactions, when caring for an older patient, the chiropractor must take sufficient time to explain procedures and give a reasonable description of the expected (and perhaps unexpected) outcomes of care. Good communication with patients, young and old, is the best way to avoid a negative doctor-patient experience in practice.

Although few absolute contraindications to chiropractic care exist, some clinical scenarios require careful consideration of the technique choices and specific maneuvers used.[11] *Normal* age-related changes may indicate the need for careful selection and administration of chiropractic adjustments (Table 17-1).

REGIONAL ADJUSTING CONSIDERATIONS

Cervical Spine

Excessive rotation and extension of patient's cervical spine must be avoided, particularly in patients who have a history of stroke, show signs and symptoms of stroke, or are at high risk for stroke.[11]

Practitioners using higher amplitude adjustments should consider altering their technique to limit rotational and extension vectors as part of the adjustive process, or else they should shift to the application of lower force procedures. The needs of patients, including geriatric patients, vary widely, and all chiropractors must evaluate

Table **17-1**   IMPACT OF AGE-RELATED CHANGES ON CHIROPRACTIC CARE

Changes in the Aging Body	Impact on Chiropractic Practice and Decision-Making	Proposed Solutions
Decreased bone density	Increased risk of fracture	Low-force techniques, broader contact points, pediatric adjusting protocols
Decreased muscle mass	Decreased resistance to adjustive force	Lighter palpation, lighter adjusting, exercise to increase muscle mass and strength, soft tissue techniques to decrease hypersensitivity
Decreased ligament and tendon elasticity	Increased risk of sprain or strain after adjustment, decreased range of motion	Techniques that do not take joints past physiologic range of motion, prone adjusting techniques
Increased capillary and skin fragility	Increased risk of abrasion and bruising from adjusting	Lighter tissue pull; care should be taken not to slide contact along skin
Increased atherosclerosis	Increased risk of clotting, stroke, and blood vessel tears	Extension, rotation, double thrusting, and high amplitude adjusting near vessels with plaque should be avoided

each patient individually, adapting their technique appropriately. For the patient in the stabilization phase of the K-W model[8] (see Chapter 16), additional strategies should be employed to maintain range of motion and enhance intrinsic muscle strength in the cervical spine.[7,8]

Thoracic Spine

The posterior-to-anterior (P-A) force of a chiropractic adjustment is unlikely to cause damage to the bodies of the thoracic vertebrae in an osteoporotic patient. Thoracic spine fractures generally result from compressive axial forces applied to the body of the vertebra, not a force vector used in specific chiropractic adjusting of the thoracic spine. Rib fractures, however, are a greater concern. Avoiding the typical **expiration thrust** may be advisable (e.g., thrusting when patients' ribs are at their most flexed or "bent" position). The chiropractor should adjust using lower force techniques in the thoracic spine of osteoporotic patients, or use manual but light thrusts with broader contact on inspiration, or both. Allowing the chiropractor's hands to contact the ribs should be avoided by keeping the adjusting hand or hands close to the spine. Although some chiropractic technique instructors recommend using spinous contacts to avoid a potential fracture of the transverse process, the spinous contact may be quite tender and uncomfortable in older patients who have decreased muscle mass and epidermal thinning. "Anterior" thoracic adjusting, wherein the adjustive forces are translated through the sternum and ribs, is not recommended by the authors in patients with osteoporosis or advanced osteoarthritis.

Lumbopelvic Region

In frail patients, those with a history of hip injury, surgery, or instability, or those with neurologic symptoms in lower extremities, the best course is *not* to use the femoral neck area as a **fulcrum** in the adjustive procedure. In addition, for patients who have had a hip replacement, the ipsilateral knee should never be forced to cross the patient's midline, because of the risk that prosthesis dislocation or injury to the hip joint

may occur. Avoiding lumbosacral side posture adjustive maneuvers altogether may be prudent in such patients. Although caution should be exercised when using lumbosacral side posture maneuvers in elderly patients, many skilled chiropractors have carefully and safely used such techniques for decades. Prone adjustments of patient's lumbar, sacroiliac, and pelvic regions may offer appropriate and effective alternate adjusting strategies and have the additional advantage of easier placement of the patient on the adjusting table.

Suggested adjusting strategies include methods such as Thompson, Logan, sacrooccipital technique (SOT), activator, or the alternate prone maneuvers taught in several manual high-velocity, low-amplitude (HVLA) techniques such as Gonstead, diversified, or segmental meric recoil procedures.

Extremities*

As with the technique considerations addressed earlier, wide variation may be found in the chiropractic profession regarding manual approaches to rib and extremity problems. Because adjustments to ribs may be simply and safely achieved with instrument adjusting, practitioners may wish to explore instrument-assisted methods, at the very least for use in cases in which more forceful methods may be contraindicated. Practitioners choosing to use more classical, or cavitating, adjustive methods need to be especially cognizant of the decreased bone density and ligament elasticity, as well as the increased pain sensitivity, of older patients.[11]

To avoid injuries to the shoulder joint, care should be taken to examine and record patient's range of motion and history. As in the evaluation of any extremity, the doctor must first allow the patient to demonstrate his or her active ranges of motion before assessing passive motion, noting any restrictions or limitations. A principal contraindication to any type of adjusting maneuver is the inability of the patient to assume to position in which the adjustment is administered. Although

---

*For a discussion of rib fractures, see the Thoracic Spine section.

this rule of thumb is particularly important in extremity adjusting, it also applies to general assessment and adjustment of the aging spine.

Low-force adjusting, including instrument-assisted adjusting, of extremities such as knees, ankles, and shoulders is often an effective strategy. Again, practitioners using more classical methods must carefully screen for contraindications. Because maintaining motion and increasing muscular integrity around the joint enhances joint functionality and integrity, patients with extremity complaints should be encouraged to participate in a carefully designed routine of physical activity involving the joint in question (see Chapter 14). Recommendations regarding physical activities must be tailored to each patient's health status and ability, subsequent to a careful examination of the patient and communication with other providers involved in the patient's care.

ADVANTAGES AND LIMITATIONS OF SELECTED TECHNIQUE SYSTEMS

Each of the following techniques may be particularly suited to certain clinical scenarios and less useful for others. Little scientific study has been conducted ranking the relative efficacy of the various techniques.[1,2] The following list of potential advantages and limitations of the various techniques is offered as a seed for discussion about appropriate care strategies.[11]

Though the highest priority must be given to patient needs, chiropractors also must remember that they, too, are aging and should therefore select adjustive methods that do not impart excessive stresses into their own musculoskeletal structures, especially the wrists and low back. Listed here are examples of potential strengths and limitations of various adjustive techniques, from both the patient and doctor's perspectives.

The following techniques are presented in alphabetical order, with no order of preference implied.

Diversified Technique

Potential advantages of **diversified technique** (Fig. 17-1):

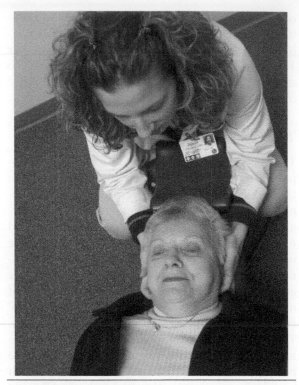

Fig. 17-1 Cervical spine adjustment.

- Multiple procedure options are available for all spinal segmental levels.
- Amount of force may be varied.
- No special equipment is needed.
- Motion is introduced into specific segmental areas.

Potential limitations:

- Side-posture adjusting in the lumbopelvic areas may be unsuitable for the aged spine or patient comfort or tolerance.
- Thoracic A-P adjustments may be contraindicated in patients with osteoporosis.
- Cervical rotation may be contraindicated in certain patients.
- Some patients may prefer noncavitating methods.

Gonstead Technique

Potential advantages of the **Gonstead technique:**

- This technique provides multiple options for patient placement, such as prone, seated, and knee-chest positions.

- Specific short-lever adjustments are incorporated.
- Force potential is variable.
- Motion into specific segmental areas is introduced.

Potential limitations:
- Knee-chest table may not be suitable for elderly patients with decreased flexibility.
- Some patients may prefer noncavitating methods.

Flexion Distraction Technique

Potential advantages of **flexion distraction technique:**
- Joint mobility may be increased.
- Pliability of soft tissues may be increased.
- Mechanically assisted table requires minimal exertion by the doctor.
- The procedure is hypothesized to promote the influx of fluid into the disk.

Potential limitations:
- Low-force procedures may have minimal appeal to some patients.
- The procedure is not a full-spine technique.
- Motorized version of the table may be uncomfortable for some patients.

Full-Spine Specific, Toggle Recoil, Meric Recoil Techniques

Potential advantages of full-spine specific, toggle recoil, **meric recoil techniques:**
- Application of the dynamic thrust adjustment with patient in prone position eliminates possible stress of side-posture positioning or rotation for patients with limited range of spinal motion.
- A full-spine technique system, applying specific short-lever adjustment procedures, allows for varying the amplitude of force to the tolerance of the patient. Quick, shallow, controlled HVLA dynamic thrust is used.
- Elderly or acute pain patients find the Hi-Lo table accessible and convenient for getting on and off.

- Double-lamina contacts or "baby meric" adjusting may offer an appropriate alternative in the care of the aging spine.

Potential limitations:
- Certain patients may initially find the abdominal suspension (thoracic extension) table mechanism uncomfortable.
- Active cervical spine rotation required in the prone positioning may be contraindicated in certain patients.
- Some patients may prefer noncavitating methods.

Instrument-Assisted Adjusting Methods

Potential advantages of instrument-assisted adjusting methods (Fig. 17-2):
- Force of dynamic thrust may be controlled.
- The technique may be applied for acute patients who are unable to tolerate a manual dynamic thrust.
- The technique is applicable for acute patients or patients who cannot tolerate distraction or rotation.

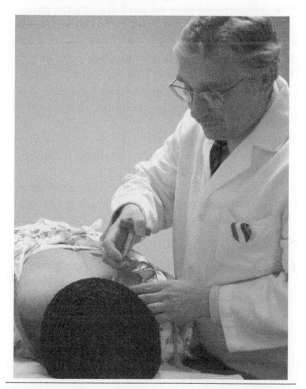

Fig. **17-2** Activator adjustment.

- Minimal bending and exertion is required of the doctor.

Potential limitations:

- Use of an instrument decreases the amount of *hands-on* care the patient will receive. Touch is an important element of the chiropractor-patient relationship.
- Low-force procedures may have minimal appeal to some patients.
- The technique imparts less motion into the spine or joints as compared with manual dynamic thrust technique procedures.

Logan Basic Technique

Potential advantages of **Logan basic technique:**

- Minimal degree of force may be a good option for patients with osteoporosis.
- The technique addresses sacrum and pelvis stability and postural distortions.
- Minimal physical exertion is required by the doctor.
- Adjustment may be performed with the doctor seated.
- The technique does not introduce rotation into spine, which may be good option for patients who are at risk for stroke.
- The technique is applicable for acute patients who cannot tolerate distraction or rotation.

Potential limitations:

- Low-force procedures may have minimal appeal to some patients.
- Patients may be uncomfortable with the sacrotuberous ligament contact point.

Sacrooccipital Technique

Potential advantages of sacrooccipital technique:

- The technique is gentle and uses gravity and the patient's weight to slowly perform the adjustment.
- The risk of fracture is minimized; the technique is a good option for patients with osteoporosis.
- Broader contact is used.
- The occipital area is addressed in depth.

- Minimal physical exertion by the doctor is required.
- Rotation into spine is not introduced, a consideration for patients who are at risk for stroke.

Potential limitations:

- Low-force procedures may have minimal appeal to some patients.
- Some patients may be unable to lie prone or supine on the pelvic blocks for the extended time required to complete the correction.
- The technique imparts less motion into spinal joints than dynamic thrust.

Thompson Technique

Potential advantages of Thompson technique:

- Drop-piece table segments are incorporated to facilitate application of dynamic thrust adjusting procedures.
- Minimal physical exertion is required by the doctor.
- Force potential for delivering adjustments is variable. Force may be controlled through changing settings on drop-piece table segments.
- A terminal point drop table enhances the effective force of thrust without increasing amount of force used on the patient.
- The technique provides for prone and supine adjusting protocols.

Potential limitations:

- Noncavitating procedures may have minimal appeal to some patients.
- Some patients may dislike the occasionally jarring effect of the drop-piece table segments.
- Leg length analysis may not be appropriate for patients with leg prostheses or anatomic leg length inequality.

Upper Cervical Techniques

Potential advantages of upper cervical techniques (Fig. 17-3):

- The upper cervical (UC) region is addressed in depth.

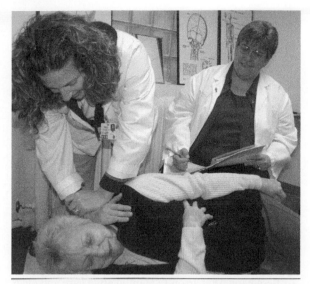

Fig. 17-3 Upper cervical toggle recoil adjustment.

- Certain UC technique procedures may be applied with low force.
- Most UC techniques do not introduce rotation into cervical spine.

- The technique allows the patient to receive chiropractic care, even when lower spinal segments cannot be adjusted.

Potential limitations:

- Limiting adjustment exclusively to the cervical spine may not appeal to some patients.
- The technique may not address thoracic, lumbar, and pelvic segments as effectively as full-spine technique procedures.
- Some UC techniques do not impart as much motion into spine as other manual full-spine adjusting techniques.

CONCLUSION

Perhaps the most important protocol for the chiropractor to implement in caring for aging patients is to perform a thorough assessment of the patient's overall health status and then to employ techniques appropriate to the patient's entire clinical picture. Evaluating a patient without a preconceived notion of which techniques to use is prudent (Table 17-2). After considering

Table **17-2**   CHIROPRACTIC TECHNIQUES COMMONLY USED FOR AGING PATIENTS

Chiropractic Technique	Core Procedure
Diversified technique	Draws from diverse sources of manual adjusting methods, short and long lever; variable force, variety of contact points
Flexion distraction technique	Axial traction on specialized tables, primarily focused on lumbar disks
Full-spine specific, Meric recoil, toggle recoil	Specific contact, short-lever, prone manual adjusting with controlled application of force; emphasis on direction of thrust in relation to articular planes; controlled depth of thrust
Gonstead technique	Specific contact, short-lever manual adjustments using multiple analytic procedures; controlled force with specific vectors; patient adjusted on specialized Gonstead bench, knee-chest table, or cervical chair
Instrument-assisted techniques	Instrument-assisted adjustment with specific application of force; force and vectors may be controlled to offer specific adjustment of any joint or bone
Logan basic technique	Cephalad pressure on sacrotuberous ligament; gentle mobilization of sacroiliac and other joints
Sacrooccipital technique	Pelvic blocking with padded wedges; uses patient weight assisted by gravity to adjust pelvic and lower lumbar joints
Thompson technique	Full-spine adjusting procedure incorporating use of specialized table with mechanical drop-piece table segments
Upper cervical techniques	Specific adjustment of atlas, axis, occiput, or any combination; may be high or low force

the patient's stage of degeneration, co-morbidities, and any special needs, an individually tailored management plan can be employed. With this strategy, patients are likely to enjoy the best possible outcomes while under chiropractic care.

Additional discussion on chiropractic techniques in the care of older patients can be found in the 2001 textbook, *Chiropractic Care of the Older Patient*.[11]

Review *Questions*

1. When adjusting an older patient with osteoporosis, what is the most important thing to remember regarding the force of the adjustment?
2. Under what circumstances should symptomatic joints not be used as fulcrums in the adjustive procedure?
3. What technique considerations are important in avoiding rib fractures?
4. What technique modifications may be helpful for cervical spine adjustments of older patients?
5. What case management considerations are necessary in older patients with decreased muscle mass?
6. How should palpation be modified for older patients with fragility of the capillaries or skin?
7. How should adjustive technique be modified for older patients with increased elasticity of tendons or ligaments?

Concept *Questions*

1. What are the possible advantages of being well versed in both standard and low-force adjusting methods?

2. Should radiography be used more frequently with older patients? Why or why not?

REFERENCES

1. Perle SM et al: Chiropractic technique procedures for specific low back conditions: characterizing the literature, *J Manipulative Physiol Ther* 24(6):407, 2001.
2. Perle SM et al: Rating specific chiropractic technique procedures for specific low back conditions, *J Manipulative Physiol Ther* 24(7):449, 2001.
3. Cooperstein R: Technique system overview: activator methods technique, *Chiropr Tech* 9:108, 1997.
4. Cooperstein R: Technique system overview: sacro-occipital technique, *Chiropr Tech* 8:125, 1996.
5. Cooperstein R: Technique system overview: Thompson technique, *Chiropr Tech* 7(2):60, 1995.
6. Bergmann TF, Larson L: Manipulative care and older persons, *Top Clin Chiropr* 3(1):56, 1996.
7. McCarthy KA: A chiropractic approach to aging, degeneration, and the subluxation, *Top Clin Chiropr* 8(1):61, 2001.
8. Kirkaldy-Willis WH, Bernard TN: *Managing low back pain*, ed 4, Philadelphia, 1999, Churchill-Livingstone.
9. Haldeman S, Kohlbeck FJ, McGregor M: Risk factors and precipitating neck movements causing vertebrobasilar artery dissection after cervical spine trauma and spinal manipulation, *Spine* 24:785, 1999.
10. Klougart N, Leboeuf-Yde C, Rasmussen LR: Safety in chiropractic practice. Part II: treatment to the upper neck and the rate of cerebrovascular incidents, *J Manipulative Physiol Ther* 19:563, 1996.
11. Cooperstein R, Killinger LZ: Chiropractic techniques in the care of the older patient. In Gleberzon B, editor: *Chiropractic care of the older patient*, Oxford, UK, 2001, Butterworth Heinemann.

Occupational Health

David P. Gilkey, DC, PhD, DACBO, DACBOH

Key Terms

ACTIVE ANALYSIS	MALINGERING	PHYSICAL REHABILITATION
ANTHROPOMETRIC	MAXIMUM MEDICAL	THORACIC OUTLET
CARPAL TUNNEL	IMPROVEMENT	SYNDROME
SYNDROME	NATIONAL INSTITUTE	VIDEO DISPLAY TERMINAL
CHRONIC PAIN SYNDROME	FOR OCCUPATIONAL	(VDT)
CUMULATIVE TRAUMA	SAFETY AND HEALTH	VOCATIONAL
DISORDER (CTD)	(NIOSH)	REHABILITATION
de QUERVAIN'S DISEASE	OCCUPATIONAL SAFETY AND	WORK HARDENING
DUPUYTREN'S CONTRACTURE	HEALTH ADMINISTRATION	WORKER'S COMPENSATION
ERGONOMICS	(OSHA)	
HYPOCHONDRIASIS	PASSIVE ANALYSIS	

"The ultimate challenge to a physician is to prevent what he treats."

JOSEPH SWEERE

Chiropractic has long played a vital role in the treatment of work-related injury and illness, compiling a solid record of clinical and cost-effectiveness. In recent years, development of a chiropractic specialty in occupational health (OH) has significantly expanded the range of work-related services that chiropractors provide. The profession's focus on treatment has been enlarged to include prevention and interdisciplinary case management.

Traditional roles of OH physicians, safety professionals, and industrial hygienists have been limited and generally separated, but the evolution of modern industry, regulatory overlap, and marketplace forces are bringing these disciplines closer together.[1] The chiropractic OH and safety specialist is well equipped to offer a broad spectrum of needed services for a wide range of industry challenges.

INJURY AND ILLNESS PREVENTION

Prevention Paradigm and Safety Philosophy

According to Heinrich, 88% of accidents are the result of human behavior and therefore preventable.[2] The American Public Health Association states that the cornerstones of prevention are anticipation of the potential for disease or injury, surveillance (accurate identification, reporting, and recording of occupational disease and injury), analysis of collected data, and control.[3]

Traditional methods of controlling or eliminating workplace hazards include engineering out or removing the hazard, using personal protective equipment (PPE), administrative interventions, and training in the proper and safe use of equipment. Engineering is frequently quite costly and therefore cannot be used in many potentially hazardous environments. If the hazard cannot be engineered out, administrative controls may limit worker exposure time through job rotation or schedule changes. Worker selection strategies may limit exposure of workers who are incapable of performing certain jobs. Job training is essential to provide workers with instruction in safe and efficient performance of required duties; workers must be trained to minimize risk of injury or illness.

Corporate realities depend on the bottom line. Companies ask: if we commit to practicing prevention, can we stay in business, make a profit, and remain competitive? If the answer is yes, prevention and safety become part of the corporate culture. If not, prevention is reduced to after-injury record keeping, accident investigations, and invoking safety regulations. This reactive posturing results in increased accident rates and costly **worker's compensation** (WC) claims.

Industrialized nations are moving toward prevention strategies. In many cases, this effort is driven by the high cost of work-related injury and illness, although in some instances, the desire to embrace prevention is an organic outgrowth of good management principles.

Chiropractor's Role in Industry

Duties of the OH physician are changing. Once largely limited to treatment services, OH physicians now perform roles ranging from purely administrative to highly interactive. Aside from treating occupational injury and illness, these roles include preemployment and preplacement examinations, return-to-work and independent medical examinations, medical monitoring, health education and counseling, work-site analysis, job analysis, specific fitness evaluation, baseline health determination, evaluation of work influence, emergency planning, rehabilitation programs, and now security and prevention of bioterrorism in the workplace. Experienced chiropractic OH specialists also participate in advising medical management, evaluating the effectiveness of medical programs, cost containment, and record management. In addition, these specialists serve as advisors to employers or insurance companies, as well as patient advocates.[4-7]

Chiropractic OH consultant Robert Lynch was contacted by SACO Defense, Inc., a Maine firearm manufacturer, to assist in reducing musculoskeletal injury and lost workdays. After 3 months of detailed ergonomic analysis, Dr. Lynch advised implementation of a broad range of prevention strategies. Ergonomic improvements were made whenever possible. Over 500 employees were trained in workplace safety measures. Included was a regime of exercises designed by Dr. Lynch, which employees performed for approximately 5 minutes two or three times a day.

Lost workdays plummeted by 66%. SACO's WC premiums dropped from $2 million in 1989 to $40,000 in 1993. In 1990, SACO experienced 44 lost-time injuries, with 913 workdays lost. In 1994, two lost-time injuries occurred, with a total of 3 days lost—an 82% improvement in lost-time injuries and a 73% reduction in WC costs per hours worked.[8]

OCCUPATIONAL ERGONOMICS

Ergonomic science is the study of people in relation to their jobs.[9,10] Included are environmental aspects of the workplace, such as temperature, light, noise, adequate airflow, and the physical arrangement of the workplace. Because ergonomics is closely associated with neuromusculoskeletal (NMS) injury and disease, emphasis is placed on the design of the workplace as it relates to physical demands placed on the worker. Individuals have different physical capabilities and limitations. A key concept in applied ergonomics is to *fit the job to the worker* rather than force the worker to fit the job.[9-11] Applied ergonomics seeks to improve worker comfort through analysis and application of ergonomic principles.

Chiropractic education and training provides an excellent foundation for understanding the biomechanical basis of applied ergonomics. Anatomy, physiology, pathophysiology, posture, and biomechanics are fundamental aspects of ergonomics. The chiropractic postgraduate OH program includes problem-solving skill development, anthropometrics, safety engineering, risk factor identification and analysis, methods for passive and **active analysis** of the workplace, safety engineering, development and implementation of control strategies, ergonomic programs, and communication skills to increase effectiveness with industry.

Anthropometrics

Anthropometric data are used ergonomically to determine reach and clearance measurements when designing the workplace. Data analysis shows variations between sexes in average heights, weights, reaches, and other parameters. The following are examples of height and weight averages reported in the U.S. populations[10-12]:

NASA: Male 70.8 inches,   Female 61.8
                   181 lb   inches, 113.5 lb
Chaffin: Male 69 inches   Female 63.7 inches
Selan: Male 69 inches   Female 63.9 inches

The *Golden Rule of Design* states that clearance allowances must be designed for the largest users and reach capabilities must be designed for the smallest users. Incorporating adjustability whenever possible is important.

Back Pain Risk Factors

Physical and emotional risk factors associated with low back pain (LBP) in the workplace are highly relevant to chiropractic practice. Correlations have been found between LBP and the following[13]:

- Lack of job satisfaction
- Duration of employment under 5 years
- Time of day (6:00 AM to noon)
- Sense of monotony on the job
- Alcohol consumption
- Drug abuse
- Smoking tobacco
- Taller stature

Cumulative Trauma Disorders Risk Factors

Key risk factors associated with **cumulative trauma disorders** (CTDs) include repetition or frequency of motion, force of exertion, posture of the body, duration of task, recovery or cycle time, exposure to cold temperatures, and exposure to vibration.[9,14-20]

Gilkey and Williams provide a detailed synopsis of key points in the proposed **Occupational Safety and Health Administration (OSHA)** ergonomic standards.[21] Of particular importance are the following signal risk factors for CTDs:

- Performance of the same motion or motion pattern every few seconds for more than 2 continuous hours or for more than 4 hours total in the 8-hour work shift
- Fixed or awkward posture for more than a total of 2 to 4 hours
- Use of a vibrating or impact tool for more than a total of 2 to 4 hours
- Using forceful hand exertions for more than a total of 2 to 4 hours
- Unassisted frequent or forceful manual handling for more than a total of 1 to 2 hours

Other risk factors associated with developing CTDs include age (50% of claimants are over age 50), hypertension, coronary heart disease, stroke, hyperlipidemia, genetic factors, alcohol and tobacco use, lack of exercise, and poor diet.[22] Researchers have recently identified a *carpal tunnel gene*, suggestive of a genetic predisposition for **carpal tunnel syndrome** (CTS) that may exist in certain populations. The MCP-1 gene might be a candidate for the genetic marker of CTS development. Individuals with this gene are at increased risk for developing CTS.[23]

Performing the Ergonomic Evaluation

Passive Analysis

The first step in ergonomic evaluation is **passive analysis** of workplace data, which should be performed every 2 years to ensure that negative trends in injury or illness are not occurring. If available, documents describing types and patterns of worker injuries and illness should be thoroughly evaluated by the OH physician. Simple review and analysis of company documents can reveal significant clues to the presence of ergonomic hazards and related injuries.

Passive analysis begins with a review of OSHA logs for incidence and details of back injuries or

CTDs.[11,24,25] This appraisal is followed by review of accident investigation reports for details about injuries and calculation of incidence rates (IR) and severity rates (SR) for CTDs and back injuries. Next comes detailed assessment of employee records and WC claims, health care costs related to CTDs and back injuries, absenteeism rates, requests for job changes, employee turnover rates, employee training records, and past safety inspections, audits, and reports. Passive analysis calls for detective skills on the part of the analyst; the goal is to search for patterns contributing to injuries.

IR calculation can provide a comparison to a known industry standard. A high IR usually indicates a need for ergonomic and prevention intervention. SR calculation indicates the serious nature of injuries and potential costs associated with lost workdays. The calculation of IR and SR can be accomplished as follows[11,24,25]:

$$IR = \frac{\text{Number of incidents for the time period} \times 200,000 \text{ hours}}{\text{Number of hours worked during the period}}$$

$$SR = \frac{\text{Number of days lost for the time period} \times 200,000 \text{ hours}}{\text{Number of hours worked during the period}}$$

Active Analysis

Work site evaluation affords the chiropractic OH physician the opportunity to observe, sample, measure, and record the presence of potential ergonomic hazards. This active analysis requires the OH physician to select the best tools for the job; no single form or checklist exists that is applicable to all workplaces.[11] The specific nature of job tasks at each workplace determines the most appropriate approach for active analysis, which may include checklists, observations, interviews, videos, photographs, sampling, measuring, and monitoring.[11,24,25] The information gleaned from these various procedures is correlated with passive analysis findings to develop ergonomic prevention strategies.[11,24]

Active analysis should emphasize surveillance for potential ergonomic hazards such as:
- Excessive force
- Frequent repetitions
- Awkward postures
- Contact stress

- Short cycle times
- Automated pace
- Monotony
- High psychologic stress
- Lack of control
- Excessive noise
- Excessive heat or cold
- Poor lighting
- Destructive work culture

Ergonomic Intervention

Implementation of ergonomic controls endeavors to fit the job to the worker. When possible, the first step is to engineer out the hazard. Today's technological marketplace offers a wide array of ergonomic devices and equipment for both manufacturing and sedentary workplaces. Design solutions are specific to each work site. Recommendations may include engineering interventions such as mechanical lift assist devices, power-driven hand tools, and adjustable workstations; ergonomic PPE such as friction-enhancing gloves, protective eye wear, and hearing-conservation wear; ergonomic training in proper work postures, proper lifting techniques, and fitness instruction; and administrative interventions, including job rotations and changes in break schedule and production rate.

Some ergonomic challenges require only simple intervention, while others entail complex and costly solutions. Communication with company management and all affected individuals is essential. Once intervention has been completed and an ergonomic program is underway, results may be measured by the same passive and active analysis methods used earlier. Programs should be monitored on an ongoing basis and audited every 2 years to document results and the need for further intervention.[11]

NEUROMUSCULOSKELETAL ILLNESS AND INJURY

Scope of the Problem

Between 60% and 80% of the general population will suffer from LBP at some point in their lives, and 5% to 30% experience LBP at any given

Varicon, a glass manufacturing company with annual sales over $60 million, was suffering from an epidemic of low back injury cases when chiropractic physician and OH diplomate Joseph Sweere was called in to provide an ergonomic assessment. Dr. Sweere's recommendations included ergonomic improvements, safety training, wellness education, and worker preplacement selection and screening.

Following implementation of Sweere's prevention plans, Varicon's incidence of low back injury decreased by 80%.[26] The Varicon case established the efficacy of the biomechanical stress index (BSI), which is now widely use by chiropractic OH consultants.

time.[27] The burden to social and financial systems is significant. Estimates suggest that 22.4 million cases of back pain occur annually, equaling a 12-month period prevalence of 17.6% in the general populations, and 65% are work related.[28] Back pain is the most frequently cited reason for worker's filing injury claims. According to the National Safety Council (NSC), low back disorders make up 30% to 40% of all WC injuries.[29] The **National Institute for Occupational Safety and Health (NIOSH)** reports that 19% to 25% of all WC claims are for back pain.[30] Back pain is the second most frequently recorded reason for lost workdays in America, the common cold being first.[31] The Bureau of National Affairs (BNA) reports that back pain accounts for more than 500 million lost workdays each year.[30] On any given day, an estimated 6.5 million people are home from work, in bed, as a result of back pain. New back pain cases are generated at a rate of 1.5 million per month.[31]

Equally significant as the prevalence of back pain and injury are the costs associated with it. The average cost of a work-related lower back injury in Ohio was $23,716 in 1990, which increased to $30,000 by 1994.[32,33] In addition, NSC reports that the total actual costs of all work-related injuries was $122.6 billion in 1999.[29] Most WC carriers agree that back injuries are the most expensive claims, comprising 65% to 90% of benefit costs.[32] The real eco-

nomic impact of back pain also includes hidden costs, bringing total back pain expenses as high as $100 billion annually.[33-35] Because of the prevalence and costs, a growing shift in awareness and concern has occurred about NMS injury and illness in the workplace. Although back pain clearly remains the number one challenge to industry, CTDs have emerged as a sleeping giant.

Cumulative Trauma Disorders

Review of the literature from the United States shows a sharp rise in the number of CTDs affecting upper extremity (UE) between 1981 and 1994:
- 1981: CTDs make up 18% of occupational illness; approximately 20,500 cases reported.[36]
- 1982: CTDs make up 21% of occupational illness; approximately 22,000 cases reported.[37]
- 1988: CTDs make up 48% of occupational illness; 115,000 cases reported.[16]
- 1990: CTDs make up 50% of occupational illness; 147,000 cases reported.[37]
- 1991: CTDs make up 56% of occupational illness; 223,000 cases reported.[38]
- 1992: CTDs make up 60% of occupational illness; 282,000 cases reported.[36]
- 1993: CTDs make up 60% of occupational illness; 302,000 cases reported.[37]
- 1994: CTDs make up 68% of occupational illness; 332,000 cases reported.[39]
- 1995: CTDs make up 62% of occupational illness; 308,000 cases reported.[40]

BLS, NIOSH, and OSHA began to consolidate the injury and illness data in 1994 by combining NMS disorders for both UE and lower back related to ergonomic risk factors such as overexertion and repetitive motion. These conditions are now identified as musculoskeletal disorders (MSDs):
- 1994: MSDs affecting UE and back; 705,800 cases reported.[39]
- 1995: MSDs affecting UE and back; 705,000 cases reported.[40]
- 1996: MSDs affecting UE and back; 647,344 cases reported.[41]
- 1997: MSDs affecting UE and back; 603,096 cases reported.[42]

- 1998: MSDs affecting UE and back; 593,000 cases reported.[43]
- 1999: MSDs affecting UE and back; 598,000 cases reported.[44]
- 2000: MSDs affecting UE and back; 577,800 cases reported.[45]

A 770% increase in CTDs was reported between 1983 and 1993, a trend attributed to increased public awareness of CTDs, broader definitions of compensable claims, increased numbers of service industry workers, and increased use of **video display terminals (VDTs)**.[38]

A decreasing trend has been evident since 1994 with nearly an 18% drop in the number of reported MSDs reported between 1994 and 2000. Explanations for this encouraging trend may include a positive response by industry to the increased emphasis by OSHA and labor organizations on curtailing the MSD epidemic in American workplaces. OSHA had allocated significant resources to developing the Ergonomic Standard, resulting in increased public awareness and concern over the number of workers affected with MSDs. The Standard, short lived as it was (discontinued in 2001), served as motivation for many businesses to engage prevention strategies to reduce ergonomic risk factors.

CTDs are reported as occupational illnesses, not injuries. CTDs make up only 4% of the reported work-related injuries but constitute approximately 60% of work-related illnesses.[46,47] Despite the alarming numbers, some experts believe that CTDs may be underreported, with IR as much as 130% higher.[46]

CTDs are not only the fastest growing workplace illness, but also one of the most expensive occupational illnesses to treat. Cost estimates have recently been established at $20 billion to $27 billion per year in the United States.[36,48,49] The National Council on Compensation Insurance has stated that the average CTD case costs $29,000, including wage loss and treatment, in the early 1990s. Litigation and settlement costs exceed the medical and lost wage expenses, averaging $50,000 per case.[50] Costs for managing MSDs have risen to an average of $84,000 for surgical cases, with basic medical management averaging approximately $23,000 per case[51] (Fig. 18-1).

RESEARCH ON CAUSAL RELATIONSHIPS

Only recently has serious research been undertaken to establish the relationship between workplace activities and exposures and specific ergonomic-related injury and illness.[20] This relationship is, of course, self-evident to many injured workers, and the existence of ergonomic hazards has long been recognized. Bernadini Ramazini, the father of occupational medicine, wrote in 1713:

So much for workers whose diseases are caused by the injurious qualities of the material they handle. I now wish to turn to other workers in whom certain morbid affections gradually arise from other causes, from particular posture of the limbs or unnatural movements of the body called for while they work. Such are the workers who all day long stand or sit, stoop or are bent double; who run or ride or exercise their bodies in all sorts of ways.[9]

Despite this nearly 300-year-old warning, no formal study in ergonomics was undertaken until 1949 when the British Admiralty held the first ergonomics symposium.[52] A recent landmark in this evolving field came in 1995, when Silverstein and colleagues, in an evaluation of the literature on work-related musculoskeletal disorders (WMSDs) prepared for OSHA's ergonomics task force,[20] stated that, "The literature shows unarguably that certain jobs and certain work-related factors are associated with the manifold risk of contracting a WMSD compared to other population groups or groups not exposed to these risk factors."

NIOSH and the National Academy of Sciences (NAS) both set forth to assess the literature in a similar fashion using the same basic criteria as that used by Silverstein. The intent was to evaluate the state of science relating to work exposures and MSD endpoints. The initial searches yielded over 2000 studies examining risk factors followed by a detailed analysis of over 600 high-quality articles. The conclusions were overwhelmingly supportive of work relatedness of MSDs.[39,53]

The literature search and evaluation process that Silverstein presented focused on cumulative trauma rather than musculoskeletal accidents or back injuries,[20] whereas the studies by NIOSH and NAS focused on all MSDs.[39,53] The basic cause-and-effect process for CTDs is described as fol-

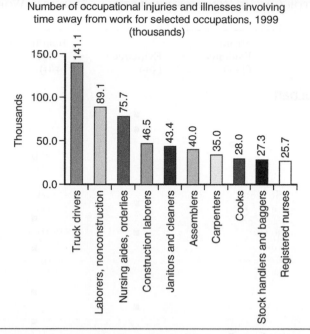

Fig. 18-1 From the Bureau of Labor Statistics *Safety and Health Statistics* program. *(Additional information is available from Department of Labor: Lost-worktime injuries and illnesses: characteristics and resulting time away from work, 1999, [news release], USDL, 01-71.)*

lows.[20,39,53] "It is assumed . . . that repeated efforts (movements, postures, etc.), static work, continuous loading of the tissue structures, or lack of recovery time trigger or cause a pathological process that then manifests itself as WMSD."

Strength of data was ranked for a variety of CTDs, based on the following criteria[20,39,53]:

1. Do the results of the studies show an association between disease and work exposure?
2. Do the results show a temporal (time-related) relationship?
3. Is there consistency in the association?
4. Can a change in disease be predicted by a change in work exposure?
5. Is there coherence of evidence?

NIOSH ranked the scientific evidence for risk factors of repetition, force, posture, and vibration as: strong, evidence, insufficient evidence, and evidence of no effect. NIOSH then offered the status of understanding to each area of the body, including neck and neck-shoulder, shoulder, elbow, hand-wrist, and back (Table 18-1).

Tendon Disorders

Tendon disorders include tendonitis/tendonosis, tenosynovitis, epicondylitis, **de Quervain's disease,** and **Dupuytren's contracture.** Silverstein's data review[20] concluded that convincing evidence of a causal relation exists between repetitive stress and tendonitis of the shoulder, hand, and wrist. It also concluded that weakly convincing evidence exists for tendonitis of the elbow and that the evidence on Dupuytren's contracture is uncertain. Finally, it concluded that the evidence for Achilles tendonitis is job specific. Associated risk factors include repetitive and overhead work for the shoulder, repetitive and forceful gripping for the hand and wrist, repetitive high-force use for the elbow, and job-specific stresses, such as ballet dancing for Achilles tendonitis.

Peripheral Nerve Disorders

Peripheral nerve disorders include CTS, **thoracic outlet syndrome** (TOS), and radiculopathy. Silverstein's data review concluded that strong evidence exists for CTS, weak evidence

Table **18-1**   EVIDENCE FOR CAUSAL RELATIONSHIP BETWEEN PHYSICAL WORK FACTORS AND MSDs

Body Part / Risk Factor	Strong Evidence (+++)	Evidence (++)	Insufficient Evidence (+/0)	Evidence of No Effect (−)
NECK AND NECK/SHOULDER				
Repetition		■		
Force		■		
Posture	■			
Vibration			■	
SHOULDER				
Posture		■		
Force			■	
Repetition		■		
Vibration			■	
Elbow				
Repetition			■	
Force		■		
Posture			■	
Combination	■			
HAND/WRIST				
Carpal Tunnel Syndrome				
Repetition		■		
Force		■		
Posture			■	
Vibration		■		
Combination	■			
Tendonitis				
Repetition		■		
Force		■		
Posture		■		
Combination	■			
Hand-Arm Vibration Syndrome				
Vibration	■			
BACK				
Lifting/forceful movement	■			
Awkward posture		■		
Heavy physical work		■		
Whole body vibration	■			
Static work posture			■	

From Bernard BP: *Musculoskeletal disorders and workplace factors*, Cincinnati, Ohio, 1997, National Institutes for Occupational Safety and Health, No. 97-141.

for TOS, and that no available evidence exists for cervical radiculopathy. Associated risk factors for CTS include repetitive and forceful gripping, repetitive movements, extreme positions, stretching, and contact pressure to the wrist. For TOS, risk factors include repetitive arm movements and manual work.

Muscle Disorders

Muscle disorders include neck tension syndrome, myalgia, and myofascial syndromes. A higher prevalence is reported related to repetitive work with constrained head and arm postures and sustained and repetitive elevation of the arms. Silverstein's review of available studies found the data to be incomplete for establishing strong association of muscle disorders and work exposure. Individual studies do support the relatedness of a portion of muscle disorders to occupational exposure. Specifically, fibromyalgia, traumatic myalgias, and muscle pain syndromes of unknown origin are excluded from work-related myalgia syndromes. Examples of occupations affected are VDT workers, typists, and assembly line workers. Associated risk factors include static loading and repetitive work.

Joint Disorders

Joint disorders include arthritis, osteoarthrosis, and spondylosis. Silverstein concluded that evidence supports a moderate association of workplace risk factors and the development of osteoarthrosis. The one associated risk factor is continuous joint compression, which produces osteoarthritic changes within joints.

Summary Conclusions for CTDs

- Ample and consistent evidence supports the association of workplace risk factors of repetition, load, posture, and vibration to the development of CTDs.
- Related signs and symptoms increase with continued exposure.
- Related signs and symptoms decrease with diminished exposure.
- Expression of signs and symptoms is related to work organization, psychosocial, and personal mediating factors.

BACK AND SPINE

Initiating Factors in Workplace Injury

NIOSH has established beyond any reasonable doubt that lifting, forceful movement, whole-body vibration, awkward posture, and heavy physical work are associated with work-related LBP.[39] The NSC identifies overexertion as the number one cause of back injury and lifting as the most frequently offending activity.[13,29]

Calculations of force are used as predictors of low back injury. The Utah Back Compressive Force Model is used to predict the compressive force brought to bear on the intervertebral disk. Evaluating factors include load, posture, frequency, and duration of lift. Assumptions are made for task characteristics and task posture. The NIOSH lifting equation considers a broad range of criteria, including[54]:

- Load weight
- Horizontal location—distance of the load away from the body relative to the feet
- Vertical location—distance of the hands above the floor
- Vertical travel distance—distance from origin to the destination
- Asymmetry angle—amount of deviation from a mid-sagittal plane
- Lifting frequency—average number of lifts per minute measured over a 15-minute period
- Lifting duration—the relative time engaged in lifting activity
- Coupling classification—the quality of load grip
- Significant control—the relative lifter control over load

Many factors are important in attempting to establish a cause-and-effect relationship between hazard exposure and a back injury. OSHA's proposed ergonomic standard identified the following signal risk factors for lifting and back injury prevention[24]:

- Load weight over 35 pounds
- Frequency of lifting more than 25 times in 2 hours
- Frequent forceful exertions greater than 10 lb in 2 hours

Epidemiologic studies of LBP show certain types of work have higher rates of incidence. Kelsey and Golden report that the highest rates of LBP occur in truck drivers, manual material handlers, nurses, and nursing aides.[13]

Treatment Protocols for Spine-Related Injury

The author proposes the following as appropriate methods and practices for work-related NMS conditions commonly seen in chiropractic practice.

Initial diagnostic procedures include history taking and physical examination, routine x-ray, and indicated laboratory tests. Follow-up diagnostic and imaging procedures are performed only if indications for further testing exist after the therapeutic trial period. This follow-up testing (some of which requires referral to other health facilities) may include computed tomography, magnetic resonance imaging, myelography, discography, surface and electrode electromyography and somatosensory evoked potentials, thermography, functional capacity evaluation, and psychologic assessment.[55-57]

Chiropractic spinal adjustment/manipulation[58] (Fig. 18-2) is the foundation of the chiropractic therapeutic approach. When appropriate, adjunctive procedures may include thermal treatments (hot and cold) and mechanically assisted traction or inversion therapy, which may be self-applied in chronic conditions. Other therapeutic options include ultrasound, electrotherapy (electronic muscle stimulation [EMS], interferential, galvanism), needle acupuncture, and nutritional therapy. The optimal therapeutic duration for these procedures is 1 to 3 months.[57,59-61]

Supervised exercise rehabilitation can play a crucial role in recovery from work-related injury or illness. The optimal therapeutic duration is 1 to 3 months as adjunct to other treatments. The patient's active participation in collagenous repair, tissue organization, and strengthening is essential.[52,62-65] Active exercise follows the acute phase of recovery and should continue through subacute to complete recovery. Patients are recommended to continue with exercise on a self-directed basis indefinitely. (See Chapter 14 for more on active care.)

The doctor's role is not limited to diagnosis and therapy. When necessary, carefully thought out work restrictions should be instituted during acute and subacute phases of recovery as adjunct to other treatments. Permanent restrictions must be judiciously applied. Workstation modification based on ergonomic analysis should also be considered.

The current consensus is that the greatest therapeutic impact is made on spinal conditions within the first 90 to 120 days and certainly by 6 to 9 months after injury.[58,66] Chronicity, characterized by lack of improvement with time and treatment, can become evident by 4 to 9 months after injury. Within the WC system, care offered for chronic somatic pain disorders, including spinal conditions, is frequently denied reimbursement because of alleged lack of appropriateness and cost-efficiency. Collaborative efforts between disciplines are the best way to achieve true maximum therapeutic value and benefit.

WORKER'S COMPENSATION
Historical Development

WC is a system of benefits designed to protect and assist workers suffering adverse health affects as a result of their employment. The first WC legislation in the United States was passed in 1910 in New York but was soon declared unconstitutional. Successful enactment of a WC law occurred in 1914,[67] and by 1948, all American states had enacted WC laws.[2] WC covers medical care, compensation for wage loss, costs for **vocational rehabilitation,** compensation for permanent disability, and death benefits for heirs.[2,6,7]

Chiropractic care is recognized in all state WC laws in the United States, but many states give employers great latitude in determining which provider will treat the injured worker. Since 1974, U.S. government employee WC law has allowed injured employees to be treated by the chiropractor of their choice. Chiropractic coverage follows Medicare language, reimbursing for manual manipulation of the spine for subluxations. Similar to Medicare, adjunctive physical therapy procedures performed in the chiropractic office are not covered. However,

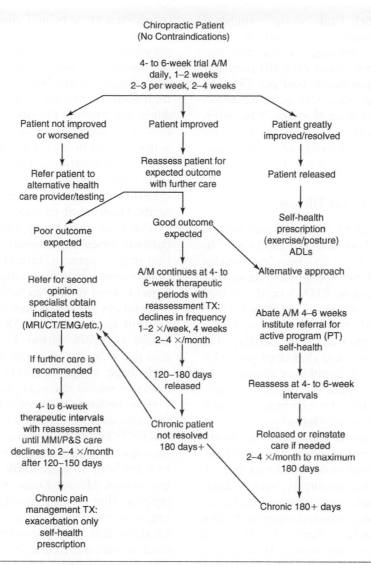

Fig. 18-2 Algorithm for chiropractic spinal adjustment/manipulation for somatic disorders. *ADLs,* Activities of daily living; *A/M,* adjustment/manipulation; *CT,* computed tomography; *EMG,* electromyography; *MMI,* maximum medical improvement; *MRI,* magnetic resonance imaging; *P&S,* permanent and stationary; *PT,* physical therapy; *TX,* treatment. *(From Sweere JJ, editor:* Chiropractic family practice—a clinical manual, *Gaithersburg, Md, 1992, Aspen Publishers.)*

unlike Medicare, federal **worker's compensation** does mandate reimbursement for x-rays, physical examinations, and appropriate laboratory tests.

Chiropractic Cost-Effectiveness

Numerous studies have provided cost comparisons between medical and chiropractic services,

with virtually all concluding that chiropractic demonstrates greater efficacy and cost-effectiveness. A 1988 Florida study[68] showed the average cost of a case managed by a doctor of chiropractic (DC) was $1204 compared with similar cases managed by a medical physician (MD), which averaged $2213. The average total temporary disability for chiropractic patients was 39 days compared with 58 for those under medical management. A 1991 Utah study[69] analyzed 3062 back injury claims for comparison of DC to MD services. DC managed cases had one tenth the lost time compared with MD managed cases. The average treatment cost per DC case was $526 compared with MD costs of $684. Additional WC studies from Montana, Wisconsin, Oregon, Iowa, California, and Kansas reiterate similar cost-efficiency benefits of chiropractic services.[68] (See Chapter 23 for further detail.)

Defining Accident and Illness

A work-related accident is an instantaneous event; anything else is considered an illness.[70] In determining eligibility for WC benefits, injuries must fit into one of two categories: those that arise out of employment (AOE) or those that arise in the course of employment (COE).[2,70] COE is the clear and simple work-related accident that is readily apparent to all parties. AOE can be an insidious disease that does not exhibit for many years.[70] Examples of illnesses are asbestosis or CTD in which the disease manifestation occurs long after the exposure. All back injuries are reported as accidents.[2]

Work-related injury cases entail significant paper work. Injuries must be reported to employers within a given statute-mandated time period. In many instances, the statute is 1-year's duration. In most instances, employers require immediate notification of work-related injury or illness. This requirement can be difficult when injury or illness is not apparent to the worker. Disputes can erupt when communications are delayed. Prompt reporting is always a good practice.

Case Management Issues

Care and management of patients has historically been the responsibility of the treating physician. With work-related injuries, however, third-party payers, administrators, employers, and consultants often usurp this decision-making role, particularly in cases that fail to resolve as quickly as expected. Physician management has become more complex in recent years.

Cost has become the prime focus of most state WC systems, with efforts to reduce costs acting as the driving force behind changes in the way OH services are provided and paid. Unfortunately, prevention is not often pursued with the same enthusiasm as other cost-containment strategies. Great efforts have been made to design treatment algorithms and standard protocols to guide the treating physician into uniform channels of service delivery, with some state WC divisions forming multidisciplinary panels of experts to develop treatment guidelines. These guidelines have empowered nonmedical personnel to question treatments that deviate from prescribed treatment protocols.

The rate of recovery varies greatly between patients based on a broad number of variables that may be present. Investigators have reported that as many as 90% of patients treated within 3 days of onset recovered within 2 weeks.[71] Other researchers have reported substantial improvement of approximately 33% of patients within 2 weeks and 66% within 7 weeks.[72,73] However, also noted is that as many as 40% of individuals with back pain are likely to have recurrent episodes within the next year.[74]

The challenge, however, is the 25%, who account for 80% to 90% of the WC treatment expenditures.[32,59] The political and economic imperative of *appropriate care at a reasonable price* is difficult to apply fairly to recalcitrant NMS injury or illness syndromes. Managed care, with its cost-sensitive policies that reward providers for undertreating, can compound the problem in these cases. Credentialing and preauthorization procedures often require adherence to WC, consensus, or proprietary guidelines. Physicians who frequently depart from the guidelines place themselves in jeopardy of losing authorization to render service.

The chiropractic profession's "Mercy Guidelines" provide a standard by which other guidelines can be measured. Although questions about frequency of visits, duration of care, and the number of treatments that will be reimbursed often receive the most attention, deeper issues are strongly emphasized in the Mercy document.[56,58] These issues include patient needs, therapeutic goals, necessity and appropriateness of care, indications and contraindications, safety, and effectiveness. Frequency and duration of care become self-evident as a by-product of good practice.

Reporting Requirements

The WC system places much of the onus for reporting on the OH physician. OH care facilities and offices must file timely reports that convey useful, accurate information[7]:

- First report of injury—usually includes injured worker identification, time, date, place, description of accident or illness, diagnosis, treatment plan, and work status.
- Employee ability to work—whether the employee is on temporary total disability, temporary partial disability, or is able to return to work unrestricted.
- Treatment plan—what services are necessary, how frequently the patient will be seen for treatment, and an estimate of the expected duration of care.
- Interval status reports—progress reports should be sent monthly and describe improvement, worsening, need for ongoing care, referral, special testing, expected release date, and ability to work.
- Modified work—the employer should be informed if permanent or temporary changes are needed in the physical demands of the injured worker's job.
- **Maximum medical improvement** (MMI)— when all available forms of care have been offered, the condition ceases to improve, and 6 to 9 months have passed; when MMI is reached, the symptomatic plateau is reported, and the nature and frequency of stationary state is described.[58,59]
- Permanent disability—persistent or recurrent pain and any permanent loss or restriction of physical activity is reported.
- Need for vocational rehabilitation—opinion is offered regarding the worker's ability to perform his or her usual and customary preinjury work and need for retraining in a less physically demanding job.
- Release from care—the WC carrier, employer, or both are notified when releasing a patient from care.

Litigation

A key indicator of workplace safety, health, and morale is the amount of litigation of WC cases. If more than 10% of WC injury cases are represented by lawyers, a problem exists in that workplace. Litigation in WC occurs within the WC system itself and not the civil courts.[60] However, evidence from a WC proceeding may be admissible in a civil action.[75] Cases of permanent disability and impairment may be litigated. Common issues in question may be:

- Causation: Is the illness or injury work related?
- Apportionment: What percentage of the illness or injury is related to this work situation?
- Benefits: Is the injured worker entitled to any or all of the WC benefits?
- Does any permanent disability or impairment exist? If so, how much?
- Is the injured worker entitled to vocational rehabilitation benefits?

Litigation generally delays benefit distribution to the injured worker while driving up the cost of its delivery. In recent years, efforts have been made to reduce the amount of litigation in the WC system. One such strategy is the use of the independent medical examiner (IME). Ideally, the IME is a physician with specialty training in OH. Reports follow special formats established by WC courts or administrators.

Independent Medical Examiner Reports

Complete IME reports should contain the following[76]:

- History of injury or illness
- Medical history
- Physical examination findings
- Review of medical records
- Diagnostic impression
- Opinion on causation and apportionment
- Opinion on MMI status
- Residual subjective complaints
- Residual objective findings
- Opinion on the worker's ability to return to work
- Residual permanent disability and impairment
- Opinion regarding the need for future chiropractic or medical care

- Discussion of any unusual or conflicting issues, disagreements with other examiners, or special concerns about which the judge should know.

WORKER REHABILITATION

Rehabilitation of workers focuses on two main areas: physical and vocational. **Physical rehabilitation** (PR) is largely addressed in the treatment paradigm. (See Chapter 14 for further detail on rehabilitation.) PR goals are intended to achieve restoration of optimal strength, stability, and integrity of the injured worker through a planned functional program. Vocational rehabilitation (VR) is the successful return to work through a planned program.

In uncomplicated cases, PR does not present a challenge; treatment leads to resolution, and the patient returns to work. Serious, disabling, and prolonged illness and injury present a formidable challenge. PR and VR may require interdisciplinary collaboration to facilitate return to work.

Strategies must be developed to overcome barriers to successful return to work. Areas to be addressed include[65]:

- Functional work capacity limits
- Musculoskeletal integrity and stability
- Behavior and attitude factors
- Cognitive factors
- Vocational status

Each component must be evaluated, measured, and assessed. This process calls for interdisciplinary referral and communication with the medical physician, occupational therapist, physical therapist, psychologist, counselors, and vocational or case management specialist. The injured worker should be encouraged to cooperate and participate actively in his or her rehabilitation. An effort should be made to involve the employer liaison and WC insurance representative. A team approach is most likely to yield optimal results.

Assessing Physical Capabilities and Limitations

The physical capabilities and limitations of workers can be assessed with numerous techniques. Useful methods include[6,77,78]:

- Static strength testing (isometric)
- Dynamic strength testing (isotonic and isokinetic)
- Job analysis
- Work simulation testing
- Manual materials handling testing
- Aerobic capacity testing
- Posture tolerance testing
- Anthropometric measures

The assessment of musculoskeletal stability and integrity is measured, in part, by the previously listed tests. Such tests are indicators of functional capacities but may not reflect the seriousness, nature, or outcome of the pathophysiologic process of the injury or disease. In cases when the chiropractic OH specialist is evaluating a patient but is not the treating physician, obtaining the opinion of the treating physicians is essential as to the patient's relative risk of injury, reinjury, exacerbation, or regression from such testing or involvement in work activities.

Specific concerns regarding behavioral and attitudinal factors may include[77]:

- Abnormal illness behavior, such as delayed recovery, **hypochondriasis** (deep anxiety about one's health that may manifest in symptoms not attributable to organic disease), hysterical neurosis, functional overlay, functional illness, nonorganic pain, and **malingering** (intentional falsification or overstatement of illness or injury)
- Abnormal treatment behavior, such as frequently changing physicians, frequent disagreements with the treating physician, self-prescription for care, self-directed use of splints, braces, and medical equipment
- **Chronic pain syndrome** development—a complex disorder following injury that is characterized by physical and mental stress, including disproportionate subjective complaints to objective findings, psychologic findings, lack of motivation, and continuing beyond 6 months
- Psychosocial stressors such as anxiety over possible reinjury, marital problems, or child-related concern at home
- Dependency and addiction to prescription, over-the-counter or illegal drugs, or to alcohol

- Employment dissatisfaction with an underlying desire to change jobs or careers or to punish the boss
- Secondary gain impeding recovery for a monetary settlement for injuries or disabilities

Vocational Status Assessment

Vocational status assessment can be a key indicator of success in PR and VR programs. Lack of job satisfaction is strongly associated with occupational injury; workers who dislike their jobs are two and one half times as likely to suffer industrial injuries.[79] Understanding how the worker feels about his or her past and potential employment is critical. Questions to be answered in this assessment process include:

- Is there job satisfaction?
- Have there been negative work appraisals from supervisors?
- Is there work available at the same company?
- What has been the length of disability?
- What type of disability status does the worker have?
- What pay scale will he or she have after return?
- Does the worker agree with the job description?
- Have there been changes in the company?
- Is this a new job or career?
- Is the job description compatible with the injured worker's physical capabilities and limitations?
- What is the relative risk of reinjury or new injury with the proposed new job?
- Are there health insurance benefits on the new job, and do they cover the injured worker's residual needs from their past injuries?

WC systems vary from state to state with respect to VR services. Some states provide VR benefits if the injured worker is not able to return to his or her usual job. Costs may be capped at levels that significantly limit resource use. Some states have entirely eliminated the VR benefit.

Return to Work

Early return to work is highly desirable. Approximately 80% to 90% of injured workers return to their employment within the first month after injury.[13] Protracted total temporary disability (TTD) drastically reduces the likelihood of ever returning to work. Only 50% of individuals remaining out of work for 6 months ever return. Of injured workers remaining out of work for more than 1 year, only 25% eventually return to work. The likelihood of return for workers off the job more than 2 years is negligible.[80]

TTD beyond 6 weeks is critical, as workers begin to decondition both physically and emotionally. Negative reinforcers associated with prolonged TTD include loss of self-esteem, tax-free disability income, attention and sympathy from family and friends, relief from responsibilities, and revenge against the employer.[81]

To authorize return to work, OH physicians should evaluate the following[77,80]:

- Are impairments stable?
- Are there potentially exacerbating work activities required?
- Is the injury or illness condition progressive?
- Is the condition characterized by remission and exacerbation of symptoms likely to cause additional TTD?
- Does the impairment cause a direct threat of new injury to the worker or his or her co-workers?

Factors Encouraging Return to Work

Aronoff and colleagues studied the characteristics of injured WC patients who returned to work in spite of their pain. Based on case analyses done retrospectively 5 years after injury, correlation was found with the following[80]:

- Early intervention and physical rehabilitation
- Positive hospital course of care
- High motivation
- Mastery of pain
- Stress-reduction strategies
- Positive work history
- Employment-centered purpose, identity, and satisfaction
- High incentive to return to work

- No psychopathologic conditions
- No medication dependency
- No secondary gain factors
- No litigation factors

Physical Improvement Strategies

Preparing a patient for return to work may include physical improvement strategies such as **work hardening** and back school.[60,62-65] The goal of increasing tolerance to work activities is based on the specific adaptation to the imposed demand (SAID) principle. This process involves 1 to 2 hours per day of physical rehabilitation, including aerobic, flexibility, and strength training.[65] Fitness evaluation techniques may also be used in conjunction with work hardening.

Back school protocols, which offer education and training in proper posture, movement, strength assessment, and work safety hygiene, can enhance the injured person's ability to accommodate actual employment. Protocols assess worker capability and increase tolerance to work activities. Goals are accomplished through work simulation in conjunction with other WC services.

DIPLOMATE PROGRAM IN OCCUPATIONAL HEALTH

Postgraduate education in OH trains chiropractors as consultants and advocates to industry with the ultimate goal of injury and illness prevention. Specific educational goals are intended to develop skills and knowledge for interdisciplinary problem solving and language development, team interaction, and application of illness and injury prevention in the workplace.

The OH diplomate program is taught as a series of postgraduate seminars at Council on Chiropractic Education (CCE) accredited chiropractic colleges. The curriculum is divided into three major phases of 100 hours each, with 24 learning modules and a year-long project-based exercise in an actual workplace in the field. After completing various topic modules, students take examinations and must achieve a minimum grade requirement. After completing all three phases of study, the students become eligible for the American Chiropractic Board of Occupational Health Diplomate examination.

Topics covered in the Occupational Health Diplomate Program include[82]:
- The Field of Occupational Health
- Preplacement-Biomechanical Stress Index
- Biomechanics-Ergonomics
- Injury Prevention
- Sitting in the Workplace
- Physical Rehabilitation
- Stress Management
- Cumulative Trauma Disorders
- Chemical and Environmental Hazards
- Chronic Pain
- Narrative Report Writing
- Occupational Multidiscipline Teams
- Legal Considerations in Occupational Health
- Independent Medical Examiner's Role
- Communications
- Safety Engineering

The diplomate program also requires a 1-academic-year class project. Projects to date have focused on ergonomic problem solving of NMS-related injury and illness in a specific industry setting.

Review *Questions*

1. What is the main reason that companies sometimes decide not to engineer out workplace hazards?
2. Name four duties of the OH physician.
3. What are the main risk factors associated with LBP?
4. What are the main risk factors associated with CTDs?
5. What is the most frequently cited reason for filing WC claims?
6. What explains the recent decrease in incidence of MSD claims?
7. What has NIOSH concluded regarding the work-relatedness of ergonomic risk factors to the development of MSDs?
8. True or false? In all states in the United States, workers injured on the job can choose to be treated by a chiropractor, with the assurance that the bill will be paid by WC insurance.

9. What are several methods of assessing physical capabilities and limitations?
10. What are several behavioral and attitudinal factors that may influence recovery from an occupational injury?

Concept *Questions*

1. How can specific training in OH expand the nature of a chiropractor's practice?
2. How can a chiropractor determine whether a patient is malingering?

REFERENCES

1. Gilkey DP, Williams HA: The comprehensive environmental, health, and safety program: a new trend in industry, *J Am Chiropr Assoc* 31:22, 1994.
2. Tiffin J, McMormick EJ: *Industrial psychology,* Englewood Cliffs, NJ, 1965, Prentice-Hall.
3. Weeks JL, Levey BS, Wagner GR, editors: *Preventing occupational disease and injury,* Washington, DC, 1991, American Public Health Association.
4. LaDou J, editor: *Occupational health and safety,* ed 2, Chicago, 1994, National Safety Council.
5. Plog BA, editor: *Fundamentals of industrial hygiene,* ed 3, Chicago, 1988, National Safety Council.
6. Herington TN, Morse LH, editors: *Occupational injuries evaluation, management, and prevention,* St Louis, 1995, Mosby.
7. Sweere JJ: Role of the chiropractic physician in occupational health. In Sweere J, editor: *Chiropractic family practice—a clinical manual,* Gaithersburg, Md, 1994, Aspen Publishers.
8. Lammert G: Maine DC works with company and union to reduce injuries, *J Chiropractic* 8:41, 1994.
9. Pheasant S: *Ergonomics, work and health,* Gaithersburg, Md, 1991, Aspen Publishers.
10. Chaffin DB, Andersson GB: *Occupational biomechanics,* ed 2, New York, 1991, John Wiley and Sons.
11. Selan J: *The advanced ergonomics manual,* Dallas, 1994, Advanced Ergonomics.
12. International Business Machines Corporation: *Ergonomics handbook,* Purchase, NY, 1987, The Corporation.
13. Kelsey JL, Golden AL: Occupational and workplace factors associated with low back pain. In Deyo RA, editor: *Occupational back pain spine: state of the art reviews,* vol 2, Philadelphia, 1987, Hanley and Belfus.
14. Carson R: Key ergonomic tips, *Occupational Hazards* 8:43, 1994.
15. Gilkey DP, Williams HA: Ergonomics and CTDs: the problems, causes, enforcement and solutions, *J Am Chiropr Assoc* 31:27, 1994.
16. Chesler L: Repetitive motion injury and cumulative trauma disorder: can the wave of products liability litigation be averted? *Computer Lawyer* 9:13, 1992.
17. Keyserling WM, Armstrong TJ, Punnett L: Ergonomic job analysis: a structured approach for identifying risk factors associated with overexertion injuries and disorders, *Applied Occupational Environmental Hygiene* 6:353, 1991.
18. Kroemer KH: Avoiding cumulative trauma disorders in shops and offices, *Am Ind Hyg Assoc J* 53:596, 1992.
19. Sandler HM: Are we ready to regulate cumulative trauma disorders? *Occupational Hazards* 6:51, 1993.
20. Hagberg M et al: *Work-related musculoskeletal disorders: a reference book for prevention,* Bristol, UK, 1995, Taylor and Francis.
21. Gilkey DP, Williams HA: Injury prevention in the workplace: a closer look at OSHA's proposed ergonomic standard, *Occupational Health Briefs* 2:1, 1995.
22. LaDou J: Cumulative injury in workers' compensation. In *Occupational medicine: state of the art reviews,* vol 3, Philadelphia, 1988, Hanley and Belfus.
23. Omri K et al: Association of MCP-1 gene polymorphism A-2518G with carpal tunnel syndrome in hemodialysis patients, *Amyloid* 9:3, 2002.
24. Occupational Safety and Health Administration: *Draft of proposed regulatory text,* ErgoWeb, [on-line] Internet, accessed on Dec. 17, 2002. URL: tucker.mech.utah.edu, 1995.
25. American National Standards Institute: *Z365—control of work related cumulative trauma disorders,* New York, 1994, The Institute.
26. Sweere JJ: Chiropractic in industry, *Today's Chiropr* 5:10, 1988.
27. Cassidy DJ, Wedge JH: The epidemiology and natural history of low back pain and spinal degeneration. In Kirkaldy-Willis WH, editor: *Managing low back pain,* ed 2, New York, 1988, Churchill Livingstone.
28. Guo H et al: Back pain prevalence in U.S. industry and estimates of lost workdays, *Am J Pub Health* 89:7, 1999.
29. National Safety Council: *Injury facts 2000 edition,* Itasca, Ill, 2000, National Safety Council.
30. Bureau of National Affairs: Ergonomics: back pain identified as major problem for U.S. workers in NIOSH study of 1988 data, *Occupational Safety and Health Reporter* 22:2068, 1993.
31. Kahlil TM et al: *Ergonomics in back pain,* New York, 1993, Van Nostrand.
32. Snook SS: The costs of back pain in industry. In Deyo RA, editor: *Occupational back pain, spine: state of the art reviews,* vol 5, Philadelphia, 1991, Hanley and Belfus.
33. Marras WS: Occupational low back disorder causation and control, *Ergonomics* 43:7, 2000.
34. Bureau of National Affairs: Statistics: back injuries blamed for half of claims filed by health care work-

ers, cab drivers, *Occupational Safety and Health Reporter* 23:484, 1993.

35. Marras WS, Ferguson SA, Waters TR: The effectiveness of commonly used lifting assessment methods to identify industrial jobs associated with elevated risk of low-back disorders, *Ergonomics* 42:1, 1999.

36. LaBar G: Ergonomics can't wait any longer, *Occupational Hazards* 4:33, 1994.

37. Bureau of National Affairs: Ergonomics: 770% increase, *Occupational Safety and Health Reporter* 24:1794, 1995.

38. Bureau of National Affairs: Ergonomics: repeated trauma claims of upper extremities most prevalent in meatpacking jobs, study says, *Occupational Safety and Health Reporter* 24:846, 1994.

39. Bernard BP: *Musculoskeletal disorders and workplace factors,* National Institutes for Occupational Safety and Health, No. 97-141, Cincinnati, Ohio, 1997.

40. NIOSH: *Facts work-related musculoskeletal disorders,* [on-line] Internet, accessed on 12/17/02. URL: http://www.cdc.gov/niosh/muskdsfs.html

41. National Archives and Records Administration: Ergonomics program; final rule, *Federal Register* 65:220, 2000.

42. NIOSH: *National occupational research agenda for musculoskeletal disorders,* NIOSH, No. 2002-117 Cincinnati, Ohio, 2001.

43. Department of Labor: *Lost-worktime injuries and illnesses: characteristics and resulting time away from work, 1998,* [on-line] Internet, accessed on 12/17/02. URL: http://stats.bls.gov/iif/oshcdnew.htm#00Supplemental%20Tables

44. Department of Labor: *Lost-worktime injuries and illnesses: characteristics and resulting time away from work, 1999,* [on-line] Internet, accessed on 12/17/02. URL:http://stats.bls.gov/iif/oshcdnew.htm#00Supplemental%20Tables

45. Department of Labor: *Lost-worktime injuries and illnesses: characteristics and resulting time away from work, 2000,* [on-line] Internet, accessed on 12/17/02. URL: http://stats.bls.gov/iif/oshcdnew.htm#00Supplemental%20Tables

46. Edril M, Dickerson OB, Glackin E: Cumulative trauma disorders of the upper extremity. In Zenz C, editor: *Occupational medicine,* ed 3, St Louis, 1994, Mosby.

47. Bureau of National Affairs: Ergonomics: focus on cumulative trauma disorders said to cause "misdirection of resources," *Occupational Safety and Health Reporter* 24:1181, 1994.

48. White L, editor: Back school. In White L, editor: *Spine: state of the art reviews,* vol 5, Philadelphia, 1991, Hanley and Belfus.

49. Occupational Safety and Health Administration: *Background on the working draft of OSHA's proposed ergonomic standard,* [on-line] Internet,

accessed 12/17/02. URL: http://www.OSHA.gov//F:\osha\sltc\ergono~1\backgr~1.htm

50. Rigdon JE: How a plant handles occupational hazards with common sense, *The Wall Street Journal*, New York, September 28, 1992.

51. National Institute for Occupational Safety and Health: *NIOSH testimony to OSHA comments on the proposed ergonomics program,* Docket #S-777, NIOSH, Cincinnati, Ohio, November 2000.

52. Oborne DJ: *Ergonomics at work,* ed 2, New York, 1992, John Wiley and Sons.

53. National Academy of Sciences: *Work-related musculoskeletal disorders: a review of the evidence. National Academy of Sciences 1998,* [on-line] Internet, accessed on 12/17/02. URL: http://books.nap.edu/books/0309063272/html/1.html

54. U.S. Department of Health and Human Services, Public Health Services: *Revised NIOSH lifting equation,* Cincinnati, 1994, CDC and NIOSH.

55. Haldeman S, Chapman-Smith D, Peterson D, editors: *Guidelines for chiropractic quality assurance and practice parameters,* Gaithersburg, Md, 1993, Aspen Publishers.

56. Vear HJ, editor: *Chiropractic standards of practice and quality of care,* Gaithersburg, Md, 1992, Aspen Publishers.

57. Division of Worker's Compensation: *Medical treatment guidelines,* Denver, 1995, Department of Labor and Employment.

58. Gilkey DP: Issues concerning chiropractic standards of practice. In Sweere JJ, editor: *Chiropractic family practice—a clinical manual, suppl,* Gaithersburg, Md, 1993, Aspen Publishers.

59. Schafer RC, editor: *Basic chiropractic procedural manual,* ed 4, Arlington, Va, 1984, Associated Chiropractic Academic Press.

60. Mayer T, Politin P: Spinal rehabilitation. In Haldeman S, editor: *Principles and practice of chiropractic,* ed 2, Norwalk, Conn, 1992, Appleton & Lange.

61. North American Spine Society: Common diagnostic and therapeutic procedures of the lumbosacral spine, *Spine* 16:1161, 1991.

62. Mooney V: Preface. In White L, editor: *Back school, spine: state of the art reviews,* vol 5, Philadelphia, 1991, Hanley and Belfus.

63. Martin L: Back basics: general information for back school participants. In White L, editor, *Back school, spine: state of the art reviews,* vol 5, Philadelphia, 1991, Hanley and Belfus.

64. Robinson R: The new back school prescription: stabilization training part I. In White L, editor, *Back school, spine: state of the art reviews,* vol 5, Philadelphia, 1991, Hanley and Belfus.

65. Bronston LJ, Gehri DJ: A return to work protocol for mechanical low back pain. In Sweere JJ, editor, *Chiropractic family practice—a clinical manual, suppl,* Gaithersburg, Md, 1993, Aspen Publishers.

66. Gilkey DP: Chiropractic care: how much is enough? *J Am Chiropr Assoc* 29:29, 1992.

67. National Safety Council: *Accident prevention manual for business and industry,* ed 10, Itasca, NY, 1992, The Council.

68. American Chiropractic Association: *How to help your employees and your company with chiropractic,* Arlington, Va, 1995, The Association.

69. Jarvis KB, Phillips RB, Morris JD: Cost per case comparison of back injury claims of chiropractic versus medical management for conditions with identical diagnostic codes, *J Occup Med* 8:847, 1991.

70. Gilkey DP, Williams HA: Occupational illness or injury, *International Academy of Chiropractic Occupational Health Consultants Newsletter* 7:4, 1994.

71. Coste J et al: Clinical course and prognostic factors in acute low back pain: an inception cohort study in primary practice, *BMJ* 308:6298, 1994.

72. Cherkin DC et al: Predicting poor outcomes for back pain seen in primary care patient's own criteria, *Spine* 21:28, 1994.

73. Croft PR et al: Outcome of low back pain in general practice: a prospective study, *BMJ* 316:7141, 1998.

74. Carey TS et al: Recurrence and care seeking acute pain: results of a long-term follow-up study, *Med Care* 37:2, 1999.

75. Railton WS: *OSHA compliance handbook,* Rockville, Md, 1992, Government Institutes.

76. Division of Industrial Accidents: *Guidelines for medical examination and report,* San Francisco, 1985, California Division of Worker's Compensation.

77. Scheer SJ, Wickstrom RJ: Vocational capacity with low back pain impairment. In Scheer SJ, editor: *Medical perspective in vocational assessment of injured workers,* Gaithersburg, Md, 1991, Aspen Publishers.

78. Tramposh AK: The functional capacity evaluation: measuring the maximal work abilities. In White L, editor: *Back school, spine: state of the art reviews,* vol 5, Philadelphia, 1991, Hanley and Belfus.

79. Bureau of National Affairs: Hand surgeon correlates disability with negative job satisfaction, anger, *Occupational Safety and Health Reporter* 24:398, 1994.

80. Aronoff GM et al: Pain treatment programs: do they return workers to the workplace? In Deyo RA, editor: *Occupational back pain, spine: state of the art reviews,* vol 2, Philadelphia, 1987, Hanley and Belfus.

81. Imbus HI: Clinical aspects of occupational medicine. In Zenz C, editor: *Occupational medicine,* ed 3, St Louis, 1994, Mosby.

82. American Chiropractic Board of Occupational Health: *American Chiropractic Board of Occupational Health curriculum learning objectives and content guidelines,* Washington, DC, 1996, American Chiropractic Association.

Sports Chiropractic

Stephen M. Perle, MS, DC, CCSP

Key Terms

ATHLETIC TRAINER
CARDINAL SIGNS
CAVITATION
CLOSED KINETIC CHAIN
CONTROLLED MOVEMENT
CRYOKINETICS
CRYOTHERAPY
ECCENTRIC LOADING
ERGOGENIC
FEAR AVOIDANCE
  BEHAVIOR

GRADE I, II, AND III SPRAIN
  OR STRAIN
ILIOTIBIAL FRICTION
  SYNDROME
INFLAMMATION
KINEMATICS
KINESIOLOGY
KINETIC CHAIN
KINETICS
OPEN KINETIC CHAIN
OVERUSE INJURIES

PATELLOFEMORAL
  ARTHRALGIA
SHOULDER IMPINGEMENT
  SYNDROME
SPORTS MEDICINE TEAM
STRESS FRACTURE
STRESS REACTION
TENDINITIS
TENDINOSIS
TRAINING VOLUME
TRIAGE

Sports chiropractic and sports medicine have grown and matured over the years. Sports medicine has its origins in the Roman Empire, when treatment was provided to help gladiators become ready for competition. In the last century, sports medicine has progressed from a hobby of some in the medical profession who dabbled in treating athletes to its current status as an area of specialization with fellowship-based training programs. A variety of professionals and paraprofessionals specialize in the care of athletes, including practitioners of medical primary care specialties (e.g., internal medicine, family practice, pediatrics, gynecology), secondary care specialties (e.g., orthopedics, neurology, endocrinology), and limited licensed professions (e.g., chiropractic, dentistry, optometry, podiatry, psychology). Certain paraprofessionals are also involved in sports medicine (e.g., athletic trainers, personal trainers, nutritionists, physical therapists). Finally, some in the research community consult with and conduct research on athletes (e.g., exercise physiologists, biomechanists).

Sports and sports medicine establishments resisted sports chiropractic for many years, and progress has been gradual. However, as more and more athletes benefited from chiropractic care, they continued to seek out chiropractic care on their own and then demanded the inclusion of chiropractors on sports medicine teams. Despite much initial and some continued resistance, team athletic trainers and medical physicians gradually began to refer players to chiropractors. Eventually, many teams included chiropractors in official capacities on their sports medicine teams.[1] Currently, sports chiropractors are members of any comprehensive sports medicine staff, from the Olympics and professional sports to collegiate, scholastic, and youth club sports.

Babe Ruth relied heavily on the treatment he received from Erle "Doc" Painter, a chiropractor who served as athletic trainer for the New York Yankees[2,3] (Fig. 19-1). The U.S. Olympic sports medicine team first included a chiropractor, George Goodheart, at the Lake Placid Winter Olympics of 1980. Eileen Haworth was the first U.S. Olympic team chiropractor to participate in the physician-training program at the U.S. Olympic Committee (USOC) Colorado Springs training center in 1982. Currently, Doctors of

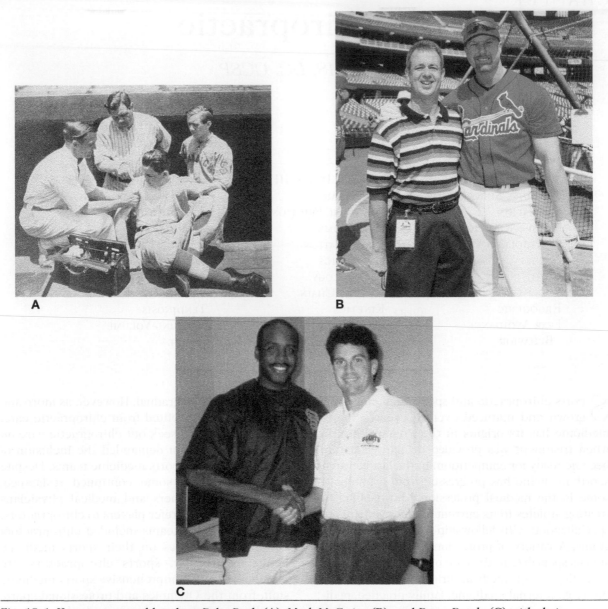

Fig. 19-1 Home run record breakers Babe Ruth (**A**), Mark McGwire (**B**), and Barry Bonds (**C**) with their respective chiropractors, Erle "Doc" Painter, Ralph Filson, and Nick Athens. (*A courtesy* NCA's Chiropractic Journal, *May 1934; B courtesy* American Chiropractic Association; *C courtesy* Today's Chiropractic.)

Chiropractic (DCs) seeking to participate in the U.S. Olympic program apply for internships at the training center where they are evaluated for the breadth and depth of their clinical competence and for their ability to work cooperatively within a multidisciplinary team.[4]

Organizationally, sports chiropractic in the United States received a major boost when Robert Hazel, Jr., was elected President of the Council on Sports Injuries and Physical Fitness (Sports Council) of the American Chiropractic Association (ACA). Under his leadership the Council's membership increased substantially, and the organization developed an indexed, peer-reviewed scientific publication, *Chiropractic Sports Medicine*, later renamed the *Journal of Sports Chiropractic and Rehabilitation*.* Relationships were established with various sports organizations, including the NFL Players Association and Pro Beach Volleyball, to provide credentialed chiropractors for sporting events or to receive referrals for the care of athletes.

The ACA Sports Council also worked to develop postgraduate board certification, with programs for Certified Chiropractic Sports Physicians (CCSP) and Diplomate of the American Chiropractic Board of Sports Physicians (DACBSP), both regulated by the American Chiropractic Board of Sports Physicians (ACBSP).† The ACBSP has worked diligently to establish high standards for competency and ethics.[5]

SPORTS INJURIES IN CHIROPRACTIC PRACTICE

In many ways, sports chiropractic differs little from general chiropractic practice. Many of the conditions treated are observed in the general population, although with different causes. Examples include (1) an ankle sprain from stepping on a toy that a child left in the hallway, rather than from landing on another player's foot when rebounding in basketball; (2) hurting the lower back from picking up a box at work, rather than from lifting a heavy weight in the gym; or (3) lateral epicondylosis from the excessive use of a screwdriver, rather than from playing tennis.

Unique Elements

Many unique elements exist in the management of the athletic patients. Dietary education is more often furnished with the intent of improving athletic performance rather than treating obesity. Added emphasis on soft tissue techniques and extremity adjustment/manipulation

Journal of Sports Chiropractic and Rehabilitation ceased publication in 2001.
†Both designations replace the term *physician* with *practitioner* for those practicing in states that deny chiropractors the use of the term *physician*.

also is provided, because injuries to soft tissues and extremities are the most common type of sports injuries. Many athletes seek chiropractic care in an effort to find a performance advantage—an **ergogenic** effect (i.e., an effect that tends to improve or enhance athletic performance). Two studies[6,7] investigated the ergogenic effects of chiropractic care; however, because of methodologic problems, any conclusions as to possible benefits are premature.

An understanding of the unique psychology of the athlete is important. In general practice, the chiropractor must be vigilant for patients with **fear avoidance behavior** who need motivation to work through the pain and effort of rehabilitation to treat their conditions.[8,9] In sports chiropractic practice, on the other hand, the practitioner must be vigilant for the athlete whose motivation to return to training or competition causes him or her to work too hard on rehabilitation or to return to a high level of activity too soon. In fact, the athlete's motivation to continue to train and compete may be the source of many injuries.[10]

Although injured workers often want their DCs to provide an excuse from work, injured athletes are fearful that the doctor will tell them to refrain from training or competition. Instructing the injured athlete to discontinue training (or competition) often leads the athlete to discontinue care instead of discontinuing training. Therefore whenever prudent, practitioners should tell athletes to reduce **training volume** (duration times intensity) and to discontinue training only if their condition does not improve at an acceptable rate. This approach often results in the athlete taking responsibility for the decision to discontinue training rather than blaming the doctor for "making" him or her stop.

Sports Medicine Team

Chiropractors seeking to integrate within a multidisciplinary **sports medicine team** must understand the roles of all the members on that team, particularly the leadership role of the **athletic trainer**. The team's goals are preventing, treating, and rehabilitating sports injuries, as well as working to enhance the performance of the healthy athlete.

At most events when an athlete is injured, the athletic trainer will conduct the initial evaluation and determine whether consultation with another professional on the sports medicine staff is needed (i.e., the trainer will **triage** the athlete). At some events a medical director controls all aspects of the involvement of the sports medicine team. Bypassing the system is not proper protocol, and such a breech may have negative consequences for the athlete or the doctor or both. When working with a team or at an athletic event, proper protocol must be clearly understood at the outset to avoid misunderstandings.

ON-FIELD EVENT PARTICIPATION

On-field event participation can be one of the most satisfying venues for sports chiropractors. There is, of course, the excitement of being at an athletic event, often with access to locations not ordinarily open to nonplayers. Watching a football game from the sidelines, a hockey game from the bench, or a marathon from the finish line provides an unequaled perspective on the sport. Depending on the event, this type of participation may be contractually paid by the team, or more often this participation occurs on a voluntary basis as a member of an event's sports medicine staff. Such work can be rewarding both from an experiential standpoint and from a marketing standpoint. However, care should be taken to avoid overstepping the bounds of the relationship. Sometimes the benefit will be to the profession and not the individual professional, particularly when working at national and international class events. In such cases, the athletes are usually not from the locale where the event is taking place and thus will not become the chiropractor's regular patients. There is value, nonetheless, as the athletes discover that chiropractic care should become part of their sports health care.

As mentioned earlier, the hierarchy of the sports medicine staff needs to be understood at the outset. Once that understanding is established, the sports chiropractor at an event has the opportunity to learn from other professionals and possibly teach them about chiropractic. Further, treating an athlete who needs to continue competing at an event is a great test of the practitioner's clinical skills. It is similar to the advertisement for automobile tires in which there are images of race cars and an announcer who says that they learn more in a day at the track about how to make tires better than they would in years of testing on the road. Similarly, the skills the practitioner learns while helping injured athletes to compete also helps improve the effectiveness and efficiency of the treatment of nonathletes. Treatment at events runs the gamut from old to new injuries to helping improve the athletes' neuromusculoskeletal function so that they may compete at a higher level.

MECHANISMS OF SPORTS INJURIES

Seven basic mechanisms of sports injuries have been characterized and may occur singularly or in combinations. They are the following:
- Contact (e.g., tackle in football)
- Impact (e.g., hitting the ground while running)
- Overuse (e.g., impingement syndrome from swimming)
- Dynamic overload (e.g., muscle strain from excessive effort)
- Inflexibility and muscle imbalance (e.g., hamstring muscle strain from tightness and weakness of the hamstrings)
- Structural vulnerability (e.g., hyperpronation of the foot or joint dysfunction)
- Rapid growth (e.g., Osgood-Schlatter disease)[11]

The degree of injury from any of these mechanisms will vary, depending on the force involved. Injuries range from the macro level (i.e., evident or acute onset injury, including **Grade II and III sprains and strains,** fractures) to the micro level (i.e., repetitive or overuse injuries including tendinosis, myofascial trigger points, **Grade I sprains and strains,** stress fractures, stress reactions). Obviously, macrotrauma more likely involves high magnitude forces. Such forces are typically associated with high-velocity sports such as skiing or those involving more massive athletes, such as football.[12] Microtrauma is common to all sports, making up to 50% of all injuries.[11] Typically called **overuse injuries,** these are the result of repetitive low-magnitude forces, causing microscopic disruption of the structure of the involved tissues.[12]

High-force injuries cause failure or rupture of the tissue to various degrees. Thus depending on the force and the rate of application of that force, when muscle, ligament, and tendon are subjected to high loads, they will tear at a microscopic level (Grade I), tear at the macroscopic level resulting in partial tear (Grade II), or suffer a complete tear (Grade III).[11]

High rates of speed or a great magnitude of load can cause bone to fracture. Repeated low-force loading may result in a stress reaction (evident on a bone scan but not on radiographic films) or a stress fracture (evident on both bone scan and in radiographic studies).[13,14] The specific tissue injured depends on the rate of loading and the age of the athlete. Younger athletes are more prone to avulsion fractures, whereas the same mechanism of injury in the older athlete will spare the bone and injure the ligament, muscle, or the tendon.[11]

Neuromusculoskeletal Dysfunction

A variety of neuromusculoskeletal (NMS) conditions affecting athletes may be classified as *dysfunction*. The primary NMS dysfunction treated by chiropractors is the subluxation complex.[16] This dysfunction includes but is not limited to spinal and extremity joint dysfunction (i.e., subluxation), myofascial trigger points (i.e., tender, neurologically hyperactive loci in muscle that can produce referred pain),[17] and adhesions (i.e., scar tissue).[18,19] These are common sequelae to training and competing.

Prevention of Sports Injuries

Understanding the rules, techniques, biomechanics and mechanisms of injuries in each sport is crucial to preventing injuries and is the minimal knowledge needed to work with athletes in any sport. Although a detailed description of injuries specific to each sport is beyond the scope of this

OVERUSE SYNDROMES

Microtrauma is typically the result of repetitive use, the so-called *overuse syndrome*. Overuse syndromes are believed to result from repeated microtrauma that overrides the body's ability to repair the injury, which may be considered analogous to fatigue failure of mechanical parts. Overuse syndromes affect athletes in all sports.[12]

Classifying these microtraumatic conditions as overuse syndromes is hazardous; if they are due to overuse, then the only treatment would be to use the injured part less. Thus it might be preferable to think of these conditions as "mal-use" syndromes. Dysfunction (both joint and muscle), improper equipment, improper sports technique, and increasing the volume of training (intensity and duration) too rapidly are all causes of overuse syndromes.

Common examples include the following:

Tendinosis. Although formerly called **tendinitis,** this appellation appears to be inappropriate. Rather than being an inflammatory condition, biopsies have shown a degeneration of a tendon.

Stress fracture. This microfracture in bone can be observed on both radiographic films and bone scans.

Stress reaction. The same condition as a stress fracture but at an earlier stage, this microfracture can only be found on bone scans.

Shoulder impingement syndrome. Also known as *swimmer's shoulder,* the greater tuberosity of the humerus impinges on the supraspinatus tendon and subacromial bursa, resulting in pain and tendon degeneration.

Patellofemoral arthralgia. In this condition also known as *runner's knee,* the patellofemoral joint becomes irritated, which is often the result of tight hamstring muscles, hyperpronation, or improper choice of running shoes.

Iliotibial friction syndrome. In this common injury in runners, a tight tensor fascia lata causes the iliotibial band to snap over the lateral femoral epicondyle.

text, an outstanding discussion of sport-specific mechanisms of sports injuries can be found in *Sports Injuries: Mechanisms, Prevention, and Treatment*.[20] For the chiropractor in particular, differentiating macrotrauma and NMS dysfunction is important.

Preventing *macro*trauma may not be possible, because these injuries are often accidental. Increased awareness of the terrain, the movements and location of other competitors, improved training, better protective equipment, and safety-based improvements in sports rules may all decrease (although never eliminate) the incidence of macrotrauma. *Micro*trauma may be avoided by improved training, better techniques, and improvements in equipment, ensuring that the intensity and duration of training does not exceed the body's ability to adapt to the demands of training.

Because dysfunction is associated with microtrauma, its prevention is dependent on preventing microtrauma. Similarly, it is reasonable to assume that correcting such dysfunction should help prevent other sports injuries by improving NMS function. Minimizing biomechanical dysfunction through spinal and extravertebral adjustment/ manipulation, as well as other adjuncts, is a central focus of the sports chiropractor.

BIOMECHANICS, PHYSIOLOGY, AND REPAIR OF SPORTS INJURIES

Kinetics, Kinematics, and Kinesiology

A complete understanding of the nature of the injury (i.e., what tissue is injured and the extent of the injury) requires understanding the biomechanics of injury. The biomechanical principles relevant to sports injuries are the **kinetics** (forces), **kinematics** (movements), and **kinesiology** (muscles causing the forces and movements) of the injury process and the material properties of the hard and soft connective tissues involved.[21] Knowing which tissues receive or generate forces during a certain movement enables the practitioner to locate the weak link in the kinetic chain.

The **kinetic chain** is the sequence of links (bones) that transmit forces (kinetics) generated

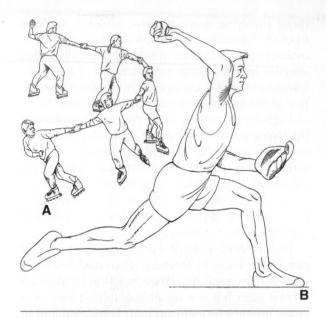

Fig. 19-2 Examples of kinetic chains. **A**, A chain of roller skaters executing a whip maneuver. **B**, The body segments of a baseball pitcher. *(From Zachazewski JE, Magee DJ, Quillen WS: Athletic injuries and rehabilitation, Philadelphia, 1996, WB Saunders.)*

by muscles (kinesiology) to create movement (kinematics). For any action, a specific sequence of the links in the kinetic chain allows for the efficient generation of forces, which causes the movement required for that activity. Problems in the sequence result in injuries somewhere along the kinetic chain.[22] Examples of the kinetic chain can be seen in Fig. 19-2. Each skater is considered a link in the chain. The forces generated by the whole chain of links (skaters) are summated, and the result is that the last person in the chain is moving faster than the first. However, a problem anywhere along this chain (dysfunction of a link) will affect the function of the "whip" (see Fig. 19-2, *A*).

Steindler[23] coined the terms **closed kinetic chain** and **open kinetic chain**. A closed kinetic chain is one in which the terminal joint of the limb that is moving is fixed to an immobile object. The classic example is running. The foot is the terminal joint, and it is on the immobile object— the ground. Forces that are generated in the leg push against the ground, causing movement. The classic example of an open kinetic chain activity is throwing a ball (see Fig. 19-2, *B*). where the arm functions as an open kinetic chain, whereas the leg functions as a closed kinetic chain.

In a baseball pitcher (see Fig. 19-2, *B*), an alteration in the function of any joint from the great toe all the way to the fingers of the hand will have an effect on some other link that affects the pitch. The classic example is what has become known as the "Dizzy Dean syndrome." Dizzy Dean, a Hall of Fame baseball pitcher, fractured his left big toe in the 1937 All-Star game. Dean returned to play too rapidly, before the toe completely healed. He altered his throwing mechanics to lessen the pain in his toe, resulting in a career-ending injury to his pitching shoulder.[21] Thus the pitcher with shoulder pain requires an examination of not only the shoulder but also all the links in the kinetic chain for the throwing motion. The practitioner must determine whether a problem in another link has caused the athlete to change throwing mechanics and, consequently, produced the shoulder problem. Even when the injury is the result of trauma, the practitioner should examine the links in the kinetic chain. Even a minimally malfunctioning link may be of the magnitude that could prevent complete recovery, despite being below the threshold necessary to cause a direct injury.

Equating pain with inflammation is a common misconception about the pathophysiology of tendon injuries (tendinopathies) (Fig 19-3). This

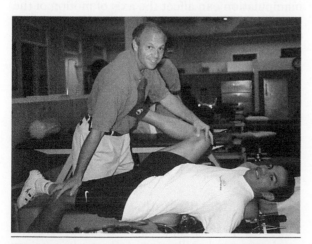

Fig. 19-3 Derek Parra, 2002 Olympic Gold Medalist in speed skating, with his chiropractor, Keith Overland. *(Courtesy Keith Overland.)*

erroneous belief has led to the misnaming and consequent improper treatment of tendinopathy. Typically, this condition has been called *tendinitis;* however, because of the relatively avascular nature of tendons, most tendinopathy is degenerative rather than inflammatory,[11] which led Puddu and colleagues to coin the currently preferred term, *tendinosis,* in 1976.[24]

Role of Inflammation in Repair

It is essential to understand the repair process. Typically, health care providers treating trauma try to minimize the inflammatory response. However, **inflammation** *is a crucial, natural step in the repair of any injury*. Although a feature of such diseases as rheumatoid arthritis, inflammation that is out of control or "purposeless" is not typical of sports injuries.[11] The current trend of treating rheumatoid arthritis with antiinflammatory medications appears to have affected the methods used to treat all injuries that start with inflammation. A commonplace assumption is that inflammation is harmful and should always be stopped. When treating injuries after the acute stage, it is important to remember that the presence of pain does not necessarily mean that inflammation is also present. Pain is only one of the four **cardinal signs** of inflammation; the others are swelling, redness, and heat.

In sports injuries, inflammation is typically "purposeful" and should be supported rather than inhibited.[11] Controlled movement and cryotherapy (therapeutic application of ice) are two ways to support purposeful inflammation.

Controlled Movement

Controlled movement is the use of braces to prevent movements that would worsen the injury, while allowing other ranges of motion. Movement stimulates blood flow, activates fibroblasts (which repairs the injury) and prevents excessive swelling. Although beneficial to ancient man as a natural, built-in splinting method, swelling is not as effective as a proper brace that allows movement. Swelling and its concomitant splinting ultimately decrease range of motion and cause more impairment than controlled movement.

Cryotherapy is the quintessential adjunctive treatment of sports injuries. It has been thought that ice reduces inflammation, but this result has not been experimentally validated. However, ice has known effects that are important in the treatment of acute sports injuries. Cold analgesia decreases pain, which allows for movement of the injured part. Movement, rather than immobilization, maintains range of motion, stimulates circulatory perfusion of the injured site, and prevents atrophy of uninjured tissues, thus speeding recovery. Icing also appears to help reduce the zone of secondary injury from posttraumatic hypoxia by slowing the metabolism of cells distal to any circulatory disruption caused by the injury.[25] This method of treatment is consistent with the fundamental philosophies of chiropractic—vitalism, naturalism, and therapeutic conservatism. In other words, the body has the ability to heal itself, and treatment should be natural and the least invasive possible.[26]

TREATMENT APPROACHES TO SPORTS INJURIES—THE CHIROPRACTIC MODEL

The chiropractic approach to the management of sports injuries often combines local and whole-system methods. The local approach involves treatment directed at the specific tissue injured, whereas the whole-system approach is directed toward tissues, which may be relatively distant from the local site of injury, whose dysfunction results in added stresses to the injured tissue. These dysfunctional tissues are either involved in the cause of the injury, or, at a minimum, they interfere with the complete and rapid recovery from the injury. Treating these dysfunctional tissues is similar to what has been termed *reducing force loads*.[27] For example, appropriate management of a knee injury may involve direct attention to the knee, but treatment may also include adjustment/manipulation of the lumbar spine or ankle or treatment of soft tissue dysfunction at the hip or ankle.

Treating Dysfunction

Chiropractic primarily concerns itself with the treatment of NMS dysfunction, termed the *sub-luxation complex*.[16] Management of sports injuries does not fundamentally differ from treating NMS dysfunction in nonathletes, except that athletes respond faster but also place more stress on the NMS system.

Treating Microtrauma

Chiropractic treatment of microtrauma is multifaceted, with a variety of local treatments to the injured tissue and distal treatments to improve overall function. Certain soft tissue treatment methods, such as postisometric relaxation (PIR),[28] Active Muscular Relaxation Techniques (AMRT),[29-31] Muscle Energy Techniques,[32] Active Release Techniques (ART),[19] and Graston Instrument–assisted Soft Tissue Mobilization (GISTM)[18] are applied directly to the injured soft tissues to assist their healing.[18,33-49] By helping to elongate the muscle, these methods may be helpful in treating myofascial trigger points or other muscular dysfunctions that cause shortening or spasm of the muscle. ART and GISTM may help break up soft tissue adhesions, which inhibit function and restrict movement. GISTM has been shown to specifically stimulate fibroblasts to both replicate and synthesize collagen, which will help heal soft tissue injury[50,51] (see Chapter 13 for greater detail on soft tissue procedures).

Pilot research has shown that ankle joint manipulation can affect the axis of motion of the ankle, knee, or hip joint.[52] This research provides some support for the common practice of manipulating joint dysfunctions kinetically associated with the injured tissue at the site of injury and proximal or distal in the kinetic chain.* As noted earlier, a whole-system approach, in which joints and other structures are seen in relationship rather than in isolation, is central to effective chiropractic case management of sports injuries.

Treating Macrotrauma

The chiropractic approach to macrotrauma emphasizes rehabilitation, improved function, and the treatment of NMS dysfunction associ-

---

*References 33, 35, 39-41, 43, 44, 49, 53-66.

ated with the injury. Manual medicine pioneer Mennel's initial introduction to extremity manipulation was in the management of post-fracture pain after the fracture had healed.[65] Adjustment/ manipulation can be the part of the treatment of macrotrauma[40,62,66] or dysfunction secondary to the trauma.[67] As described in greater detail in Chapter 23, scar formation and a disorganized connective tissue matrix are likely to develop unless appropriate postinjury rehabilitation is provided, in which adjustment/manipulation may play an important role. Early exercise and joint motion in rehabilitation produces a better concentration of collagen, resulting in a more organized scar tissue, with better tensile strength and function compared with soft tissue not rehabilitated soon after injury.

Comparison of Medical and Chiropractic Approaches

As previously described, the chiropractic model primarily addresses the biomechanical and neurophysiologic dysfunction of the NMS. It is a whole-system approach in which treatment addresses the overall functioning of the body and does not necessarily solely focus on the specific site of injury. For example, a patient with plantar fasciitis may be treated by adjusting the ankle or knee joint, along with stretching or other myofascial treatments, to correct the biomechanics of gait,[44] thus theoretically minimizing stress on the plantar fascia.

Commonly, the medical approach is more locally focused, with treatment often exclusively directed to the site of injury. Once again considering the patient with plantar fasciitis discussed in the previous paragraph, medical treatment would be directed at the plantar fascia, with either physical therapy modalities or medication (or both) used to relieve the symptoms along with rest to allow for healing.

Depending on the circumstances, chiropractors may decide to use a local treatment in addition to their traditional whole-system approach. With the plantar fasciitis case, the practitioner might also adjust the joints in the leg and also use physiotherapeutic modalities or procedures

similar to ART[19] or GISTM[18] to have a direct effect on the plantar fascia.

MANAGEMENT OF SPECIFIC TYPES OF DISORDERS

A thorough discussion of the management of specific sports injuries is beyond the scope of this text. For such a discussion the reader is referred to *Conservative Management of Sports Injuries*.[68] Currently, the research literature on chiropractic management of sports injuries consists of one clinical trial[62] and a substantial number of case reports. The following is a basic introduction to the general principles of management for injuries of muscles, tendons, and ligaments.

Fundamental Clinical Approach

Acute management typically includes standard first aid using rest, ice, compression, and elevation (RICE).[69] Rest, compression, and elevation all reduce swelling. Swelling can have the beneficial effect of naturally splinting the injured part, but it is detrimental if the athlete has the ability to stabilize the injured part appropriately. With appropriate stabilization (e.g., Air-Cast), controlled mobility will speed recovery.[70,74]

As noted earlier, ice is commonly believed to be antiinflammatory; however, its mode of action is to increase blood flow, decrease pain, and decrease metabolism. The increased blood flow augments the supply of nutrients to injured areas, thus helping to speed recovery. As an analgesic, ice allows the athlete to commence early self-mobilization, which speeds healing, prevents a loss of range of motion, and stimulates blood flow. Finally, ice may prevent secondary necrosis, which is the death of cells not injured in the original trauma. This cell death is due to hypoxia distal to the injury site from the disruption of circulation. By decreasing metabolism, ice prevents secondary necrosis. As soon as tolerated, cryotherapy (application of ice) or **cryokinetics** (ice plus motion) is helpful. Icing is followed by controlled stretching and accommodative resistance exercises (the doctor provides the resistance).[25,75]

Muscle

Muscle dysfunction requires treatment appropriate to the type of dysfunction as follows: (1) myofascial trigger points would be treated with PIR[28] or trigger point pressure release[76]; (2) chronic muscle shortening would be treated with PIR[28] or postfacilitation stretches[77,78]; and (3) adhesions would be treated with ARTs[19] or GISTM.[18] Although spinal adjustment/manipulation has often been used as part of the treatment for muscle strains, only one study has found that it speeds recovery from muscle strain. In Cibulka's[79] study, adjustment/manipulation of the sacroiliac joint increased the strength and speed of recovery from a hamstring injury. Current research is equivocal on the effects of adjustment/manipulation on muscle strength in uninjured people, with two studies finding increased muscle strength and two finding no change.[80-83]

Tendon

Because most tendinopathies are not associated with inflammation, treatment should stimulate repair of the degeneration and promote healing by stimulating inflammation and collagen deposition.[11] **Eccentric loading** (i.e., where a muscle lengthens during the contraction) of tendons[84-87] and longitudinal massage[50,51] such as GISTM has been shown to stimulate tendon regeneration.

Ligament

Because ligaments are structurally weakened by immobilization[88] and strengthened by movement and exercise,[89] early controlled movement is important in the treatment of sprains. Early controlled movement has been found to result in the complete recovery of Grade III medial collateral ligament sprains to the extent that a blinded examiner could not determine whether the ligament had ever been injured.[73,74,90]

Joint Dysfunction

Some chiropractors restrict their treatment of joints to adjustment/manipulation of the spine only. However, it should be noted that as far back as September 1896, the founder of chiropractic, Daniel David Palmer, wrote in a letter that he performed adjustment/manipulation of the foot, 1 year after he discovered chiropractic. Palmer proposed that this method should be used for foot conditions. In the 1930s, other chiropractors and osteopaths wrote about the influence of foot adjustment/manipulation on the function of the rest of the body.[91] Thus extremity adjustment/manipulation and spinal adjustment/manipulation have often been used not only for problems local to the symptomatic joint but also for conditions elsewhere along the kinetic chain. Extremity motion palpation, as well as adjustment/manipulation, are fundamental to chiropractic management of athletic injuries and are included in the programs leading to eligibility for the Certified Chiropractic Sports Physician (CCSP) and Diplomate of the American Chiropractic Board of Sports Physicians (DACBSP) examinations (see Chapters 10 and 12 for details on extremity palpation and adjustment/manipulation).

The few studies of extremity adjustment/manipulation in the peer-reviewed literature have been primarily basic rather than applied in nature.[92-98] The first biomechanical studies related to adjustment/manipulation were actually conducted on extremities.[94,95] Roston and Wheeler-Haines[94] appear to be the first to use the term **cavitation** to refer to the cracking sound associated with joint adjustment/manipulation, and they identified the gas released during cavitation as more than 80% carbon dioxide.

Very few clinical trials have been conducted on the effects of extremity adjustment/manipulation. Studies on asymptomatic healthy subjects have shown no effect of ankle adjustment/manipulation on range of motion.[98,99] However, in subjects with Grade I or Grade II ankle sprain, Pellow and Brantingham[62] found that ankle manipulation reduced pain and increased ankle range of motion and ankle function compared with sham treatment. For a more complete discussion of extremity adjustment/manipulation, the reader is referred to Peter Gale's "Joint Mobilization" chapter in *Functional soft tissue examination and treatment by manual methods: the extremities.*[100]

Rehabilitation

The purpose of rehabilitation is to return the athlete to preinjury status as rapidly as possible, which involves restoration of flexibility, both in terms of joint range of motion and the flexibility of the overall musculotendinous system. Muscles must be conditioned to restore their strength, power, and endurance. The aerobic capacity of the cardiovascular system must be restored, although it is prudent when treating an injury to maintain cardiovascular function with an activity that is safe for the injured athlete (e.g., using an upper body ergometer with a lower extremity injury). Proprioception, functional activities, and sport-specific skills must be retrained. If there were errors in technique that led to the injury, these, too, must be corrected. Finally, an often overlooked part of the rehabilitation is restoration of a proper attitude about training and competition, which is a role for the sports psychologist.[69] (Rehabilitation is discussed in depth in Chapter 14.)

Review *Questions*

1. What features of sports chiropractic practice differentiate it from general chiropractic practice?
2. When working as part of a sports medicine team, why is it crucial to understand the whole sports medicine team?
3. What are the seven basic mechanisms of sports injuries?
4. What distinguishes Grade I, Grade II, and Grade III injuries?
5. Why might an overuse syndrome be called a mal-use syndrome?
6. What are some common overuse syndromes? Describe.
7. What can be done to prevent sports injuries?
8. What is the kinetic chain?
9. Why is tendonitis an uncommon and often misdiagnosed condition? What is the more common cause of tendinopathy?
10. Discuss the overall management of muscle, tendon, and ligament injuries.

Concept *Questions*

1. What is the rationale for the treatment of sports injury–related inflammation?
2. What is the treatment for tendinopathy?
3. What differentiates the chiropractic model from the medical model for the management of sports injuries?

REFERENCES

1. Stump J, Redwood D: The use and role of sport chiropractors in the National Football League: a short report, *J Manipulative Physiol Ther* 25(3):E2, 2002.
2. Dintenfass J: Dr. Erle Painter, pioneer sports chiropractor, presents his experiences with Boston Braves and New York Yankees, *Chiropr Sports Med* 1(3):114, 1987.
3. Rehm W: "Doc" Painter and the "Mighty" New York Yankees . . . Ruth, DiMaggio, and Gehrig were his patients, *Chiropr Hist* 12(1):10, 1992.
4. Danchik JJ: *History of chiropractic involvement in the Olympics.* In Haley R, editor, Olympic Sports Chiropractic Symposium: 2002, May 18-19, East Rutherford, NJ, 2002, New Jersey Chiropractic Society Sports Council.
5. Moreau WJ: *Development of an ethics policy and procedures in a chiropractic specialty*, ACC X/RAC VIII Conference, 2002, New Orleans, La, 2002, Association of Chiropractic Colleges.
6. Lauro A, Mouch B: Chiropractic effects on athletic ability, *J Chiropr Res Clin Invest* 6(4):84, 1991.
7. Schwartzbauer J et al: Athletic performance and physiological measures in baseball players following upper cervical chiropractic care: a pilot study, *J Vertebral Subluxation Res* 1(4):33, 1997.
8. Waddell G et al: A fear-avoidance beliefs questionnaire (FABQ) and the role of fear-avoidance beliefs in chronic low back pain and disability, *Pain* 52(2):157, 1993.
9. Waddell G: *The back pain revolution*, New York, 1998, Churchill Livingstone.
10. Stanish WD: Overuse injuries in athletes: a perspective, *Med Sci Sports Exerc* 16(1):1, 1984.
11. Leadbetter WB: Soft tissue athletic injury. In Fu FH, Stone DA, editors: *Sports injuries: mechanisms, prevention, and treatment*, ed 2, Philadelphia, 2001, Lippincott–Williams & Wilkins.
12. Perle SM: The biomechanics and physiology of nontraumatic soft tissue injury and repair: a literature review, *Top Clin Chiropr* 4(2):1, 1997.
13. Jackson DW et al: Stress reactions involving the pars interarticularis in young athletes, *Am J Sports Med* 9(5):304, 1981.
14. Jones BH et al: Exercise-induced stress fractures and stress reactions of bone: epidemiology, etiology, and classification. In Pandolf KB, editor: *Exercise*

and sport science reviews, Baltimore, 1989, Williams & Wilkins.

15. Lachmann S, Jenner JR: Soft tissue injuries in sport, ed 2, London, 1994, Blackwell Scientific Publications.

16. Lantz CA: The vertebral subluxation complex, ICA Inter Rev Chiropr (Oct):37, 1989.

17. Mennell JM: The musculoskeletal system: differential diagnosis from symptoms and physical signs, Gaithersburg, Md, 1992, Aspen Publishers.

18. Carey MT: The Graston technique instruction manual, ed 2, Indianapolis, 2001, TherapyCare Resources.

19. Leahy PM: Active Release Techniques: logical soft tissue treatment. In Hammer WI, editor: Functional soft tissue examination and treatment by manual methods: the extremities, ed 2, Gaithersburg, Md, 1999, Aspen Publishers.

20. Fu FH, Stone DA, editors: Sports injuries: mechanisms, prevention, and treatment, ed 2, Philadelphia, 2001, Lippincott–Williams & Wilkins.

21. Whiting WC, Zernicke RF: Biomechanics of musculoskeletal injury, Champaign, Ill, 1998, Human Kinetics.

22. Kibler WB: Determining the extent of the functional deficit. In Kibler WB et al, editors: Functional rehabilitation of sports and musculoskeletal injuries, Gaithersburg, Md, 1998, Aspen Publishers.

23. Steindler A: Kinesiology of the human body under normal and pathological conditions, Springfield, Ill, 1955, Charles C. Thomas.

24. Puddu G, Ippolito E, Postacchini F: A classification of Achilles tendon disease, Am J Sports Med 4(4):145, 1976.

25. Knight KL: Cryotherapy in sport injury management, Champaign, Ill, 1995, Human Kinetics.

26. Coulter ID: Chiropractic: a philosophy for alternative health care, Oxford, UK, 1999, Butterworth-Heinemann Medical.

27. Nirschl RP: Elbow tendinosis/tennis elbow, Clin Sports Med 11(4):851, 1992.

28. Lewit K: Post-isometric relaxation in combination with other methods of muscular facilitation and inhibition, Man Med 2:101, 1986.

29. Liebenson C: Active muscular relaxation techniques. Part I. Basic principles and methods, J Manipulative Physiol Ther 12(6):446, 1989.

30. Liebenson C: Active Muscular Relaxation Techniques. Part II. Clinical application, J Manipulative Physiol Ther 13(1):2, 1990.

31. Liebenson C: Manual resistance techniques and self-stretches for improving flexibility/mobility. In Liebenson C, editor: Rehabilitation of the spine: a practitioner's manual, Baltimore, 1996, Williams & Wilkins.

32. Chaitow L: Muscle energy techniques, New York, 1996, Churchill Livingstone.

33. DeFranca GG: The snapping hip syndrome: a case study, Chiropr Sports Med 2(1):8, 1988.

34. Leahy PM, Mock LE III: Altered biomechanics of the shoulder and the subscapularis, Chiropr Sports Med 5(3):62, 1991.

35. BenEliyahu DJ: Conservative chiropractic management of patellofemoral pain syndrome: a case study, Chiropr Sports Med 6(2):57, 1992.

36. Hammer WI: Meniscotibial (coronary) ligament sprain: diagnosis and treatment. Chiropr Sports Med 2(2):48, 1988.

37. Schneider MJ: Snapping hip syndrome in a marathon runner: treatment by manual trigger point therapy—a case study, Chiropr Sports Med 4(2):54, 1990.

38. Horrigan JM: Resolution of a groin injury in a professional hockey player by soft tissue mobilization: a case report, Chiropr Sports Med 6(4):151, 1992.

39. Wood A: Conservative management of patellofemoral pain syndrome, J Sports Chiropr Rehabil 12(1):1, 1998.

40. Ames R: Weightlifting injuries and their chiropractic management: a clinical review. Part 2: Injury and management overview, J Sports Chiropr Rehabil 12(2):71, 1998.

41. Glasco G, Glasco W: Conservative evaluation and intervention of a sport-related injury: turf toe, J Sports Chiropr Rehabil 12(2):82, 1998.

42. Baer JM: Iliotibial band syndrome in cyclists: evaluation and treatment: a case report, J Sports Chiropr Rehabil 13(2):66, 1999.

43. Pollard H, Quodling N: Management of hamstring injury: a review and case report, J Sports Chiropr Rehabil 13(3):98, 1999.

44. Pollard H, So V: Management of plantar fasciitis: a case report, J Sports Chiropr Rehabil 13(3):93, 1999.

45. Buchberger DJ: Posterior-superior glenoid impingement of the throwing shoulder: evaluation and management, J Sports Chiropr Rehabil 14(2):5, 2000.

46. Hammer WI, editor: Functional soft tissue examination and treatment by manual methods: the extremities, ed 2, Gaithersburg, Md, 1999, Aspen Publishers.

47. Leahy PM: Active Release Techniques soft tissue management system for the upper extremity, Colorado Springs, Colo, 1996, Active Release Techniques.

48. Leahy PM: Active Release Techniques soft tissue management system for the upper extremity, Colorado Springs, Colo, 1998, Active Release Techniques.

49. Moreau CE, Moreau SR: Chiropractic management of a professional hockey player with recurrent shoulder instability, J Manipulative Physiol Ther 24(6):425, 2001.

50. Gehlsen GM, Ganion LR, Helfst R: Fibroblast responses to variation in soft tissue mobilization pressure, Med Sci Sports Exerc 31(4):531, 1999.

51. Davidson C et al: Rat tendon morphologic and functional changes resulting from soft tissue mobilization, Med Sci Sports Exerc 29(3):313, 1997.

52. Ball KA, Perle SM: *Effect of a single manipulation of the tibiotalar (ankle) joint upon lower extremity joint alignment*. In Rosner AL, editor: 2002 International Conference on Spinal Manipulation, 8th Annual Conference on Advancements in Chiropractic, CCCRC Biannual Research Symposium, 2002, Toronto, Ontario, Canada, The Foundation for Chiropractic Education and Research.

53. Michaud TC: Recurrent lower tibial stress fracture in a long-distance runner: a case report, *Chiropr Sports Med* 2(3):78, 1988.

54. Michaud TC: Pathomechanics and treatment of hallux limitus: a case report, *Chiropr Sports Med* 2(2): 55, 1988.

55. Morley JJ: Treatment of chronic athletic injuries of the low back and lower extremity utilizing manipulation, *Chiropr Sports Med* 3(1):4, 1989.

56. Souza TA: Evaluating lateral knee pain, *Chiropr Sports Med* 3(4):103, 1989.

57. Gerber JM, Pierson VL: Long thoracic nerve injury in a high jumper: a case report, *Chiropr Sports Med* 7(1): 9, 1993.

58. Williams BD, Brockholn JL: Subacromial impingement syndrome: a case series, *Chiropr Sports Med* 8(3):104, 1994.

59. Baker GJ: iliotibial band and tibialis posterior syndromes resulting from a fixed talus: a case report, *Chiropr Sports Med* 8(4):119, 1995.

60. Gelfound CJ, Devore JW: Manipulation and rehabilitation in the treatment of patellofemoral tracking dysfunction: a single-subject experiment, *Chiropr Sports Med* 9(4):131, 1995.

61. Stoddard JK, Johnson CD: Conservative treatment of a patient with a mild acromioclavicular joint separation, *J Sports Chiropr Rehabil* 14(4):118, 2000.

62. Pellow JE, Brantingham JW: The efficacy of adjusting the ankle in the treatment of subacute and chronic grade I and grade II ankle inversion sprains, *J Manipulative Physiol Ther* 24(1):17, 2001.

63. Kaufman RL: Conservative chiropractic care of lateral epicondylitis, *J Manipulative Physiol Ther* 23(9):619, 2000.

64. Meyer JJ et al: Effectiveness of chiropractic management for patellofemoral pain syndrome's symptomatic control phase: a single subject experiment, *J Manipulative Physiol Ther* 13(9):539, 1990.

65. Mennell JM: *Joint pain: diagnosis and treatment using manipulative techniques*, Boston, 1964, Little Brown.

66. Buchberger DJ: Scapular-dysfunctional impingement syndrome as a cause of grade 2 rotator cuff tear: a case study, *Chiropr Sports Med* 7(2):38, 1993.

67. Buchberger DJ: Use of Active Release Techniques in the postoperative shoulder: a case report, *J Sports Chiropr Rehab* 13(2):60, 1999.

68. Hyde T, Gengenbach M, editors: *Conservative management of sports injuries*, Baltimore, 1997, Williams & Wilkins.

69. Brukner P, Khan K: *Clinical sports medicine*, ed 2, Sydney, 2001, McGraw-Hill.

70. Kern-Steiner R, Washecheck HS, Kelsey DD: Strategy of exercise prescription using an unloading technique for functional rehabilitation of an athlete with an inversion ankle sprain, *J Orthop Sports Phys Ther* 29(5):282, 1999.

71. Kannus P: Immobilization or early mobilization after an acute soft-tissue injury? *Phys Sportsmed* 28(3): 55, 2000.

72. Kamps B et al: The influence of immobilization versus exercise on scar formation in the rabbit patellar tendon after excision of the central third, *Am J Sports Med* 22(6):803, 1994.

73. Reider B et al: Treatment of isolated medial collateral ligament injuries in athletes with early functional rehabilitation: a five-year follow-up study, *Am J Sports Med* 22(4):470, 1994.

74. Eiff MP, Smith AT, Smith GE: Early mobilization versus immobilization in the treatment of lateral ankle sprains, *Am J Sports Med* 22(1):83, 1994.

75. Knight KL: Cold as a modifier of sports-induced inflammation. In Leadbetter WB, editor: *Sports-induced inflammation*, Park Ridge, Ill, 1990, American Academy of Orthopaedic Surgeons.

76. Simons DG, Travell JG, Simons LS: *Travell and Simons' myofascial pain and dysfunction: the trigger point manual, upper half of body*, vol 1, Baltimore, 1999, Williams & Wilkins.

77. Hammer WI: Muscle imbalance and postfacilitation stretch. In Hammer WI, editor: *Functional soft tissue examination and treatment by manual methods: the extremities*, ed 2, Gaithersburg, Md, 1999, Aspen Publishers.

78. Liebenson C: Manual resistance techniques and self stretches for improving flexibility and mobility. In Liebenson C, editor: *Rehabilitation of the spine: a practitioner's manual*, Baltimore, 1996, Williams & Wilkins.

79. Cibulka MT et al: Hamstring strain treated by mobilizing the sacroiliac joint, *Phys Ther* 66(8):1220, 1986.

80. Bonci A et al: Strength modulation of the spinal erector muscles immediately following manipulation of the thoracolumbar spine, *J Chiropr Res Clin Invest* 6(2):29, 1990.

81. Bonci A, Ratliff C: Strength modulation of the biceps brachii muscles immediately following a single manipulation of the C4/5 intervertebral motor unit in healthy subjects; a preliminary report, *Am J Chiropr Med* 3(1):14, 1990.

82. Pollard H, Ward G: Strength change of quadriceps femoris following a single manipulation of the L3/4 vertebral motion segment: a preliminary investigation, *J Neuromusculoskel Sys* 4(4):137, 1996.

83. Suter E et al: Decrease in quadriceps inhibition after sacroiliac joint manipulation in patients with anterior knee pain, *J Manipulative Physiol Ther* 22(3): 149, 1999.

84. Jensen K, Di Fabio RP: Evaluation of eccentric exercise in treatment of patellar tendonitis, *Phys Ther* 69:211, 1989.

85. Stanish WD, Rubinovich RM, Curwin S: Eccentric exercise in chronic tendonitis, *Clin Orthop* July(208):65, 1986.

86. Fyfe I, Stanish WD: The use of eccentric training and stretching in the treatment and prevention of tendon injuries, *Clin Sports Med* 11(3):601, 1992.

87. Alfredson H et al: Heavy-load eccentric calf muscle training for the treatment of chronic Achilles tendinosis, *Am J Sports Med* 26(3):360, 1998.

88. Hargens AR, Akeson WH: Stress effects on tissue nutrition and viability. In Hargens AR, editor: *Tissue nutrition and viability*, New York, 1986, Springer-Verlag.

89. Cabaud HE et al: Exercise effects on the strength of the rat anterior cruciate ligament, *Am J Sports Med* 8(2):79, 1980.

90. Buss D et al: Nonoperative treatment of acute anterior cruciate ligament injuries in a selected group of patients, *Am J Sports Med* 23(2):160, 1995.

91. Keating JC Jr et al: A brief history of manipulative foot care in America, 1896-1960, *Chiropr Tech* 4(3):90, 1992.

92. Méal GM, Scott RA: Analysis of the joint crack by simultaneous recording of sound and tension, *J Manipulative Physiol Ther* 9(3):189, 1986.

93. Mierau D et al: Manipulation and mobilization of the third metacarpophalangeal joint: a quantitative radiographic and range of motion study, *Man Med* 3:135, 1988.

94. Roston JB, Wheeler-Haines R: Cracking in the metacarpo-phalangeal joint, *J Anat* 81:165, 1947.

95. Unsworth A, Dowson D, Wright V: Cracking joints: a bioengineering study of cavitation in the metacarpophalangeal joint, *Ann Rheum Dis* 30(4):348, 1971.

96. Watson P, Kernohan WG, Mollan RAB: A study of the cracking sounds from the metacarpophalangeal joint, *Proc Instn Mech Engrs* 203:109, 1989.

97. Watson P, Mollan RAB: Cineradiography of a cracking joint, *Br J Radiol* 63:145, 1990.

98. Nield S et al: The effect of manipulation on range of motion at the ankle joint, *Scand J Rehabil Med* 25:161, 1993.

99. Fryer GA, Mudge JM, McLaughlin PA: The effect of talocrural joint manipulation on range of motion at the ankle, *J Manipulative Physiol Ther* 25(6):384, 2002.

100. Gale P: Joint mobilization. In Hammer WI, editor: *Functional soft tissue examination and treatment by manual methods: the extremities*, ed 2, Gaithersburg, Md, 1999, Aspen Publishers.

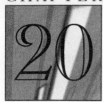

Wellness: A Lifestyle

Jennifer Jamison, MB BCh, PhD, EdD, FACNEM

Key Terms

ACTIVE COPING	HYPOTHALAMIC-PITUITARY	PRUDENT DIET
AEROBIC FITNESS	AXIS	PSYCHOSOCIAL
ANTIOXIDANTS	LACTO-OVO-VEGETARIAN	RECONCEPTUALIZING
BONE DENSITY	LEGUMES	REFINED SUGARS
CALORIES	LEUKOTRIENES	RELAXATION RESPONSE
COGNITIVE THERAPY	LIFESTYLE INTERVENTIONS	RELAXATION TRAINING
CORTISOL	MAINTENANCE CARE	SELF-CARE CONTRACT
DEEP BREATHING	OSTEOPOROSIS	THROMBOCYTE
EICOSANOIDS	PASSIVE COPING	VEGAN
FIBROMYALGIA	POLYUNSATURATED FATS	VEGETARIAN
HEME IRON	PRIMARY CONTACT	WEIGHT-BEARING EXERCISE
HOLISTIC	PRACTITIONER	WELLNESS
	PROSTAGLANDINS	WHOLE GRAINS

The chiropractic roles of the **primary contact practitioner** and expert in pain management require that chiropractors become instruments of healing. Successful chiropractors function as skilled manual practitioners and communicators, understanding people at both biomechanical and **psychosocial** levels.

Chiropractic's acceptance within the health care system and its recognition as a unique profession has, however, largely paralleled its successful management of musculoskeletal pain. The chiropractor's primary strategy in clinical management is manual intervention primarily through the spinal adjustment. Although acute pain may be primarily a physical problem, chronic pain is clearly a psychobiologic phenomenon. Chronic pain management requires recognition that the psyche and soma and the mind and body are inseparable. Psychosocial factors are among the best predictors of whether acute pain will become chronic.[1]

Therefore clinical management of chronic pain requires that intervention not be limited to physical measures. Research consistently demonstrates that patients are better able to cope with painful stimuli when they have some personal control over their situations.[2] Such findings suggest that successful pain management goes beyond purely manual intervention and that chiropractic's success in this field involves more than osseous adjustments and soft tissue work. Interventions as diverse as **cognitive therapy** (i.e., mental approaches designed to improve problem-solving skills) and **relaxation training** (i.e., physical approaches such as exercises to release muscular tension) have been reported to influence self-reported pain.[3]

Chiropractors can enhance their own **wellness** and that of their patients through a variety of **lifestyle interventions**. The most common of these self-care measures involve diet, exercise, movement, and relaxation. Adding these options to chiropractic manual methods provides a sound foundation upon which to base the content of contemporary chiropractic practice.

ACTIVE VERSUS PASSIVE APPROACHES

Active coping strategies, in which patients make an effort to function in spite of pain, are associated with better adaptive functioning than **passive coping** strategies, in which reliance may be placed on drug intervention. In contrast to passive coping strategies, which rely largely on the efforts of others, active coping strategies encourage increased patient responsibility in health care and substantially enhance the sense of personal control.[4] Chiropractors have long encouraged active patient involvement through therapeutic and preventive exercise regimens. This approach is consistent with the community's trend toward self-care and the requirement that chiropractors, similar to other health professionals who practice as a portal of entry into the health care system, promote health, screen for the early manifestations of disease, and either treat or refer patients as required.

MAINTENANCE CARE: MORE THAN PERIODIC ADJUSTMENTS

An American study found that chiropractors overwhelmingly agree that **maintenance care** to optimize health, prevent disorders, provide palliative care, and minimize recurrences should include exercise, adjustments, dietary recommendations, and patient education about lifestyle changes.[5]

Such a wide-ranging approach maximizes the preventive potential of chiropractic care. The clinical management of headaches offers an excellent example. Spinal adjustment/manipulation has been shown to decrease the frequency and intensity of both migraine and tension headaches (see Chapter 24 for further details on headaches), but there are many causes of headaches. Emotional, dietary, physical, environmental, and hormonal factors have been reported to be equally likely to precipitate a migraine, tension, or combined headache episode.[6] Using a variety of lifestyle interventions to modify emotional responses, dietary choices and physical and environmental stimuli may avert such headache attacks. An example of an active approach available to chiropractors as a supplement to manual adjustments is progressive muscle relaxation, which has been shown to improve tension headache and is most effective for those who receive home-practice instructions.[7]

An exploratory study in Australia confirmed that many chiropractic patients are likely to benefit from additional personalized health information messages.[8] The chiropractor's role as primary contact practitioner, which involves functioning as a trustworthy source of health information, counselor, and clinician, can be time consuming. Therefore strategies that facilitate effective time management of the primary contact role are highly relevant to the chiropractic practice. Selective use of health information brochures provides one cost-effective option whereby chiropractors may enhance patient awareness of health issues.[9] With the shift to increased personal responsibility in health care, it is timely that chiropractors use various user-friendly tools to establish themselves as **holistic** primary contact practitioners in conventional health care.[10]

PRUDENT DIET

Essentials of Healthy Eating

A *prudent dietary pattern* is characterized by high intakes of vegetables, fruits, **legumes, whole grains**, fish, and poultry. It carries a lower risk than the *Western dietary pattern*, which is characterized by high intakes of red meat, processed meat, refined grains, sweets and desserts, fried foods, and high-fat dairy products.[11] A **prudent diet** is also a balanced diet. It involves eating a variety of foods and includes foods from each of the five major food groups. Dairy products are an important source of calcium, riboflavin, and protein. Animal products (meat, poultry) provide protein, iron, and B_{12}. Grains and cereals provide carbohydrates, proteins, thiamin, and potentially niacin. Fruits and vegetables are important sources of **antioxidants**, vitamins, and minerals, whereas fats are a major source of energy and vitamin A. Astute food selection enables **vegetarians** to eat a healthy diet. **Lacto-ovo-vegetarians**, by including milk and eggs in their diet, avoid most nutrient deficiencies. but they need to be aware of iron deficiency. **Vegans** who exclude all animal products need to exercise even greater care and are also at risk of zinc, calcium, and vitamin B_{12} deficiencies. Dietary combinations of legumes and grains can obviate any risk of protein deficiency.

Vitamins, Minerals, Fats, and Oils

Adequate intake of vitamins and minerals is important for normal metabolism. *The minerals most likely to be deficient in the average diet are zinc, calcium, and iron.* Examples of food sources of these minerals are oysters and nuts for zinc, dairy products and sardines for calcium, and lean red meat for **heme iron,** fish for iron, and the less well-absorbed nonheme form of iron found in nonanimal products.

Vegetarians can avoid animal products rich in these minerals by selecting vegetable options. Alternate sources of calcium include dark green vegetables, broccoli, and sesame seeds, and iron can be obtained from pumpkin, cabbage, citrus fruits, and pawpaw. The concentration and biologic availability of these minerals in vegetables is lower than in animal products. Food combinations can enhance absorption. Foods rich in vitamin C increase the amount of inorganic iron absorbed from cereals and vegetables. As little as 50 mg of vitamin C can double the absorption of iron from other components in a meal.

A good diet is preferable to nutritional supplements because the ratios of nutrients in whole foods are likely to be more consistent with metabolic needs. Furthermore, both nutrient and nonnutrient components in foods have important physiologic effects. Only relatively recently has the potential of lycopene (the red carotenoid pigment in tomatoes, various berries, and other fruits) to reduce the risk of certain cancers been identified[12] or the immunologic influence of phytosterols.[13] Dietary supplements may inadvertently omit important food constituents and may under supply or over supply various nutrients.

Although dietary fats, particularly saturated fats, should be limited, an adequate intake of unsaturated fat (e.g., linoleic and linolenic acids), the essential unsaturated fatty acids, is necessary. Essential unsaturated fatty acids serve as dietary precursors for the formation of **eicosanoids,** which are powerful regulators of cell and tissue functions. They are the precursors of various **prostaglandins** and **leukotrienes** that enhance **thrombocyte** aggregation, vascular constriction and dilation, and bronchial and uterine contraction.

Vegetable oils and fish are important dietary sources of **polyunsaturated fats**. In fact, to prevent cardiovascular and other chronic disease, it has been suggested that fish should be eaten two to three times a week.[14] For vegetarians and vegans, alternative sources of omega-3 fatty acids are spinach, flaxseeds, rapeseeds (rapeseed oil is also known as *canola*), walnuts, and navy or baked beans. Nonetheless, no more than 25% of dietary energy should be derived from fat. At low intakes of fat, the type of fat appears to be less significant,[15] but the total daily cholesterol intake should be restricted to less than 300 mg, and saturated fat should be reduced to less than 10% of the total **calories**.

A diet rich in whole-grain products, vegetables, and fruits is highly recommended. Although the benefits of fruit and vegetable intake may become evident with the consumption of as few as three servings per day,[16] a daily intake of at least five servings of fruits and vegetables and at least six servings of breads, cereals, or legumes are recommended.[17] A serving is one slice of bread, one-half cup of cereal or pasta, a medium piece of fruit, or one-half cup of legumes. Eating fresh whole foods is another important dietary principle. Although processing may occasionally enhance the bioavailablity of nutrients, it usually reduces the nutrient value of foods. Eating whole foods, including whole grains, is necessary to approximate the recommended intake of 25 grams of fiber per day.

Foods to Avoid

Refined sugars should be limited, as should salt and sodium. A sodium intake of less than 2.5 grams or 100 micromolars per day requires that no salt be added during or after food preparation and that heavily or visibly salted items be excluded.

Alcoholic beverages should be consumed in moderation or not at all.[17] One-half pint of beer, one measure of spirits, or one glass of sherry or wine is considered one unit. The consumption of alcohol by men should not exceed 4 units or 40 grams of absolute alcohol per day on a regular basis or 28 units per week. Drinking is considered hazardous when 4 to 6 units are consumed per day or 28 to 42 units are consumed per week. Women should consume no more than 2 units of alcohol per day on a regular basis or 14 units per week. Drinking is harmful to women when 4 or more units per day or 28 or more units per week are consumed. Abstinence during pregnancy is highly recommended.

Fig. 20-1 provides a template for helping patients acquire good dietary habits.[10] Although a good diet can promote general health, specific dietary changes can target particular conditions. Prevention of cardiovascular disorders, **osteoporosis,** and even cancer may be facilitated by careful dietary choices. Fig. 20-2 demonstrates how this basic diet may be altered to reduce specifically the risk of cancer.[10] A prevalent theme is to limit energy consumption.

Keeping Weight within a Normal Range

Excess calorie consumption has emerged as the major dietary health hazard of modern industrialized society. Maintaining a normal body weight and keeping the body mass index (BMI) between 20 and 25 is advocated.

$$BMI = Wt(kg)/Ht(m^2)$$

(Body mass index is the weight in kilograms divided by the height in meters squared.)

All foods are a source of energy, but gram-for-gram fat is twice as energy-dense as carbohydrates and proteins. It is, however, not only

			NUTRITIONAL WELLNESS PROTOCOL
CURRENT	INTENDED	ACHIEVED	DIETARY AIM
			I eat fresh fruit or raw vegetables twice or more daily.
			I eat two or more servings of vegetables each day.
			I eat nuts, legumes, fish or chicken without the skin each day.
			I eat nuts, legumes, fish or chicken in preference to red meat.
			I eat yellow/orange and cruciferous vegetables each day.
			I eat from a calcium source, e.g., low fat milk or yogurt, sardines, sesame seeds, etc. each day.
			I eat liquid vegetable oils in preference to animal fats or solidified vegetable oils.
			I avoid excess salt.
			I eat wholegrain/wholemeal products in preference to refined products.
			I limit my sugar intake.
			I limit my fat intake.
			I limit my alcohol intake.
			I avoid charred, barbecued food.
			I avoid cured or smoked food.
			I maintain my ideal body weight.*
Insert details of present activity.	Insert date at which intended activity will be achieved.	Insert progress report on new dietary behavior.	

*To maintain an ideal body weight ingest 15 kcal for every pound of ideal body weight; to lose weight ingest 10 kcal for every pound of desired body weight; to gain weight ingest 20 kcal for every pound of desired body weight.

Fig. 20-1 Nutritional wellness protocol.

energy intake that influences body weight. In fact, the trend toward an increasingly sedentary lifestyle in the United States is believed to explain the growing prevalence of obesity, despite a shift toward consumers purchasing reduced fat and low-calorie food products.[18]

EXERCISE

Longevity and Cardiovascular Effects

Exercise promotes wellness. Physical activity has even been found to lengthen life.[19] Compared with active persons, sedentary men are over two and one-half times more likely to die from any cause and over three and one-half times more likely to die from cardiovascular disease.[20] A prospective study of over 12,000 American men found that 10 to 36 minutes each day of leisure-time physical activity of moderate intensity significantly reduced premature mortality.[21] A significantly lower death rate was also reported in individuals who performed an average of 47 minutes versus 15 minutes of activity per day.[22]

Epidemiologic studies indicate that a physically inactive lifestyle is associated with twice the risk of developing coronary artery disease.[23] The scientific evidence from 75 trials implies a strongly positive protective relationship between cardiovascular fitness and coronary heart disease.[24] Regular exercise modifies a number of the major modifiable risk factors for heart disease,[23] including the blood lipid profile,[25] blood pressure levels,[26] and fibrinogen levels.[27]

DIETARY MINIMIZATION OF CANCER RISK			
CURRENT	INTENDED	ACHIEVED	DIETARY AIM
			Overall I eat 400–800 grams (5 or more serves) of vegetables and fruits each day.
			Overall I eat 600–800 grams (7 or more serves) of cereals, pulses and roots each day.
			I eat cauliflower, cabbage, brussels sprouts, asparagus, or other cruciferous vegetables each day.
			I limit red meat to no more than 80 g on any one day.
			I limit my intake of processed or refined foods.
			I eat at least two servings each day of green leafy or yellow vegetables or yellow/orange fruit.
			I eat potatoes, bananas or resistant starch enriched products, wheat, or corn/maize each day.
			I eat soy and alfalfa sprouts, soy products, legumes, and lentils each day.
			I eat complex carbohydrates in preference to refined processed foods.
			I use olive oil but limit my fat intake avoiding animal fats and margarine.
			I eat fish in preference to meat.
			I limit my alcohol intake.
			I limit my salt intake using herbs and spices to season foods.
			I avoid burnt, charred, barbecued food.
			I avoid cured or smoked food.
			I maintain my ideal body weight.*
Insert details of present activity.	Insert date at which intended activity will be achieved.	Insert progress report on new dietary behavior.	

*Ideal body weight=wt(kg)/ht(m^2)=20–25

Fig. 20-2 Dietary minimization of cancer risk.

Musculoskeletal Effects

Musculoskeletal health also requires adequate physical activity. Physical activity, **aerobic fitness**, and muscle strength all influence **bone density**. A lifestyle that combines a moderate level of physical activity with an adequate calcium intake promotes a competent skeleton.[28] Older people with osteoporosis can benefit from moderate weight-bearing exercises.[29] Exercise not only protects against bone loss but also prevents fractures by reducing the risk of falls through improved strength, flexibility, balance, and reaction time.[30-32] Appropriate physical activity in older osteoporotic individuals decreases pain and improves fitness and the overall quality of life.[30]

Additional Benefits of Exercise

Evidence is accumulating that suggests that physical activity may help reduce the risk of cancer.[32,33] Physically active people have been shown to have a decreased rate of all-cancer mortality, and the incidence of colon, breast, and perhaps prostate cancer is lower in active individuals when compared with sedentary persons. Mental health and standard body weight are also more likely in groups who regularly exercise.[34] Exercise is a recognized strategy for stress reduction and is also a form of relaxation.

Health gains result both from high activity–high fitness exercises and from high activity–low fitness procedures. Leisure-time physical activity that fails to achieve cardiovascular fitness will, nonetheless, provide a health benefit. Older adults achieve a similar health benefit from high activity–high fitness exercises (e.g., squash, running) as they do from high activity–low fitness procedures (e.g., walking, gardening). Increased physical activity may be beneficial in preventing and managing disorders as diverse as hyperlipidemia, hypertension, obesity, nicotine addiction, diabetes mellitus, emotional disorders, cancer, osteoporosis, and age-related declines in muscular strength.[35,36] It has even been suggested that the principal focus for exercise health should be physical activity rather than physical fitness.[37] Leisure-time physical activity

rather than strenuous training is increasingly believed to be directly related to the high-density lipoprotein cholesterol level and inversely related to levels of total cholesterol, triglycerides, fibrinogen, and blood pressure.[38]

How Much Exercise is Needed?

Although it has been clearly established that exercise is beneficial, the intensity, duration, frequency, type, and time period during life when exercise is important have yet to be determined. Whereas the gross intensity of work effort needed for health benefits seems to be 20 kJ/minute[39] (achieved by cycling or ballroom dancing for 50 seconds, climbing stairs for 40 seconds, or sprinting uphill for 30 seconds), identifying the desirable threshold intensity of leisure activities for individuals is problematic.

Particular health benefits have nonetheless been linked with helping particular disorders (Table 20-1). Walking or cycling at least three times per week for 20 minutes is associated with reduced mortality from heart disease and all causes in men over the age of 64 years.[40] Compared with individuals who have no regular vigorous exercise, the risk of cardiovascular disease is reduced in those who exercise three times a week.[41] Aerobic exercise, performed 3 to 5 days per week for 20 to 60 minutes at an intensity of 55% to 90% of maximum heart rate and 40% to 85% of maximum oxygen intake reserve, is recommended to maintain cardiovascular fitness and weight control.[42] Improvement in the lipid profile is proportional to the amount of exercise performed, and benefits are most noted after walking or jogging approximately 15 km (9.3 miles) per week. Approximately 30 minutes of aerobic exercise three times a week may achieve a blood pressure reduction in individuals with elevated blood pressure. For weight loss, five to seven sessions per week of low-intensity exercise, such as walking for 30 to 40 minutes per session, is recommended.

For certain conditions, the amount of time involved in the activity appears to have a greater impact than the number of days per week that the activity is performed.[43] Men who exercise for more than 2 hours a day decrease their inci-

Table **20-1** ACTIVITY QUOTIENT FOR SPECIFIC HEALTH BENEFITS

Aim	General Health	Fitness	Fitness	
OBJECTIVE	Establish a regular physical activity pattern	Cardiovascular and muscle fitness	Muscle strength and endurance	
ACTIVITY	Physical activity	Exercise	Exercise	
MODE	Aerobic activity	Aerobic activity	Resistance exercises	Flexibility exercises
FREQUENCY	Most days	3-5 days/wk	2-3 days/wk	2-3 days/wk
DURATION	30 min over a day	20-60 min continuous	8-10 exercises; 1-3 sets as tolerated	4 or more repetitions per muscle group
INTENSITY	50%-70% MHR; 3-4 RPE	60%-80% MHR; 3-6 RPE	8-12 lifts of a load that produces fatigue in 8-12 repetitions	Static stretches; proprioceptive neuromuscular facilitation; ballistic stretch

MHR, Maximal heart rate (220 minus age); *RPE*, rating of perceived exertion (0-10).

dence of colorectal cancer by 50%, compared with men who participate in regular physical exercise for less than 1 hour per day. Men who walk 2 to 3 hours per week may reduce their risk of benign prostatic hypertrophy by up to 25%.[44]

For other conditions, the nature of the exercise is important. For example, osteoporosis prevention requires **weight-bearing exercises**. The prevention and control of osteoporosis may be facilitated by endurance weight-bearing activities, which stresses the femur and spine, for 20 to 40 minutes three times a week. Daily activity that includes a complete active range of motion, as well as weight-bearing and non–weight-bearing exercises, is optimal for cartilage viability.[45] The outcome of exercise is not limited to musculoskeletal or somatic benefits. Regular exercise, regardless of its nature or duration, enriches mental health and provides an invaluable aid in managing psychosocial stress.

STRESS MANAGEMENT
Physical and Psychosocial Stressors

Physical and psychosocial stimuli share a common stress response. Although the physiologic adaptation evoked by the stress response is well suited to acute physical stressors, the stress response is less well suited to the chronic psychosocial stressors encountered in modern life.

The hypothalamus receives and responds to emotional, cognitive, and physical information. It sets muscle tone through its control of the autonomic nervous and endocrine systems. The apparent discrepancy between the physiologic stress reaction and the socially sanctioned behavioral response is believed to hold the potential for adverse health repercussions. The physiologic response to danger is fight or flight, but socially acceptable behavior requires a calm response and suppression of anger or fear. However, although interactive biologic signaling has been clearly demonstrated, a causal link between psychosocial stress and immune function and disease has yet to be clarified.[46] Nonetheless, the literature leads to the conclusion that stress and pain are interactive and that diagnosis and management of neck-shoulder, back, and noncardiac chest pain should include consideration of psychologic factors.[47-49]

Strategies for Dealing with Stress

Failure to cope with psychosocial stress may result in persistent vigilance, an ongoing state of alert. This may be exhibited as insomnia and fatigue or in physical repercussions such as backache, tension headaches, or **fibromyalgia.**[47] It is, however, the individual's response, rather than the stimulus itself, that ultimately determines the stress response.[50] Any behavior plan or coping strategy should, consequently, be rational, flexible, and farsighted. Approaches to stress management include psychosocial and physical measures. Helpful strategies include the following:

- Identify and eliminate lifestyle variables that are perceived as stressful. Example: Leave for work before rush hour, rather than drive at the peak of traffic.
- Change perceptions of potentially stressful situations by converting threats to challenges. Example: View an examination as an opportunity to demonstrate knowledge rather than an ordeal.
- Reduce target organ damage. The physical response to a perceived threat can be dulled and sometimes eliminated by changing the arousal of the target organ. Example: Become aware of tense muscles, and consciously relax them.

Consistent with contemporary thinking in mind-body medicine is the realization that the mind does not clearly discriminate between physical life events and imagination or visual images. The body attributes validity to both psychologic and physiologic triggers. Both psychologic and physiologic arousal is influenced by the patient's perception of events as bland or threatening, as manageable or uncontrollable. When an event

is perceived as stressful, the body mobilizes its resources to deal with the threat.

Neural and Hormonal Pathways of Stress Response

The stress response is largely mediated through the autonomic nervous system and the **hypothalamic-pituitary axis.** Sympathetic nervous system domination increases respiratory and heart rates, elevates blood pressure levels, mobilizes fat stores, and increases cellular metabolism through direct neural stimulation and epinephrine release from the adrenal medulla. The hypothalamus simultaneously induces release of pituitary hormones that stimulate secretion of adrenal cortical hormones. **Cortisol,** the most important of these hormones, enhances the availability of glucose from protein and glycogen. In the long-term, this availability suppresses the immune system and results in muscle wasting.

In contrast, if an event is not perceived as stressful, it is unnecessary for the body to mount a stress response. Belief systems or wellness strategies that change mental images may serve to modulate the stress response. A number of strategies can be recruited to change perceptions—to convert a threat to a challenge. One approach is to mobilize and deploy coping resources effectively by undergoing a change of attitude. Another is to refine problem-solving skills. The first approach requires that the situation and the patient's self-concept be reviewed by examining the facts from a different perspective. The second approach necessitates improved task-oriented coping skills. Although chiropractors can in some cases counsel patients to enable them to use these approaches, referral to health professionals specializing in these areas may also be appropriate.

Reconceptualizing

Reconceptualizing a situation and the individual's ability to cope can be particularly helpful, because much of modern-day stress results from individuals responding primarily to mental representations of their environment rather than its objective reality. The situation can be reviewed by looking for the plusses rather than focusing on the minuses. This approach essentially involves changing from the pessimistic view of the "glass as half empty" to the optimistic version of the "glass as half full." Replacing defeatist self-talk with assertive affirmations can help modify self-concept and develop a positive outcome expectation. Replacing negative "can't do" reinforcement with positive "can do" self-talk reduces the likelihood of an unwanted stress response.

Although altering one's visual imagery may be a useful interim response, changing current coping strategies ultimately provides a more productive outcome, because the emphasis is shifted from thought to action. An effective technique for reaching a balanced appreciation and undertaking effective problem solving is to view the situation from diverse perspectives.[51]

De Bono's approach lists the advantages, disadvantages, possibilities that a situation offers, and possible consequences of taking various actions.[51] He also advocates canvassing other views of the situation. Having gathered such additional information, the patient becomes aware of the possible impact of the problem on his or her situation, not only in terms of its possible negative impact but also with respect to opportunities it may offer. In addition, to potentially change the patient's attitude toward the problem, this strategy enhances the patient's awareness of the options for problem solving.

Relaxation Methods

In addition to cognitive emotional strategies, stress can be managed at a more physical level. When people habitually respond to stressful situations with a **relaxation response,** their stress arousal threshold is raised. This higher threshold can be achieved by strategies as diverse as regular exercise or a relaxation program. Results of 34 studies suggest that aerobically fit subjects have a reduced psychosocial stress response when compared with either their baseline values or to control groups.[52] Even a 5-minute walk or 3-minute jog can help relieve acute tension.

In addition to exercise, relaxing tense muscle groups can reduce stress. Although massage is a good option, simple tasks such as stretching both vertically and horizontally—stretching tall and wide—can induce relaxation.

Specific areas of the body can be relaxed. Moving the head forward and back and from side to side can ease tense neck muscles. To minimize any risk of vascular compromise, it is prudent to avoid neck rotation, especially in older adults. Slowly bending forward to rest the chin on the chest, then backward pointing the chin skyward, and finally leaning the right ear toward the right shoulder followed by a similar action on the left side, are movements that are both safe and relaxing. Each position is held for approximately 7 seconds. Similarly, exercises that take large joints through their ranges of motion can be used to relax other muscle groups.

The fundamental principle, when feeling stressed, is to move joints that are surrounded by tight muscles and to repeat the exercise 8 to 10 times. Becoming aware of tense muscles and deliberately relaxing them is a handy approach.

Although any stress management technique is helpful, given the plethora of stress management options, attempting to match the intervention with a particular patient's response is sometimes useful.[10] Patients experiencing acute stress respond well to techniques such as slowing down, breathing, and muscle relaxation. Talking, walking, and breathing slowly provides somatic feedback that suggests reduced tension.

Deep breathing is a powerful relaxation strategy. Abdominal breathing reduced to a rate of less than 12 cycles per minute is relaxing. Sighing is also conducive to tension reduction. Individuals who tend to experience a physical response to stress may benefit most from focusing on their breathing, relaxing their muscles, and using specific techniques such as massage to achieve muscle-trigger release.

Individuals whose dominant response is emotional may try detached observation and thought stopping. Thought stopping involves recognizing intrusive thoughts, deliberately putting them aside, and focusing on something positive.

Detached observation involves assuming a physically relaxed posture while mentally distancing oneself from the problem. The aim is to view the situation as an observer rather than an active participant. Recognizing stressful thoughts and deliberately replacing stress-provoking thoughts with positive expectations reduces the intensity of the stress experience. Diverse strategies for helping patients reduce and control stress are readily available.[10] An Australian pilot study suggests that some chiropractic patients believe they would benefit from chiropractic care that included information about stress-management strategies.[53] Use of such strategies in the chiropractic management of stress may be effectively complemented by referral to a counseling professional (e.g., psychiatrist, psychologist, clinical social worker, pastoral counselor).

HEALTH CONTRACT

Patients in pain are often prepared to implement demanding lifestyle changes as long as there is a likelihood that these changes will result in noticeable pain relief. Convincing patients to persist with beneficial, although inconvenient, lifestyle changes once pain has resolved usually evokes a very different response. Similarly, getting well patients to change risky habits and adopt wellness behaviors creates a clinical challenge for primary practitioners. One approach to overcoming obstacles to lifestyle change is the use of a **self-care contract**[10] (Box 20-1).

The steps involved in developing a self-care contract are the following:

- Make the patient aware of his or her health needs. Patient awareness of the discrepancies between his or her current health status and optimal health provides a template for formulating a personal wellness program. Optimal health is the best health an individual can achieve, given their genetic composition. Discrepancies that the patient identifies between his or her current and optimal health status can be reworded as health needs and then used as the wellness goals for the self-care program.
- Identify various strategies that can be used to meet wellness goals and fulfill health needs. An awareness of various strategies for meeting individual health needs will enable the patient to select the options that are most compatible with his or her lifestyle. Adherence to the self-care program is greatly enhanced by selecting interventions that are least disruptive and most acceptable to the patient.

Box 20-1 STEPS FOR FORMULATING A SELF-CARE CONTRACT

STEP I
Identify objective and subjective health needs.

STEP II
Prioritize health needs through negotiation.

STEP III
Delimit agreed health goals, based on health needs assessment.

STEP IV
List possible intervention options to achieve health goals.

STEP V
Select preferred interventions.

STEP VI
Formulate a self-care contract specifying goals, interventions, time lines, and rewards.

STEP VII
Monitor progress, and modify specifications as necessary.

- Formulate the contract. The health goals are ranked with respect to both the clinician's professional assessment and the patient's health perceptions. The health program is then negotiated, based on selected health goals. The patient chooses the intervention strategies that are to be included in the program. Goals, interventions, and timelines are clearly specified. Adherence to proposed changes is greatly enhanced by patient commitment to the contract.
- Monitor the outcome. Although it is the patient's responsibility to implement a self-care wellness contract, the clinician contributes by monitoring the patient's outcome. Such monitoring may be at the level of measuring physiologic changes or observing whether the patient has managed to implement the entire program or needs help to modify particular interventions or formulate more realistic goals. The clinician's

ongoing commitment is to motivate the patient and provide a reliable resource for information.

Chiropractors can use handouts as templates for increasing patient awareness of lifestyle hazards, ascertaining personal risk of various disorders, and developing self-care health promotion programs (available at www.jamisonhealth.com). Regular use of such tools could transform the tendency of consumers to overlook chiropractors as sources of comprehensive wellness information.[54,55]

CONCLUSION

Good chiropractic care is not limited to treating the patient's problem; it also seeks to promote lifelong wellness by addressing the patient's lifestyle. As mind and body are two aspects of a single, indivisible entity, physical changes have psychosocial repercussions and vice versa. Disease and wellness are influenced by a variety of physical, chemical, microbial, and psychosocial triggers. In many instances, exposure to potentially deleterious triggers is a matter of personal choice. Increasing patient awareness of the possible repercussions of lifestyle decisions is an increasingly important aspect of competent primary care professional practice.

Review *Questions*

1. Is pain a purely physical phenomenon? If not, how does this affect the role of the chiropractor in working with patients with chronic and acute pain?
2. What are the four major self-care measures that chiropractors can recommend to patients?
3. What are active coping strategies, and how do they differ from passive coping strategies? Why is it important to use active coping strategies in addition to passive approaches?
4. Aside from chiropractic adjustment and manipulation, what other approaches are frequently included in maintenance care?
5. What are the essentials of a healthy diet?
6. Which nutrients must vegetarians make particular efforts to include in their diets?

7. Which minerals are most likely to be deficient in the average Western diet? Which types of foods should be maximized, and which should be minimized?
8. What is one animal and one plant source of omega-3 fatty acids? What major illness do they help to prevent?
9. Does processing more often increase or decrease the nutrient value of foods?
10. What are the benefits of regular exercise? Which types of exercise yield what benefits?

Concept *Questions*

1. In your experiences as a chiropractic patient, to what extent have lifestyle interventions such as diet, exercise, and stress management been part of your chiropractic care? To what extent do you wish to include these interventions in your work with patients?
2. A patient comes to you upset that his 14-year-old son has announced that he is becoming a vegetarian. What helpful information can you provide?

REFERENCES

1. Deyo R, Tsui-Wu YJ: Functional disability due to back pain: a population based study indicating the importance of socio-economic factors, *Arthritis Rheum* 30:1, 1987.
2. Kaplan RM: Coping with stressful medical examinations. In Friedman HS, DiMatteo MR, editors: *Interpersonal issues in health care*, New York, 1982, Academic Press.
3. Turner JA, Jensen MP: Efficacy of cognitive therapy for chronic low back pain, *Pain* 52:169, 1993.
4. Jensen MP, Turner JA, Romano JM: Self-efficacy and outcome expectancies: relationship to chronic pain coping strategies and adjustment, *Pain* 44:263, 1991.
5. Rupert RL: A survey of practice patterns and the health promotion and prevention attitudes of U.S. chiropractors. Maintenance care: part I, *J Manipulative Physiol Ther* 23(1):1, 2000.
6. Scharff L, Turk DC, Marcus DA: Triggers of headache episodes and coping responses of headache diagnostic groups, *Headache* 35(7):397, 1995.
7. Blanchard EB et al: The role of regular home practice in the relaxation treatment of tension headache, *J Consult Clin Psychol* 59:467, 1991.
8. Jamison JR: Identifying non-specific triggers in chiropractic care, *Chiropr J Aust* 28:65, 1998.
9. Jamison JR: The health information brochure: a useful tool for chiropractic practice? *J Manipulative Physiol Ther* 24(5):331, 2001.

10. Jamison JR: *Maintaining health in primary care*, Edinburgh, 2001, Churchill Livingstone.

11. Hu FB et al: Prospective study of major dietary patterns and risk of coronary heart disease in men, *Am J Clin Nutr* 72(4):912, 2000.

12. Gerster H: The potential role of lycopene for human health, *J Am Coll Nutr* 16(2):109, 1997.

13. Bouic PJD, Lamprecht JH: Plant sterols and sterolins: a review of their immune-modulating properties, *Altern Med Rev* 4(3):170, 1999.

14. Uauy R, Mena P, Valenzuela A: Essential fatty acids as determinants of lipid requirements in infants, children and adults, *Eur J Clin Nutr* 53(Suppl 1):S66, 1999.

15. Wynder EL, Weisburger JH, Ng SK: Nutrition: the need to define "optimal" intake as a basis for public policy decisions, *Am J Public Health* 82:346, 1992.

16. Huang HY, Helzlsouer KJ, Appel LJ: The effects of vitamin C and vitamin E on oxidative DNA damage: results from a randomized controlled trial, *Cancer Epidemiol Biomarkers Prev* 9(7):647, 2000.

17. National Health & Medical Research Council: *Is there a safe level of daily consumption of alcohol for men and women?* Canberra, 1987, Australian Government Publishing Service.

18. Heini AF, Weinsier RL: Divergent trends in obesity and fat intake patterns: the American paradox, *Am J Med* 102(3):259, 1997.

19. Lee IM, Paffenbarger RS Jr, Hennekens CH: Physical activity, physical fitness and longevity, *Aging (Milano)* 9(1-2):2, 1997.

20. Haapanen N et al: Characteristics of leisure time physical activity associated with decreased risk of premature all-cause and cardiovascular disease mortality in middle-aged men, *Am J Epidemiol* 143(9):870, 1996.

21. Leon AS, Myers MJ, Connett J: Leisure time physical activity and the 16 year risk of mortality from coronary heart disease and all-causes in the MRFIT, *Int J Sports Med* 18(Suppl 3): S208, 1997.

22. Paffembarger RS et al: Physical activity, all-cause mortality, and longevity of college alumni, *N Engl J Med* 314:605, 1986.

23. Miller TD, Balady GJ, Fletcher GF: Exercise and its role in the prevention and rehabilitation of cardiovascular disease, *Ann Behav Med* 19(3):220, 1997.

24. Eaton CB: Relation of physical activity and cardiovascular fitness to coronary heart disease, part II: cardiovascular fitness and the safety and efficacy of physical activity prescription, *J Am Board Fam Pract* 5(2):157, 1992.

25. DeCourcy SN, Moore K, Ratcliffe C: Effects of exercise on serum cholesterol: a review, *Am J Chiropractic Med* 3:111, 1989.

26. Arroll B, Beaglehole R: Does physical activity lower blood pressure: a critical review of clinical trials, *J Clin Epidemiol* 45:439, 1992.

27. Ernst E: Regular exercise reduces fibrinogen levels: a review of longitudinal studies, *Br J Sports Med* 27(3):175, 1993.

28. Uusi-Rasi K et al: Associations of physical activity and calcium intake with bone mass and size in healthy women at different ages, *J Bone Miner Res* 13(1):133, 1998.

29. Kohrt WM, Ehsani AA, Birge SJ Jr: Effects of exercise involving predominantly either joint-reaction or ground-reaction forces on bone mineral density in older women, *J Bone Miner Res* 12(8):1253, 1997.

30. Prior JC et al: Prevention and management of osteoporosis: consensus statements from the Scientific Advisory Board of the Osteoporosis Society of Canada, 5, physical activity as therapy for osteoporosis, *Can Med Assoc J* 155(7):940, 1996.

31. Province MA et al: The effects of exercise on falls in elderly patients. A preplanned meta-analysis of the FICSIT Trials. Frailty and injuries: cooperative studies of intervention techniques, *JAMA* 273(17):1341, 1995.

32. Kiningham RB: Physical activity and the primary prevention of cancer, *Prim Care* 25(2):515, 1998.

33. Oliveria SA, Christos PJ: The epidemiology of physical activity and cancer, *Ann N Y Acad Sci* 833:79, 1997.

34. Hiraoka J et al: A comparative epidemiological study of the effects of regular exercise on health level, *J Epidemiol* 8(1):15, 1998.

35. Burnham JM: Exercise is medicine: health benefits of regular physical activity, *J La State Med Soc* 150(7):319, 1998.

36. Bauman A, Owen N: Physical activity of adult Australians: epidemiological evidence and potential strategies for health gain, *J Sci Med Sport* 2(1):30, 1999.

37. Teague ML, Hunnicutt BK: An analysis of the 1990 Public Health Service physical fitness and exercise objectives for older Americans, *Health Values* 13:15, 1989.

38. Assanelli D et al: Effect of leisure time and working activity on principal risk factors and relative interactions in active middle-aged men, *Coron Artery Dis* 10(1):1, 1999.

39. Shephard RJ: What is the optimal type of physical activity to enhance health? *Br J Sports Med* 31(4):277, 1997.

40. Bijnen FC et al: Physical activity and 10-year mortality from cardiovascular diseases and all causes: the Zutphen elderly study, *Arch Intern Med* 158(14):1499, 1998.

41. Fraser GE, Shavlik DJ: Risk factors for all-cause and coronary heart disease mortality in the oldest-old, the Adventist health study, *Arch Intern Med* 157(19):2249, 1997.

42. Morey SS: ACSM revises guidelines for exercise to maintain fitness, *Am Fam Phys* 59:473, 1999.

43. Slattery ML et al: Physical activity and colon cancer: a public health perspective, *Ann Epidemiol* 7(2):137, 1997.

44. Platz EA et al: Physical activity and benign prostatic hyperplasia, *Arch Intern Med* 158(21):2349, 1998.

45. Minor MA: Exercise in the treatment of osteoarthritis, *Rheum Dis Clin North Am* 25:397, 1999.

46. Ader R, Cohen N, Felten D: Psychoneuroimmunology: interactions between the nervous system and the immune system, *Lancet* 45:99, 1995.

47. Linton SJ: An overview of psychosocial and behavioral factors in neck-and-shoulder pain, *Scand J Rehabil Med* 32:67, 1995.

48. Minocha A, Joseph AS: Pathophysiology and management of noncardiac chest pain, *J Ky Med Assoc* 93(5):196, 1995

49. Waddell G: Biopsychosocial analysis of low back pain, *Baillieres Clin Rheumatol* 6(3):523, 1992.

50. Antonovsky A: *Health, stress and coping*, San Francisco, 1979, Jossey-Bass Publishers.

51. De Bono E: *Serious creativity*, London, 1992, Harper Collins.

52. Crews DJ, Landers DM: A meta-analytic review of aerobic fitness and reactivity to psychosocial stressors, *Med Sci Sports Exerc* 19(Suppl 5):S114, 1987.

53. Jamison JR: Stress management: an exploratory study of chiropractic patients, *J Manipulative Physiol Ther* 23(1):32, 2000.

54. Jamison JR: Chiropractic patient-centred care: suggestions from an international case study, *Chiropr J Aust* 31:92, 2001.

55. Jamison JR: Perceptions: a case study of chiropractic patients in eastern Australia, *Chiropr J Aust* 30:2, 2000.

A Patient's Introduction to Chiropractic

Louis Sportelli, DC

Key Terms

ALLOPATHIC
KINESTHETIC
PATIENT EMPOWERMENT
REPORT OF FINDINGS

This is an era of **patient empowerment** in which informed consumers seek to play an active role in their health care. Because no television programs feature chiropractors as health care heroes and no entity in chiropractic has the economic viability to compete with multimillion-dollar pharmaceutical company advertising budgets, the responsibility for conducting an educational program falls upon the individual chiropractor. Great opportunities await those who can communicate with confidence, conveying a message credible in content and congruent with the expectations of the patient.

Most doctors of chiropractic who survive and flourish even in challenging economic times do so because of a systematic program of patient education, coupled with well-organized office management procedures that incorporate an effective clinical and business system that is understood by the doctor and staff. Although this should be an ongoing process, the initial visit and **Report of Findings** are crucial in educating patients about the benefits of chiropractic care. The long-term benefits of time spent educating patients are immeasurable: ease of patient management through enhanced cooperation, increased referrals, and reduced risk of malpractice exposure because doctor-patient bonding has been established.

PRECONCEPTIONS

Patients seeking chiropractic services enter the office with a variety of perspectives:
- Some have been referred by an enthusiastic, satisfied patient who understands the health benefits of chiropractic. "Word of mouth" referral is the way most people seek chiropractic services.
- Others have not been satisfied with conventional medical care for their condition but are also skeptical about chiropractic.
- Many have little knowledge about chiropractic and no strong negative or positive preconceptions about it.

It is important to remember that new chiropractic patients are not seeking to determine what is wrong with medicine but what is right about chiropractic. They want to know whether chiropractic can help restore and maintain their health. To meet this need, they must be provided with a factual and believable Report of Findings.

Patients need their basic questions answered:
- Can you help me?
- How long will it take?
- How much will it cost?

These questions must be answered in a way that removes fear. Patients may fear that they are not in the right office or that the chiropractor cannot diagnose or does not refer. Discussing not only the chiropractic approach to the problem but also the other possible options creates patient confidence. Learning that the chiropractor is cooperative and will work with the patient's medical physician or other health care provider offers necessary reassurance.

IMPORTANCE OF PATIENT EDUCATION

Communicating clearly and warmly with every patient is imperative. Doctors must be conscious to make all that they say meaningful, informative, empowering, and educational. Patients who have grown up with the **allopathic** (i.e., traditional medical) model and have now opted to seek nonallopathic (i.e., complementary, alternative) care have taken a giant step and need to be supported in their decision. Effective communication by the chiropractor can bridge the gap between the cold, sterile health care system of the past and the new, humanistic system of the future.

How the message is conveyed is as important as the message itself. The nuances of presentation help the patient understand the message. Most communication will be verbal. The clinician should be certain that it is a dialogue, not a monologue; allow time for questions by the patient; and periodically inquire about the patient's thoughts about what has been said. The questions will help to identify any underlying beliefs that the patient may not initially mention.

In addition, including visual and **kinesthetic** forms of delivery can enhance the effectiveness of verbal communication. Patients often provide clues to their preferred mode of communication by the very language they use: "I *hear* what you're saying" or "I can *see* that" or "I *feel* that you understand." Understanding patients' communication styles enables the clinician to "touch" them with the presentation. For those patients who are primarily kinesthetic, a brief, reassuring hand on the shoulder when delivering a report or when they leave is received well. For others with a more visual style, providing charts

and written material is ideal. Communicating in the fashion preferred by the patient will enable the clinician to effectively present the message and have it understood.

Patient education can be accomplished through a variety of methods. Some doctors use audio or videotaped materials to educate patients, whereas others give patient lectures or spinal health classes. Whatever additional methods the chiropractor may choose, the most personal relationship doctors can develop with their patients comes from direct one-to-one interaction. The most critical time to develop this relationship is during the initial Report of Findings.

REPORT OF FINDINGS

The first visit offers an opportunity to establish a bond with the patient that is unlikely to be afforded at any other time during the health care encounter. The case history, physical examination, diagnostic evaluation, and Report of Findings can provide the foundation for a long-standing relationship. Doctors must take the necessary time and use a well-documented, easy to understand, consumer-oriented program to educate patients. Providing a booklet or pamphlet to patients with their Report of Findings can substantially strengthen this effort. The material should be personalized and correlated to the findings, thereby becoming a document to which the patient can refer and show to friends and family to increase understanding of chiropractic care.

After the initial welcome, case history, physical examination, diagnostic testing, clinical review, and acceptance of the individual as a patient, the clinician should choose a special place in the office where the Report of Findings may be presented. This will help to develop a consistent, dependable process; it will also convey to the office staff the significance the doctor places on patient education. As with other aspects of chiropractic practice, over time the clinician will grow more comfortable with this routine and more effective in presenting reports.

It is very important that the doctor become familiar with the content of the written material used in the Report of Findings. The tenth edition of Sportelli's *Introduction to Chiropractic* is specifically designed for this purpose, but the process and concepts discussed here apply, regardless of the material used. Other pamphlets, such as those published by the Foundation for Chiropractic Education and Research (FCER) or William Esteb's Patient Media, Inc. may be suitable for patient educational purposes, depending on the clinician's practice style and personal preference.

Personalizing the Booklet

The patient's name should be written in the booklet to personalize the document. It can then be tailored to match the patient's specific needs. When personalized, patients are unlikely to discard this material. Often, when patients return for their second or third visit, they will ask for another copy of the booklet for a neighbor or friend; it should be provided gladly. One of the most significant opportunities for patient education and referral is immediately after the very first visit. The patient's interest in the particular condition is very strong, as are compliance and commitment.

Family, friends, and neighbors are anxious to know what the doctor said. The patient, using the highlighted and personalized booklet, can confidently answer this question. The clinician may take advantage of blank space in the booklet (e.g., the inside of the front cover) to write specific patient advice and recommendations to encourage patient compliance. These instructions are also an excellent way to help provide informed consent by way of illustration and instruction.

Black and red felt tip pens, highlighters, and tape flags are valuable tools for marking specific pages for emphasis. Of course, findings from the patient's history and physical examination related to the presenting complaint should be noted in the patient's booklet. In addition, the doctor should determine whether any preexisting lumbar or cervical problems or whiplash injuries exist that are *not* specific to the patient's reason for the current visit. The clinician should be certain to highlight these past problems as well, because they represent chronic injuries that may delay progress or impede full recovery.

CAUTION SIGNS

Either verbally or in the booklet used for the Report of Findings, patients should be informed about symptoms serious enough to warrant an immediate call to the doctor.

This caution could be conveyed as follows: "If blurred vision, dizziness, severe headaches, ringing in ears, or nausea are experienced, contact the chiropractic office immediately. If any of the previously mentioned symptoms persist, avoid putting the neck in a position that will require extension of the neck (i.e., looking up), rotation (i.e., looking over the shoulder), or both. If symptoms worsen and the doctor cannot be contacted, the nearest hospital emergency room should be consulted."

This important advice may be significant in the event of litigation, because it will enable the clinician to provide evidence that the patient has been properly advised concerning symptoms that may be a potential problem, helping to mitigate a failure to provide informed consent.

Connections between a current condition and a childhood accident or a decades-old automobile accident are rarely something patients have previously considered. However, when they are pointed out and highlighted in the Report of Findings, patients become sensitized to the potentially long-lasting effects of past traumas to the spine and nervous system.

Emphasizing Fundamental Concepts

The power of the body to heal itself is a key concept for the patient to understand. Health and wellness come from within, and the role of the doctor of chiropractic is to promote self-healing of the body. Through chiropractic's more than 100-year history, practitioners have emphasized the body's ability to adapt to its environment and the need to maintain the nervous system free from neurologic irritation. Although these ideas are second nature to chiropractors, they are new concepts to most chiropractic patients. Therefore it is essential for clinicians to mention them to patients at the first visit, because they form the foundation for all that follows.

Aside from emphasizing the significance chiropractic places on the role of the nervous system, it is important to note the importance of nutrition, water, rest, clean air, exercise, and a positive mental attitude. All are consistent with the patient's current knowledge base and the increasingly holistic view of health care being reported in most popular publications. Regardless of practice style, if the doctor is determined to develop long-term relationships with patients and help them understand the value of chiropractic, they need to feel that the clinician is someone they can trust. One way to do this is to help patients understand the wellness and prevention concepts that can be supported by evidence.

DEFINING CHIROPRACTIC

What is chiropractic? The clinician's ability to answer this question clearly, in nontechnical language that patients can readily comprehend, is crucial. Clinicians should be able to explain that chiropractic is a natural healing art emphasizing the relationship between the body's structure (especially the spine) and its various functions, and that chiropractors correct spinal imbalances and/or dysfunctions called "subluxations" with specifically applied adjustments, also commonly called "spinal manipulations."

It may be helpful to let the patient know that the spine is the chiropractor's "avenue of approach" in dealing with various conditions. The medical physician who injects a drug into an arm is using the arm as an avenue of approach to affect other areas of the body. Because the spine houses the spinal cord and the nervous system is influenced by spinal manipulations (i.e., adjustments), the doctor of chiropractic pays special attention to the vertebral column in diagnosing, evaluating, and analyzing the condition of the patient. The clinician should mention that a variety of adjustments exist in the chiropractor's repertoire, that the type of adjustment most appropriate to the individual patient's needs is always chosen, and that adjustments may occasionally cause some soreness or stiffness but are rarely uncomfortable.

Informing the patient of this possibility in advance will significantly offset any apprehension or concerns.

Because back pain, neck pain, and headaches represent 90% of all patient visits to a doctor of chiropractic, the clinician should tell patients, "Chiropractic is best known for its success with back pain, neck pain, and headaches." For patients with any of these conditions, this offers assurance that they have come to the right place. For patients with other conditions that might also respond to chiropractic care but for which less research documentation exists, it is appropriate to mention (in cases where this is accurate) that chiropractic can sometimes be helpful in cases such as theirs. At the same time, the clinician should be certain to assure them that if other methods of health care are indicated, they will be referred to a medical physician or other health care practitioner.

Correlating Spinal Problems with Symptoms and Signs

Chiropractic booklets generally include an illustration of the spinal column that can be used to reinforce the importance of the spine and nervous system. The clinician should use a red felt tip pen to circle areas of the spine where problems were found during the examination (e.g., muscle spasm, spinal curvature, degenerative joint disease as seen on a radiograph). Writing down the initial working diagnosis—spasm, osteoarthritis, spurring, curvature, restricted joint motion—will make the report more relevant. This visual demonstration supports verbal communication (Fig. 21-1).

It should not be assumed that the patient understands how a spine looks; the clinician should allow time for questions and to determine if the patient understands the information presented.

In cases where the patient has radiating pain or paresthesia in an extremity, a highlighter should be used in the booklet to trace and illustrate that the patient's arm or leg pain stems from a cervical or lumbar involvement. Although simple to the doctor, this is difficult for some patients to fully

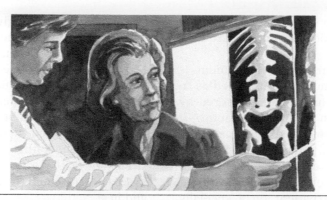

Fig. **21-1** A patient Report of Findings showing radiographs. *(From Sportelli L:* Introduction to chiropractic, *ed 9, Palmeton, Pa, 2000, Practicemakers Products, Inc.)*

grasp. Once patients see the connection, fear is reduced and compliance increases.

In cases involving a visceral organ problem, it is important to explain that the spine connects to visceral organs without making unrealistic claims. Clinicians should explain that "disorders involving organs and internal glands of the body may also, in some cases, respond to chiropractic care." If asked whether scientific evidence supports this, it is important to be truthful. The chiropractor might say, "At this time far less research exists concerning chiropractic's effect on internal organ problems than exists concerning its effect on back pain, neck pain, and headaches," adding, "but virtually every chiropractor has seen at least some cases in which internal organ problems appear to have responded positively to chiropractic care." It is important to understand that clinical results achieved by a chiropractor with a single patient may be different from results achieved with groups of patients in clinical trials. The individualized program between doctor and patient benefits from being monitored at each visit and changed where necessary.

Avoiding Exaggerated Claims

Much of the criticism launched at chiropractic has hit hard at unsubstantiated claims. C.O. Watkins, a pioneer in chiropractic education, addressed this problem perfectly: "Let's be bold in what we hypothesize, but cautious and humble in what we claim." Although it is legitimate

to use unproven methods (all health care providers do so), it is never permissible to make inaccurate claims about these methods, despite the fact that the clinician may have seen individual patients who appeared to have a similar condition successfully treated with chiropractic. Care should be taken not to extrapolate from a single patient encounter—no matter how spectacular—to an entire class of patients or disorders.

Furthermore, doctors of chiropractic need to rethink the explanations of chiropractic's pioneers and reframe them in the universal language of science. Clinicians must rid themselves of quasireligious rhetoric and abandon supernatural suppositions that isolate the profession from science. Instead, they must explain what is done using reasoned analysis and a professional demeanor.

EXPLAINING THE ADJUSTMENT

For most new patients, the chiropractic adjustment is unlike anything they have previously experienced. Strange as it may seem to the chiropractor, some new patients may have heard false accounts of chiropractors jumping from ladders and landing on the patients' spines, walking on people's backs, or other equally exaggerated stories. It is crucial to bear in mind that the very idea of the click or audible pop after an adjustment can be frightening to a new patient. Clinicians should adopt the motto, "The best surprise is no surprise." The better chiropractors can explain in advance to patients what to expect during each step in the process, the less likely they are to be anxious about the care they seek (Fig. 21-2).

A simple explanation of the adjustment is essential. Adjustment should be described as "a very skilled procedure usually administered by hand in a precise fashion by the chiropractor." If the clinician uses instrument adjusting as a central part of the practice, patients should be told how this is done. In either case, clinicians should explain that the chiropractic adjustment consists of placing the patient on a specially designed adjusting table, chair, or other equipment, and then applying pressure using specific chiropractic techniques to the areas of the spine that are not functioning properly or that do not move properly within their normal range of motion.

In preparing patients for a course of care, it is helpful to mention that although some cases

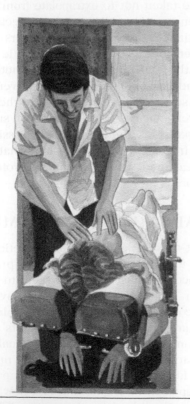

Fig. 21-2 An adjustment. *(From Sportelli L: Introduction to chiropractic, ed 9, Palmeton, Pa, 2000, Practicemakers Products, Inc.)*

show a dramatic, positive response to the first adjustment, in the typical case improvement is gradual, because it usually takes time for the body to incorporate the changes brought about by the adjustment. Clinicians should emphasize that the goal of treatment is for the patient "to get as well as possible as fast as possible." Analogies are often helpful, such as the time it takes for orthodontic procedures to ultimately straighten teeth. Braces do not straighten teeth in 1 day. Nature and the body need time to adapt and heal.

Mild soreness after adjustments is common and should be mentioned at the first visit. By alerting patients in advance, they are less prone to worry and better able to withstand adverse comment or misinformation from well-meaning friends.

Trial of Care and Ongoing Care

Although chiropractic can be a valuable part of an ongoing health care program, it is often best implemented initially as a short-term trial. Placing patients in the position of making a long-term commitment before they have experienced positive results from care is truly putting the cart before the horse. Patients who do not attain noticeable improvement during the trial of care (current practice guidelines and research published in the literature have generally limited this initial clinical trial to a range of 2 to 6 weeks) should be referred to another practitioner. Most experienced doctors have reached this conclusion on their own. Generally, practitioners will suggest that if a patient is under care for 2 weeks and has not shown any demonstrable change (the change need not be dramatic), a reevaluation of the patient is needed to determine whether some additional underlying condition is present.

The many patients who do experience improvement under the care of a chiropractor will want to know what they can do to sustain their newfound wellness or "sense of well being." For these patients, the Report of Findings can lay the groundwork for ongoing wellness care by incorporating concepts of health maintenance.

Complementary and Supportive Procedures

If the clinician's practice style and the patient's condition warrant supportive care, nutritional counseling, dietary advice, or other lifestyle guidance, this should be addressed in the Report of Findings. Supportive care often includes common procedures in physical therapy such as heat, cold, ultrasound, traction, or other procedures and devices intended to help promote the healing process. Although the clinician may choose to leave some of the details for a later visit, it is advisable to at least introduce these issues in the initial Report of Findings and to emphasize in detail areas of nonadjustive care that should be put into practice immediately.

If the informational booklet or pamphlet the clinician is using covers this material, it provides a good opportunity to highlight certain specific areas to explain in greater detail what is being recommended and why and how this is important to the patient. This can become a very individualized area of the booklet, keyed to the needs of this specific patient in the areas of diet, nutrition, water intake, regularity, and lifestyle interventions (Figs. 21-3 and 21-4).

Posture

Proper self-care should include attention to posture. In the Report of Findings, it is most helpful to target the discussion of posture in relation to the patient's specific spinal patterns. For example, in a patient with slumping posture and respiratory problems, the clinician might note, "Poor posture compromises movements of the rib cage so that the lungs may not function at maximum efficiency to bring oxygen to the tissues and eliminate carbon dioxide wastes. Other vital organs of the body may be restricted when posture is improper, producing structural stress." In this case the clinician can use the specific recommendation to make the general point about the need for proper posture.

Children

It is helpful to point out the potential value of chiropractic care for children, because various

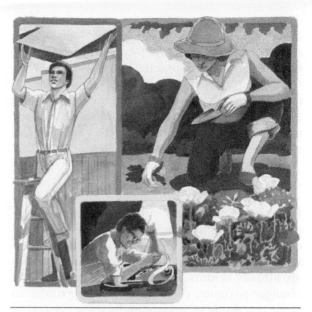

Fig. 21-3 A collage of daily work activity. (*From Sportelli L:* Introduction to chiropractic, *ed 9, Palmeton, Pa, 2000, Practicemakers Products, Inc.*)

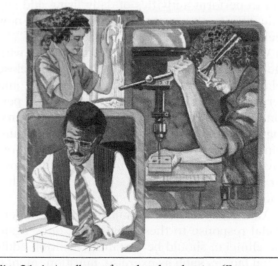

Fig. 21-4 A collage of work-related pain. (*From Sportelli L:* Introduction to chiropractic, *ed 9, Palmeton, Pa, 2000, Practicemakers Products, Inc.*)

childhood activities, such as learning to walk, can affect spinal structures. Parents often do not associate chiropractic care with children. Removing any barriers to providing chiropractic care will ultimately have a positive effect on the clinician's practice. Clinicians have noted historically that children with colic, otitis media, and other common childhood ailments may be responsive to chiropractic care. Working with children represents a unique opportunity to demonstrate the value of chiropractic intervention. However, care must be exercised to balance patient needs, parental concerns, and clinical utility.

Seniors

With the growing senior population, the Report of Findings should emphasize that chiropractic care can play an integral role in the health and well-being of the senior citizen. For patients who are already seniors, the relevance is obvious. For younger patients, this affords an opportunity to plant the seeds of understanding, for referral of older friends and relatives, and eventually for their own care as the younger patients grow older. It is easy to establish the health care value for an aging population. The ability to ambulate and to perform activities of daily living add significantly to the quality of life people are now seeking.

When describing the changes that come with age, chiropractors should emphasize the close relationship among the muscles, vertebrae, and nerves. The clinician should note that "as a person ages, the muscles that help maintain spinal alignment start to lose the tone needed to maintain balance. When this occurs, spinal vertebrae have a greater tendency to misalign or move erratically. This affects the spinal nerves that lead to vital parts of the body."

Although chiropractic adjustments are a beneficial response to these challenges, once again the clinician should be certain to mention additional factors such as exercise, nutrition, mental attitude, and lifestyle, because all of these strongly affect the overall health of the individual. Consistent with the clinician's own practice philosophy and knowledge of these areas, the patient should be advised on these helpful adjuncts.

To the extent that the clinician is able to offer helpful information (the word "doctor" originally meant "teacher") the idea is reinforced that the clinician, as a doctor of chiropractic, can serve as a primary health care advisor, a "health care coach," on a range of health care matters.

Discussing Surgery

For patients whose conditions (particularly lumbar and cervical disk syndromes) might require surgery, it is exceedingly helpful to use a Report of Findings booklet that includes a section on indications for surgery. This is crucial, because malpractice litigation frequently involves charges of failure to refer, failure to diagnose, or failure to inform. As part of this discussion, it is advisable to share with patients the signs and symptoms that are red flags for surgical referral. It is not unusual for patients to experience these signs yet not understand their significance or discuss them with the doctor early enough.

Among the signs for a possible surgical referral are intractable pain (i.e., pain that cannot be relieved); recurrent crippling attacks of pain and immobility that affect the livelihood of the individual and his or her quality of life; and any sig-

ROLE OF BOOKLET IN RISK MANAGEMENT

In some cases, neck muscles may be in such severe spasm that the head cannot be turned from side to side to see oncoming traffic. In this case, the chiropractor may recommend that the patient not drive. If the clinician records this recommendation in the Report of Findings and the patient's chart, it may prevent any blame being placed upon the chiropractor should the patient fail to heed the advice. For example, if a patient has been warned by the chiropractor not to drive until advised to do so because of severe torticollis, but the patient ignores this recommendation and has a collision while driving home from the chiropractor's office, it is unlikely that the patient or the patient's family would hold the chiropractor responsible for the accident if the warning has been recorded appropriately.

Taking such preventive steps helps to risk proof the clinician's practice. Patients also see these steps as an indication of high-quality, personalized care.

nificant neurologic deficit (i.e., loss) in ability to walk, properly balance, or control bowel or bladder. Patients should be told that the clinician is aware that some cases require surgery and that referral to a surgeon for a consultation, evaluation, or both will be provided if chiropractic fails to bring sufficient improvement in a reasonable period of time.

Self-Care at Home

Instructions for self-care at home are an essential part of comprehensive chiropractic case management. These instructions, which should be individualized for each patient, play an important role in preventing the patient from interfering with the healing process by engaging in activities that may be harmful. Many patients, for example, need to be given recommendations such as, "Do not apply heat. Do not sleep in a soft bed. Do not walk on rough terrain."

Exercises should be personalized, assigning the number of sets and repetitions the patient is to do for each exercise. While praising the benefits of exercise, it is also important to point out that it is possible to do too much of a good thing. Patients should be advised to be on the lookout for any negative reactions to their exercise programs. Caution should be strongly emphasized when recommending an exercise program. Particularly with cervical spine exercises, the clinician should note (in writing) that if the patient experiences a negative reaction, the program should be stopped and the problem reported to the chiropractic office immediately. In particular, patients should be told, "Do not forcefully move the head when doing any of these movements. If pain, dizziness, loss of balance, or similar symptoms are experienced, stop the movement or exercise immediately and contact the office."

Addressing Potential Problems

The clinician's role in educating patients should not be confined to addressing only their presenting symptoms. By briefly describing the role of chiropractic care for other conditions, clinicians can lay the groundwork for future health challenges that patients may experience. This can be done either verbally or with written materials. For instance, it is certainly worthwhile to provide written information on the effects of whiplash injury on the cervical spine, in addition to a list of possible postaccident signs and symptoms (e.g., soreness, headaches, dizziness, limitation of motion, muscle spasm). Although the patient may not be currently seeking care for an automobile accident injury, it is likely that at some point a friend or acquaintance will do so. By providing this information, the clinician provides the patient with a basis on which to make a helpful referral.

Keeping Proper Records

The doctor should note the Report of Findings discussions in the patient's chart and record the fact that an instructional booklet was given to the patient outlining the major issues surrounding the patient's condition and proposed care. A checklist form is appended to use as an instructional guide and as proof of instruction.

The form and content of the clinician's spoken and written communication with patients will strongly influence the success of his or her practice. The need to be personal is of increasing importance, because many people feel depersonalized, disenfranchised, and distant from many health care providers. Chiropractic can become the health care profession that provides both personal human touch and high-tech diagnostic technologic sophistication. Permitting patients to be heard, enabling them to maintain a sense of personal dignity, and delivering high-quality health care services are essential to this goal.

Review *Questions*

1. Why do chiropractors need to educate patients about chiropractic care?
2. What are three basic questions that patients need to have answered in the Report of Findings?
3. Explain how a chiropractor might apply the visual, auditory, and kinesthetic modes of communication in a Report of Findings.

4. What are some benefits of giving regular spinal health care classes?

5. What are some advantages of using a booklet or pamphlet to supplement the verbal Report of Findings?

6. How can instructional booklets aid in risk management?

7. Briefly define the following terms in language easy for patients to understand: chiropractic, subluxation, and adjustment.

8. How can chiropractors decrease patients' fears about chiropractic adjustment/manipulation?

9. Why is it important not to extrapolate from a single patient encounter—no matter how spectacular—to an entire class of patients or disorders?

10. What particular considerations are appropriate in presenting a Report of Findings to an elderly patient?

Concept *Questions*

1. How might a chiropractor who is shy when speaking in public prepare to give an effective Report of Findings or spinal care class?

2. C.O. Watkins said, "Let's be bold in what we hypothesize, but cautious and humble in what we claim." What problems for the profession as a whole can develop as a result of individual chiropractors making inaccurate or excessive claims?

SUGGESTED READING

Sportelli L: *Introduction to chiropractic,* ed 10, Palmeton, Pa, 2000, Practicemakers Products, Inc.

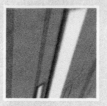

PART FIVE

RESEARCH

Research Essentials

Daniel Redwood, DC and William C. Meeker, DC, MPH

Key Terms

ACTIVE CONTROL	FALSE NEGATIVE	PREVALENCE
ABNORMALITY	FREQUENCY	PROGNOSIS
ANECDOTE	GOLD STANDARD	PROSPECTIVE STUDIES
BASIC SCIENCE RESEARCH	HAWTHORNE EFFECT	RANDOM ERROR
BIAS	HEALTH SERVICES	RANDOMIZED CLINICAL
BLINDING	RESEARCH	TRIALS (RCTs)
CASE SERIES	INCIDENCE	RANDOMIZED CONTROLLED
CASE STUDY	INTERNAL VALIDITY	TRIALS (RCTs)
CLINICAL EPIDEMIOLOGY	INTEROBSERVER RELIABILITY	RELIABILITY
CLINICAL RESEARCH	INTERVENTION	RETROSPECTIVE STUDIES
CLINICAL TRIALS	INTRAOBSERVER	RISK
COHORT	RELIABILITY	SAMPLE
CONFOUNDING BIAS	LONGITUDINAL STUDIES	SELECTION BIAS
CONTROL GROUP	MAGNITUDE	SELF-CARE
CORRELATION	MEASUREMENT BIAS	SENSITIVITY
COST-EFFECTIVENESS	META-ANALYSES	SHAM ADJUSTMENT/
CROSS-SECTIONAL STUDIES	NATURAL HISTORY	MANIPULATION
DIAGNOSIS	OBSERVATIONAL STUDY	SINGLE-BLIND STUDY
DOUBLE-BLIND STUDY	OPERATIONAL DEFINITION	SPECIFICITY
EVIDENCE-BASED HEALTH	OUTCOME MEASURES	STATISTICAL SIGNIFICANCE
CARE	P-VALUES	SYSTEMATIC ERROR
EXPERIMENTAL GROUP	PLACEBO	SYSTEMATIC REVIEWS
EXTERNAL VALIDITY	POPULATIONS	TRIPLE-BLIND STUDY
FALSE POSITIVE	PRETEST POSTTEST DESIGN	VALIDITY

Fueled by a spirit of exploration, research is an ongoing quest for greater understanding. The most important purpose of chiropractic research is to provide chiropractors with accurate information so that they can be more helpful to their patients. Researchers have a responsibility to ask the questions that matter most. Students and practitioners also have a responsibility: to keep current with newly emerging information by being avid consumers of research.

Ideally this means subscribing to one or more scholarly journals and reading them on a regular basis. At the very least, it means reading detailed summaries and discussions of current research and searching MEDLINE and other databases when necessary for evidence-based answers to questions that arise in the course of daily practice. Every profession that holds science in high esteem expects all of its practitioners to stay well informed throughout their careers. For chiropractic to occupy a respected place among the health professions, this is absolutely essential.

Aside from its practical value in improving the quality of patient care, research also has a broader sociologic purpose; this purpose is related to the credibility and cultural authority that chiropractic derives from generating new knowledge. Without exception, the professions that thrive are those that are perceived as being the experts in a particular field. Although expertise has various components, none is more essential than generating new knowledge. If the chiropractic profession fails to do so in its areas of specialty, others will fill the gap.

Chiropractic research has three main divisions: (1) clinical, (2) basic science, and (3) health services research. **Clinical research** addresses issues directly related to patient care, as in a study by Boline and colleagues,[1] which found that chiropractic outperformed the medication amitriptyline for tension headache patients. **Basic science research** explores underlying struc-

tures and mechanisms, as in a study by Dishman and Bulbulian,[2] which investigated reflexes in the gastrocnemius muscle after spinal adjustment/manipulation and offered support for the theory that manual spinal procedures may lead to short-term inhibitory effects on the human motor system. **Health services research** studies chiropractic's role in society, as in a study by Hawk and Long[3] that evaluated use of chiropractic in several Midwestern states and reported that over 40% of workers with low back pain use chiropractic, that use increases with age, and that it is more common for rural compared with nonrural residents.

For chiropractic as for other health professions, all three types of research are important. The focus of this chapter is clinical research.

RESEARCH TERMINOLOGY

Active control—A procedure that may have therapeutic effects, performed on the control group in a clinical trial.

Abnormality—A condition that is not normal. Abnormality may be defined either statistically or in terms of adverse health consequences.

Anecdote—A story about a clinical event or case.

Basic science research—Research that explores structures and mechanisms.

Bias—A process tending to produce results that depart systematically from true values.

Blinding—Shielding the subject, the person administering the treatment, or the person assessing the outcome from knowledge that might compromise the integrity of a study.

Case series—A written report on the details of a series of related cases.

Case study—A written report on the details of a single case.

Clinical epidemiology—The application of epidemiologic principles to clinical case management (see definition of epidemiology).

Clinical research—Research that addresses issues directly related to patient care.

Clinical trial—A prospective longitudinal experiment designed to assess the comparative efficacy or effectiveness of a treatment, often labeled a randomized clinical trial (RCT) if random assignment of subjects is made to each of the comparison treatment groups (see definition of randomized clinical trial).

Cohort—A defined group of people observed over a period of time.

Confounding bias—Bias that results from the interaction of two or more factors in a cause-and-effect relationship such that the presence of one factor makes it difficult to evaluate the true effect of the other factors.

Control group—A comparison group assignment in a clinical trial that receives no treatment, a placebo treatment, or an alternative treatment (see definitions of placebo and active control).

Correlation—A consistent statistical relationship between two variables such that one variable tends to predict the other. It may suggest but not prove a causal relationship.

Cost-effectiveness—The relative health value of an intervention compared with its financial cost.

Cross-sectional studies—Measurements taken at one moment in time.

Diagnosis—The identification and measurement of an abnormality in a particular patient that has clinical ramifications.

RESEARCH TERMINOLOGY—CONT'D

Double-blind study—An experiment in which patients and either doctors or outcome assessors are blinded.

Evidence-based health care—A health care system in which, to the greatest extent possible, procedures used by health care providers have been subjected to rigorous standards of scientific observation, experimentation, and documentation.

Experimental group—The group in a clinical trial that receives the intervention being tested.

External validity—The degree to which the results of a study can be expected to hold true in other settings.

False positive—(1) A test that is positive despite the absence of the disease or condition being tested; (2) a situation in which Intervention A is no better than Intervention B, but errors in the data or its interpretation lead one to reasonably conclude that Intervention A actually *is* better than Intervention B. Also called *Type I error.*

False negative—(1) A test that is negative despite the presence of the disease or condition being tested; (2) a situation in which Intervention A is actually superior to Intervention B, but errors in the data or its interpretation lead one to reasonably conclude that it is *not* superior to Intervention B. Also called *Type II error.*

Frequency—A general or statistical expression of how often a condition or disease occurs. Statistical expressions of frequency take two forms: (1) prevalence and (2) incidence (see definitions of prevalence and incidence).

Gold standard—A measure of agreed upon accuracy and validity.

Hawthorne effect—The tendency of people in a research study to change their behavior, compromising the validity of the data.

Health services research—Research that studies the structure, process, and outcomes of the health delivery system and its role in society.

Incidence—The proportion of a clearly defined group (i.e., population) initially free of a condition, that develops it over a given period of time.

Internal validity—The degree to which the results of a study are correct for the methods and sample of patients included in the study (see definitions of validity and external validity).

Interobserver reliability—The consistency of measured results between different practitioners evaluating the same thing (see definition of intraobserver reliability).

Intervention—A procedure used for treatment or prevention of illness.

Intraobserver reliability—The consistency with which one practitioner can consistently arrive at the same result (see definition of interobserver reliability).

Longitudinal—Involving serial measurements taken over time.

Magnitude—The size of an effect.

Measurement bias—Systematic error in data resulting from poor methods of observation.

Meta-analysis—A systematic review that usually includes a ranking of the quality of each study, plus statistical pooling of the data from all studies to determine the average effect of treatment (see definition of systematic review).

Natural history—The usual progression of an illness in the absence of intervention.

Observational study—A study in which the researcher observes events as they occur naturally or in the course of normal practice, without attempting to influence them.

Operational definition—A description of the methods, tools, and procedures required to make an observation (i.e., a definition that is specific and allows objective measurement).

Outcome measures—Parameters that indicate a change in health status, used in studies of treatment effectiveness. These must be specifically defined at the beginning of the study.

P-values—A statistical statement generally representing the probability of a false-positive conclusion, or Type I error. They are used to account for the possibility of random error and to measure the statistical significance of a finding.

Placebo—An intervention designed to mimic a "real" treatment and performed on a control group in a clinical trial. Its purpose is to control for the nonspecific therapeutic effects of care so that the specific effects of an actual treatment can be measured.

Continued

RESEARCH TERMINOLOGY—CONT'D

Population—A group meeting a specific set of criteria.

Pretest posttest design—A study design in which baseline (i.e., pretreatment) and outcome (i.e., posttreatment) measurements are performed.

Prevalence—The proportion of a population having a particular condition or outcome at a given moment.

Prognosis—The predicted course of an illness.

Prospective study—A study that generates new data based on events that occur after the study begins (see definition of retrospective).

Random error—The influence of chance variation.

Randomized controlled trial—A prospective, longitudinal study in which patients are divided into two or more groups on a randomized basis (see definition of clinical trial).

Reliability—The consistency of a measurement when repeated.

Retrospective study—A study that reviews events that have already occurred (see definition of prospective).

Risk—The likelihood of an adverse event or outcome. Risk is determined by measuring the relationship between the presence of possible risk factors and the subsequent incidence of particular conditions.

Sample—A subset of a population.

Selection bias—Bias that occurs when the group selected for study differs in significant ways from the true population.

Self-care—Methods used by individuals to enhance their own health.

Sensitivity—The proportion of times a diagnostic procedure is correct in patients without a specific diagnosis (see definition of specificity).

Sham adjustment/manipulation—A manual intervention used for research purposes that must be convincing enough for research subjects to believe it is a real adjustment/manipulation, although it has none of the specific physiologic or therapeutic effects of a real adjustment/manipulation. Also called *placebo adjustment/manipulation*.

Single-blind study—A study in which the patients are blinded as to whether they are in the experimental group or the comparison group.

Specificity—The proportion of times a diagnostic procedure is correct in patients without a specific diagnosis (see definition of sensitivity).

Statistical significance—A statement based on inferential statistics indicating that a good probability exists that a conclusion is not wrong because of random error. The magnitude of a therapeutic effect and the size of the sample are two key factors influencing statistical significance.

Systematic error—Error reflecting bias (see definition of bias).

Systematic review—A summary of scientific knowledge in an area accomplished by a review of published research, in which explicit objective methods are used to evaluate the methodological quality and the results.

Triple-blind study—A study in which patients, doctors, and outcome assessors are blinded.

Validity—The degree to which an observation or measurement provides an indication of the true state of the phenomena being measured. Also called *accuracy*.

CLINICAL EPIDEMIOLOGY

To be an intelligent reader of research papers, one must be familiar with the basic concepts and terminology of **clinical epidemiology,** because these form the basic structure of clinical research in the health sciences. Epidemiology is the study of the **incidence** and progression of diseases in **populations.** Clinical epidemiology, which is the application of epidemiological principles to patient case management, represents an attempt to bring order and quantitative methodology to the process of answering specific clinical questions that arise during patient care.

Decision Making in Practice

The questions addressed in clinical epidemiology are mostly the same questions that practitioners consciously or unconsciously ask themselves when evaluating patients and determining the most appropriate courses of action. As described in Fletcher, Fletcher, and Wagner's classic text, *Clinical Epidemiology: The Essentials,*[4] these questions can be grouped into the following categories: **abnormality, diagnosis, frequency, risk, prognosis,** treatment, prevention, cause, and cost. In applying research to case management, it helps to break down the process into these various components, to learn how to use the scientific literature to help answer the questions that arise each step along the way.

Abnormality

The concept of abnormality is a foundation for all health care practice, including chiropractic, because if no abnormality exists there may be no need for the **intervention** of a health care practitioner. To know whether something is abnormal presumes that one knows what is normal, but defining normal is not as simple as it first appears. A purely statistical approach defines normal as any condition that occurs most of the time in most people. However, this assumes that "usual" is the equivalent of "good" (i.e., that no disease or dysfunction occurs in the majority of a population). This is an unwise assumption, as demonstrated by the fact that most American adults have plaque deposits in their arteries, which are related to heart attacks and early deaths. In addition, some phenomena that are unusual are known to be positive health indicators. For example, very low cholesterol levels are rare in the population of the United States, but they tend to confer greater protection against heart disease than do statistically average (i.e., normal) cholesterol levels.

Far better than the statistical definition of abnormality is a model that defines abnormality in terms of a relation to negative health consequences. Using this model, normal means *good* and abnormal means *bad*, which is consistent with the way most people use these terms. To demonstrate whether a particular parameter is normal or abnormal (i.e., whether it is associated with adverse health consequences) can require extensive epidemiologic research. High blood pressure is a good example. Research has demonstrated that very high blood pressure in combination with other factors is closely related to stroke and other problems. Even mild hypertension has been shown to increase the risk of future cardiovascular disease. The key point here is that clinicians consider a certain range of blood pressure to be normal, *not because most people have it, but because a threshold level exists beyond which negative health consequences begin.*

Fletcher, Fletcher, and Wagner offer one other possible definition of abnormality. According to this model, a measurement is considered abnormal only if treatment of the condition represented by the measurement leads to a better outcome. They note that to "label people abnormal can cause adverse psychologic effects that are not justified if treatment cannot improve the outlook."[4]

Diagnosis

Diagnosis involves further application of the concept of abnormality. Diagnosis is the identification and measurement of an abnormality in a particular patient. This could be a medical physician looking for an infection or a chiropractor looking for clinical manifestations of subluxation or joint dysfunction. The purpose of reaching a diagnosis is to determine a course of action. Different diagnoses lead to different interventions, because experience, theory, common sense, and (in some cases) scientific evidence, suggest that specific clinical problems generally (but not always) respond better to specific interventions.

Like all measurements, good diagnostic procedures should be reliable and valid. **Reliability** is defined as the consistency of a measurement when repeated. **Interobserver reliability** refers to the consistency of measured results between different practitioners evaluating the same thing, whereas **intraobserver reliability** measures the consistency with which one practitioner can consistently arrive at the same result.

Motion palpation procedures have been subjected to inter- and intraobserver reliability studies, with mixed results.[5-8] This in turn has led different chiropractors to different conclusions: Troyanovich and colleagues[9] suggests abandoning the method, whereas Cooperstein[10] proposes that the palpation procedure itself may alter the motion characteristics of the tested joints, thus causing the lack of consistent agreement.

Another study tested interexaminer reliability among students, clinicians, radiology residents, and radiologists from both the chiropractic and medical professions in their interpretation of abnormal lumbar spine radiographs. The researchers found no significant difference between the scores of chiropractic radiologists and skeletal radiologists or between chiropractic and medical clinicians. The data also showed that the chiropractic radiologists, chiropractic radiology residents, and chiropractic students scored significantly higher than the corresponding medical categories (general medical radiologists, medical radiology residents, and medical students, respectively).[11]

Validity, or accuracy, is the degree to which an observation or measurement provides an indication of the true state of the phenomena being measured. For example, an oral thermometer provides a measurement of body temperature, but if not used in the proper fashion the reading may not be true. Another possibility is that the thermometer was not manufactured properly. As a result a fever may be missed, or alternatively, a fever may be diagnosed when none exists. Either kind of mistake could have major clinical implications. Thus all diagnostic procedures or tools should be subjected to research to determine not only reliability but also accuracy.

Diagnostic validity is further evaluated for the characteristics of **sensitivity, specificity,** and predictive value. Sensitivity is the proportion of times a diagnostic procedure is correct in patients without a specific diagnosis, whereas specificity is the proportion of times a diagnostic procedure is correct in patients without a specific diagnosis. To establish the sensitivity, specificity, and predictive value of a procedure, the procedure must be compared with a **gold stan-**

dard, which is a measure of agreed upon accuracy and validity.

To determine the sensitivity and specificity of a diagnostic procedure for identifying vertebral subluxation complex (VSC), a gold standard must establish two groups of subjects: (1) those with VSC and (2) those without VSC. Because of variations in criteria for assessment and identification of VSC, no such broadly accepted gold standard for subluxation exists, making this kind of research a major challenge.[12]

Frequency

Knowing how frequently a condition or disease occurs is important in determining its importance in health care policy making; it is also helpful to the clinician as one factor in determining whether a particular patient has this condition. If the frequency of a suspected condition is one in 20 million patients, stronger evidence is necessary for making that diagnosis than for a condition where the frequency is 1 in 20. For example, the frequency of low back pain of mechanical origin is much more common in chiropractic practice than low back pain as the result of prostate cancer. Thus if prostate cancer is suspected, additional diagnostic testing is necessary.

When frequency is expressed with words like *often, sometimes,* or *occasionally,* the meaning is imprecise. Such imprecise language can be appropriate when it accurately reflects honest uncertainty, as is often the case in clinical situations. However, when numeric expressions of frequency are possible, they are certainly preferable. In the research context, they are essential.

Numeric expressions of frequency take two forms: (1) **prevalence** and (2) incidence. Prevalence is the proportion of a group of people having a particular condition or outcome at a given moment. Incidence is the proportion of a group initially free of a condition that develops it over a given period of time.[4]

At a lecture one of the authors (DR) presented to a group of fourth year medical students, a class member asked, "What proportion of the population has a subluxation?" The answer is that data on the prevalence of subluxation does not yet exist. In part this is because the chiropractic profession has not yet formulated a uniform and widely accepted **operational definition** (i.e., one that is specific and allows objective measurement) of the neuromusculoskeletal condition chiropractors call subluxation.

Risk

Recognition of risk factors is an important part of chiropractic clinical practice. Estimates of risk are based on measuring the relationship between the presence of possible risk factors and the subsequent incidence of particular conditions.[4] Much of the scientific literature on risk deals with infectious disease, but risk factors such as smoking and high-fat diets have also been well explored. Chiropractors have always emphasized avoiding or minimizing lifestyle risk factors, as well as musculoskeletal risk factors such as improper lifting methods or lack of appropriate exercise.

Because the human body's structure and function are complex, a direct, one-to-one relationship between a specific risk factor and a particular condition does not usually exist. More often, the interaction of several factors is involved. Because of this complexity, it is usually quite difficult to accurately estimate risk based solely on first-hand experience from one's own practice. A far more complete understanding of risk factors can be obtained by consulting the scientific literature.

It is worth noting here that **correlation** does not necessarily imply causation. Correlation is a consistent statistical relationship between two variables. To demonstrate causation, however, one must show both correlation and a reasonable physiologic mechanism through which this occurs. Correlation without causation would be present in a study that finds that 99 out of 100 people lying on a stretcher in an ambulance are subsequently treated in hospitals but concludes that the ambulances are not the cause of the hospitalizations. An example of correlation *with* causation would be found in a study that correlates tuberculosis (TB) with the presence of the TB bacillus and concludes that this bacillus is causally related to TB, because it disrupts lung function.

Prognosis and Intervention

Prognosis is the predicted course of an illness. Accurate prognosis depends on the **natural history** of an illness, which is the usual progression of an illness in the absence of clinical intervention. Generally if the natural history of an illness involves full recovery within a limited period, irrespective of intervention by a health care provider, such intervention is not needed unless it is likely to improve the patient's quality of life during the recovery period.

The clinician, after arriving at a diagnosis and prognosis, decides whether to intervene in the patient's life and if so to what degree. The point of any intervention is to change the patient's health status for the better. In acute situations such interventions may be termed *treatments*, but intervention can also take the form of preventive measures in which the doctor encourages the patient to engage in **self-care** activities (e.g., exercise, healthy diet, meditation) that promote health.

Implicit in any clinical intervention is the expectation that it will improve upon the natural history of the problem. Evidence supporting the value of an intervention must demonstrate that it is superior to doing nothing, to a **placebo** treatment, and perhaps to some competing intervention. Evidence for the value of chiropractic interventions comes from clinical experience, case studies, observational **cohort** studies, and **randomized clinical trials (RCTs)**. These types of evidence are described later in this chapter, and the evidence from research on chiropractic is presented in Chapters 23, 24, and 25.

Cost

Although most people would prefer that cost not be a factor, it is a key determinant in seeking health care services; **cost-effectiveness** is demanded of all health care providers and their interventions. Those individual practitioners and professions that can demonstrate maximum results at a minimum cost are a valuable commodity in the economics of health care. Studies by Manga[13,14] and Stano and Smith[15-17] stand out as the foremost efforts thus far in demonstrating the cost-effectiveness of chiropractic care. Manga's study for the provincial government of Ontario, Canada, concluded that doubling the use of chiropractic services from 10%

to 20% could realize savings of as much as $770 million annually in direct costs and $3.8 billion in indirect costs[14] ; Stano concluded from an extensive review of insurance records that mean total costs were $1000 for each medical episode and $493 per chiropractic episode.[17]

STUDY DESIGNS

Useful evidence comes in many forms. Evidence evaluating the effectiveness of chiropractic interventions comes from clinical experience, case studies, observational cohort studies, and RCTs. To understand the nature and value of these forms of evidence, some additional terms must be defined.

First, the distinction between **retrospective** and **prospective studies** must be understood. Retrospective studies review events that have already occurred, as in a "retrospective review of records," whereas prospective studies seek to generate new data based on events that occur after the study begins. Readers of clinical research papers will also need to distinguish between **cross-sectional** and **longitudinal studies.** Cross-sectional studies involve measurements taken at one moment in time, whereas longitudinal studies involve serial measures taken over time. Finally, **blinding** (i.e., shielding the subject, the person administering the treatment, or the person assessing the outcome from knowledge that might compromise the integrity of a study) plays an important role in enhancing the validity of **clinical trials.** Because subjects in a study might alter their behavior depending on whether they believe they are receiving a real treatment or a placebo, efforts are made to blind patients to this information. Similarly, because doctors or assessors of the outcome may feel a stake in a particular result, they are also blinded when possible. In a **single-blind study,** it is usually the patients who are blinded; in a **double-blind study,** patients and either the doctors or outcome assessors are blinded; in a **triple-blind study,** patients, doctors, and outcome assessors are all blinded.

Anecdote

The oldest and simplest form of transmitted data is the **anecdote,** which is a story about a clinical event. The story of Daniel David Palmer's adjustment of Harvey Lillard in 1895 (in which Lillard's hearing reportedly improved) is an anecdote that has been passed down through the years. When a chiropractor verbally describes a satisfying case to a friend, a colleague, or a class of students, this is anecdotal material. The fact that a particular story is anecdotal does not indicate whether it is accurate or inaccurate.

However, anecdotes are considered to be the lowest level in the hierarchy of evidence (see Table 23-2 in Chapter 23 for a chart showing this hierarchy of evidence). This is because they are generally based on a single case, involve an incomplete recitation of the facts, and do not involve specific measurements or efforts at replication. Anecdotes are, however, often useful as a basis for further research.

Case Study and Case Series

A **case study** is a written report on the details of a particular case and should include the history, examination findings, diagnosis, treatment, and outcome. Case studies are published in virtually all research journals. Despite their limited generalizability, case studies are an important part of the research literature, because they often provide the first published evidence about a particular potential benefit of a treatment. Moreover, thought-provoking case studies sometimes represent a first step on the road toward more rigorous research on a topic.

A **case series** moves one step beyond the case study, in that it is a written report on the details of a series of cases. An instructive model of practice-based research (reported as both case studies and case series) is the work of Browning on chiropractic management of pelvic pain.[18-25] In this work the clinician demonstrates relief from pelvic pain after chiropractic adjustment/manipulation.

Observational Cohort Studies

An **observational study** is one in which the researcher studies events as they occur naturally or in the course of normal practice, without any attempt to influence them. A example of a large observational study on chiropractic is Cox and Feller's report on 424 consecutive cases of low back pain,[26] in which the patient cohort (i.e., a defined group of people who are observed over a period of time) was treated by participating chiropractors who were permitted to deliver care as they normally would in practice. In this study, 83% of 331 lumbar disc syndrome patients completing care (13% of whom had previous low back surgeries) had good to excellent results. (Excellent was defined as >90% relief of pain and return to work with no further care required. Good was defined as 75% relief of pain, return to work, with periodic manipulation or analgesia required.) There was a median of 11 treatments and 27 days to attain maximal improvement.

When baseline (i.e., pretreatment) and outcome (i.e., posttreatment) measurements are performed, this is often called a **pretest posttest design.**

Experimental Studies and Controlled Trials

Observational studies differ from experimental studies, in which the investigator alters or controls some of the circumstances in which the intervention occurs. The so-called gold standard of experimental studies is the **randomized controlled trial (RCT).** An RCT is a prospective, longitudinal study in which patients are randomly assigned to two or more groups in an effort to avoid **bias** that can occur if the groups differ significantly from one another at the beginning of the trial.

The **experimental group** receives the treatment being tested, whereas the **control group,** for purposes of comparison, receives no treatment, a placebo treatment, or an alternative treatment. A prime example of an RCT on chiropractic care for tension headaches is the previously mentioned study by Boline and colleagues,[1] in which one group received chiropractic adjustment/manipulation, while another group received amitriptyline. Both groups fared about the same in terms of headache pain relief during the period of treatment; however, afterwards the group receiving medication reverted back to prestudy

status, whereas the chiropractic group maintained their levels of improvement.

One significant controversy in experimental design in chiropractic research is that in some studies the participating chiropractors are specifically instructed regarding the methods with which they may intervene. For example, in the Cherkin and colleagues[27] study on low back pain, chiropractic care was somewhat limited compared with the wider range of adjustive and adjunctive treatment (i.e., physiotherapy) procedures available in most chiropractic offices. Some have claimed that because such limits do not reflect the daily reality of chiropractic practice, the generalizability of such studies is open to question.[28] In the Cherkin and colleagues[27] study, both chiropractic and physical therapy were found to be only marginally more effective than reading a book about back pain.

The generalizability of a study is also known as its **external validity,** defined as the degree to which the results can be expected to hold true in settings other than the study setting.[4] **Internal validity** is the degree to which the results of a study are correct (i.e., true) for the **sample** of patients actually studied. In evaluating the quality and value of a research study, both internal and external validity are crucial. Without internal validity, the conclusions are truly meaningless or even misleading. Without external validity, the results of the study cannot be generalized beyond the specific situation of the study.

One of the challenges for clinical scientists is to balance the need for internal validity against the desire for external validity. For example, the Meade study[29,30] concluded that chiropractic care for low back pain was more effective than medical care delivered within British hospitals. External validity was high, because both forms of care were studied in settings with practitioners who did not alter their care for the purposes of the study. However, internal validity was questioned, because the study was not designed to determine the reason that chiropractic was more effective for back pain. Some critics suggested that the difference was due to chiropractor and patient rapport and greater attention being paid to chiropractic patients, rather than to the effectiveness of spinal adjustment/manipulation.

Systematic Reviews and Meta-Analyses

To evaluate the effectiveness of an intervention for a particular condition (e.g., spinal adjustment/manipulation for low back pain), it is necessary to survey the full range of studies that have addressed the topic, giving due consideration to the strengths and weaknesses of the various studies in the literature. This is done through rigorous **systematic reviews** and **meta-analyses,** which can exert a very strong influence on the credibility of the intervention they address, in some cases catapulting a procedure into much more widespread use and in other cases causing a procedure to be dropped from standard practice.

Both systematic reviews and meta-analyses evaluate each study for methodological quality based on criteria, including the size of the sample, randomization, blinding of patients and investigators, controls and placebos, the nature of the treatment, duration and frequency of treatment, outcomes, and effect sizes. A meta-analysis is a systematic review that usually includes a ranking of the quality of each study, plus a statistical pooling of the data from all studies to determine the average effect of treatment.

In general, systematic reviews and meta-analyses on adjustment/manipulation for low back pain tend to agree that such procedures are appropriate for many acute and chronic low back pain cases[31,32] Although far fewer randomized trials exist than for low back pain, systematic reviews have also been conducted on adjustment/manipulation for neck pain and headache. Most have drawn only cautious conclusions in favor of this intervention based on the current state of the evidence[33,34]

Placebo Controversy

Placebo, which means *I shall please* in Latin, is the linchpin of experimental design in pharmaceutical research. In that context, the placebo, or "dummy pill," is a tablet designed to appear identical to the tablets containing the medication being studied. Its purpose is to remove, to the greatest extent possible, knowledge on the part of the research subjects as to whether they are in the experimental group (which receives the medication) or the placebo group (which receives the sugar pill).

All treatments have nonspecific effects, said to be the result of the act of giving (and receiving) care. Physician and author Andrew Weil refers to this phenomenon as the "healing effect."[35] Thus any effect of a placebo treatment is credited to the nonspecific category. The challenge in research is to determine whether the experimental treatment will have specific (i.e., "real") effects against the targeted health complaint, disorder, or pathology.

For drug research, the placebo pill is a brilliant investigative device. For nonpharmaceutical methods such as chiropractic, acupuncture, massage, and physical therapy, finding a proper placebo has proved far more problematic. A white tablet cannot be used as an effective placebo in a trial on spinal adjustment/manipulation, because all participants would know that it is a pill and not a manual intervention. A valid chiropractic placebo, or **sham adjustment/ manipulation,** must be convincing enough for research subjects to believe it is a true adjustment/manipulation, while at the same time having none of the physiologic or therapeutic specific effects of a real adjustment. Proposed examples have included using a spring-loaded chiropractic adjusting instrument with the tension set to zero,[36,37] delivering a manual thrust to a drop-piece rather than a spinal structure,[38] and light massage combined with passive motion applied to the limbs.[39] The problem with most proposed adjustment/manipulation shams is that to be believable some touch or manual contact with the body is necessary. From a bioengineering perspective, however, such manual interventions or contacts are likely to produce at least some physiologic reaction that might be therapeutic.

Thus far, efforts to find a valid chiropractic placebo have raised as many questions as they have answered. The current consensus in the research community is that finding a workable placebo adjustment/manipulation remains a high priority, although some have proposed that a legitimate chiropractic placebo might be an impossibility and that resources devoted to finding and using placebos would be more fruitfully devoted to direct, head-to-head comparisons between chiropractic and conventional medical approaches.[40]

Controls and Active Controls

In the absence of a validated placebo adjustment/manipulation, investigators have used various manual methods as control interventions. These noncavitating procedures (in which no audible joint release takes place) generally involve some form of touch, manual pressure, or massage. A key advantage of this strategy is that many research subjects in these control groups, particularly those who have not previously had chiropractic care, believe that they have had a real adjustment/manipulation. A potential disadvantage is that the nontherapeutic nature of these noncavitating procedures has not been established. An emerging body of evidence exists on the therapeutic effects of massage,[41-45] as does a long history within the chiropractic and osteopathic professions of using noncavitating, "low force" manual procedures.

An alternative construction, the **"active control,"** was used by Bove and Nilsson in a study on episodic, tension-type headache published in the *Journal of the American Medical Association*.[46] These chiropractic researchers randomized subjects into two groups, one receiving soft tissue therapy plus spinal adjustment/manipulation and the other receiving soft tissue therapy (i.e., light massage) and a placebo laser treatment. By identifying the soft tissue therapy as an active control, the investigators avoided the implication that these noncavitating manual methods function as a nontherapeutic placebo.

In this study, both the experimental and control groups experienced significant reductions in mean daily headache hours and use of analgesic medication, but there was no statistically significant difference between the groups in the degree of the improvement. Thus the researchers accurately reported that "as an isolated intervention, spinal manipulation does not seem to have a positive effect on episodic tension-type headache." Unfortunately the subtleties of this carefully worded conclusion were misunderstood by the press, which incorrectly interpreted these findings to mean that chiropractic care (which frequently includes adjustment/manipulation *and* soft tissue procedures) does not help headaches. In fact, the authors of the study have noted that adjustment/manipulation is beneficial for cervicogenic headache (see Chapter 24).

EVIDENCE-BASED HEALTH CARE

The push for **evidence-based health care** has gathered great momentum in recent years. Health services research has demonstrated that much in modern medicine lacks a strong evidence base, and that some widely used procedures have never been subjected to any scientific testing. A fully evidence-based system would be one in which all procedures used by health care providers have been subjected to rigorous standards of scientific observation, experimentation, and documentation. Although this may remain an unattainable ideal, it serves as a central guiding principle in contemporary health care policy.

The evidence used as the basis of an evidence-based health care policy must be screened to eliminate potential sources of error in the documentation process so that experts reach a strong consensus and consumers are confident that each procedure does what it is intended to do.

For the student or practitioner seeking to evaluate the accuracy of evidence, a basic knowledge of certain measurement and documentation procedures is essential. In addition to validity and reliability, which were discussed earlier, it is important to consider issues related to numbers and probability, populations and samples, **statistical significance,** bias, ranking, and random and **systematic error.**

Populations and Samples

One can never assume that results in one successful case can be broadly generalized to other cases. Factors other than the primary clinical intervention may play an important role in a particular patient's recovery. However, if the intervention is studied in a larger group of people and produces similar positive results in a substantial proportion of cases, the evidence becomes stronger. Thus the size of the sample group being studied is a critical factor in evaluating the importance of a particular study. A study with six subjects carries far less weight than one with 300 subjects. A sample is a subset of a population, with a population defined as a group of people meeting a specific set of criteria (e.g., low back pain, one-sided headaches).[4]

Statistical Significance

Clinical research relies on measures of probability to determine the statistical significance of a finding. The key factors influencing statistical significance (i.e., the power of the finding) are the size of the sample and the degree of change in the primary **outcome measures,** which are the key parameters the study seeks to measure and must be defined at the beginning of the study. For example, outcome measures in headache studies often include intensity, duration, and frequency of pain, as well as changes in medication dose used by subjects.

Standards of reporting research require that some results be expressed in terms of **p-values,** which are designed to take into account the potential influence of **random error** (i.e., the influence of chance). Typically, most reported p-values represent the probability of a **false positive,** or Type I error; although p-values are also reported for other types of statistics. False-positive errors are situations where Intervention A is no better than Intervention B, but errors in the data or its interpretation lead one to reasonably conclude that Intervention A *is* actually better than intervention B. This is in contrast to a false-negative, or Type II error. In the case of a **false negative,** Intervention A is actually better than Intervention B, but errors in the data or its interpretation lead one to reasonably conclude that it is *not* better than Intervention B.

P-values less than 0.05 are considered statistically significant, because researchers generally agree that if the likelihood of error is less than 1 in 20, the results are probably not the result of chance. The 0.05 cutoff point for statistical sig-

Is it Clinically Significant?

Statistical significance is not necessarily equivalent to clinical significance. Particularly in studies with large samples, a relatively small change in an outcome measure may achieve statistical significance without representing a difference that truly matters in terms of the patient's health and well-being. To properly interpret the results of a clinical trial, one must examine the **magnitude** of the treatment effect, often known as the *effect size*. Statistical testing determines if the results are valid; the magnitude of the effect determines clinical significance. For example, in a blood pressure study of several thousand hypertensive patients, it may not be unusual to achieve statistical significance for a therapy that decreases patients' blood pressure by an average of 1 mm Hg or even less. Although real, it is questionable that such small decreases in blood pressure have clinical significance.

When evaluating the true value of interventions for which statistically significant results have been attained, it is crucial to consider not just statistical significance but the degree to which patients are likely to be helped or harmed by the intervention.

nificance is customary, but it is also arbitrary. Some research articles report any statistically significant result as p-values less than 0.05, whereas others report the exact probability (0.02) and allow readers to interpret the degree of significance. Lower p-values (0.03, 0.01) carry greater statistical significance, whereas higher p-values (0.1, 0.3) carry less. P-values greater than 1 in 5 (0.20) are customarily reported as p-values greater than 0.20 because of general agreement that a probability of error above this level is too high.

Bias

Although random error reflects the role of chance, systematic error reflects bias. Fletcher, Fletcher, and Wagner define *bias* as "a process at any stage of inference tending to produce results that depart systematically from the true values."[4] Generally, bias results from errors in observation or errors in measurement if the observations have been quantified. Types of bias include **selection bias, measurement bias,** and **confounding bias**.

Selection bias occurs when the groups being studied differ in significant ways other than those that are the focus of the study. This could involve differences in age, gender, the severity of the disease, the presence of different diseases, or differences in lifestyle factors such as diet or exercise. Measurement bias occurs when different or inconsistent methods are used to evaluate the different groups being studied.

Confounding bias occurs when two or more factors interact in the causation of a disease or health condition so that the presence of one factor makes it difficult to evaluate the true effect of the other factors. Confounding bias and selection bias may overlap one another. An example of confounding bias is situation in which a doctor delivering two experimental drugs in a clinical trial favors one over the other. Unless the doctor is blinded as to which drug is being administered, the patient may be able to detect the doctor's bias, thus endangering the fairness of the comparison.

Another potential source of error comes from the **Hawthorne effect,** which is the tendency of people in a research study to change their behavior, perhaps because of the special attention they receive or their own increased awareness of the health effects of their behaviors. This kind of bias endangers external validity. For example, a treatment may look good under study conditions, but fail to perform as well in routine clinical practice.

FUTURE RESEARCH HORIZONS

The modern era of chiropractic research dates from the mid-1970s when the U.S. government convened a conference on "the research status of spinal manipulation,"[47] under the auspices of the National Institute of Neurological and Communicable Diseases and Stroke (NINCDS), a division of the National Institutes of Health (NIH). Responding to the recommendations of the conference report, the chiropractic profession substantially strengthened its research capacity. During the 1990s this effort came to

fruition with the establishment of several funding programs at the national level. Since 1994 the Chiropractic Demonstration Grants program at the U.S. Health Resources and Services Administration has funded a number of clinical trials, demonstration projects, and the annual Research Agenda Conference.

In 1997, NIH established the Consortial Center for Chiropractic Research to build research capacity, bolster the profession's research infrastructure, and initiate pilot studies. The consortium has involved 13 chiropractic institutions and universities in 20 basic and clinical science projects and other efforts. It also aims to develop an environment for training future scientists and to encourage collaboration between basic and clinical scientists and between the chiropractic and conventional medical communities.

The future of chiropractic science is in the profession's hands. The number of sophisticated chiropractic researchers is growing, and training programs for developing future scientists are being established. Chiropractors, many with PhDs in specific disciplines, have been able to compete successfully for grants and have had publications accepted in major scientific journals. The advent and the popularity of the emerging field of complementary and alternative medicine have opened additional doors for chiropractic science. It is an exciting time; there has been much progress. Although chiropractic research is still in its early stages, it will have an increasingly important role in defining the profession's future.

Review *Questions*

1. What are the best ways for chiropractic students and practitioners to stay current with new research developments?
2. What are the most important purposes of health sciences research?
3. What are the three different definitions of abnormality?
4. What is the difference between sensitivity and specificity?
5. What is the difference between correlation and causation?
6. Why is it important to consider the natural history of an illness in determining the

effectiveness of an intervention for patients with that illness?

7. What difficulties arise in trying to blind doctors and patients during studies on nonpharmacologic interventions such as chiropractic, acupuncture, massage, and physical therapy?

8. What are some examples of procedures that have been used as placebo or control interventions in studies on chiropractic?

9. What are the key findings of the study by Boline and colleagues on tension headaches?

10. Does statistical significance sometimes differ from clinical significance? How?

Concept *Questions*

1. How might the chiropractic profession arrive at an operational definition for subluxation? What might be the components of this definition?

2. Should RCTs be considered the gold standard in clinical research on chiropractic? Why?

REFERENCES

1. Boline P et al: Spinal manipulation vs. amitriptyline for the treatment of chronic tension-type headaches: a randomized clinical trial, *J Manipulative Physiol Ther* 18(3):148, 1995.

2. Dishman JD, Bulbulian R: Spinal reflex attenuation associated with spinal manipulation, *Spine* 25(19):2519, 2000.

3. Hawk C, Long CR: Factors affecting use of chiropractic services in seven Midwestern states of the United States, *J Rural Health* 15(2):233, 1999.

4. Fletcher RH, Fletcher SW, Wagner EH: *Clinical epidemiology: the essentials*, ed 3, Philadelphia, 1988, Lippincott, Williams & Wilkins.

5. Love RM, Brodeur RR: Inter- and intra-examiner reliability of motion palpation for the thoracolumbar spine, *J Manipulative Physiol Ther* 10(1):1, 1987.

6. Herzog W et al: Reliability of motion palpation procedures to detect sacroiliac joint fixations, *J Manipulative Physiol Ther* 12(2):86, 1989.

7. Keating JC et al: Interexaminer reliability of eight evaluative dimensions of lumbar segmental abnormality, *J Manipulative Physiol Ther* 13(8):463, 1990.

8. Mootz RD et al: Intra- and interobserver reliability of passive motion palpation of the lumbar spine, *J Manipulative Physiol Ther* 12(6):440, 1989.

9. Troyanovich SJ, Harrison DD, Harrison DE: Motion palpation: it's time to accept the evidence, *J Manipulative Physiol Ther* 21(8):568, 1998.

10. Cooperstein R: The sacral leg check: destructive orthopedic test par excellence, *J Am Chiropr Assoc* 39(8):20, 2002.

11. Taylor JAM et al: Interpretation of abnormal lumbosacral radiographs: a test comparing students, clinicians, radiology residents, and radiologists in medicine and chiropractic, *Spine* 20:1147, 1995.

12. Meeker WC: Concepts germane to an evidence-based application of chiropractic theory, *Top Clin Chiropr* 7(1):67, 2000.

13. Manga P et al: *The effectiveness and cost-effectiveness of chiropractic management of low-back pain*, Richmond Hill, Ontario, Canada, 1993, Kenilworth.

14. Manga P: *Enhanced chiropractic coverage under OHIP as a means for reducing health care costs, at obtaining better health outcomes and achieving equitable access to health services*, Report to the Ontario Ministry of Health, Ontario, Canada, 1998.

15. Stano M, Smith M: Chiropractic and medical costs of low back care, *Med Care* 34(3):191, 1996.

16. Smith M, Stano M: Costs and recurrences of chiropractic and medical episodes of low back care, *J Manipulative Physiol Ther* 20(1):5, 1997.

17. Stano M: The economic role of chiropractic: further analysis of relative insurance costs for low back care, *J Neuromusculoskeletal Sys* 3(3):139, 1995.

18. Browning JE: Pelvic pain and organic dysfunction in a patient with low back pain, response to distractive manipulation: a case presentation, *J Manipulative Physiol Ther* 10:116, 1987.

19. Browning JE: Chiropractic distractive decompression in the treatment of pelvic pain and organic dysfunction with evidence of lower sacral nerve root compression, *J Manipulative Physiol Ther* 11:426, 1988.

20. Browning JE: The recognition of mechanically induced pelvic pain and organic dysfunction in the low back pain patient, *J Manipulative Physiol Ther* 12:369, 1989.

21. Browning JE: Chiropractic distractive decompression in treating pelvic pain and multiple system pelvic organic dysfunction, *J Manipulative Physiol Ther* 12:265, 1989.

22. Browning JE: Uncomplicated mechanically induced pelvic pain and organic dysfunction in low back pain patients, *J Can Chiropr Assoc* 35:149, 1991.

23. Browning JE: Distractive manipulation protocols in treating the mechanically induced pelvic pain and organic dysfunction patient, *Chiropr Tech* 7:1, 1995.

24. Browning JE: The mechanically induced pelvic pain and organic dysfunction syndrome: an often overlooked cause of bladder, bowel, gynecologic and sexual dysfunction, *J Neuromusculoskeletal Syst* 4:52, 1996.

25. Browning JE: Mechanically induced pelvic pain and organic dysfunction in a patient without low back pain, *J Manipulative Physiol Ther* 13:406, 1990.

26. Cox JM, Feller JA: Chiropractic treatment of low back pain: a multicenter descriptive analysis of presentation and outcome in 424 consecutive cases, *J Neuromusculoskel Syst* 2:178, 1994.

27. Cherkin DC et al: Comparison of physical therapy, chiropractic manipulation, and provision of an educational booklet for the treatment of patients with low back pain, *N Engl J Med* 339(14):1021, 1998.

28. Rosner AL: Musculoskeletal disorders research. In Redwood D, Cleveland CS III, editors: *Fundamentals of chiropractic,* St Louis, 2003, Mosby.

29. Meade TW et al: Low back pain of mechanical origin: randomized comparison of chiropractic and hospital outpatient treatment, *BMJ* 300:1431, 1990.

30. Meade TW et al: Randomized comparison of chiropractic and hospital outpatient management for low back pain: results from extended follow-up, *BMJ* 311:349, 1995.

31. Bigos S, Bowyer O, Braen G: *Clinical practice guideline No 14,* AHCPR, Pub No 95-0643, Rockville, Md, 1994, Agency for Health Care Policy and Research, Public Health Service, US Department of Health and Human Services.

32. Bronfort G: Spinal manipulation: current state of research and its indications, *Neurol Clin* 17:91, 1997.

33. Aker PD et al: Conservative management of mechanical neck pain: systematic overview and meta-analysis, *BMJ* 313:1291, 1996.

34. Hurwitz WL et al: Manipulation and mobilization of the cervical spine. A systematic review of the literature, *Spine* 21:1746, 1996.

35. Weil A: *Spontaneous healing,* New York, 1995, Alfred A Knopf.

36. Hawk C et al: Issues in planning a placebo-controlled trial of manual methods: results of a pilot study, *J Altern Comp Med* 8(1):21, 2002.

37. Redwood D: Methodological changes in the evaluation of complementary and alternative medicine: issues raised by Sherman et al and Hawk et al, *J Altern Comp Med* 8(1):5, 2002.

38. Waagen GN et al: Short-term trial of chiropractic adjustments for the relief of chronic low back pain, *Man Med* 2:63, 1986.

39. Balon J et al: A comparison of active and simulated chiropractic manipulation as adjunctive treatment for childhood asthma, *N Engl J Med* 339:1013, 1998.

40. Redwood D: Same data, different interpretation, *J Altern Comp Med* 5(1):89, 1999.

41. Field T et al: Chronic fatigue syndrome: massage therapy effects on depression and somatic symptoms in chronic fatigue syndrome, *J Chronic Fatigue Syndr* 3:43, 1997.

42. Field T et al: Juvenile rheumatoid arthritis: benefits from massage therapy, *J Pediatr Psychol* 22:607, 1997.

43. Ferrell-Torry AT, Glick OJ: The use of therapeutic massage as a nursing intervention to modify anxiety and the perception of cancer pain, *Cancer Nurs* 16(2):93, 1993.

44. Shulman KR, Jones GE: The effectiveness of massage therapy intervention on reducing anxiety in the work place, *J Appl Behav Sci* 32:160, 1996.

45. Nixon M et al: Expanding the nursing repertoire: the effect of massage on post-operative pain, *Aust J Adv Nurs* 14:21, 1997.

46. Bove G, Nilsson N: Spinal manipulation in the treatment of episodic tension-type headache: a randomized controlled trial, *JAMA* 280(18):1576, 1998.

47. Goldstein M, editor: *The research status of spinal manipulation,* Monograph No 15, Washington, DC, 1975, US Department of Health, Education, & Welfare.

Musculoskeletal Disorders Research

Anthony L. Rosner, PhD

Key Terms

Agency for Health Care
  Policy and Research
  (AHCPR)
Algorithm
Carpal Tunnel
  Syndrome
Cervicogenic Headache
Clinical Trial
Co-Morbid Diseases
Cost-Effectiveness
Disk Herniation

Duke Headache Evidence
  Report
Gold Standard
Iatrogenic
International
  Classification of Disease
  Codes
Meta-Analyses
Migraine Headache
Mobilization
Osteopathic Manipulation

RAND
Repetitive Stress
  Disorders
Sham
Systematic Review
Tension Headaches
Transcutaneous
  Electrical Nerve
  Stimulation
Whiplash

Notwithstanding the fact that chiropractic has existed as a formal profession for over a century, most of the rigorous, systematic research that has been recognized to support this form of health care has emerged in just the past 25 years. In 1975—a turning point for chiropractic research—Murray Goldstein of the National Institute of Neurological and Communicable Diseases and Stroke (NINCDS) conducted and published an assessment of the research status of spinal manipulation; the results were not encouraging. Goldstein's report concluded that there was little rigorous outcomes research in support of chiropractic intervention for back pain and other musculoskeletal disorders.[1]

In addition to the insufficient numbers of randomized clinical trials (RCTs) or observational studies of sufficient quality published in the established medical journals, early outcomes trials suffered from any number of significant design flaws, such as the following:

- Often lacking an adequate description of adjustment/manipulation, these trials commonly described **mobilization** (i.e., noncavitating manual movements of joints) rather than manipulation. Furthermore, the methods often lacked adequate descriptions to permit their precise replication.
- Ambiguity existed in the clinical characterizations of the sample population.
- Qualifications of those administering treatment were not reported, whether they were chiropractors, osteopaths, physical therapists, or medical physicians.
- Physician-patient contact times were not uniform across compared groups.
- Sample sizes were often too small to approach statistical significance.
- Failure to observe or control baseline characteristics was common.
- Experimental bias was often introduced into the trial and was often implicit in the recruitment process.
- In a laboratory setting, under tightly controlled conditions, the interventions

tended to be very individualized and as such were difficult if not impossible to generalize to the clinical situation.

Nearly 30 years after the NINCDS conference, dramatic changes are in evidence regarding data demonstrating the efficacy of spinal adjustment/manipulation. Regarding low back pain as assessed by government agencies in the United States,[2] Canada,[3] Great Britain,[4] Sweden,[5] Denmark,[6] Australia,[7] and New Zealand,[8] one could argue that chiropractic care appears have vaulted from last place to first as a treatment option.

For example, *Clinical Practice Guideline 14—Acute Low Back Problems in Adults*, a 1994 assessment of low back pain by the **Agency for Health Care Policy and Research (AHCPR)**, an agency of the U.S. government, placed adjustment/manipulation in the first two treatment options (among 22 different types of interventions) to be considered, together with the use of analgesics and nonsteroidal antiinflammatory drugs (NSAIDs).[2] Commenting on this landmark report in an *Annals of Internal Medicine* editorial, Marc Micozzi stated:

The Agency for Health Care Policy and Research (AHCPR) recently made history when it concluded that " . . . spinal manipulation hastens recovery from acute low back pain and recommended that this therapy be used in combination with or as an alternative to nonsteroidal anti-inflammatory drugs . . . . " Perhaps most significantly, the guidelines state that " . . . spinal manipulation offers both pain relief and functional improvement."[9]

The British guidelines lauded that "there is considerable evidence that manipulation can provide short-term symptomatic benefits" in certain patients[4]; the Danish report echoed this sentiment by declaring that "manual treatment can be recommended for patients suffering from acute low back symptoms and functional limitations of more than 2 to 3 days' duration."[6]

This chapter describes the more recent evolution of musculoskeletal disorders research, with primary emphasis on back and neck pain, most types of headache, and pain in the extremities. The focus is on research since the defining moment of the 1975 NINCDS conference. Key events influencing the profession's reversal of

fortune are identified, and recent studies, which on balance clearly demonstrate the benefits of chiropractic intervention are discussed.

HISTORICAL PERSPECTIVE

Through the 1920s the chiropractic profession remained largely unfamiliar with research methodology, relying primarily upon testimonials from cured patients to document its effectiveness.[10] This was the era when allopathic medicine was just beginning to follow an experimental research regimen that had been proposed by Claude Bernard in 1865.[11] Chiropractic research was significantly hampered at this time and for many decades thereafter by staunch opposition from the American Medical Association (AMA).[12]

In the early years of the profession, most chiropractic professional schools were proprietary and depended upon tuition and clinical fees for survival. Under those conditions, little research was possible except for some case studies, many of which provided invaluable clinical insights. Many of these early investigations followed the interests of B.J. Palmer and the Palmer School of Chiropractic, beginning with the establishment of a "spinographic" laboratory in 1910, in which it was believed that radiographs would provide the opportunity for detecting spinal displacements.[13] After the introduction of this technology, it was asserted by some that patient recovery increased dramatically.[14] Palmer proposed that, "spinography does more than read subluxations, it proves the existence, location, and degree of exostosis, ankylosis, abnormal shapes and forms, all of which may prevent the early correction to normal position of the subluxation."[15] The growing interest in radiography was reflected by the introduction of full-spine radiography by Thompson,[15] later refined in 1931 by the use of a single film.[13]

H.E. Crowe's description of the term **"whiplash"** in 1928 introduced the importance of the soft tissue injury. Whiplash refers to soft tissue injuries in the vicinity of the cervical spine, often caused by automobile accidents.[16] Although now accepted as a medical term, the condition is often associated with litigation[17] and suffers from a scanty literature base.[18]

Largely through the efforts of Joseph Janse and Fred Illi, the sacroiliac joint became the next key focus in chiropractic research. Starting in 1943 in the laboratory at the Institute for the Studies of Statistics and Dynamics of the Human Body in Geneva, Switzerland, Illi's ongoing work provided insight into the functioning of the sacroiliac joint as a synovial articulation required for fully upright bipedal locomotion.[19]

During World War II, European chiropractic researchers developed the practical spinal analysis, called *motion palpation*, as a collective work. A group of Belgian chiropractors, including Marcel and Henri Gillet, Maurice Lickens, Fenande De Mey, Henri Poeck, and Paul de Borchgrave, drew upon chiropractic pioneer O.G. Smith's theory that the vertebral joint has both a circumscribed field and center of motion that become offset when a subluxation occurs.[20] Publications began to describe the methods available to help the practitioner find and demonstrate the evident changes in mobility of the vertebral and sacroiliac articulations before and after an adjustment.[21,22]

By the mid-1970s chiropractic adjustment/manipulation began to be covered under Medicare in response to political efforts by chiropractic practitioners and patients. In a 1974 report, a Senate subcommittee recommended that "this would be an opportune time for an 'independent, unbiased' study of the fundamentals of the chiropractic profession." Consequently, Congress authorized up to $2 million of the 1974 Department of Health Education and Welfare (DHEW) appropriation for that purpose.[10]

Organized and chaired by osteopathic physician Murray Goldstein, Associate Director of NINCDS, the conference topic was termed *spinal manipulation* in order to emphasize the common ground shared by the multidisciplinary group of leading clinicians and scientists who met for 3 days in Washington. Although the conference failed to deliver a consensus as to the indications, contraindications, and precise scientific basis for the results obtained by manipulation of the spine,[1] it did produce the following comments by its organizer, which set the stage for the next 25 years of chiropractic research:

But perhaps of most far reaching importance, the workshop documented that although there are a number of meaningful basic and clinical research questions about manipulative therapy and vertebral biomechanics that are amenable to investigation, there was relatively little quantitative data either in support or in opposition to the several clinical hypotheses . . . . I suspect the NINCDS Workshop cleared the air by demonstrating that there are precise scientific issues relevant to manipulative therapy that deserve research attention.[23]

In the years since 1975, the chiropractic profession has heeded this call, producing an extensive body of research.

BACK PAIN RESEARCH

Methods of Measurement

As in other clinical outcomes research, chiropractic investigations require both reproducible and verifiable measurements from multiple points of view involving both the patient and clinician. Box 23-1 illustrates five such perspectives: (1) the results of physical examinations; (2) functional abilities; (3) patient perception regarding pain, satisfaction, duration of complaint, and use of medications; (4) general health and psychosocial assessments; and (5) direct and indirect costs of treatment. All the indices listed have been verified in the literature; use of the measures represented on this list helps to ensure that an outcome study achieves sufficient construct validity.

At the same time, outcomes research (particularly involving physical methods) is tarnished by what appears at first glance to be a conundrum. Table 23-1 lists outcome studies in order of decreasing rigor, from the most fastidious, demanding (and costly) RCT to anecdotes arising from everyday clinical experiences. At first glance, one might assume that the most controlled investigation (the **clinical trial**) would yield the most useful information. Indeed, the clinical trial is often referred to as the **"gold standard"**[24] in clinical research. Paradoxically, because the double-blind study is so controlled, this most rigorous member of the clinical research hierarchy presents its own difficulties in its generalizability:

Box **23-1** CLINICAL OUTCOMES INSTRUMENTS IN CHIROPRACTIC RESEARCH

PHYSICAL EXAMINATION

Neuologic deficits
Straight-leg raises

FUNCTIONAL OUTCOME ASSESSMENTS

Oswestry back disabllity index
Roland-Morris low back pain disability questionnaire
Neck disability index
Range of motion
Muscle strength

PATIENT PERCEPTION OUTCOME ASSESSMENTS

Pain

Visual analog scale (VAS)
Verbal rating scale (VRS)
Behavioral rating scale (BRS)
McGill pain questionnaire (MPQ)
West Haven-Yale multidimensional pain inventory (WHYMPI)
Patient satisfaction
Patient diary; duration of episode
Use of medications

GENERAL HEALTH AND PSYCHOSOCIAL ASSESSMENTS

Health-related quality of life
Medical outcomes study short-form general health survey
Sickness impact profile
SF-36
Dartmouth primary care cooperative information project (COOP)
Million behavioral health inventory (MBHI)
Modified Zung depression index

COSTS (DIRECT AND INDIRECT)

All visits to provider
Prescription and nonprescription drugs or supplements
Laboratory costs
Diagnostic imaging
Referral to specialists
Hospital costs
Workdays lost by patient
Retraining for replacement labor
Caregiver to assist in domestic duties
Iatrogenic events
Legal and malpractice costs

Table **23-1** Hierarchy of Clinical Research Designs in Decreasing Rigor

Design Classification	Definition
1. Randomized clinical trial	Defined treatment to one group; placebo or sham to second (placebo)
2. Prospective (cohort) study	Defined treatment to one group, no control; blank or sham group
3. Retrospective study	Study performed after treatment (many cases)
4. Cross-sectional study	Study of all subjects performed at one point of time
5. Case control study	After response of one case and matched control(s) over time
6. Single-subject case series	After response of one case over time
7. Case report	Detailed report on one single case
8. Anecdotes	Recollections of case responses, lacking details of case reports

- The characteristics of its own experimental patient base (including co-morbidities*) may differ significantly from those of the individual presenting complaints in the doctor's office.
- Potentially important ancillary treatments are restricted, screening out conceivably significant and perhaps unidentified elements that occur in the natural setting of the patient's visit to the physician.
- Outcome results chosen may not necessarily be those used to evaluate a patient's welfare under care of an actual physician.
- Experimental groups may not be large enough to reach statistical significance, even though the clinical effect may be real in many individuals.

Thus experimental designs at the "low" end of the spectrum (i.e., anecdotes, single case reports) offer their own form of generalizability, although they are of an uncontrolled and often confounded nature. Again, this does not mean that they fail to provide clinical significance.

Ideally, to support a particular type of intervention, what is needed are research results from *both* ends of the hierarchy shown in Table 23-1, to capture both the rigor and generalizability sought in clinical documentation. It is, after all, material from the anecdotes and clinician's office that provide the impetus—the inspiration—to design and conduct a RCT in the first place (see Chapter 22).

*Co-morbidities are conditions existing simultaneously in a patient.

Clinical Trials on Back Pain

Approximately 50 clinical trials including spinal adjustment/manipulation can be identified; a minimum of 25 published in English were confirmed by 1992,[25] the number increasing to at least 34 by 1997,[26] and the balance thereafter. Suffering from the design flaws mentioned previously, the earlier trials tended to suggest only short-term benefits for spinal therapy, eliciting a widespread belief from many quarters that it was beneficial in the alleviation of acute pain, but that there existed insufficient documentation of its efficacy with either severe problems or long-term complications.[2,25,27]

Nineteen of the strongest and most prominent clinical trials addressing the role of spinal adjustment/manipulation in the management of low back pain are summarized in Table 23-2. Those published through 1997 were of sufficient validity to be included by Bronfort in the evidence supporting spinal manipulative therapy for back pain[26]; four remaining trials published after 1997 are listed as well. Collectively, these trials indicate the following:

1. In recent years, there has been a proliferation of publications addressing *chronic* low back pain, offering sufficient refutation to previous assertions that the benefits of adjustment/manipulation are limited to acute cases.
2. Increasing recognition is given to using more objective, reproducible outcome measures such as those proposed in Box 23-1.
3. The difference between manipulation and mobilization seems to have been

Table **23-2** SUMMARY OF LEADING ACUTE AND CHRONIC LOW BACK PAIN CLINICAL TRIALS INVOLVING SPINAL MANIPULATION

Author	Branches	No of Subjects	Subject Complaints	Outcomes	Follow-Up
Hadler[28]	SMT (MD)	26	LBP (acute)	Disability	2-4 weeks
	Mobilization (MD)	28			
Glover[29]	SMT (MD) and diathermy	43	LBP (acute)	Pain	7 days
	Detuned ultrasound	41			
Matthews[30]	SMT (PT)	165	LBP (acute)	Recovery	2 weeks
	Heat	126			
MacDonald[31]	SMT (DO) and back school	49	LBP (acute)	Disability	1-3 weeks
		46			
Farrell[32]	SMT (PT) and mobilization	24	LBP (acute)	Recovery	1-3 weeks
	Diathermy, exercises, and ergonomic instructions	24		Pain	
Koes[33,34]	SMT (PT) and mobilization	36	LBP (chronic)	Severity main complete	6 weeks-12 months
	Massage, exercise, heat, and PM	36		Physical functioning	
	Analog, MD advice	32		Perceived global efficiency	
	Detuned modalities	40			
Pope[35]	SMT (DC)	70	LBP (chronic)	Pain	3 weeks
	Massage	36		Disability	
	TENS	28			
	Corset	30			
Waagen[36]	SMT (DC)	11	LBP (chronic)	Pain	2 weeks
	Sham SMT (DC)	18			
Coxhead[37]	SMT (DC)	Factorial study with 16 different combinations	LBP (chronic)	Pain	4 weeks-4 months
	Traction				
	Exercise				
	Corset				
	No treatment				
Triano[38]	SMT (DC)	70	LBP (chronic)	Pain	2-4 weeks
	Sham SMT (DC)	70		Disability	
	Back school	69			
Giles[39]	SMT (DC)	36	LBP (chronic)	Pain	1 month
	Acupuncture	20		Disability	
	Medication	21			

Table **23-2**   SUMMARY OF LEADING ACUTE AND CHRONIC LOW BACK PAIN CLINICAL TRIALS
INVOLVING SPINAL MANIPULATION—CONT'D

Author	Branches	No of Subjects	Complaints	Subject Outcomes	Follow-Up
Andersson[40]	SMT (DO)	83	LBP (subacute)	Pain	1-12
	MD therapy	72		Disability	weeks
				Range of motion	
				Straight-leg raising	
Skargren[41]	Chiropractic	219	LBP (chronic;	Pain	6-12
	Physiotherapy	192	includes	Disability	months
			patients with	General health	
			neck pain	Cost	
			and those		
			with acute		
			undefined		
			problems		
			excluded		
			from study)		
Meade[42,43]	SMT (DC)	384	LBP (acute and	Disability	6 weeks-
	SMT (PT)	357	chronic)	Pain	3 years
				Analgesics	
Bronfort[44]	SMT (DC)	11	LBP (acute and	Improvement	1 month
	GP (MD)	10	chronic)	Work loss	
Zylbergold[45]	SMT (PT) and heat	8	LBP (acute	Pain	1 month
	Heat and exercise	10	and chronic)	Disability	
	Ergonomic	10			
	instruction				
Doran[46]	SMT (MD)	116	LBP (acute	Improvement	3 weeks-
	Physiotherapy	114	and chronic)		3 months
	Corset	109			
	Analog	113			
Hoehler[47]	SMT (MD)	56	LBP (acute	Pain	3 weeks
	Soft tissue massage	39	and chronic)	Improvement	
Cherkin[48]	SMT (DC)	122	LBP (acute	Bothersomeness	4-12
	McKenzie (PT)	133	and chronic)	Disability	weeks
	Booklet (MD)	66		Cost	

DC, Doctor of chiropractic; *DO,* doctor of osteopathy; *LBP,* low back pain; *MD,* doctor of medicine; PM, patient modalities; *PT,* physical therapist; *SMT,* spinal manipulative therapy; *TENS,* transcutaneous electrical nerve stimulation.

appreciated, with the inclusion of mobilization as a discrete arm of the clinical trial, often called a **"sham"** or "mimic" procedure. (The reader should note that "manipulation" and "chiropractic management" have often been used synonymously, sometimes causing serious confusion, in ways outlined in the following section.)

4. In recent studies a trend exists toward specifically identifying practitioners as chiropractors with proper training in adjustment/manipulation, often having the liberty to treat as they would in actual clinical practice. In this manner, the research becomes more pragmatic and gains external validity, helping to solve the conundrum proposed in Table 23-1.

(A conspicuous exception to this trend, however, is the Cherkin study,[48] to be discussed later.)

Beginning with the publication of a prospective study by Kirkaldy-Willis and Cassidy in 1985, which represented the first time a chiropractor (Cassidy) coauthored an article published in a medical journal,[49] there has been a consistent trend suggesting that improvement in the main complaint produced by manual therapy at least equals that achieved by standard medical treatment. Moreover, this is accomplished without side effects such as intestinal tract ulcers, erosions of the stomach or intestinal tract lining,[50] or liver and kidney damage associated with the prolonged use of analgesics and NSAIDs.[51]

A rather startling result from a trial by Koes and colleagues[33] suggests that improvement in the main complaint produced by manual therapy was not only superior to standard medical treatment but also that the latter intervention even failed to keep pace with the placebo group, in which no intervention took place (see Table 23-2; Fig. 23-1).

One of the most important current trends is that, in contrast to earlier trials in which the relief provided by spinal adjustment/manipula-tion appeared to be *short-lived* (less than 3 weeks),[28,29,47] some of the more recent, larger trials demonstrate that the beneficial effects of spinal manipulative therapy are uniquely *long-lived*, persisting for as much as 12 months[34,41,42] to 3 years.[42] One problem that has been raised regarding the Meade study, however, is that only 28% of its patients were randomized into the chiropractic branch of treatment.[42]

The RAND Appropriateness and Utilization Study

A second facet of musculoskeletal disorders research with regard to back pain and chiropractic can be credited to the **RAND** Corporation, a nonprofit research and development company that first gained prominence with research for the U.S. military during World War II. In addition to defense, RAND's research fields include the health sciences, education, applied economics, sociology, and civil justice.

Several years and millions of dollars in the making, the RAND Appropriateness and Utilization Study has sought to provide "a comprehensive set of indications for performing spinal manipulation with low back pain,"[52] the guide-

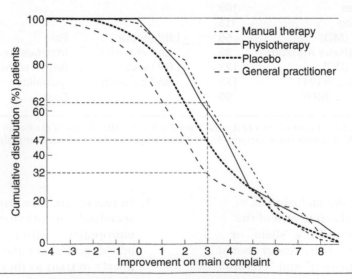

Fig. 23-1 Low back pain outcomes after various treatments in randomized clinical trial (RCT). Improvement in the main complaint at 6-week follow-up (intention-to-treat analysis). *(From Koes BW et al: The effectiveness of manual therapy, physiotherapy, and treatment by the general practitioner for nonspecific neck and back complaints: a randomized clinical trial,* Spine *17(1):28, 1992.)*

lines being based upon a review of the literature, appropriateness ratings by both multidisciplinary and all-chiropractic panels of experts, and field studies abstracted from five geographic sites: (1) Portland, Ore; (2) Minneapolis, Minn; (3) Miami, Fla; (4) San Diego, Calif; and (5) Toronto, Ont.

RAND's literature review of 67 articles and 9 books published between 1952 and 1991 established that chiropractors within the United States performed 94% of all the adjustments/manipulations for which reimbursement was sought, with osteopaths delivering 4% and general practitioners and orthopedic surgeons accounting for the remainder.[52] Support was consistent for the use of spinal adjustment/manipulation as a treatment for patients with acute low back pain and an absence of other signs or symptoms of lower limb nerve root involvement. If minor lower limb neurologic findings or sciatica was present, the evidence was deemed to be either insufficient or conflicting. There was no systematic report on the frequency of complications.

The appropriateness of chiropractic spinal adjustment/manipulation was assessed by two expert panels, one multidisciplinary and one all chiropractic, each rating a comprehensive array of over 1500 clinical scenarios for appropriateness or inappropriateness of chiropractic intervention. These scenarios varied according to length of symptoms; clinical course of pain; presence of co-morbid diseases; history in response to previous treatments for back pain; findings on physical examination; and findings on lumbosacral radiographs, computed tomography (CT), and magnetic resonance imaging (MRI).

Among the appropriate conditions recognized by the *multidisciplinary* panel[53] for chiropractic intervention were acute (less than 3 weeks' duration) back pain with the absence of neurologic findings and acute back pain with minor neurologic findings and uncomplicated lumbosacral neurologic radiographs. In the final ratings, panelists rated 7% of all conditions as appropriate for spinal adjustment/manipulation, although these conditions represent the majority of back pain patients. As might be anticipated, the *all-chiropractic* panel[54] rated a higher

percentage (27%) of all conditions as appropriate. Inappropriate ratings by the multidisciplinary and all-chiropractic panels were 60% and 48%, respectively. On the all-chiropractic panel, there was a higher level of intrapanel agreement than was achieved on the multidisciplinary panel (63% versus 36%).

Depending upon the criteria for assessment, the RAND field studies have reported varying levels of appropriateness of chiropractic intervention. For one site (San Diego), the level of appropriateness varied between 38% and 74%; the level of inappropriateness ranged from 19% and 7%, depending upon whether the criteria of the multidisciplinary or the all-chiropractic panel were applied. Data from other geographic areas of the United States is required before inferences for the national population can be drawn; it has been demonstrated that such a study is feasible.[55]

Systematic Reviews, Meta-Analyses, and Trial Ratings for Low Back Pain

In an effort to filter out low-quality studies, systems rating trial quality have abounded as an attempt to ensure the legitimacy of the evidence used to support various therapeutic approaches. These ratings form the cornerstone of both systematic literature reviews and **meta-analyses**. *Systematic review* is defined as a comprehensive and rigorous review of the peer-reviewed scientific literature requiring a predetermined threshold of graded quality in order to be included. In meta-analyses, on the other hand, actual effect sizes are calculated from pooled results of different clinical trials using a variety of statistical procedures, taking into account the size of each study.

An excellent example of a rating system for trial quality is the scoring mechanism shown in Fig. 23-2, taken from an earlier meta-analysis addressed to the concept of spinal manipulative therapy in the treatment of low back pain. In Anderson's study of 23 RCTs, in most cases spinal manipulative therapy was compared with other therapies rather than true no-treatment placebos. Although the effectiveness of spinal adjustments per se could not be clearly evaluated, they

METHODOLOGY QUALITY CODING FOR META-ANALYSIS[54]

Study #

Discussion of Research Question/Hypothesis
_____ (3) Yes
_____ (0) No

Randomization Performed
_____ (12) Adequate randomization
_____ (6) Partial—not adequately described
_____ (0) Inadequate or no randomization

Analysis of Randomization Efficacy
_____ (6) Adequate—table showing distribution of major prognostic factors
_____ (3) Partial—reported successful but no data
_____ (0) No information

Selection Description/Discussion of Inclusion/Exclusion Criteria
_____ (12) Adequate = reproducible (pt. source, inclusion/exclusion, diagnosis)
_____ (6) Partial—2 of 3 above
_____ (0) Inadequate—1 of 3 above

Patient Characteristics
_____ (6) Standard reporting (e.g., age, sex) + other possible
_____ (3) Standard
_____ (0) Substandard (not even minimal characteristics)

Blinding of Patients
_____ (12) Yes
_____ (6) Unsuccessful or results not stated
_____ (0) No

Blinding of Evaluators
_____ (12) Yes (successful)
_____ (6) Partial (blinding not rigorous or not completely successful)
_____ (0) No

Description of Interventions
_____ (12) Adequate—clear/reproducible + definitions
_____ (6) Partial—some description/not well defined
_____ (0) Inadequate—broad description/no definition

Intervention Controls
_____ (12) No contamination/ideal control
_____ (6) Some contamination (confounding variables) but minor
_____ (0) Significant contamination/results in question

Discussion of TX Number, Frequency, Duration
_____ (12) Protocol + actual numbers for all
_____ (9) Protocol + actual numbers for 2 of 3
_____ (6) Protocol + actual numbers for 1 of 3
_____ (3) Protocol only/no actual
_____ (0) No actual/protocol insufficient to reproduce

Outcome Measures
_____ (12) Subjective + objective + other (e.g., MMPI)
_____ (6) Subjective + objective
_____ (3) Objective only
_____ (0) Subjective only

Compliance
_____ (6) Exact report of data
_____ (3) Qualitative description
_____ (0) Not mentioned

Discussion of Bias
_____ (6) Yes
_____ (0) No

Withdrawals
_____ (6) Mentioned
_____ (3) Mentioned, disregarded in analysis or unclear how they were handled
_____ (0) Not mentioned

Discussion of Alpha/Beta Errors
_____ (6) Yes (explicit)
_____ (3) Brief mention of small sample size
_____ (0) No

Total Score _____
Denominator for percentage calculation will be based on only those questions applicable to paper evaluated. If all questions apply, then 135 points are possible.

Fig. 23-2 Methodology quality coding for meta-analysis. *(From Shekelle PG et al:* The appropriateness of spinal manipulation for low back pain: indications and ratings by an all-chiropractic expert panel, *monograph no R-4025/3-CCR/FCER, Santa Monica, 1992, RAND.)*

consistently proved more effective in the treatment of low back pain than any of the comparative interventions.[56]

Shekelle's meta-analysis, noteworthy in that it represented the first time a chiropractor (Alan Adams) coauthored an article in the *Annals of Internal Medicine*, retrieved 58 articles representing 25 trials. The authors concluded that the data supported the short-term

benefit of spinal manipulation in some patients, particularly those with uncomplicated, acute low back pain. Data regarding *chronic* low back pain at the time of this publication were judged insufficient to evaluate the efficacy of spinal manipulation in managing this particular condition.[25]

This qualification may no longer stand. The evidence supporting the use of spinal adjustment/manipulation in managing chronic low back pain is now substantial. In a systematic review of 16 randomized controlled trials involving manipulation and adjustment for chronic low back pain, van Tulder and colleagues identified two of high-quality, only one of which was judged to be of sufficient quality by Bronfort and shown in Table 23-3.[31,57] Here, the evidence supporting manipulation for chronic low back pain is found to be actually *stronger* than that for acute conditions. There is limited evidence that manipulation is more effective than a placebo treatment for acute low back pain (level 3).

There is no evidence that manipulation is more effective than [other] physiotherapeutic applications . . . or drug therapy . . . . There is strong evidence that manipulation is more effective than a placebo treatment for chronic LBP [low back pain] (level 1). There is moder-

ate evidence that manipulation is more effective for chronic LBP than usual care by the general practitioner, bed-rest, analgesics, and massage (level 2).[*58]

A somewhat different interpretation was reached in Bronfort's systematic review.[26] Here, the evidence supporting spinal adjustment/manipulation for managing either acute or chronic low back pain was judged to be "moderate," whereas the evidence supporting spinal adjustment/manipulation for managing a *mix* of chronic and

*In the van Tulder review, Level 1 refers to "strong" evidence, with multiple, relevant, high-quality RCTs; Level 2 refers to "moderate" evidence, with one relevant, high-quality RCT and one (or more) relevant, low-quality RCT; and Level 3 refers to "limited" evidence, with one relevant, high-quality RCT or multiple relevant, low-quality RCTs.

Table **23-3** SCORING THE QUALITY OF CLINICAL TRIALS: VARIABILITY OF WEIGHTS GIVEN TO KEY METHODOLOGIC DOMAINS[59]

Scale	No of Items	Randomization	Blinding	Withdrawals
Andrew, 1984	11	9.1	9.1	9.1
Beekerman et al, 1992	24	4.0	12.0	16.0
Brown, 1991	6	14.3	4.8	0.0
Chalmers et al, 1990	3	33.3	33.3	33.3
Chalmers et al, 1981	30	13.0	26.0	7.0
Cho, Bero, 1994	24	14.3	8.2	8.2
Colditz et al, 1989	7	28.6	0.0	14.3
Deltsky et al,1992	14	20.0	6.7	0.0
Evans, Pollack, 1995	33	3.0	4.0	11.0
Goodman et al, 1994	34	2.9	2.9	5.9
Gotzsche, 1989	16	6.3	12.5	12.5
Imperiale/McCullough, 1990	5	0.0	0.0	0.0
Jadad et al, 1996	3	40.0	40.0	20.0
Jonas et al, 1993	18	11.1	11.1	5.6
Kjeijnen et al, 1991	7	20.0	20.0	0.0
Koes et al, 1991	17	4.0	20.0	12.0
Levine, 1991	29	2.5	2.5	3.1
Linde et al, 1997	7	28.6	28.6	28.6
Nurmohamen et al, 1992	8	12.5	12.5	12.5
Onghena/van Houdenhove, 1992	10	5.9	5.9	2.9
Poynard, 1988	14	7.7	23.1	15.4
Reisch et al, 1989	34	5.9	5.9	2.9
Smith et al, 1992	8	0.0	25.0	12.5
Spitzer et al, 1990	32	3.1	3.1	9.4
ter Riet, 1990	18	12.0	15.0	5.0

acute low back pain was considered "inconclusive." Furthermore, all but *one* of the back pain studies considered to be of sufficient validity were eliminated by the criteria invoked by van Tulder, whereas the latter study included one trial[58] that had been rejected by Bronfort.

The fact that systematic reviews may conflict in both their conclusions and their acceptance of particular studies is troublesome. A recent study dramatically illustrates how meta-analyses can be reduced to subjective value scales, with disastrous results. In their efforts to compare two different preparations of heparin for their respective abilities to prevent postoperative thrombosis, Juni and colleagues demonstrated that diametrically opposed results could be obtained in different meta-analyses, depending upon which of 25 scales is used to distinguish between high- and low-quality RCTs. The root of the problem is evident from the variability of weights given to three prominent features of RCTs (randomization, blinding, and withdrawals) shown in Table 23-3 by the 25 studies that have compared the two therapeutic agents. In one study (Jadad et al, 1996), one third of the total weighting of the quality of the trial is afforded to both randomization and blinding, whereas in another (Imperiale and McCullogh, 1990), *none* of the quality scoring is derived from these two features.

Widely skewed intermediate values for the three aspects of RCTs under discussion are apparent from the 23 other scales presented. The astute reader will immediately suspect that sharply conflicting conclusions might be drawn from these different studies—and these are amply borne out by the statistical plots shown in Fig. 23-3. Here each of the meta-analyses listed resolve the 17 studies they have reviewed into high- and low-quality strata, based upon their respective scoring systems. It can be seen that 10 of the authors selected scored a statistically superior effect of one heparin preparation (i.e., the low-molecular–weight heparin [LMWH]) over the other (but only for the *low*-quality studies). Seven other studies reveal precisely the *opposite* effect, in which the *high*- but not the low-quality studies display a statistically significant superiority of LMWH.

Therefore depending upon which scale is used, the clinician can either demonstrate or refute the clinical superiority of one clinical treatment over the other. In this manner, all the rigor and labor-intensive elements of the RCT and its interpretation by the meta-analysis are simply reduced to subjective value judgment through the arbitrary assignment of numbers in the weighting of experimental quality.[59]

Returning to the discussion on low back pain, yet another systematic review of RCTs cites adequate follow-up periods, avoidance of cointerventions (i.e., additional therapies used with adjustment/manipulation), and avoidance of dropouts as frequent strengths. Recurrent weaknesses, however, include randomization procedures, sample sizes, and blinded assessments of outcomes (the latter being virtually impossible to perform in a trial involving manual therapy, because the physical nature of adjustment/manipulation is so difficult to disguise).[60] Moreover, a meta-analysis of 51 literature reviews of spinal manipulative therapy suggests that, although the overall methodologic quality was low, 9 of the 10 methodologically best reviews reached positive conclusions regarding spinal adjustments.[61]

One key point bears repeating: *The results of systematic reviews and meta-analyses are completely dependent on the criteria chosen by the authors of the reviews.* Consumers of such literature are therefore well advised to read the text, not just the conclusions in the abstract, to understand and properly evaluate the validity of a study's conclusions.

Lumbar Disk Herniation Research

The options for treating disk herniations are surgery or conservative care, the latter often involving spinal adjustment/manipulation. With no controlled trials to date that directly compare these two options, it is perhaps helpful to mention that, during a 30-year career, one leading orthopedic surgeon never encountered a patient with a **disk herniation** that was aggravated by manipulation.[62]

Two randomized trials currently support the wisdom of considering spinal adjustment/manipulation as a treatment option for this condition.

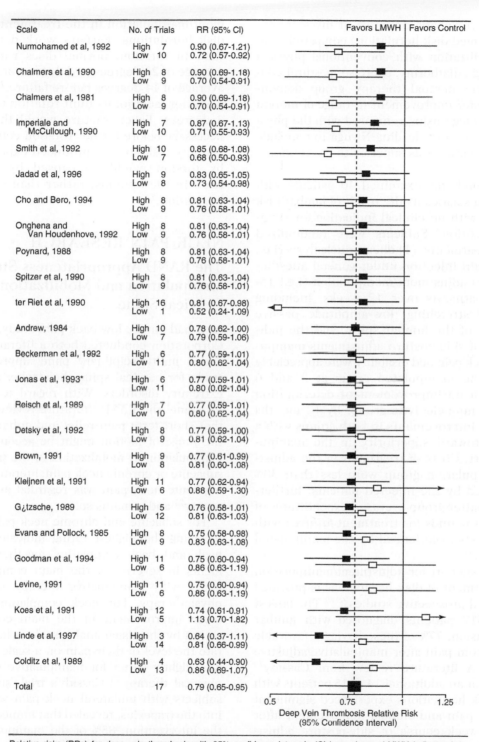

Scale		No. of Trials	RR (95% CI)
Nurmohamed et al, 1992	High	7	0.90 (0.67-1.21)
	Low	10	0.72 (0.57-0.92)
Chalmers et al, 1990	High	8	0.90 (0.69-1.18)
	Low	9	0.70 (0.54-0.91)
Chalmers et al, 1981	High	8	0.90 (0.69-1.18)
	Low	9	0.70 (0.54-0.91)
Imperiale and McCullough, 1990	High	7	0.87 (0.67-1.13)
	Low	10	0.71 (0.55-0.93)
Smith et al, 1992	High	10	0.85 (0.68-1.08)
	Low	7	0.68 (0.50-0.93)
Jadad et al, 1996	High	9	0.83 (0.65-1.05)
	Low	8	0.73 (0.54-0.98)
Cho and Bero, 1994	High	8	0.81 (0.63-1.04)
	Low	9	0.76 (0.58-1.01)
Onghena and Van Houdenhove, 1992	High	8	0.81 (0.63-1.04)
	Low	9	0.76 (0.58-1.01)
Poynard, 1988	High	8	0.81 (0.63-1.04)
	Low	9	0.76 (0.58-1.01)
Spitzer et al, 1990	High	8	0.81 (0.63-1.04)
	Low	9	0.76 (0.58-1.01)
ter Riet et al, 1990	High	16	0.81 (0.67-0.98)
	Low	1	0.52 (0.24-1.09)
Andrew, 1984	High	10	0.78 (0.62-1.00)
	Low	7	0.79 (0.59-1.06)
Beckerman et al, 1992	High	6	0.77 (0.59-1.01)
	Low	11	0.80 (0.62-1.04)
Jonas et al, 1993*	High	6	0.77 (0.59-1.01)
	Low	11	0.80 (0.02-1.04)
Reisch et al, 1989	High	7	0.77 (0.59-1.01)
	Low	10	0.80 (0.62-1.04)
Detsky et al, 1992	High	8	0.77 (0.59-1.00)
	Low	9	0.81 (0.62-1.04)
Brown, 1991	High	9	0.77 (0.61-0.99)
	Low	8	0.81 (0.60-1.08)
Kleijnen et al, 1991	High	11	0.77 (0.62-0.94)
	Low	6	0.88 (0.59-1.30)
Gøtzsche, 1989	High	5	0.76 (0.58-1.01)
	Low	12	0.81 (0.63-1.03)
Evans and Pollock, 1985	High	8	0.75 (0.58-0.98)
	Low	9	0.83 (0.63-1.08)
Goodman et al, 1994	High	11	0.75 (0.60-0.94)
	Low	6	0.86 (0.63-1.19)
Levine, 1991	High	11	0.75 (0.60-0.94)
	Low	6	0.86 (0.63-1.19)
Koes et al, 1991	High	12	0.74 (0.61-0.91)
	Low	5	1.13 (0.70-1.82)
Linde et al, 1997	High	3	0.64 (0.37-1.11)
	Low	14	0.81 (0.66-0.99)
Colditz et al, 1989	High	4	0.63 (0.44-0.90)
	Low	13	0.86 (0.69-1.07)
Total		17	0.79 (0.65-0.95)

Favors LMWH | Favors Control

Deep Vein Thrombosis Relative Risk
(95% Confidence Interval)

Relative risks (RRs) for deep vein thrombosis with 95% confidence intervals (CIs) are shown. LMWH indicates low-molecular-weight heparin. Black squares indicate estimates from high-quality trials and open squares indicate estimates from low-quality trials. Arrows indicate that the values are outside the range of the x axis. Broken line indicates combined estimate from all 17 trials. Solid line indicates null effect line. The scales are arranged in decreasing order of the RRs in trials deemed to be of high quality. Asterisk indicates unpublished scale.

Fig. 23-3 Results from sensitivity analyses of studies on heperin, dividing trials in high- and low-quality strata, using 25 different quality assessment scales. Note the wide range in conclusions about the value of the medication being studied. *LMWH,* Low molecular weight heparin. *(From Juni P et al: The hazards of scoring the quality of clinical trials for meta-analysis, JAMA 282(11): 1054, 1999.)*

One study (involving 51 cases of myelographically confirmed disk herniation) compared rotational mobilization with conventional physical therapy (e.g., diathermy, exercise, postural education). The manual therapy group demonstrated greater improvement in range of motion and straight leg raising compared with the physical therapy cohort, leading Nwuga to conclude that manipulation was superior to conventional treatment.[63]

The second trial examined 40 patients with unremitting sciatica as the result of lumbar disk herniation with no clinical indication for surgical intervention. Subjects were randomized into two treatments: (1) chemonucleolysis (i.e., chymopapain injection under general anesthesia) and (2) adjustment/manipulation (i.e., 15-minute treatments over 12 weeks, including soft tissue stretching, low-amplitude passive maneuvers of the lumbar spine, and the judicious use of side-posture adjustments/manipulations). Back pain and disability were appreciably lower in the manipulated group at 2 and 6 weeks, with no improvement or deterioration in the chemonucleolytic group. By 12 months there were improvements in both groups with a tendency toward superiority in the manipulated cohort. Costs of treatment in the adjustment/manipulation group were less than 30% encountered by the injected patients; furthermore, the latter group averaged expenditures of 300 British pounds for treatment *failures* with no such costs experienced by the manipulated population.[64]

Further support for adjustment/manipulation in the treatment of disk herniations is provided from several prospective studies.[65-69] The largest involved 517 patients diagnosed with lumbar disk protrusion, 77% of these having a favorable response from pain after manipulative/adjustive therapy.[68] A literature review from Cassidy[70] suggests that an additional 14 of 15 patients with lumbar disk herniations experienced significant relief from pain and clinical improvement after a 2- to 3-week course of side-posture adjustment/manipulation.

Cassidy,[70] who disputes the assertion by Farfan that rotational stress causes disk failure, supports the safety of rotational adjustment/manipulation in the treatment of lumbar disk herniations. Farfan's work demonstrates that, in rotation, normal discs withstand an average of 23 degrees and degenerated discs an average of 14 degrees before failure.[71] However, posterior facet joints limit rotation to only 2 to 3 degrees. Facet fracture would therefore be necessary before further rotation could occur,[72] and any disk failures produced experimentally by torsion would be caused by peripheral tears in the annulus, rather than prolapse or herniation.[72]

NECK PAIN RESEARCH

The RAND Appropriateness Study: Manipulation and Mobilization of the Cervical Spine

As it had for the low back pain study, the RAND Corporation conducted both a literature review and a multidisciplinary panel appropriateness study for cervical spine, headache, and upper-extremity disorders. With regard to the cervical spine, the RAND literature review suggested that short-term pain relief and enhancement of the range of motion might be accomplished by manipulation or mobilization in the treatment of subacute or chronic neck pain; literature describing acute neck pain was regarded as extremely scanty[73] and remains so.

For subacute and chronic neck pain, the trial receiving the highest rating indicated that, for neck and back complaints together, improvements in severity of the main complaint were larger with manipulative therapy rather than physiotherapy. For neck complaints only, the mean improvement in the main complaint as shown by the visual analog scale (where patients rate the level of their pain on a scale of 0 to 10) was slightly better for manipulative rather than physical therapy.[74] Cassidy's trial, studying 100 subjects with unilateral neck pain with referral into the trapezius, revealed that immediately after the intervention, 85% of the manipulated group and 69% of the mobilized group reported pain improvement. The decrease in pain intensity was more than 1.5 times greater in the manipulated group.[75] The literature regarding upper extremities, headache, and complications is referred to in the following appropriate sections.

As in the earlier low back study by RAND,[55] the appropriateness of chiropractic cervical spinal manipulation was assessed by an expert multidisciplinary panel, rating an array of more than 1400 clinical scenarios for appropriateness of chiropractic intervention. In the final ratings, panelists rated 41% of all conditions as appropriate and 43% as inappropriate for chiropractic, with disagreement on only 2% of all conditions.[76] An example of a condition deemed appropriate was morning neck stiffness with radiographic findings of early degenerative changes in the cervical spine. An example considered inappropriate was possible or definite radiculopathy with no advanced imaging studies.

It is important to remember that ratings of appropriateness depend on data available at the time the ratings are performed. As further research emerges, future ratings may change accordingly.

Other Studies

Despite the lack of investigations involving acute neck pain, a trend toward improvement exists—at least in the main complaint shown in the clinical trials displayed in Table 23-4. The effects seem to be particularly dramatic in the studies of Koes[34,77] and Sloop.[78] Improvements of 44% in the visual analogue scale and 41% in head repositioning are apparent in the manipulated group in the Rogers study, as opposed to the respective values of 9% and 12% in the control group. Rogers suggests that there may be a possible effect of adjustment/manipulation on proprioception (i.e., position sense) in patients with chronic neck pain.[79]

Although improvements were observed, differences between the four interventions specified in the Skargren study[41] or between the three interventions used by Jordan[80] could not be detected. Similarly, both the cervical rotary and supine lateral break manipulative procedures used by van Schalkwyk demonstrated improvements during the course of treatment but could not be differentiated from each other in terms of effect magnitudes.[81]

In a retrospective study by McMorland and Suter involving 119 patients, those with neck pain were shown to have average reductions of 57% and 48% in their chronic pain and disability, respectively. Because this was not a clinical trial, it is not possible to account for the natural history of this condition; therefore no claims of treatment efficacy can be made.[82]

Whiplash Research

The problem facing both diagnosticians and victims of whiplash is that most moderate to severe cases are invisible upon standard medical examination. As elusive as the causative "smoking gun" might be regarding this condition, it involves a broader array of soft tissue, neurologic, and temporomandibular joint problems than presumed only a decade ago.[83] In Quebec alone, the fact that whiplash in 1989 accounted for 20% of all traffic injury insurance claims with an average compensation period of 108 days,[84,85] led a multidisciplinary task force to conclude that "neck pain is to the automobile what low back pain is to the workplace."[86]

The elusiveness of a definitive, reproducible pathology for whiplash-associated disorders (WAD) has often led the legal, insurance, and medical communities to erroneously conclude that the symptoms of WAD have no physical or organic basis. This has produced charges that WAD patients are malingering or overly influenced by litigation neurosis on the part of the patient, leading to the overlaying of psychologic factors that compound the problem. One indication of the increasing societal concern about whiplash is reflected by the fact that in a 1995 revision of a 1988 text on WAD, Stephen Foreman and Arthur Croft increased the number of references cited from 600 to over 1250.[83]

Also known as *cervical acceleration-deceleration syndrome*,[83] whiplash has often been misunderstood as having the spontaneous recovery rate of 90% often associated with low back pain victims.[2] In a review of the literature, Bannister and Gargan[87] document recoveries from cervical injury cited in 12 published studies, ranging

Table **23-4**   SUMMARY OF LEADING NECK PAIN CLINICAL TRIALS INVOLVING SPINAL MANIPULATION

Author	Branches	No of Subjects	Subject Complaint	Outcome	Follow-Up
Koes[33,34]	SMT (PT) and mobilization	21	Neck pain (chronic)	Severity main complete	6 weeks-12 months
	Massage, exercise, heat, and PM	13		Physical functioning	
	Analog, MD advice	17		Perceived global efficiency	
	Detuned modalities	14			
Sloop[78]	Diazepam, SMT (MD)	21	Neck pain (chronic)	Pain	3 weeks
	Physiotherapy	18		Improvement	
Skargren[41]	Chiropractic	219	Neck pain (chronic; includes patients with low back pain and those with acute undefined problems excluded from study)	Pain	6-12 months
	Physiotherapy	192		Disability General health Cost	
Rogers[79]	SMT	10	Neck pain (chronic)	Pain	?
	Exercise	10		Repositioning	
Jordon[80]	Chiropractic	40	Neck pain (chronic)	Pain	4-12 months
	Physiotherapy	40		Disability	
	Intensive training	39		Medication use Perceived effect Physician global assessment	
van Schalkwyk[81]	Cervical rotary SMT	10	Neck pain (acute and chronic)	Pain	1 month
	Lateral break SMT	10		Disability Range of motion	

DC, Doctor of chiropractic; *DO,* doctor of osteopathy; *LBP,* low back pain; *MD,* doctor of medicine; *PM,* patient modalities; *PT,* physical therapist; *SMT,* spinal manipulative therapy; *TENS,* transcutaneous electrical nerve stimulation.

from 12% to 86% (averaging 57%). Stabilization or resolution of pain occurs with an unweighted average of 7.3 months.[87] A review of 15 additional studies by Arthur Croft,[88] who documents the persistence of symptoms after WAD injuries for periods exceeding 18 years, provides even more dramatic evidence.

From a morphologic point of view, immobilization of the neck after the soft tissue trauma that accompanies WAD is indefensible. Severe soft tissue injury (rupture of muscles, joint capsules, and synovial folds) may occur around the cervical spines of accident victims.[89] Consequently, scar formation, cross-linking of collagen fibers, and adhesions might be expected to result in traumatized soft tissues that were not rehabilitated soon after injury. Specifically:

1. Healing without proper motion will cause a disorganized connective tissue matrix to appear, with adhesions and unnecessary scar formation.[90,91]

2. Early exercise and joint motion in rehabilitation produces a better collagen concentration, which is superior to scar tissue.[92]

3. Improved tensile strength is observed in the collagen deposit when proper rehabilitation takes place after injury.[93,94]

4. If venous blood supply to paraspinal muscles is depressed for 2 hours (which might be anticipated in some soft tissue injuries), irreversible muscle damage occurs.[95] With decreased vascularization, rapid degeneration of the muscle spindles occurs—with subsequent revascularization changing their shape and neural innervation.[96]

Regarding manual therapy in the management of whiplash patients, two larger studies have been reported in the literature. One demonstrated that, in subjects displaying significant cervical lateral-flexion passive end–range asymmetries and a history of neck trauma and frequent episodic neck stiffness, a single unilateral lower cervical adjustment delivered to the side of most restricted end-range of motion is capable of reducing the magnitude of asymmetry, but only transiently (for periods less than 48 hours).[97] A second study involving 93 patients in a retrospective review by structured telephone interviews indicated that those with restricted range of neck movement after whiplash injury were the most likely to improve after chiropractic adjustment/manipulation. Many patients had received previous treatments, particularly physiotherapy.[98]

The abundance of literature on the cause, diagnosis, treatment, and sociology of whiplash led a multidisciplinary group (the Quebec Task Force) to collect 10,382 titles and abstracts, of which 1204 met the criteria for preliminary screening before 294 (3% of the initial sample) were ultimately rated; 21% of the latter (0.6% of the initial sample) were ultimately accepted.[86] Of the 10 randomized controlled trials pertaining to WAD accepted by the Quebec Task Force, only one addressed spinal adjustment/manipulation. This was the investigation by Cassidy[75] previously described.

The accomplishments of the Quebec Task Force are as follows[86]:

1. *New classification of WAD*: WADs were classified on two scales. The first, based on clinical presentation, specified five grades based on the presence of musculoskeletal signs (i.e., decreased range of motion, point tenderness), neurologic signs (i.e., decreased or absent deep tendon reflexes, weakness, sensory deficits), or fracture and dislocation. The second scale specified five grades based on the duration of the injury, ranging from 4 days to more than 6 months.

2. *Management advice and **algorithm*** (i.e., a step-by-step problem-solving procedure): Even though mobilization and manipulation are distinguished from each other, they were both classified as active treatments. In the precise language of the task force, the "consensus is that manipulation treatments by trained persons for the relief of pain and facilitating early mobility can be used in WAD. All such treatments should . . . discourage extended dependence upon the health professional . . . . Long-term, repeated manipulation without multidisciplinary evaluation is not justified."

3. *Directives for education and research*: In defining the skills and knowledge needed for the effective management of WAD patients, the task force concluded that the primary interventionist "must possess the qualities of a clinical anatomist" and the

fundamental knowledge of rehabilitation of the musculoskeletal system and clinical epidemiology. Research was found to be extremely scanty, with the therapeutic interventions requiring immediate further investigation, including manipulation and specific physiotherapeutic interventions. It praised the research of both David Cassidy in Saskatchewan and Ake Nygren in Sweden as ideals for international, interdisciplinary research.

The work of the Quebec Task Force, however, is not without criticism. Freeman[99] has raised several objections to the Task Force Guidelines, including the following:

1. *Near total elimination of relevant literature*: The fact that 97% of all articles were eliminated before consideration raises a strong possibility that both instructive and useless data were discarded.
2. *Arbitrary recommendations*: In the resulting absence of literature to consider, the task force gave its own opinion equal weight with primary research data, lending a misleading sense of robustness to its recommendations.
3. *Propagation of the myth that most WAD patients recover in 6 to 12 weeks*: Upon closer examination, this length of time has no basis in primary research. In fact,

considerable data already cited contradicts this impression and paints a far bleaker picture.[87-96]

4. *The undertaking was sponsored by an insurance industry*: Societe d'assurance automobile du Quebec (SAAQ) as the sponsoring organization of the entire project would be expected to have a vested interest in its outcome, possibly compromising the objectivity of the literature research, evaluation, and ultimate recommendations of the task force.

A major need exists for more data (from both clinical trials and case series) to be provided about this complex and elusive condition. One encouraging note is that Cassidy's group is conducting a 5-year study addressing both the incidence and management of whiplash injuries, including controlled trials to assess both the clinical and **cost-effectiveness** of chiropractic and other interventions.[100]

HEADACHE RESEARCH

The treatment of headaches with spinal adjustment/manipulation has generated a proliferation of research in the peer-reviewed literature, reflected in part by the multiple outcomes research designs shown in Table 23-5. At least

Table **23-5**   Headache Outcomes Research Using Spinal Manipulation

Type of Headache	Author	No of Patients	Arms	Outcomes	Design
Tension[101]	Boline	126	SMT Amitriptyline	Frequency Total pain OTC drugs Global health	RCT
Tension[102]	Bitterli		SMT No treatment	Pain	RCT
Tension[103]	Hoyt	22	Palpation Palpation, SMT No treatment	Intensity EMG	RCT
Tension[104]	Bove	75	SMT Laser	Analgesic use Frequency Intensity	RCT

Table **23-5** HEADACHE OUTCOMES RESEARCH USING SPINAL MANIPULATION—CONT'D

Type of Headache	Author	No of Patients	Arms	Outcomes	Design
Cervicogenic[105]	Nilsson	54	SMT Laser	Analgesic use Frequency Intensity	RCT
Cervicogenic[107]	Whittingham	105	SMT toggle	Sickness impact Neck disability index Pain drawings and diaries	RCT
Migraine[108]	Nelson	209	SMT Amitriptyline SMT and Amiltript	Frequency Intensity OTC use Functional capacity	RCT
Migraine[109]	Tuchin	123	SMT Detuned ultrasound	Frequency Intensity Duration Disability Associated symptoms Medications	RCT
Migraine[110]	Parker	85	Mobilization SMT by DC SMT by MD	Frequency Intensity Duration	RCT
Posttraumatic[111]	Jensen	19	SMT Cold packs	Pain index ROM Adjunctive symptoms	RCT
Tension[112]	Mootz	11	SMT Cold packs TP	Frequency Intensity Duration	CS
Tension[113]	Droz	332	SMT	Pain	RS
Cervicogenic[114]	Vernon	33	SMT	Frequency Intensity Duration	PS
Migraine[115]	Wight	87	SMT	Pain	CS
Cervical migraine[116]	Stodolny	31	SMT	Pain ROM Dizziness	PS
Chronic[117]	Turk	100	SMT	Analgesic use	PS

CS, Case studies; *EMG,* electromyography; *OTC,* over-the-counter; *PS,* prospective studies; *RCT,* randomized clinical trial; *ROM,* range of motion; *RS,* retrospective studies; *SMT,* spinal manipulative therapy; *TP,* trigger point therapy.

10 RCTs are indicated,[101-105,107-111] the remainder being case series, retrospective series, or prospective series.[112-117] These have been amply summarized by five literature reviews,[118-122] four of them systematic.[118-121] Additional basic research[123,124] (see following discussion) describes a possible mechanism of **cervicogenic headache** and provides compelling support for considering chiropractic intervention as a key strategy for the management of headaches. (For detailed definitions of the various classifications of headaches, see Chapter 24).

Published studies have generally classified headaches into three major groups, as recommended by the International Headache Society[125]: (1) tension, (2) cervicogenic, and (3) migraines and unclassified headaches.

Tension Headache

The most dramatic of the trials pertaining to **tension headaches** was the 1995 study by Boline and colleagues.[101] A group of 70 patients who were administered chiropractic health care over a 6-week period displayed parity with a cohort of 56 patients who were administered amitriptyline (a leading medical intervention for headache treatment) over the same period, in terms of four primary outcome measures (i.e., headache frequency, total headache pain, OTC medication use, global health). More significantly, during the 4-week follow-up period, patients undergoing spinal adjustment/manipulation maintained their improvements, whereas medicated patients reverted to baseline values (Fig. 23-4). Of profound importance is the fact that the Boline and colleagues study was rated the highest in quality of all trials compared in the three independent systematic literature reviews mentioned earlier.[118-120]

This prolonged improvement seen with chiropractic patients compared with those under medication is reminiscent of the randomized trials pertaining to low back pain, in which the superior effects of chiropractic intervention were apparent for up to 3 years after treatment, as previously discussed.[42] The enhanced consequences of chiropractic management in the treatment of tension headaches is supported by two other randomized controlled trials,[102,103] although sample sizes were smaller so as to blunt the statistical analyses. High-velocity thrusting did not seem to confer additional benefits on patients given massage and trigger point therapy, as shown in a trial by Bove and Nilsson.[104] Although this particular investigation would suggest that high-velocity thrusting confers no additional benefits for managing tension headache, both groups of patients who had been administered massage (which is commonly included in chiropractic management) showed significant and indistinguishable improvements over baseline values in all the outcome measures observed. The danger of misinterpretation arises when chiropractic health care is equated with only one of its elements—high-velocity adjustment/manipulation.

Cervicogenic Headache

Studies pertaining to the effect of adjustment/manipulation on cervicogenic headache are compelling. In comparing patient groups given either high-velocity cervical spinal adjustment/manipulation or low-level laser treatments as a nontherapeutic control, Nilsson observed improvements of the manipulated group in terms of pain experienced, headache hours per day, and need for less analgesic medication to alleviate discomfort. Statistically significant recoveries in all categories shown in Table 23-5 (analgesic use, frequency, intensity) were obtained with those patients subjected to high-velocity adjustments, although both the control and the experimental groups had been subjected to massage.[105] Nilsson's investigation speaks eloquently to the importance of using large enough groups to achieve statistical significance (an earlier report by Nilsson showed a statistically insignificant tendency toward improvement, because the experimental and control groups of patients were not large enough).[106] A less astute investigator would have become victimized by what is known as a Type II error (i.e., wrongly accepting the null hypothesis and therefore incorrectly concluding that there has been no effect). Other robust responses to adjustment/manipulation were reported elsewhere.[107]

Migraines and Unclassified Headaches

Using a very similar design to that used in Nelson's investigations with tension headache,[101] the clinician observed comparable results in a clinical trial involving patients with **migraine headache.** There was no advantage to combining amitriptyline and spinal adjustment/manipulation for treatment. Clinically important improvements were observed in all 3 study groups over time, but once again during the follow-up period, significant differences emerged—with reductions of the headache index amounting to 24% for the amitriptyline group, 42% for the spinal adjustment/manipulation group, and 25% for the combined group.[108] In comparing adjustment/manipulation to detuned ultrasound for treating migraine patients, Tuchin reported statistically

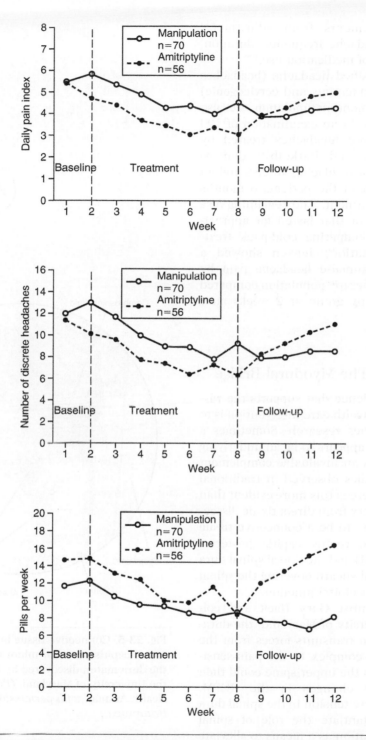

Fig. 23-4 Pain, frequency, and over-the-counter (OTC) medication use of tension headache patients undergoing either spinal manipulation or use of common headache medication (i.e., amitriptyline). *(From Boline P et al: Spinal manipulation vs. amitriptyline for the treatment of chronic tension-type headaches: a randomized clinical trial,* J Manipulative Physiol Ther *18(3):148, 1995.)*

significant improvements from adjustment/manipulation in headache frequency, duration, disability, and level of medication use.[109]

Studies of unclassified headache (headaches other than tension, migraine, and cervicogenic) responses to adjustment/manipulation are also shown in Table 23-5. In an examination of 100 patients with chronic headaches treated by manipulation, Turk and Ratkolb[117] demonstrated an absence of headaches in 25% and an improvement in 40% of the patients 6 months after completing treatment. The remaining 35% reported improvement that lasted for approximately 1 month. Comparing cold-pack treatment with mobilization, Jensen showed a reduction of posttraumatic headache pain by 43% in the manual therapy population compared with the cold therapy group at 2 weeks after treatment.[111]

Basic Research: The Myodural Bridge

Not all research evidence that supports the wisdom of a particular health care intervention is to be found in outcomes research. Sometimes a clarification of what appears to be an underlying mechanism provides an invaluable complement to effectiveness studies observed in traditional clinical trials. Nowhere is this more evident than in the recent discovery from direct tissue dissections of what appears to be a connective tissue bridge between the rectus capitis posterior minor muscle (RCPM) and the dorsal spinal dura (the outer meningeal sheath covering the spinal cord) at the atlantooccipital junction.

According to dentist Gary Hack and colleagues at the University of Maryland, the dura-muscular connection transmits forces from the cervical spine joint complex to the pain-sensitive dura. Trauma to the upper spine could then result in atrophic changes in the RCPM. Consequently, adverse tension in the spinal dura could further substantiate the role of spinal adjustment/manipulation as a means to alleviate this tension and support its effectiveness as a viable treatment for cervicogenic headache. These structural relationships are demonstrated in Fig. 23-5.[126]

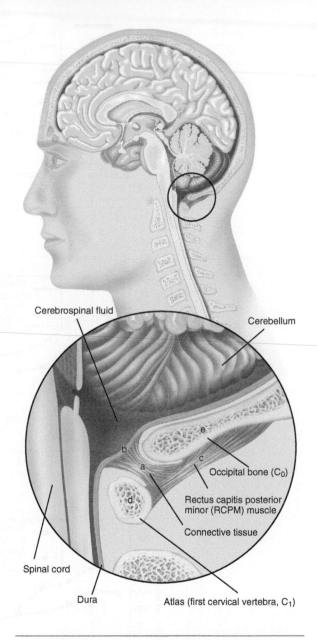

Cerebrospinal fluid

Cerebellum

e

b

a   c

Occipital bone (C_0)

d

Rectus capitis posterior minor (RCPM) muscle

Connective tissue

Spinal cord

Dura

Atlas (first cervical vertebra, C_1)

Fig. 23-5 Connective tissue bridge between the rectus capitis posterior minor (RCPM) muscle and the dura mater, discovered by Hack and colleagues at the University of Maryland. *(From 1998* Medical and Health Annual, *with permission from Encyclopedia Britannica.)*

Support for this model is shown in a parallel study in which 31 out of 39 consecutive patients who underwent plastic surgical forehead rejuvenation procedures encompassing resection of the corrugator supercilli muscle displayed total elimination or improvement of migraine headache, with improvements lasting at least 47 months.[124] Thus it is quite possible that various types of headache are at least in part triggered by tension of various muscular bridges, the relaxation of which (presumably by spinal adjustment/manipulation) could bring about substantial relief from the original complaint.

The Duke Headache Evidence Report

To verify the clinical outcomes evidence supporting spinal manipulation and a variety of other physical and behavioral interventions in the management of headache, in 1994 the **Agency for Health Care Policy and Research** (AHCPR) began a process of systematic review of the literature that was essentially identical to the review completed with the release of guidelines pertaining to low back pain, as discussed earlier.[2] Unfortunately, funding cuts to the agency caused this process to be aborted after the headache literature review had begun, and the work of the multidisciplinary committee charged with performing the literature evaluation and developing ratings of the evidence was ultimately shipped to the Duke Center for Health Policy Research and Education for safekeeping.

The Foundation for Chiropractic Education, with funds from the National Chiropractic Mutual Insurance Company, then funded an updated systematic literature review of tension and cervicogenic headache, taking into account the rapid proliferation of new literature and combining this with the work of the disbanded AHCPR headache committee. The staff at the Duke Center screened citations from the literature, abstracted the data into evidence tables, analyzed the quality and magnitude of results from these studies, and drafted an evidence report with peer review from a broad, multidisciplinary panel of 19 health care experts.

Starting with over 2500 citations from such databases as MEDLINE, MANTIS, CRAC, CINAHL, PsychoINFO, the Cochrane Controlled Trials Register, and additional articles, the panel obtained bibliographies of both physical and behavioral options for treating headache. These were either prospective studies or controlled trials, aimed at either relief from or prevention of tension-type or cervicogenic headache.

Among the physical interventions reviewed in this report were cervical spine manipulation; low-force techniques, such as cranial sacral therapy and massage (including trigger point release); mobilization; stretching; heat therapy; ultrasound; **transcutaneous electrical nerve stimulation** (TENS); surgery; and exercise (including those that are postural). Among the behavioral interventions reviewed were relaxation, biofeedback, cognitive-behavioral (stress management) therapy, and hypnosis.

The final report, which recognized the chiropractic research headache literature cited earlier,* was significant in that it concluded that nonpharmacologic treatments (including adjustment/manipulation) are of growing importance and, "if effective and available . . . [they] may be the first choice for most patients." Furthermore, it indicated that drug treatments are not suitable for all patients, may produce undesired side effects, and are not universally effective.[127] The high credibility of this document lay in the facts that Duke University is one of 12 research centers given trademark status by the U.S. Department of Health and Human Services, the 19-member interdisciplinary panel that performed the literature review was of extremely high caliber; and the evidence review was comprehensive, encompassing all behavioral and physical treatments for both tension and cervicogenic type headaches.

REPETITIVE STRESS DISORDERS RESEARCH

Adjustment/manipulation of the musculoskeletal system for treatment of pain and reduced motion is not limited to the back or neck. Over the past decade the extremities (most commonly the wrists) have become increasingly

*References: 101, 103-106, 118, 119, 122.

recognized as an area responsive to manual therapy. Compression of the median nerve within the vicinity of the wrist may lead to unilateral or bilateral paresthesia in the fingers, with or without pain in the wrist, palm, or forearm (or a combination) proximal to the area of compression. This condition, known as *carpal tunnel syndrome* (CTS), presents a variety of symptoms and is commonly confused with tendonitis. One of its major causes is the protracted strain on an extended or flexed wrist caused by repetitive stress, often found in the workplace and therefore having the potential to affect a significant population.

The rationale for adjustment/manipulation is to take pressure off the transverse carpal ligament and add adjustments of the lunate to help decompress the tunnel. It represents a departure from traditional spinal adjustment; in its application to the extremities instead, it provides a conservative, noninvasive alternative to surgery.[128,129]

Although few in number at the present, the RCTs addressing the extremities shown in Table 23-6 offer encouragement in that discrete improvements in all outcome measures shown

(physical and mental distress scores, nerve conduction, vibrometry, and pain scores) in patients compared with their initial conditions are noted in all groups undergoing manipulative therapy.[130,131] Their improvements are comparable to those achieved by the other interventions shown; in two of the three trials listed, manipulative therapy displayed the potential to accelerate improvement in certain groups of patients,[131,132] although corticosteroid injections produced more rapid improvements in patients with diagnosed disorders in synovial structures as opposed to functional disorders of the cervical spine, upper thoracic spine, or the upper ribs (i.e., the shoulder girdle).[131]

Case control studies supporting chiropractic intervention in the management of CTS suggest that, in 38 subjects, a broad array of dietary, exercise, and manipulative interventions result in statistically significant improvements in several strength measures of up to 25% over pretreatment values[133]; improved objective pain and distress levels were observed in 22 returning subjects and persisted for at least 6 months after treatment.[134]

Osteopathic manipulation has also been shown to be effective in two case series studies by

Table **23-6** SUMMARY OF LEADING CLINICAL TRIALS INVOLVING REPETITIVE STRESS DISORDERS AND SPINAL MANIPULATION

Author	Branches	No of Subjects	Complaint	Outcomes	Follow-Up
Davis[130]	SMT, splints	45	CTS	Physical or mental distress	9 weeks- 1 month
	Ibuprofen, splints	46		NCS Vibrometry	
Winters[131]	SMT	29	Shoulder pain (girdle)	Pain scores	11 weeks
	PT	29	Shoulder pain (synovial)		
	SMT	32			
	PT	35			
	Corticosteroid injection	47			
Strait[132]	TCT, OMT	13	CTS	EMG, NCS	2 months
	TCT	10			

CTS, Carpal tunnel syndrome; *EMG,* electromyography; *NCS,* nerve conduction studies; *OMT,* osteopathic manipulative therapy; *PT,* physiotherapy; *SMT,* spinal manipulative therapy; *TCT,* traditional conservative therapy.

Benjamin Sucher. The first, involving four patients with CTS, showed both clinical improvement and changes in MRI imaging that revealed that the anteroposterior and transverse dimensions of the carpal canal increased significantly after treatment. Electromyography/nerve conduction studies (EMG/NCS) measurements documented electrical improvement consistent with the clinical recovery.[135] Both clinical and electrical improvement were subsequently observed in a larger group of 16 patients with CTS.[136]

The research described for this condition is only in its preliminary stages. However, in light of the fact that CTS occurs on an epidemic scale in the workplace, with a tenfold increase in the number of lost-time cases between 1981 and 1991[137] because of this condition, health care professionals licensed and authorized to administer adjustment/manipulation should consider it to be a significant problem of critical importance (see Chapter 18).

COST-EFFECTIVENESS

An essential part of evaluating the future of any health care modality is its cost. Comparisons of the costs encountered in medical or chiropractic treatment for low back pain are common in the literature. They generally fall into one of three categories: (1) retrospective analyses of data from workers' compensation claims, (2) comparative costs obtained from the data of insurers, and (3) evaluations of the existing literature by economists. None have addressed chronic conditions per se, although one needs to recall from the introduction of this report that conditions believed to be acute and self-limiting have the strong potential to become chronic.[138] As clinicians witness the rapid rise of managed care in the United States, the issue of management costs of chronic conditions (including headache and back pain) has become one of primary importance.

Workers' Compensation Data

Representative data from compensation studies within four states are summarized in Table 23-7.[139-144] From all these findings in which there has been an attempt to match diagnoses for, if not actual severity of, disabling conditions of patients in doctors of medicine (MD) and doctors of chiropractic (DC) provider groups, a number of trends are evident:

- Days lost from work by chiropractic patients are fewer than those of patients under the care of an MD;
- Costs from compensation pools are less for chiropractic patients (as much as tenfold less in Utah[139]);
- Costs of health care expenses monitored for chiropractic patients are usually lower by a substantial margin;
- Costs per visit for chiropractic patients as compared with medical patients are lower; and
- Lengths of treatment vary.

Databases from Insurers

Insurance companies often use larger databases, which are less prone to possible skewing by regional workers' compensation data. A nationwide longitudinal survey of medical care usage and costs from 6000 randomly selected households displayed a significant cost savings for chiropractic.[145] The best design elements for providing clear episode definitions and matching severity between chiropractic and medical patients, however, have been provided by the studies of Stano and Smith.[146-148]

A key conceptual breakthrough launching Stano's research is the "bundling" of the full costs of episodes (i.e., the careful inclusion of all relevant treatment costs, not solely the costs of out-patient doctor visits) associated with either the medical or chiropractic care of patients. This was first accomplished by assigning one or more commonly used **International Classification of Disease** (ICD) **codes** to patients initially complaining of those conditions, from a total cohort of 43,476. Stano's program tracked various categories of total inpatient and outpatient payments over each episode, factoring in key patient demographic and insurance characteristics and case mix severity differences. The final cost comparisons were run in a total of 6799 patients out of a total database of over 400,000. Stano's conclusions were

Table **23-7**   Cost Comparison Analysis from Representative American States: Chiropractic versus Medical Care for Work-Related Injuries

Determinant	Utah, 1991[139]	Oregon, 1991[140-142]	Iowa, 1989[143]	Florida, 1988[144]
Similar diagnoses in patient population	ICD9 codes back only	Categories of injury, back only	Strain or sprain, back only	DRG, medical back diagnosis
Number of days lost from work (comp time)*				
DC	2.4	—	11.76	39.00
MD	20.7	—	14.08	58.00
Cost from compensation*				
DC	$68.38	—	$263.00	
MD	688.39	—	627.00	
Cost of health care expenses				
DC	$526.80	$1712.00	$222.70	$1204.00
MD	684.15	1112.00	351.90	2352.00
Cost per visit*				
DC	$40.00	$41.70	—	—
MD	133.00	111.20	—	—
Length of treatment				
DC	34.3 days	53 weeks	—	—
MD	54.5 days	19 weeks	—	—

*Represents average number per episode.

straightforward and dramatic. When all episodes of care are considered, the mean total costs are $1000 for each medical episode and $493 per chiropractic episode.[148]

Follow-up studies indicated lower costs in cases where chiropractors served as first-contact providers. Together with favorable satisfaction and quality indicators, these data suggest that chiropractors should receive careful consideration for gatekeeper status by employers and third-party payers to control health care spending.[146] In the analysis of multiple episodes, patients who move among provider groups are more likely to return to chiropractic rather than medical providers. Because this suggests that chronic patients may gravitate to chiropractic care over time, the role of the chiropractor in managing chronic low back pain as a primary provider should not be underestimated.[146]

In contrast are two recent studies, which suggest that chiropractic services are more, rather than less, expensive for medical treatments for low back conditions.[149,150] However, these two reports are fraught with weaknesses that have been addressed elsewhere by this author.[151] Seven of these weaknesses are (1) the effects of severity of illness are virtually ignored; (2) the degree of recovery does not receive adequate attention; (3) matching of services with provider type may be irregular; (4) compliance has been disregarded; (5) types of medications and their side effects are not specified; (6) medical expenses are capped by managed care, whereas those of chiropractors are allowed to seek free market levels; and (7) episodes are poorly defined or poorly contained. These shortcomings all illustrate the complexity with which meaningful, actual cost analyses must be constructed; otherwise, the types of data obtained in Table 23-5 or elsewhere[149,150] are subject to misinterpretation.

An Economist's Evaluation of Existing Literature

Pran Manga, an economist at the University of Ottawa, has been twice commissioned by the Provincial Government of Ontario to assess the effectiveness and cost-effectiveness of chiropractic management of low back pain. After assessing the comparative cost data in a first report, Manga reached the following conclusion:

There is an overwhelming body of evidence indicating that chiropractic management of low back pain is more cost-effective than medical management. We reviewed numerous studies that range from very persuasive to convincing in support of this conclusion. The lack of any convincing argument or evidence to the contrary must be noted and is significant to us in forming our conclusions and recommendations.[3]

The cost advantages for chiropractic for matched conditions appear to be so dramatic that Manga, in a second report, concluded that doubling the use of chiropractic services from 10% to 20% may realize savings as much as $770 million annually in direct costs and $3.8 billion in indirect costs. Four out of five patients of chiropractors have endured their problems for more than 6 months, typically undergoing medical care, physiotherapy, or both before consulting the chiropractor.[152]

To date, no cost studies have reviewed **iatrogenic** effects (i.e., adverse consequences of health care interventions) or calculated legal burdens, which would be expected to be heavily advantageous for chiropractic care compared with the medical alternative. Because neuromuscular disorders cause a disproportionate amount of chronic illness and disability, their effective and efficient management by chiropractic intervention clearly points toward a strategy of health care cost containment, which is likely to be aided by affording the chiropractor first-contact privileges in the provision of quality health care.

Review *Questions*

1. What were the major events in chiropractic research before 1950?
2. What is the significance of the 1975 Conference on Research sponsored by the NINCDS?
3. What is the difference between a clinical trial and a prospective study?
4. What is the difference between the appropriateness and utilization portions of the recent study on back pain by the RAND Corporation?
5. What were the strengths and weaknesses of the randomized clinical trials involving a chiropractic component cited by Koes?
6. What were the accomplishments of the Quebec Task Force, and what were its weaknesses as discussed by Croft?
7. Why is disk herniation unlikely to be caused by rotational manipulation?
8. From a morphologic point of view, immobilization of the neck after soft tissue trauma accompanying whiplash-associated disorders is indefensible. Why?
9. What is the incidence of cerebrovascular accidents, and what is their mechanism?
10. Name at least three major classes of headache as defined by the International Headache Society.

Concept *Questions*

1. What are the limitations of the randomized clinical trial, and what types of research offer data that help to answer these deficiencies?
2. What are the weaknesses of the two studies cited that suggest that chiropractic interventions are more, rather than less, expensive for medical treatments for back conditions.

REFERENCES

1. Goldstein M, editor: *The research status of spinal manipulation*, Monograph No 15, Washington, DC, 1975, US Department of Health, Education, & Welfare.
2. Bigos S et al: *Clinical practice guideline No 14—acute lower back pain in adults*, AHCPR Pub No 95-0642, Rockville, Md, 1994, Agency for Health Care

Policy and Research, Public Health Service, US Department of Health and Human Services.

3. Manga P et al: *The effectiveness and cost-effectiveness of chiropractic management of low-back pain*, Richmond Hill, Canada, 1993, Kenilworth.

4. Rosen M: *Back pain: report of a clinical standards advisory group committee on back pain*, London, 1994, HMSO.

5. Commission on Alternative Medicine, Social Departementete: *Legitimization for vissa kiropraktorer*, Stockholm, 12:13, 1987.

6. Danish Institute for Health Technology Assessment: Low-back pain, frequency, management, and prevention from an HTA perspective, *Danish Health Tech Assess* 1(1), 1999.

7. Thompson CJ: *Second report, Medicare benefits review committee*, Canberra, 1986, Commonwealth Government Printer.

8. Hasselberg PD: *Chiropractic in New Zealand: report of a commission of inquiry*, Wellington, NZ, 1979, Government Printer.

9. Micozzi MS: Complementary care: when is it appropriate? *Ann Intern Med* 129:65, 1998.

10. Wardwell WI: *Chiropractic: history and evolution of a new profession*, St Louis, 1992, Mosby.

11. Bernard C: *An introduction to the study of experimental medicine*, New York, 1927, Macmillan. (Translated by HC Greene.)

12. Fishbein M: *The medical follies*, New York, 1925, Boni & Liveright.

13. Canterbury R, Krakos G: Thirteen years after Roentgen: the originals of chiropractic radiology, *Chiropr Hist* 6:25, 1986.

14. Dye AA: *The evolution of chiropractic: its discovery and development*, Philadelphia, 1939, AA Dye.

15. Thompson EA: *Text on chiropractic spinography*, Davenport, Iowa, 1919, Palmer School of Chiropractic.

16. Crowe HE: *Injuries to the cervical spine*. San Francisco, 1928, paper presented at the meeting of the Western Orthopedic Association.

17. Foreman SM, Croft AC: *Whiplash injuries: the cervical acceleration/deceleration syndrome*, ed 2, Baltimore, 1995, Williams & Wilkins.

18. Spitzer WO et al: Scientific monograph of the Quebec Task Force on whiplash-associated disorders: refining "whiplash" and its management, *Spine* 20(8S):1S, 1995.

19. Illi FWH: *The vertebral column, life line of the body*, Chicago, 1951, National College of Chiropractic.

20. Smith OG, Langworthy SM, Paxon M: *Modernized chiropractic*, Cedar Rapids, 1906, Solon M Langworthy.

21. Gillet H: Clinical measurements of sacro-iliac mobility, *Ann Swiss Chiropr Assoc* 6:59, 1976.

22. Gillet H: Spinal and related fixations, *Dig Chiropr Econ* 1:25 (summary lesson), 2:22 and 3:26 (lessons), 1964.

23. Goldstein M: Foreword. In Korr IM: *The neurobiologic mechanisms in manipulative therapy*, New York, 1978, Plenum.

24. *Report of the US Preventive Services Task Force*, Baltimore, 1989, Williams & Wilkins.

25. Shekelle PG et al: Spinal manipulation for low-back pain, *Ann Intern Med* 117:590, 1992.

26. Bronfort G: *Efficacy of manual therapies of the spine*, Amsterdam, 1997, Thesis Publishers.

27. Jayson MIV: A limited role for manipulation, *BMJ* 293:1454, 1986.

28. Hadler NM et al: A benefit of spinal manipulation as adjunctive therapy for acute low-back pain: a stratified controlled trial, *Spine* 12:702, 1987.

29. Glover JR, Morris JG, Khosla T: Back pain. A randomized clinical trial of rotational manipulation of the trunk, *Br J Ind Med* 31:59, 1974.

30. Matthews JA et al: Back pain and sciatica: controlled trials, traction, sclerosant and epidural injections, *Br J Rheumatol* 26(6):416, 1987.

31. MacDonald RS, Bell CM: An open controlled assessment of osteopathic manipulation in nonspecific low-back pain, *Spine* 15:364, 1990.

32. Farrell JP, Twomey LT: Acute low back pain. Comparison of two conservative treatment approaches, *Med J Aust* 1:160, 1982.

33. Koes BW et al: The effectiveness of manual therapy, physiotherapy, and treatment by the general practitioner for nonspecific neck and back complaints: a randomized clinical trial, *Spine* 17(1):28, 1992.

34. Koes BW et al: Randomized clinical trial of manipulative therapy and physiotherapy for persistent back and neck complaints: results of one year follow up, *BMJ* 304:601, 1992.

35. Pope MH et al: A prospective randomized three-week trial of spinal manipulation, transcutaneous muscle stimulation, massage and corset in the treatment of subacute low back pain, *Spine* 19:2571, 1994.

36. Waagen GN et al: Short term trial of chiropractic adjustments for the relief of chronic low back pain, *Man Med* 2:63, 1986.

37. Coxhead CE et al: Multicentre trial of physiotherapy in the management of sciatic symptoms, *Lancet* 1:1065, 1981.

38. Triano JJ et al: Manipulative therapy versus education programs in chronic low back pain, *Spine* 20:948, 1995.

39. Giles LGF, Muller R: Chronic spinal pain syndrome: a clinical pilot trial comparing acupuncture, a nonsteroidal anti-inflammatory drug, and spinal manipulation, *J Manipulative Physiol Ther* 22(6):376, 1999.

40. Andersson GBJ et al: A comparison of osteopathic spinal manipulation with standard care for patients with low back pain, *N Engl J Med* 341(19):1426, 1999.

41. Skargren EI et al: Cost and effectiveness analysis of chiropractic and physiotherapy treatment for low back and neck pain, *Spine* 22:2167, 1997.

42. Meade TW et al: Low back pain of mechanical origin: randomized comparison of chiropractic and hospital outpatient treatment, *BMJ* 300:1431, 1990.

43. Meade TW et al: Randomized comparison of chiropractic and hospital outpatient management for low back pain: results from extended follow-up, *BMJ* 311:349, 1995.

44. Bronfort G: Chiropractic versus general medical treatment of low back pain: a small scale controlled clinical trial, *Am J Chiropr Med* 2:145, 1989.

45. Zylbergold RS, Piper MC: Lumbar disc disease: comparative analysis of physical therapy treatments, *Arch Phys Med Rehabil* 62:176, 1981.

46. Doran DM, Newell DJ: Manipulation in the treatment of low back pain: a multicentre study, *BMJ* 2(5964):161, 1975.

47. Hoehler FK, Tobis JS, Buerger AA: Spinal manipulation for low back pain, *J Am Med Assoc* 245:1835, 1981.

48. Cherkin DC et al: Comparison of physical therapy, chiropractic manipulation, and provision of an educational booklet for the treatment of patients with low back pain, *N Engl J Med* 339(14):1021, 1998.

49. Kirkaldy-Willis WH, Cassidy JD: Spinal manipulation in the treatment of low back pain, *Can Fam Physician* 31:535, 1985.

50. Hayllar J, Macpherson A, Bjarnason I: Gastro protection and nonsteroidal anti-inflammatory drugs (NSAIDs): rationale and clinical implications, *Drug Saf* 7(2):86, 1992.

51. Silverstein FE et al: Gastrointestinal toxicity with celecoxib vs nonsteroidal anti-inflammatory drugs for osteoarthritis and rheumatoid arthritis, *J Am Med Assoc* 284(10): 1247, 2000.

52. Shekelle PG et al: *The appropriateness of spinal manipulation for low back pain: project overview and literature review,* monograph no R-4025/1-CCR/FCER, Santa Monica, 1991, RAND.

53. Shekelle PG et al: *The appropriateness of spinal manipulation for low back pain: project overview and literature review,* monograph no R-4025/2-CCR/FCER, Santa Monica, 1991, RAND.

54. Shekelle PG et al: *The appropriateness of spinal manipulation for low back pain: indications and ratings by an all-chiropractic expert panel,* monograph no R-4025/3-CCR/FCER, Santa Monica, 1992, RAND.

55. Shekelle PG et al: The appropriateness of chiropractic spinal manipulation for low back pain: a pilot study, *J Manipulative Physiol Ther* 18(5):265, 1995.

56. Anderson R et al: A meta-analysis of clinical trials of spinal manipulation, *J Manipulative Physiol Ther* 15(3):181, 1992.

57. Sanders GE et al: Chiropractic adjustive manipulation on subjects with acute low-back pain: visual analog scores and plasma beta-endorphin levels, *J Manipulative Physiol Ther* 13:391, 1990.

58. van Tulder MW, Koes BW, Bouter LM: Conservative treatment of acute and chronic nonspecific low back pain: a systematic review of randomized controlled trials of the most common interventions, *Spine* 22(18):2128, 1997.

59. Juni P et al: The hazards of scoring the quality of clinical trials for meta-analysis, *J Am Med Assoc* 282(11):1054, 1999.

60. Koes BW, Bouter LM, van der Jeijden GJMG: Methodological quality of randomized clinical trials on treatment efficacy in low back pain, *Spine* 20:228, 1995.

61. Assendelft WJJ et al: The relationship between methodological quality and conclusions in reviews of spinal manipulation, *J Am Med Assoc* 274(24):1942, 1995.

62. Kirkaldy-Willis WH, Cassidy JD: Manipulation. In Kirkaldy-Willis WH, editor: *Managing low-back pain,* New York, 1988, Churchill Livingstone.

63. Nwuga VCB: Relative therapeutic efficacy of vertebral manipulation and conventional treatment in back pain management, *Am J Phys Med* 61(6):273, 1982.

64. Burton AK, Tillotson KM, Cleary J: Single-blind randomized controlled trial of chemonucleolysis and manipulation in the treatment of symptomatic lumbar disc herniation, *Eur Spine J* 9:202, 2000.

65. Henderson RS: The treatment of lumbar disk intervertebral disk protrusion: an assessment of conservative measures, *BMJ* 2:597, 1952.

66. Mensor MC: Non-operative treatment, including manipulation, for lumbar intervertebral disc syndrome, *J Bone Joint Surg Am* 37:925, 1955

67. Chrisman OD: A study of the results following rotary manipulation in the lumbar intervertebral disc syndrome, *J Bone Joint Surg Am* 46:517, 1964.

68. Kuo PP-F, Loh Z-C: Treatment of lumbar intervertebral disc protrusions by manipulation, *Clin Orthop* 215:47, 1987.

69. d'Ornano J et al: Effets des manipulations vertebrales sur la hernie discale lombaire, *Rev Med Orthop* 19:21, 1990.

70. Cassidy JD, Thiel HW, Kirkaldy-Willis KW: Side posture manipulation for lumbar disc herniation, *J Manipulative Physiol Ther* 16(2):96, 1993.

71. Farfan HF et al: The effects of torsion on the lumbar intervertebral joints: the role of torsion in the production of disc degeneration, *J Bone Joint Surg Am* 52:468, 1970.

72. Adams MA, Hutton WC: Mechanics of the intervertebral disc. In Ghosh P, editor: *The biology of the intervertebral disc,* vol 2, Boca Raton, 1988, CRC Press.

73. Coulter I et al: *The appropriateness of spinal manipulation and mobilization of the cervical spine: literature review, indications and ratings by a multidisciplinary expert panel,* monograph no DRU-982-1-CCR, Santa Monica, 1995, RAND.

74. Koes BW et al: A randomised clinical trial of manual therapy and physiotherapy for persistent back and neck complaints: subgroup analysis and relationship between outcome measures, *J Manipulative Physiol Ther* 16(4):211, 1993.

75. Cassidy JD, Lopes AA, Yong-Hing K: The immediate effect of manipulation versus mobilization on pain and range of motion in the cervical spine: a randomized

controlled trial, *J Manipulative Physiol Ther* 15(9): 570, 1992.

76. Coulter I et al: The use of expert panel results: the RAND panel for appropriateness of manipulation and mobilization of the cervical spine, *Top Clin Chiropr* 2(3):54, 1995.

77. Koes BW et al: A blinded randomized clinical trial of manual therapy and physiotherapy for chronic back and neck complaints: physical outcome measures, *J Manipulative Physiol Ther* 15(1):16, 1992.

78. Sloop PR et al: Manipulation for chronic neck pain. A double-blind controlled study, *Spine* 7:532, 1982.

79. Rogers RG: The effects of spinal manipulation on cervical kinesthesia in patients with chronic neck pain: a pilot study, *J Manipulative Physiol Ther* 20(2):80, 1997.

80. Jordan A et al: Intensive training, physiotherapy, or manipulation for patients with chronic neck pain: a prospective, single-blinded, randomized clinical trial, *Spine* 23(3):311, 1998.

81. van Schalkwyk R, Parkin-Smith GF: A clinical trial investigating the possible effect of supine cervical rotatory manipulation and the supine lateral break manipulation in the treatment of mechanical neck pain: a pilot study, *J Manipulative Physiol Ther* 23(5):324, 2000.

82. McMorland G, Suter E: Chiropractic management of mechanical neck and low-back pain: a retrospective, outcome-based analysis, *J Manipulative Physiol Ther* 23(5):307, 2000.

83. Foreman SM, Croft AC: *Whiplash injuries: the cervical acceleration/deceleration syndrome,* ed 2, Baltimore, 1995, Williams & Wilkins.

84. Girard N: *Statistiques descriptives dur la nature des blessures. Quebec. Regie de l'assurance automobile du Quebec. Direction des services medicaux et de la readaption.* Internal document, Quebec, 1989.

85. Giroux M: *Les blessures a la colonne cervicale. Importance du probleme.* Paper presented at Le Medicin du Quebec, Montreal, September 22-26, 1991.

86. Spitzer WO et al: Scientific monograph of the Quebec Taskforce on Whiplash Associated Disorders: redefining "whiplash" and its management, *Spine* 20:1S, 1995.

87. Bannister G, Gargan M: Prognosis of whiplash injuries: a review of the literature, *Spine* 7:557, 1993.

88. Croft AC: A proposed classification of cervical acceleration-deceleration [CAD] injuries with a review of prognostic research, *Palmer J Res* 1(1):10, 1994.

89. Jonsson H et al: Hidden cervical spine injuries in traffic accident victims with skull fractures, *J Spinal Disord* 4(3):251, 1991.

90. Akeson WH et al: Collagen cross-linking alterations in joint contractures. Changes in the reducible cross-links in periarticular connective tissue after nine weeks of immobilization, *Connect Tissue Res* 5:15, 1977.

91. Frank C et al: Medical collateral ligament healing—a multidisciplinary assessment in rabbits, *Am J Sports Med* 11:379, 1983.

92. Long ML et al: The effects of motion on normal healing ligaments, *Proc Orthop Res Soc* 7:43, 1982 (abstract).

93. Fronek J et al: The effects of intermittent passive movement [IPM] in the healing of medical collateral ligament, *Proc Orthop Res Soc* 8:31, 1983 (abstract).

94. Gelberman RH et al: Flexor tendon repair, *J Orthop Res* 4:119, 1986.

95. Crock H: *Low back surgery.* Paper presented at the International Chiropractic Conference, London, September 1987.

96. Baker D: Development and regeneration of mammalian muscle spindles, *Sci Prog* 69:64, 1984.

97. Nansel D et al: Time course considerations for the effects of unilateral lower cervical adjustments with respect to the amelioration of cervical lateral-flexion passive end-range asymmetry, *J Manipulative Physiol Ther* 13(6):297, 1990.

98. Khan S et al: A symptomatic classification of whiplash injury and the implications for treatment, *J Orthop Med* 21(1):22, 1999.

99. Freeman MD, Croft AC, Rossignol AM: Whiplash-associated disorders: redefining whiplash and its management, *Spine* 23(9):1043, 1998.

100. Chapman-Smith D: Redefining whiplash and its management, *Chiropr Report* 9:1, 1995.

101. Boline P et al: Spinal manipulation vs. amitriptyline for the treatment of chronic tension-type headaches: a randomized clinical trial, *J Manipulative Physiol Ther* 18(3):148, 1995.

102. Bitterli J et al: Zur objektivierung der manualtherapeutischen beeinflussbarket des spondylogenen korpschemerzes (objective criteria for the evaluation of chiropractic treatment of spondylotic headache), *Nervenarzt* 48(5):159, 1977.

103. Hoyt WH et al: Osteopathic manipulation in the treatment of muscle-contraction headache, *J Am Osteopath Assoc* 78:322, 1979.

104. Bove G, Nilsson N: Spinal manipulation in the treatment of episodic tension-type headache, *J Am Med Assoc* 280(18):1576, 1998.

105. Nilsson N: A randomized controlled trial of the effect of spinal manipulation in the treatment of cervicogenic headache, *J Manipulative Physiol Ther* 18(7):435, 1995.

106. Nilsson N, Christensen HW, Hartvigsen J: The effect of spinal manipulation in the treatment of cervicogenic headache, *J Manipulative Physiol Ther* 29(5):326, 1997.

107. Whittingham W: Randomized placebo controlled clinical trial of efficacy of chiropractic treatment for chronic cervicogenic headaches, *Symposium Proceedings*, 6th Biennial Congress, World Federation of Chiropractic, Paris, May 21-26, 2001.

108. Nelson CF et al: The efficacy of spinal manipulation, amitriptyline and the combination of both therapies in the prophylaxis of migraine headache, *J Manipulative Physiol Ther* 21(8):511, 1998.

109. Tuchin PJ, Pollard H, Bonello R: A randomized controlled trial of chiropractic spinal manipulative therapy for migraine, *J Manipulative Physiol Ther* 23(2):91, 2000.

110. Parker G, Tupling H, Pryor D: A controlled trial of cervical manipulation for migraine, *Aust N Z J Med* 8:589, 1978.

111. Jensen IK, Nielsen FF, Vosmar L: An open study comparing manual therapy with the use of cold packs in the treatment of post-traumatic headache, *Cephalalgia* 10:243, 1990.

112. Mootz RD et al: Chiropractic treatment of chronic episodic tension-type headache in male subjects: a case series analysis, *J Can Chiropr Assoc* 38(3):152, 1994.

113. Droz JM, Crot F: Occipital headaches: statistical results in the treatment of vertebrogenic headache, *Ann Swiss Chiropr Assoc* 8:127, 1985.

114. Vernon HT: Spinal manipulation and headaches of cervical origin, *J Manipulative Physiol Ther* 5(3):109, 1982.

115. Wight JS: Migraine: a statistical analysis of chiropractic treatment, *Chiropr J* 12:363, 1978.

116. Stodolny J, Chmielewski H: Manual therapy in the treatment of patients with cervical migraine, *Manual Med* 4:49, 1989.

117. Turk Z, Ratkolb O: Mobilization of the cervical spine in chronic headaches, *Man Med* 3:15, 1987.

118. Hurwitz EL et al: Manipulation and mobilization of the cervical spine: a systematic review of the literature, *Spine* 21(15):1746, 1996.

119. Kjellman GV, Skargren EI, Oberg BE: A critical analysis of randomised clinical trials on neck pain and treatment efficacy: a review of the literature, *Scand J Rehabil Med* 31: 139, 1999.

120. Bronfort G et al: Efficacy of spinal manipulation for chronic headaches: a systematic review, *J Manipulative Physiol Ther* 24(7):457, 2001.

121. Vernon H: The effectiveness of chiropractic manipulation in the treatment of headache: an exploration of the literature, *J Manipulative Physiol Ther* 18(9):611, 1995.

122. Vernon H, McDermaid CS, Hagino C: Systematic review of randomized clinical trials of complementary/alternative therapies in the treatment of tension-type and cervicogenic headache, *Complement Ther Med* 7:142, 1999.

123. Hack GD et al: Anatomic relation between the rectus capitis posterior minor muscle and the dura mater, *Spine* 20:2484, 1995.

124. Gayuron B et al: Corrugator supercilli muscle reaction and migraine headaches, *Plast Reconstr Surg* 106:429, 2000.

125. International Headache Society: Classification and diagnostic criteria for headache disorders, cranial neuralgias and facial pain, *Cephalalgia* 8(suppl 7):1, 1988.

126. Hack G, Dunn G, Toh MY: The anatomist's new tools. In *The 1998 medical and health annual*, Chicago, 1997, Encyclopedia Britannica.

127. McCrory DC et al: *Evidence report: behavior and physical treatments for tension-type and cervicogenic headaches*, Des Moines, 2001, Foundation for Chiropractic Education and Research.

128. Karpen M: Treating carpal tunnel syndrome, *Altern Complement Ther* 1(5):284, 1995.

129. Davis PT, Hulbert JR: Carpal tunnel syndrome: conservative and nonconservative treatment: a chiropractic physician's perspective, *J Manipulative Physiol Ther* 21(5):356, 1998.

130. Davis PT et al: Comparative efficacy of conservative medical and chiropractic treatments for carpal tunnel syndrome: a randomized clinical trial, *J Manipulative Physiol Ther* 21(5):317, 1998.

131. Winters JC et al: Comparison of physiotherapy, manipulation, and corticosteroid injection for treating shoulder complaints in general practice: randomised, single blind study, *BMJ* 314:1320, 1997.

132. Strait BW, Kuchera ML: Osteopathic manipulation for patients with confirmed mild, modest, and moderate carpal tunnel syndrome, *J Am Osteopath Assoc* 94(8):673, 1994.

133. Bonebrake AR et al: A treatment for carpal tunnel syndrome: evaluation of objective and subjective measures, *J Manipulative Physiol Ther* 13(9):507, 1991.

134. Bonebrake AR et al: A treatment for carpal tunnel syndrome: results of a follow-up study, *J Manipulative Physiol Ther* 16(3):125, 1993.

135. Sucher BM: Myofascial manipulative release of carpal tunnel syndrome. Documentation with magnetic resonance imaging, *J Am Osteopath Assoc* 93(12):1273, 1993.

136. Sucher BM: Palpatory diagnosis and manipulative management of carpal tunnel syndrome, *J Am Osteopath Assoc* 94(8):647, 1994.

137. Webster BS, Snook SH: The cost of compensable upper extremity cumulative trauma disorders, *J Occup Med* 36:713, 1994.

138. Croft PR et al: Outcome of low back pain in general practice: a prospective study, *BMJ* 316:1356, 1998.

139. Jarvis KB, Phillips RB, Morris EK: Cost per case comparison of back injury claims of chiropractic versus medical management for conditions with identical diagnostic codes, *J Occup Med* 33(8):847, 1991.

140. Nyiendo J, Lamm L: Disability low back Oregon workers' compensation of claims. I. Methodology and clinical categorization of chiropractic and medical cases, *J Manipulative Physiol Ther* 14(3):177, 1991.

141. Nyiendo J: Disability low back Oregon workers' compensation of claims. II. Time loss, *J Manipulative Physiol Ther* 14(4):231, 1991.

142. Nyiendo J: Disability low back Oregon workers' compensation of claims. III. Diagnostic and treatment procedures and associated costs, *J Manipulative Physiol Ther* 14(5):287, 1991.

143. Johnson MR: A comparison of chiropractic, medical and osteopathic care for work-related sprains/strains, *J Manipulative Physiol Ther* 12(5):335, 1989.

144. Wolk S: An analysis of Florida workers' compensation medical claims for back-related injuries, *J Am Chiropr Assoc* 27(7):50, 1988.

145. Dean H, Schmidt R: *A comparison of the cost of chiropractors versus alternative medical practitioners,* Richmond, 1992, Virginia Chiropractic Association.

146. Stano M, Smith M: Chiropractic and medical costs of low back care, *Med Care* 34(3):191, 1996.

147. Smith M, Stano M: Costs and recurrences of chiropractic and medical episodes of low-back care, *J Manipulative Physiol Ther* 20(1):5, 1997.

148. Stano M: The economic role of chiropractic: further analysis of relative insurance costs for low back care, *J Neuromuscloskel Sys* 3(3):139, 1995.

149. Carey TS et al: North Carolina Back Pain Project. The outcomes and costs of care for acute low back pain among patients seen by primary care practitioners, chiropractors, and orthopedic surgeons, *N Engl J Med* 333(14):913, 1995.

150. Shekelle PG, Markovich M, Louie R: Comparing the costs between provider types of episodes of back pain, *Spine* 20(2):221, 1995.

151. Rosner A: Comparing the costs between provider types of episodes of back pain, *Spine* 20(23):2595, 1995 (letter to the editor).

152. Manga P: *Enhanced chiropractic coverage under OHIP as a means for reducing health care costs, attaining better health outcomes and achieving equitable access to health services.* Report to the Ontario Ministry of Health, Ontario, 1998.

Headaches

Howard Vernon DC, FCCS

Key Terms

ABORTIVE THERAPY
ACTIVITIES OF DAILY
  LIVING
ANALGESIC
ANESTHETIC BLOCKADE
AURA
CERVICOGENIC HEADACHE
CLUSTER HEADACHE
COPENHAGEN NECK
  FUNCTIONAL DISABILITY
  SCALE
DIZZINESS HANDICAP
  INVENTORY
ERGOTAMINE
GONIOMETERS

HEADACHE DIARY
HYPOMOBILITY
ISCHEMIA
KAPPA COEFFICIENT OF
  RELIABILITY
MIGRAINE-TYPE HEADACHE
MIGRAINEURS
NAPROXEN
NECK DISABILITY INDEX
OSWESTRY LOW BACK PAIN
  DISABILITY INDEX
OVER-THE-COUNTER
  MEDICATIONS
PHONOPHOBIA
PHOTOPHOBIA

PREMONITORY
PROPHYLAXIS
PSYCHOMETRIC
REPETITIVE STRAIN
SEROTONIN
SUBSTANCE P
TENSION-TYPE HEADACHE
TRIGEMINOVASCULAR REFLEX
TRIGGER POINTS
TRIPTANS
VASOCONSTRICTION
VASODILATION

The most common forms of benign headaches are **tension-type headache** (TTH), **cervicogenic headache** (CH), and **migraine-type headache.** For each headache type, basic epidemiology, pathophysiologic mechanisms, and clinical manifestations are reviewed in this chapter. The middle portion of the chapter describes mechanisms and clinical procedures applicable to the cervical spine that have implications for chiropractors and apply to all three headache types. These mechanisms and procedures form a coherent manual therapy approach to the understanding and assessment of these most common forms of headaches. The final portion of the chapter presents the available evidence from randomized controlled clinical trials of spinal manipulation/adjustment for these headache types.

TENSION-TYPE HEADACHE

TTH is the most prevalent form of benign, primary headache.[1-4] The terminology of this category of headache has evolved from the earliest classification of the National Institutes of Health (NIH) Ad Hoc Committee.[5] It has been called "tension headache" and "muscle contraction headache." The most recent definitions derive from the Classification of the International Headache Society (IHS),[6] where the term TTH was proposed. TTH has been described as a bilateral headache of mild-to-moderate intensity experienced with an aching, tightening, or pressing quality of pain; it may last from 30 minutes to 7 days, is not accompanied by nausea or vomiting, and either **photophobia** or **phonophobia** (but not both) may be experienced.

The IHS introduced two forms of TTH: (1) episodic and (2) chronic. The distinction between the two forms is based solely on the frequency of headache days. In episodic tension-type headaches (ETTHs), headaches are experienced no more than 180 days per year; in chronic tension-type headaches (CTTHs), headaches occur more than 180 days per year.

Epidemiology of Tension-Type Headache

Prevalence and Incidence

A small body of population-based studies on TTH exists, the most recent of these reporting on Canadian,[7] U.S.,[8] Danish,[9] German,[10] and Finnish[11] populations. These studies have used various survey methods, including telephone interviews,[7,8] subject interviews,[9] and mail surveys.[10,11] All but one of the most recent of these studies have used the IHS criteria for TTH described previously. With one exception,[9] these studies have involved large, randomly selected samples with good response rates (Table 24-1).

Several studies reported a slightly higher rate of TTH in females than in males[7-9,11] but Gobel, Peterson-Braun, and Soyka[10] failed to confirm this. Similarly, some studies reported an increased prevalence in those aged 25 to 45,[7] whereas others found no increasing trend with age.[8-11] Schwartz and colleagues[8] reported higher prevalence rates in whites and those with higher education.

In summary, the reported prevalence rates vary from approximately 10% to 65%, depending on the classification, description, and severity of headache features. In general, these rates derive from large, randomly selected, well-representative samples. The consistency of findings is notable, particularly among urban populations, leading to the conclusion that slightly more than one third of the adult population suffers from this problem.

Frequency of Tension-Type Headache

The findings of several studies,[7,10,11] agree that only 3% of TTH sufferers experience headaches more than 180 times yearly, thus being classified as CTTH. Rasmussen[9] reported that of this 3%, the percentage that suffers TTH more than once weekly (over 52 times per year) is 20% to 30%. Gobel, Peterson-Braun, and Soyka[10] reported that only 28% suffer TTH more than 36 times yearly. Honskaalo and colleagues[11] reported an increasing yearly frequency with age, varying from 7.3 and 13.5 per year for males and females younger than 30 years of age to 27.7 per year for both genders older than 65 years. This increase appears to be linear from one decade of adulthood to the next.

Table **24-1** PREVALENCE OF TENSION-TYPE HEADACHE: RECENT STUDIES

Authors	Location	Survey Method	Sample Size	Prevalence Rate
Pryse-Phillips et al, 1992[7]	Canada	Telephone	2905	Lifetime prevalence for HA, 58%; for TTH, 21%
Honskaalo et al, 1993[11]	Finland	Mail	22,809	Prev. for once-weekly TTH, 7%-17%
Gobel, Peterson-Braun, and Soyka, 1994[10]	Germany	Mail	5000	Lifetime prevalence for TTH, 38.3%
Rasmussen et al, 1995[9]	Denmark	Interview	1000	Lifetime prevalence for all TTH, 66%; for once-weekly TTH, 20%-30%
Schwartz et al, 1998[8]	United States	Telephone	13,345	Lifetime prevalence for TTH, 38.3%

HA, Headache; *TTH*, tension-type headache.

Severity of Headaches

TTH is, by definition, a milder, less severely painful form of headache than migraine or other primary categories (i.e., **cluster headache,** CH). Gobel, Peterson-Braun, and Soyka[10] reported that in TTH sufferers, headache severity was mild in 22%, moderate in 68%, and severe in 10%. Rasmussen[9] reported that 58% of subjects in a TTH sample had "mild, infrequent conditions." Adding these subjects to the study produced the highest reported prevalence rate. Schwartz and colleagues[8] used a pain-rating scale and reported mean (standard deviation) headache severities as 4.98 (1.99)/10 for ETTH and 5.55 (2.10)/10 for CTTH. In their sample, 62% were classed as moderately severe, whereas 25% were mild and 13% severe, closely matching Gobel, Peterson-Braun, and Soyka's figures.

In summary, it appears that at least 50% of TTH sufferers rate their headaches as moderately or severely painful.

Psychosocial Influence

The psychosocial effects of all varieties of headache are substantial and highly relevant to patient management. In a follow-up study of the Canadian sample, Edmeads and colleagues[12] reported that a high proportion of TTH sufferers endured adverse effects on their relationships: 89% reported TTH adversely affected their families, 71% reported it adversely affected their friends and colleagues, and 80% reported it adversely affected their physical activities. The full range of psychosocial influence of TTH includes adverse disturbances of daily activities, disturbed quality of life, lost or disturbed workdays, as well as the costs of these disruptions. In Pryse-Phillips and colleagues' study,[7] 44% of TTH sufferers reported a significant reduction in **activities of daily living** (ADL) because of headache (with a mean duration of 18 hours per year), whereas 8% reported taking at least 1 day off work because of their last TTH.

According to Rasmussen,[9] 60% of TTH sufferers reported an adverse effect on work capacities, with 12% missing 1 or more workdays per year. Nine percent (9%) of subjects had missed work in the previous year, with an interval of 1

to 7 days lost. They estimated a work-loss rate of 820 days/1000 people per year, for a total of 2,300,000 annual workdays lost in Danish society. In Schwartz and colleagues' U.S. sample,[8] 8.3% of subjects reported lost workdays (with a mean of 9 days per year), whereas 43.6% reported "reduced effectiveness" days (mean: 5 days).

Treatment of Tension-Type Headache

Treatment of TTH varies widely within both medical and nonmedical circles. In addition, the patterns of health care use by TTH sufferers are variable. According to Edmeads and colleagues,[12] 45% of their sample of TTH sufferers had consulted with a physician; 32% of these patients were subsequently referred to a specialist. These figures are lower than those for migraine sufferers. In contrast, the Danish results reported by Rasmussen[9] are much lower, with only 14% attending a physician and 4% receiving specialist referrals. Cultural and psychosocial variables may have an influence on treatment-seeking behavior and therapy delivery in different countries.

Medical Approaches

Medications remain the mainstay of the medical approach to managing TTH. Two basic medication approaches exist: (1) symptom relief, or **abortive therapy** (given every time a headache occurs), and (2) prophylactic therapy (given on a regular basis for headache prevention). Edmeads and colleagues[12] reported that 90% of their TTH sample used **over-the-counter** (OTC) **medications,** typically **analgesic** or antiinflammatory drugs. Twenty-four percent (24%) used prescription medications, which typically include stronger doses of the OTC drugs, muscle relaxants, and combination drugs. Only 3% were on prophylactic medications, which include low-level antidepressants and **serotonin**-enhancing agents.

Wober-Bingol and colleagues[13] reported on 210 headache sufferers referred to two Austrian specialist centers. Thirty-nine percent (39%) of subjects were on some form of prophylactic regimen; however, this was a medication regimen in only 9%. Of the 19 cases that were receiving anti-depressants, 11 reported them to be effective.

Nonmedical Approaches

Considerable variety exists in the nonmedical approaches to the treatment of TTH. Edmeads and colleagues[12] reported that 34% of their headache sample had used nonmedical forms of treatment, although these may have included a broad spectrum from psychology-based treatments to physical therapies to nonpharmacologic medications. Rasmussen[9] reported that 5% to 8% of headache respondents had sought care from physiotherapists or chiropractors. Wober-Bingol and colleagues' study[13] of specialist-level patients reported that 29% had received prophylactic physiotherapy, with only one quarter reporting that it was effective. In an earlier study, Graff-Radford, Reeves, and Jaeger[14] reported that 35% of their specialist level headache subjects (U.S. sample) had previously received chiropractic treatment.

The question of the percentage of chiropractic patients who complain of headache is an important one. Unfortunately, to date no study has accurately determined this percentage or used the IHS criteria to determine the percentage of TTH versus migraine sufferers. Several studies from chiropractic college clinics estimate that between 5% and 10% of patients report to chiropractors with a primary complaint of headache.[15] According to Kelner and Wellman,[16] 10% of the chiropractic patients in their small survey of alternative health practitioners (i.e., chiropractors, naturopaths, massage therapists, reflexologists, acupuncturists) reported that headache was their primary complaint. Interestingly, this figure was the largest among the five complementary/alternative medicine (CAM) practitioners surveyed and was considerably larger than the percentage reported for the family physicians who were also surveyed.

In a recent study by Hurwitz and colleagues,[17] only 2.3% of patients sought chiropractic treatment for headache; however, 13.5% sought treatment for neck pain that may have included headache.

Clinical trial evidence for the chiropractic treatment of TTHs is presented later in this chapter (see p. 509).

CERVICOGENIC HEADACHE

Description and Epidemiology

The role of the cervical spine in headache has become increasingly well acknowledged. Despite the wealth of writing in chiropractic, osteopathic, physiotherapy, and manual medicine circles[18-22] (see reviews in references 18 through 22), as recently as the late 1980s CH was poorly recognized in orthodox medical circles. Although numerous labels for the condition already existed, such as "headache of cervical origin," "cervical headache," "vertebrogenic headache," and "spondylitic headache," Sjaastad[23-25] coined the diagnostic label of *cervicogenic headache (CH)* in 1983.

As Pollmann, Keidel, and Pfaffenrath[26] and Vincent and Luna[27] have noted, reports dating from 1926 (with the cases of Barre) to those of Bartschi-Rochaix[28] and Hunter and Mayfield[29] in 1949 to Campbell and Hoyd[30] in 1954 likely involved cases of supposed CH. From 1983 to 1987 many researchers[23,25,31,32] expanded on the topic; they provided sufficient basis for the IHS classification[6] to include CH as a distinct entity (category number 11). The criteria for this category, shown in Box 24-1, were broader and more inclusive than Sjaastad's original description, because Sjaastad's description was challenged by some[18,19,33-35] as being so restrictive as to relegate this headache type to a rare variant. Recognizing this situation, Bogduk, one of the most prominent writers in this field, has proposed a new definition of CH, which has been adopted by the North American Cervicogenic Headache Society: "Referred pain perceived in any region of the head caused by a primary nociceptive source in the musculoskeletal tissues innervated by cervical nerves" (Bogduk N, personal communication).

Furthermore, a recent classification from the International Association for the Study of Pain (IASP)[36] adds the additional criterion of successful abolishment of headache by **anesthetic blockade** of the various upper cervical nerves as a diagnostic factor. The confusion in applying these various classification or diagnostic schemes is exemplified in two recent studies. Persson and Carlsson[37] reported on 81 subjects with cervical or radicular arm pain (or pain in both areas); 67% of these subjects also reported

Box **24-1** FEATURES OF CERVICOGENIC HEADACHE

1. Unilateral pain that does not change sides
2. Reduced range of neck motion
3. Provocation of pain by neck movements, awkward neck positions, or suboccipital pressure
4. Associated neck or nonradicular shoulder/arm pain
5. Pain radiates from neck to anterior head (particularly frontal and ocular)
6. Moderate pain intensity (no throbbing pain)
7. Varying durations of pain including continuous fluctuating pain
8. Minor associated symptoms and signs (which may or may not be present) including:
   - Nausea, vomiting, dizziness
   - Photophobia and phonophobia
   - Difficulty swallowing
   - Blurred vision in ipsilateral eye

Modified from International Headache Society: Classification and diagnostic criteria for headache disorders: cranial neuralgias and facial pain, *Cephalalgia* 8(suppl 7):1, 1988.

experiencing headache. When they applied the IHS criteria, 81% of those cases were classified as having CH. However, when using Sjaastad, Fredriksen, and Pfaffenrath's 1990 criteria,[38] only 28% received the same diagnosis. They concluded that "cervical headache has no unique features that differ from those of TTH, and it would perhaps be appropriate that the diagnosis of CH is incorporated in the diagnosis of TTH."[37]

Leone and colleagues[39] applied all of the differing classification schemes to 940 primary headache cases and found very few subjects who manifested any unique features of CH that could not be subsumed in either TTH or migraine diagnoses. In fact, the boundaries between CH, TTH, and migraine headache were and continue to be quite blurred, particularly on the issue of bilaterality. Another conundrum that confuses the diagnostic picture is that many of the features of CH cited in Box 24-1 are physical signs that the astute clinician must obtain from careful physical examinations.

If the headache pain pattern is not so distinct as to point to the diagnosis immediately (as in cluster headache or, perhaps, migraine with **aura**) and the less astute clinician does not include examination of the neck in the assessment, then those features *critical* to the CH diagnosis will be absent in the clinical equation. An erroneous diagnosis of tension-type or migraine without aura might then be imposed, and the opportunity to address the possible cervicogenic cause of the headache will be lost. In this way, the prevalence of CH is very likely underestimated.

Given the diagnostic confusion previously cited, it is understandable that studies of the prevalence of CH (in either the general population or in headache samples) are fraught with difficulties and variations. A wide range of frequencies is reported in the literature. As cited previously, Leone and colleagues[39] found CH in only 0.7% of their headache sample, whereas Pffafenrath and Kaube[40] found CH in 13.8% of their larger headache sample, with 6% suffering exclusively from CH. Using the IHS criteria, along with careful questioning about cervical dysfunction, Nilsson[41] found an annual prevalence of CH in a Scandinavian population to be approximately 15%. This is roughly at the lower end of prevalence estimates for TTH[8,9] and is identical to the prevalence of migraine headaches cited in these reports. This is far from the rare variant that CH was judged to be in the early 1980s.

Mechanisms of Cervicogenic Headache

According to Bogduk[34] the cervical source of headache may lie in any of the structures innervated by the first three cervical nerves. As such, a thorough knowledge of upper cervical innervation patterns is required. Before considering these patterns, it is convenient to categorize these somatic tissues according to localization (see box, Structural Model of Cervicogenic Headache).

Clinical Mechanisms

Numerous mechanical and arthritic processes affect the region and may give rise to upper cervical pain (i.e., develop into a "pain generator").

STRUCTURAL MODEL OF CERVICOGENIC HEADACHE

EXTRASEGMENTAL STRUCTURES

Long occipitothoracic muscles are relatively superficial in the neck; they include trapezius, sternoclei-domastoid, and splenius cervicis. The occipitofrontalis muscle is also an important consideration related to cranial pain. Other important structures lying extrasegmentally include the vertebral artery (implicated in the Barre-Lieou syndrome[22,42,43] and vertebrobasilar ischemic syndrome), the ascending sympathetic chain, and the superior cervical ganglion. Older theories implicated compression or irritation of these sympathetic structures in the generation of cranial pain and cranial vasomotor dysregulation; these theories have fallen out of favor, having been replaced by sensorimotor theories of pain.

INTERSEGMENTAL STRUCTURES

These structures include the classic spinal joints and deep spinal muscles (i.e., the semispinalis occiput and cervicis, multifidus, and suboccipital muscles [posterior, lateral, and anterior]). The clinician should remember that no intervertebral disk exists between C0-C1 and C1-C2. The suboccipital articulations include the bilateral atlantooccipital joints, the bilateral atlantoaxial joints, the atlantodental joint, Joints of Luschka, and the C2-C3 intervertebral disk. The suboccipital region contains a large number of specialized ligamentous structures (see Kapandji[44] for an excellent review).

INTRASEGMENTAL STRUCTURES

This category involves the neural and vascular structures contained in the intervertebral environment of C1-C2 and the intervertebral foramina of C2-C3 (specifically, the anterior and posterior rami of C1 and C2, the C2 dorsal root ganglion, and the C3 posterior nerve root). Bogduk's reviews of upper cervical anatomy[33,34,45] are particularly extensive.

INFRASEGMENTAL STRUCTURES

This category includes the spinal cord and lower brainstem. Of particular importance is the spinal tract of the trigeminal nerve, which contains descending afferents from the trigeminal sensory ganglion that terminate as far caudally as C3 in the spinal nucleus of the V nerve. The descending tract contains three components: (1) the pars oralis (upper), (2) the pars intermedialis, and (3) the pars or subnucleus caudalis (lowest). These afferent fibers terminate on the same second-order neurons as do the afferents from the upper three cervical roots. The second-order neurons form a continuous column of cells called the *trigeminocervical nucleus* by Bogduk and Marsland[33] and the *medullary dorsal horn* by Gobel.[46] This *neural anastomosis* of converging afferents is the fundamental neuroanatomic basis by which painful structures in the upper cervical region might generate referred pain to the cranium (see following).

INNERVATION PATTERNS FOR CERVICAL HEADACHES

C1 and C2 Anterior Ramus:

- Deep anterior suboccipital muscles
- Posterior dura
- Posterior cranial vessels

The C2 anterior ramus contains the sensory fibers of the hypoglossal nerve that run in the ansa hypoglossus.

C1 Posterior Rramus:

C1 posterior ramus is very small, but Kerr[47] proved its existence decades ago.

C1 Anterior Ramus:

- Superior oblique muscle

C2 Posterior Ramus:

The C2 posterior ramus has two branches: (1) medial and (2) lateral. The medial branch becomes the lesser occipital nerve and innervates rectus capitis posticus major and minor and the medial C1-C2

STRUCTURAL MODEL OF CERVICOGENIC HEADACHE—CONT'D

joint and ligaments. The lateral branch is the largest posterior ramus of the spine and is also known as the *greater occipital nerve (GON)*. The GON gives off an articular branch to the lateral C1-C2 joint and a muscular branch to the inferior oblique. It then courses posteriorly and superior to pierce between the semispinalis capitis and trapezius muscle insertions, where it becomes cutaneous and innervates the skin of the posterior skull to the midline.

Bogduk[33,34] has called the C3 posterior ramus the "third occipital nerve." It innervates the C2-C3 zygapophyseal joint (Z-joint) and deep muscles and provides a recurrent meningeal nerve that innervates the C2-C3 intervertebral disk (IVD).

This discussion will omit mention of the many pathologic processes that can afflict the region and give rise to pain.

Extrasegmental Processes

Postural strain and microtrauma or macrotrauma can create myofascial dysfunction. **Trigger points** in the large regional muscles have been charted by Travell and Simons[48] and create typical referred pain patterns. Stress and occupational **repetitive strain** can produce static overload of these muscles, predisposing to local and referred pain.

Intersegmental Processes

Painful disorders of the C0-C3 joint structures are currently thought to be the most common disorder in cervical headaches. Pain patterns, both local and referred, have been mapped by provocation and anesthetic procedures in humans for the C0-C1 joint by Dreyfuss, Michaelsen, and Fletcher[49] and the C1-C2 and C2-C3 by Feinstein and colleagues[50] (for both joints) and others.[51-53] Researchers[54,55] have used double-blind anesthetic blockades to identify the C2-C3 zygapophyseal joint (Z-joint) as the primary pain generator in over 50% of a group of whiplash sufferers with headaches.

Trigger points have also been mapped in the deeper intersegmental and suboccipital muscles. Tenderness in the deep suboccipital muscles is the most commonly reported finding in the large number of clinical reports (see review by Vernon and colleagues[22]). In a 1992 study[56] at least one tender point was identified in at least 84% of a sample of tension-type and migraine sufferers, with most having two or more. Sjaastad,

Fredrickson, and Stolt-Neilsen[24] reported on the high prevalence of paraspinal tenderness at the C2-C3 level. *This finding has eventually become a hallmark of CH.* Bouquet and colleagues[57] reported on 24 CH sufferers, 21 of whom had an ipsilateral trigger point at C2-C3. They also commented on a frequently noted finding of what they called an "enlarged C2 spinous process." The prominence of this spinous process was proposed to result from rotational misalignment at that level. In Jaeger's report on 11 CH patients,[58] tenderness and misalignment around the transverse process of C1 were the most frequently noted findings.

Several authors have reported on standardized methods of measuring tender points in the craniocervical region. In 1989, Langemark and colleagues[59] developed a method of rating manual palpation for muscular tenderness. Tender points are rated on a three-point scale to a standardized manual pressure. It was determined that the pressure sufficient to blanch the examiners thumbnail was sufficient to elicit tenderness, which is then rated as follows:

0—No reaction
1—Slight reaction, no vocalization indicating pain, no movement
2—Moderate reaction with vocalization
3—Severe reaction with vocalization and flinching or other movements

Scores for a variety of muscles are added up bilaterally for a Total Tenderness Score (TTS). TTS in 50 TTH subjects was found to be highly reproducible on two examinations separated by 3 weeks. Comparison of findings in 24 healthy controls indicated significantly higher TTS in headache subjects. Numerous replications of this methodology have verified its reliability and validity.[60,61] Although the manual palpation method has been used in subjects with both neck pain and headache and has been found to be very reliable, no study has yet investigated the role of tenderness in cranial, suboccipital, *and* neck and scapular muscles in TTH sufferers. In an unpublished study, the author used pressure algometry, another method frequently reported to measure tender points,[62-70] in a comparison of 14 headache and 14 control subjects. There was a significant trend toward multiple tender points to be found in headache subjects (four or more). Overall values for each of eight tender points were lower in the headache as compared with control subjects.

Intrasegmental Processes

Entrapment of the greater occipital nerve (GON) and its ganglion has long been purported to cause greater occipital neuralgia. Recent evidence by Bogduk[34,71] casts more doubt on this theory, because anesthetization of the GON would reduce pain from any of the tissues it innervates. Irritation of the sensory fibers in the anterior ramus of C2 by inflammation or osteophytic outgrowths from the C1-C2 lateral joint has been implicated as a cause of the uncommon "neck-tongue syndrome,"[72] in which upper cervical pain is accompanied by "numbness" or shooting pains into one side of the tongue.

Infrasegmental Processes

Only two direct mechanisms related to mechanical disturbances have been identified for the upper cervical cord. The first concerns a controversial mechanism reported by Hack and Koritzer[73] (see Chapter 23, p. 486 for further details) involving a ligamentous connection between the rectus capitis posticus minor and the dural lining at the foramen magnum. In a small number of reported cases, surgical ligation of this ligament has resulted in improvement in headache.

The second mechanism involves a herniation of the C2-C3 intervertebral disk (IVD). This is relatively rare and until recently only Elvidge and Choh-Luh[74] had reported on it. Recently the use of C2-C3 discograms and disk fusion surgery has resurrected this idea.

The most important role for the spinal cord in CH lies in the phenomenon of afferent convergence of the upper cervical and trigeminal systems, as described previously.[22,75] This mechanism is undoubtedly the explanation for referred pain to the cranium resulting from upper cervical deep-tissue pain. It should be remembered that the same convergence phenomenon explains why posterior intracranial pathologies result in referred upper cervical pain. This may be one of the mechanisms underlying the creation of upper cervical pain and myofascial dysfunction in migraine. Painful and inflamed posterior cranial vessels can refer pain to the suboccipital region—one more cause of diagnostic confusion!

MIGRAINE HEADACHE

The topic of migraine headaches is so vast that only a summary of the essentials necessary for students or primary care practitioners will be given here. The reader is encouraged to delve more deeply into major texts and articles for more information on the many theories regarding the cause of migraines, the many clinical variants, and the many types of treatments, both acute and prophylactic.[76-79]

Definitions and Classification

Since the 1960s, migraines had been understood according to the theory of Wolff,[80] who proposed a two-phase vascular model. In the 1940s, Wolff had proposed that, in the first phase, **vasoconstriction** of the cerebral arteries produced cerebral **ischemia** that was the basis for the aura or **premonitory** (i.e., warning) phase of migraine that may include transient, nonpainful visual or sensory symptoms. The clinician then proposed that the autoregulatory mechanisms of cerebral blood flow would become hyperactive and a "rebound **vasodilation**" would occur, resulting in the stretching of the cerebral arteries with the typical pounding pain of migraine. As such, the NIH Ad Hoc Committee[5] used the following classification for the two major types of migraine headaches: *Classic migraine* included the typical migraine headache *with* the premonitory aura; *common migraine* was defined as migraine headache *without* the aura.

In 1988 the IHS published a new classification of headaches and cranial pains.[6] The IHS promoted a simpler terminology that has since become widely accepted: migraine with aura (for classic migraine) and migraine without aura (for common migraine). The characteristics of these two migraine types, which together make up the vast majority of migraine diagnoses, are shown in Box 24-2.

A common feature of migraine headache is that various factors appear to act as triggering

mechanisms.[81-84] Often, individual patients will be able to identify which factors from the common group of triggers appear to affect them the most. These include *biochemical factors*, particularly from foods rich in tyramine such as chocolate, cheese, red wine, and possibly any sort of alcohol; *environmental factors*, such as changes in barometric pressure, ambient odors, loud or harsh sounds, and certain kinds of lighting; *psychosocial factors*, particularly those associated with stress and anxiety; and *hormonal factors*, where menstruation may aggravate migraine and pregnancy may relieve it.

Epidemiology

In 1975 a landmark study, the "Pontypridd Study,"[3] confirmed several key features of the epidemiology of migraine in the Western world. Overall, the prevalence of migraine is about 15% of the population. A female-to-male ratio exists of between 2:1 and 3:1, depending upon age. Migraine headaches can begin in childhood and adolescence, peak in the third and fourth decades of life, and diminish thereafter. Table 24-2 gives data from the Pontypridd study on age and sex prevalence of migraines.

In 1992, Rasmussen and Olesen[85] published an important study of the Danish population. Seventy-four percent (74%) of their random sample had headaches during the previous year, with 16% of these being migraines. This represented a total population prevalence figure of 12%. The gender differential was confirmed with 25% of the female population reporting migraine (in males only 8% did so). Over half (56%) of

---

Box **24-2** FEATURES OF MIGRAINE

A. Migraine without aura:
 - At least five attacks lasting 4 to 72 hours
 - Headache has at least two of the following characteristics:
   Unilateral location
   Pulsating quality
   Moderate or severe intensity
   Aggravation by routine physical activity
 - At least one of the following during a headache:
   Nausea and/or vomiting
   Photophobia and phonophobia
 - Normal neurologic examination and no evidence of organic disease
B. Migraine with aura:
 - At least two attacks
 - Aura must exhibit at least three of the following:
   Fully reversible and indicative of focal cerebral cortical and/or brain stem dysfunction
   Gradual onset
   Duration less than 60 minutes
   Followed by headache with a free interval of less than 60 minutes, or headache may begin before or simultaneously with the aura
 - Normal neurologic examination and no evidence of any organic disease

Modified from International Headache Society: Classification and diagnostic criteria for headache disorders: cranial neuralgias and facial pain, *Cephalalgia* 8(suppl 7):1, 1988.

Table **24-2** MIGRAINE PREVALENCE DATA FROM THE PONTYPRIDD STUDY

Age	% Males	% Females
21-34	16.8	30.1
35-54	16.4	26.0
55-74	12.5	16.6
75 and older	4.9	10.3

Modified from Waters WE: The Pontypridd headache survey, *Headache* 14:81, 1974.

migraineurs had seen their general medical practitioner and 16% had seen a specialist. Only 7% confirmed that they had been prescribed prophylactic medication, meaning that the vast majority of migraineurs resorted only to abortive or symptomatic medications. A large percentage of migraineurs (43%) reported that they had missed 1 or more workdays in the past year because of migraine, resulting in a projected loss of 270 days/1000 people.

The most recent large-scale population-based study comes from the United States. In 2001, Lipton and colleagues[86] reported on a very large sample of just fewer than 30,000 respondents. The prevalence of migraine in this sample was 18.2% for females and 6.5% for males. Of these, 53% confirmed that they had experienced substantial impairment or the need for bed rest with their condition, and 31% reported taking at least 1 day off work in the past 3 months because of a migraine headache.

With regard to the frequency and pattern of migraine headaches, these are remarkably individuated. Migraineurs typically report their own pattern of triggering, headache development, and its subsequent course. A thorough history from each patient will elicit these details as they pertain to the individual triggering factors, the timing of the attacks during the day, their relationship to many different environmental factors, their typical presentation (i.e., which side of the head; whether an aura or prodrome is present and how often; whether some of the less common features of migraine, such as dizziness, abnormal sensations, and motor weaknesses or gastric pains are present), their response to various medications and other nonmedical measures, and their typical course.

In Stewart and colleagues' first large report,[87] 59% of females and 50% of males reported one or more severe headaches per month. Typically, migraine headaches are less frequent than TTHs and CHs. In addition, the frequency can wax and wane throughout life, particularly when women experience hormonal changes, such as during pregnancy or when receiving hormonal treatments. Finally, migraine frequency and severity appear to diminish in the latter decades of life.[88-91]

Pathogenesis

Ever since the work of Wolff, migraine has been thought to be a disorder related to the cerebral vasculature. Wolff's theory emphasized vasomotor processes, including vasoconstriction, as the basis of the "aura" or prodromal phase and vasodilation as the basis of the headache phase. This latter mechanism appeared intuitively correct given that migraine headaches are so often described as "pounding" in character. However, this theory did not explain several important features, including the following: The majority of migraine sufferers do not experience an aura or prodromal phase; migraine is unilateral, and a vascular theory is difficult to apply to this feature; vasodilation of the external cerebral vessels is common in fever, yet is not accompanied by migraine headaches, per se. The typical accompanying features of nausea and vomiting are not accounted for in an exclusively vascular theory.

In the 1980s several attempts were made to develop a neuronal theory of migraine. These models focused on hyperactivation of several cerebral or brainstem centers. Using special imaging procedures, the phenomenon of "spreading depression," originated by Leao,[92] was applied to the observation of spreading vasoconstriction from the occipital lobe of the cortex forward, particularly in time with the development of headache in migraineurs.[93,94] Other investigators focused on the role of the locus ceruleus, a brainstem nucleus associated with the central sympathetic system, as the "central generator" of the migraine cascade.[95] Additional brainstem mechanisms associated with central antinociception and involving the periaqueductal gray (PAG) matter and the nucleus raphes magnus (RPM) have been proposed. The beneficial effect of various medications popular at that time, including methysergide and propranolol, were thought to point to these sort of central mechanisms.[76]

Most recently, with the work of Moskowitz and colleagues[96-98] and others,[99-103] a combined "peripheral-central" mechanism has been advanced that has led to the development of the most powerful antimigraine medications currently available. These investigators have developed a model based on the **"trigeminovascular reflex."** In this theory, antidromic stimulation from the trigeminal sensory ganglion, which provides the nociceptive (not the autonomic) innervation of the cerebral vasculature, is thought to stimulate the peripheral nociceptive terminals on these vessels, stimulating the release of serotonin and **substance P** (SP). These two neurochemicals, in combination with others subsequently released (particularly histamine), evoke a peripheral or "neurogenic" inflammatory response, producing both pain and vasodilation. This inflammation may be sustained by other local biochemicals, and nitric oxide is currently under intense investigation in this role. Once inflamed, these vessels are rhythmically irritated by the pulse wave, producing the pounding characteristic of migraine pain. Central synaptic connections with the locus ceruleus (and with nuclei in the vestibular system) appear responsible for the associated nausea, leading to vomiting. Precisely why this mechanism operates only unilaterally is still unclear. As in past theories, trigger factors such as stress, hormonal, barometric, and biochemical mechanisms can operate at various levels, including cortical and brainstem levels, to initiate the cascade of processes eventuating in a migraine headache.[96]

The success of medications that block a particular cerebral vascular serotonin receptor subtype, the 1Ad receptor, and which are known as the *tryptans,* underscores the validity of this theory.[97,102]

Genetic predisposition has been a commonly recognized feature of migraine. This is particularly so through the maternal line. A number of genetic markers for various types of migraine in various population subgroups have been identified.[104,105] At present it appears that genetic factors likely interact with environmental factors, lowering the threshold for the incipient dysfunctions in pain modulation and cerebral vascular regulation that underlie the migraine phenomenon and that are based in potentially numerous neurologic foci.

Medical Treatment of Migraines

This section on medical treatment of migraine will focus on pharmacologic and psychologic therapies, emphasizing pharmacologic treatments. The purpose is to give the reader a cursory review of the major medications used by family doctors, headache specialists, and emergency room physicians in the management of both acute migraine attacks and the long-term condition of recurrent migraines. Evidence on the effectiveness of each of these medications should be sought in the clinical trial literature and in the many reviews of these studies in the literature. Clinical texts on the management of migraine are too numerous to mention; the reader is encouraged to use those that are most current, because migraine therapy is constantly changing.[78,79]

The pharmacologic treatment of migraine headaches is essentially divided into three main approaches: (1) abortive, (2) analgesic, and (3) prophylactic. The goal of abortive therapy is to intervene as early as possible in the migraine episode so as to abort its eventual development.[79,106-108] For many years, **ergotamine** tartrate was the drug of choice in this regard. Ergotamine is a powerful drug with the potential for many side effects and the potential to aggravate nausea, which can be counterproductive in the management of migraine headaches. It is contraindicated in numerous conditions, particularly those involving the cardiovascular system and during pregnancy. The effect of ergotamine may be enhanced by the use of caffeine. If so, the dose of ergotamine may be reduced so as to preclude the development of side effects. A safer form of ergotamine is dihydroergotamine (DHE). The side effects appear to be less severe, allowing for more potent dosing. Abortive medications are often used in the emergency room, where adjunctive therapies such as antinauseants, anxiolytics, and analgesics can be used as well.

In the last decade a new class of drugs (the triptans) has emerged that appears to target the peripheral neurogenic inflammation in the cerebral vasculature rather than induce vasoconstriction, such as ergotamine appears to do.[78,79,97,108] The first of the triptans to be made available was sumatriptan. Initially it was only available for parenteral use, as in hospital emergency rooms. In more recent years it (and other forms of the triptan family) have been made available in pill form for oral self-medication. The adverse effect of sumatriptan on the peripheral vascular system is much less than with ergotamine. The triptans have rapidly emerged as the most widely used medication for the abortive treatment of acute migraine headaches.

Analgesic therapies are probably the most commonly used medications for self-management of the majority of migraine attacks. Simple analgesics include aspirin, acetaminophen, and the nonsteroidal antiinflammatory drugs (NSAIDs) such as ibuprofen, **naproxen**, diclofenac sodium, and ketorolac.[109,110] A more powerful class of analgesics is those given in combination with sedatives and caffeine, including fiorinal and esgic. More powerful narcotics can be used in more severe bouts of acute headaches; in addition to compounds with codeine, these include the following: propoxyphene (Darvon), oxycodone (Percodan, Percocet), and meperidine (Demerol). Each of these medications has powerful side effects and the potential for abuse and addiction.

The third class of medications is used for **prophylaxis.**[110,111] Long-term, regular use of these medications may prevent migraine attacks from developing in the first place. These medications include beta-adrenergic blocking agents (e.g., propranolol), calcium channel blockers (e.g., verapamil, nifedipine), antidepressant medications (e.g., the tricyclics), monoamine oxidase (MAO) inhibitors, serotonin reuptake inhibitors, NSAIDs, and specialized medications (e.g., methysergide, lithium). Methysergide is thought to act at the same serotonin receptors as the triptans, only on a more long-term basis.[79]

Nonpharmacologic approaches to the management of migraine include self-help and lifestyle measures and specific nondrug therapies.[112,113] Migraineurs often learn which of the typical triggering factors precipitate their headaches. Dietary changes to reduce the intake of trigger foods such as chocolate, red wine, or other foods containing aggravating substances can be helpful. Avoidance of environmental or lifestyle factors such as smoking, excessive exercise, stressful situations, and alterations in the sleeping pattern can all make a difference in individual patients' conditions. Finally, awareness of the effects of various medications on a patient's migraine pattern needs to be pursued.

Nonpharmacologic therapies for migraine include chiropractic, biofeedback (thermal and electromyographic [EMG]–based); relaxation training; psychotherapies including cognitive therapy; and physical therapies such as myofascial therapy, heat and ice therapy, postural exercising, and acupuncture.[112-119]

CHIROPRACTIC TREATMENT OF HEADACHE

Treatment for headaches was recognized by the earliest chiropractors, and statistics on the success of this treatment were compiled as early as the 1920s. Numerous case studies and case series were published in the chiropractic literature,[18-22] but as of the late 1970s more rigorous clinical trials have been conducted and reported in the English and non-English biomedical literature.

To describe more fully the mode of treatment of headache by the majority of chiropractors, Vernon and McDermaid[120] conducted a survey of Canadian chiropractic specialists, Fellows of the College of Chiropractic Clinical Sciences (FCCS). The overwhelming majority of these specialists endorsed the use of spinal adjustment/manipulation, along with soft tissue therapies and postural exercises as the most commonly used and most valuable therapies.

Table 24-3 provides the relevant data from the body of randomized clinical trials published since the late 1970s on the treatment of headache by spinal adjustment/manipulation. It should be noted that several studies of neck pain treated by spinal adjustment/manipulation have also reported relief of headaches in large percentages of the subjects.

CERVICAL ASSESSMENT OF HEADACHE

Box 24-3 lists the procedures and their purported pathophysiologic mechanisms associated with chiropractic assessment in headache.

Table **24-3** EVIDENCE TABLE FOR STUDIES OF SPINAL ADJUSTMENT/MANIPULATION FOR HEADACHES

Authors	Headache Type	Sample Size	No of Times	Treatment Groups (n)	Results	Side Effects	Quality Scores
Hoyt et al[121]	Muscle contraction	22	1	(1) MANIP, 10 (2) MOB, 6; (3) REST, 6	Post-Tx S: (1) −48%‡ (2) 0 (3) 0	Not mentioned	56
Jensen, Nielsen, and Vosmar[122]	Post-traumatic	19	2	(1) MANIP, 10 (2) Ice, 9	Post-Tx S: (1) −30.7/100† 2) +6.7/100	Not mentioned	60
Nilsson[123]	Cervicogenic	39	6	(1) MANIP, 20 (2) STT, 19	Post-Tx F: (1) −3.4 (−59%) (2) −2.1 (−45%) Post-Tx S: (1) −15 (−45%) (2) −10 (−24%)	Not mentioned	64
Nilsson, Christensen, and Hartvigsen[124]	Cervicogenic	53	6	(1) MANIP, 28 (2) STT, 25	Post-Tx F: (1) −3.2* (−69%) (2) −1.6 (−37%) Post-Tx S: (1) −17* (−36%) (2) −4.2 (−17%).	Not mentioned	72

Continued

Table **24-3** Evidence Table for Studies of Spinal Adjustment/Manipulation for Headaches—cont'd

Authors	Headache Type	Sample Size	No of Times	Treatment Groups (n)	Results	Side Effects	Quality Scores
Boline et al[125]	Tension-type headache (IHS)	126	12	(1) MANIP, 70 (2) AMIT, 56	Post-Tx F: (1) −3.8/28 (2) −4.0/28 Follow-up F: (1) −1.0[†] (2) +5.0 Post-Tx S: (1) −1.3/20 (2) −1.8/20[†] Follow-up S: (1) −0.5[†] (2) +2.0	(1) 4.3% neck stiffness (2) 82.1% dry mouth, drowsy, or weight gain	75
Bove and Nilsson[126]	Tension-type headache (IHS)	75	8	(1) MANIP + STT, 38 (2) SHAM + STT, 37	Post-Tx F: (1) −1.5 hr (2) −1.9 hr Post-Tx S: (1) No change (2) No change	Not mentioned	80
Parker, Tupling, and Pryor[127]	Migraine	85		(1) CMT, 30 (2) MT, 27 (3) MOB, 28	Pre-Post F: (1) 8.5, 5.1 (2) 11.4, 9.9 (3) 8.7, 5.7 Pre-Post DUR (hours): (1) 30.5, 19.4 (2) 12.2, 11.2 (3) 14.9, 11.9 Pre-Post DIS (0-5): (1) 2.8, 1.8 (2) 2.7, 2.6 (3) 2.8, 2.2 Pre-Post S (0-10): (1) 4.9, 2.8* (2) 5.0, 4.4 (3) 5.3, 4.4	Not mentioned	

Parker, Pryor, and Tupling[128]					Post-Tx–Fl/up F (20 months): (1) 5.1, 3.8 (2) 9.9, 8.0 (3) 5.7, 4.9	
Nelson et al[129]	Migraine	218	14	(1) CMT, 77 (2) AMIT, 70 (3) CMT + AMIT, 71	Headache Index (0-70) (1) Pre: 18.6 (9.6) Post: 11.1 (8.6) Fl/up: 10.8 (9.6) (2) Pre: 16.5 (8.7) Post: 8.4 (9.0) Fl/up: 12.5 (8.3) (3) Pre: 15.1 (6.5) Post: 8.9 (7.5) Fl/up: 11.3 (7.5) Pre-Post S (0-10): (1) Pre: 5.3 (1.3) Post: 4.3 (1.5) Fl/up: 4.4 (1.7) (2) Pre: 4.6 (1.1) Post: 4.3 (1.6) Fl/up: 4.5 (1.3) (3) Pre: 4.4 (1.1) Post: 4.1 (1.4) Fl/up: 4.3 (1.4)	0% 10%

Continued

Table **24-3** Evidence Table for Studies of Spinal Adjustment/Manipulation for Headaches—cont'd

Authors	Headache Type	Sample Size	No of Times	Treatment Groups (n)	Results	Side Effects	Quality Scores
Tuchin, Pollard, and Bonello[130]	Migraine	123	16	(1) CMT, 83 (2) PLA, 40	Pre-Post F (no/mo): (1) 7.1 (7.0) −4.1 (6.6)[‡] (2) 7.3 (6.5) −6.9 (6.6) Pre-Post S: (0-10): (1) 7.9 (1.4) 6.9 (1.8) (2) 7.9 (1.2) 6.2 (1.7) Pre-Post DUR (hours): (1) 22.3 (28.3) 14.8 (19.8)[†] (2) 22.6 (27.4) 19.8 (17.7) Pre-Post DIS (hours): (1) 19.8 (21.2) 13.0 (18.2) (2) 18.9 (21.2)* 15.6 (18.2) Pre-Post Meds (no/mo): (1) 21.3 (28.4) 9.8 (12.4)[§] (2) 20.1 (28.4) 16.2 (12.4)	Not mentioned	68
TOTAL OR AVERAGE		712	7				68

MANIP, Chiropractic spinal manipulation; *MOB*, mobilization; *REST*, rest; *Tx*, treatment ; *S*, severity; *STT*, soft tissue therapy; *F*, frequency; *IHS*, inclusion based on criteria of the International Headache Society; *AMIT*, amitriptyline; *SHAM*, sham placebo treatment; *CMT*, chiropractic manipulative therapy; *MT*, manual therapy; *DIS*, disability; *DUR*, duration; *Fl/up*, follow-up; *PLA*, placebo.

Box **24-3** METHODS OF CLINICAL ASSESSMENT IN CERVICOGENIC AND TENSION-TYPE HEADACHE

REGIONAL	**MECHANISM**
Plumb line and postural observation	Anterior head carriage
	Lateral or rotational craniocervical distortion
Range of motion (ROM)	Reduced ROM
Radiography (plain film)	Visualization of neutral regional postural configuration
SEGMENTAL	
Static palpation	Segmental alignment
	Myofascial tender or trigger points
Algometry	Quantification of myofascial tenderness
Motion palpation	Detection of joint fixation or hypomobility
	Appreciation of myofascial tissues during movement
Dynamic radiographs	Detection of intersegmental motion abnormalities

These procedures and their associated dysfunction targets are described in depth in the following sections.

Physical Assessment

Regional Considerations

General posture. Anterior head posture has been correlated with increased incidence of headache and neck pain.[131-134] Many sedentary occupational postures in our modern world predispose to anterior head posture. Watson and Trott[133] provide a theoretic explanation as follows: Shortened anterior neck and shoulder muscles induce an anterior shift of the head and neck. To compensate for this and maintain optimal horizontal alignment of the cranium, the suboccipital and long occipital extensors would tighten. This would induce suboccipital joint compression and pain and would create myofascially generated pain in the affected muscles.

In their study, 30 cervical headache subjects were found to have significantly greater forward head posture than a similar number of control subjects. However, Treleaven, Jull, and Atkinson[134] failed to confirm this in a smaller group of posttraumatic headache sufferers.

Grimmer, Blizzard, and Dwyer[135] recently reported that CH sufferers have significantly longer anterior neck length measurements than do nonheadache sufferers, implying that ante-

rior head shift may be present. Placzek and colleagues[136] found no difference in head posture between chronic headache sufferers and normal controls.

Two radiographic studies[56,137] have demonstrated higher levels of straightened lordotic curves in headache subjects, which is likely associated with forward head posture. Anterior head carriage can be assessed by using a plumb line and by photographic analysis.[135,136]

Range of motion. Reduced active range of motion (AROM) in the neck has been reported frequently in subjects with neck pain and headaches. Several devices for measuring AROM and passive range of motion in the neck have been reported, including cap **goniometers**[138,139] and magnetic inclinometers,[140-143] with findings of good test-retest and interexaminer reliability.

Several studies have reported on AROM in headache subjects. Stodolny and Chmielewski[144] used a goniometer to measure cervical AROM as an outcome of manipulation therapy in patients with cervical migraine. After several treatments, AROM values increased in subjects. Kidd and Nelson[145] used a simplistic visual assessment of cervical AROM in benign headache subjects, reporting that two or more ranges were reduced in headache subjects more frequently than in controls.

Sandmark and Nisell[146] studied the degree to which active rotations and flexion and extension reproduced pain in neck pain subjects as compared with healthy controls. No actual measure of the range of motion (ROM) was taken. The sensitivity and specificity of rotations and flexion and extension in correctly identifying symptom status were 77% and 92% for rotations and 27% and 90% for flexion and extension. The high specificity values indicate that relatively little error exists in identifying nonpainful subjects when AROM is not painful.

Recently, Placzek and colleagues[136] reported significantly lower values for cervical extension in chronic headache sufferers as compared with controls. This implicates increased shortness of the anterior cervical musculature as part of the postural adaptation associated with chronic headache. Stolk-Hornsveld and colleagues[147] reported significant reductions in all cervical ROM, with the exception of forward flexion in CH subjects versus those with other types of headache. This corroborates the validity of "reduced ranges of neck motion" as a criterion of CH diagnosis.

On the other hand, Persson and Carlsson[37] found no differences in cervical ROM between groups of neck pain patients with or without headache. However, these subjects may all have had reduced ROM, thereby leaving little room for differences between the subgroups. Grimmer, Blizzard, and Dwyer[135] reported reduced extension in frequent versus infrequent female CH subjects; however, this difference was not significant after age adjustment. It is important for clinicians to keep in mind that AROM has been shown to reduce progressively after the third decade of life.[148]

Several classic prognosis studies[149-151] have reported that AROM is reduced in chronic whiplash-injured patients. Osterbauer and colleagues[152] recently reported that 10 whiplash-associated disorder (WAD) cases had a combined AROM of 234 degrees, considerably less than the normal 360 degrees. After 6 weeks of conservative treatment, total AROM increased to 297 degrees. Hagstrom and Carlsson[153] compared 30 WAD cases with 30 normal subjects and found reduced AROM in all ranges.

In a recent study, Vernon[154] objectively measured AROM in a sample of 44 chronic WAD patients (all of whom reported headache symptoms) and found moderately high correlations (p = 0.001 to 0.0001) between all ROM scores and the subjects' self-rated disability scores using the **Neck Disability Index** (NDI) (see following). This is the first demonstration of a link between validly measured aspects of WAD-related impairments with levels of disability suffered by these patients. Interestingly, AROM scores were not correlated with age and duration of complaint, once again suggesting that chronic WAD sufferers reach a stable plateau of self-rated disability and impaired ranges of neck motion. In contrast, Jordan and colleagues[155] compared self-rated disability scores using the **Copenhagen Neck Functional Disability Scale** (CNFDS) (see following) with active neck extension and found no significant correlation.

Cervical muscular function. Cervical strength testing has recently been reported for neck pain and headache subjects. Vernon and colleagues[156] reported significantly lower strength values in all cervical ranges among chronic neck pain and whiplash sufferers (almost all of whom also complained of headaches) as compared with controls. Most importantly, the ratio of flexion/extension strength was much lower (28% versus 69%) in the pain group, implicating the importance of flexor muscle weakness in this condition.

Grimmer, Blizzard, and Dwyer[135] reported that reduced cervical extensor and flexor strength predicted increasing headache frequency in women but not in men. Placzek and colleagues[136] reported reduced extensor and flexor strength and reduced endurance of the anterior cervical musculature in women with chronic headaches as compared with controls.

To summarize, it is hypothesized by many of these authors that the separate factors of chronic pain, postural decompensation, reduced ROMs, and reduced muscular strength and endurance of the cervical spine as a whole interact in a self-promoting or vicious cycle of progressive mechanical dysfunction, resulting in greater persistence of neck pain. It is also hypothesized that the focus of these regional dysfunctions is the intersegmental tissues, the dysfunction of which is discussed in the following sections.

Segmental Considerations

Static palpation for tenderness and misalignment. Conventional manual palpation can provide the clinician with information about myofascial and joint dysfunction. Careful manual assessment can identify misalignments between upper cervical segments (particularly the position of the C1 transverse processes, the C2 spinous process, and the C0-C3 posterior articulations). Tissue texture changes include tightened muscles; rotated spinous process of C2[33]; and the taut, tender bands of trigger points. Tender points can be located by pressure over any of the soft tissues and bony insertion sites. Tenderness on palpation of the tissues of the craniovertebral and paraspinal region is the most commonly reported sign of cervical dysfunction in headache subjects. Virtually every relevant author has reported on the subject, from Lewit,[157] who reported on "pain over the posterior arch of atlas," to Sachse and Erhardt,[158] who reported similar findings of suboccipital and scapular tenderness, to Graff-Radford, Reeves, and Jaeger[14] and Jaeger,[58] who reported on the numerous cervical tender points that they proposed served to perpetuate myofascial head pain.

Other researchers[6-8] reported on the high prevalence of tenderness at C2-C3. This finding eventually became a hallmark of CH. Bouquet and colleagues[57] reported on 24 CH sufferers, 21 of whom had an ipsilateral trigger point at C2-C3. The report also commented on a frequently noted finding of a prominent spinous process of C2, which they proposed was due to static rotational misalignment at that level. In Jaeger's report on 11 CH patients, tenderness and misalignment around the transverse process of C1 were the most frequently noted findings.

The findings of more recent reports have used the standardized methods of tender point analysis in headache subjects (described previously and listed in Table 24-4).

Although procedures for manual palpation permit the location (i.e., identification) of tender points and, to some degree, an assessment of the severity of tenderness present there, they are limited in the degree to which such quantification of severity can be accomplished. To address this deficiency, numerous instruments have been devised that allow the clinician to apply a controlled, measurable force, thereby permitting discrete quantification of the degree of tenderness. Because the deeper somatic tissues are of greatest concern in myofascial and joint dysfunction, devices that permit pressure stimuli (i.e., pressure algometers) have become widely used. Fischer's

Table **24-4** STUDIES OF MANUAL TENDERNESS ASSESSMENT IN NECK PAIN AND HEADACHES

Authors(s)	Findings	Location
Lebbink, Spierings, and Messinger[189]	Neck muscle soreness, stiffness, and prior neck injury more common in 164 headache sufferers than 108 controls	Neck muscles
Jensen et al[190]	Studied 14 muscle sites bilaterally in normals; used Langemark et al method of scoring; norms reported; older subjects had lower TTS values, females had higher TTS scores	Cranial and large neck muscles
Jensen et al[191]	TTS scores in TTH and migraine headache sufferers compared; TTHs had lower overall scores; TTHs with headache that day had higher TTS than matched non-HA group	Cranial and large neck muscles

Continued

Table **24-4**   Studies of Manual Tenderness Assessment in Neck
Pain and Headaches—cont'd

Authors(s)	Findings	Location
Jensen, Nielsen, and Vosmar[192]	In 19 PTHAs, 42% had tenderness at C2-C3, 89% at C3-C4 and 63% at C4-C5	Neck paraspinal muscles
Hatch et al[193]	HA subjects had at least one tender muscle more often than controls; TTS in HAs greater than controls; EMG findings not correlated to tenderness	4 cranial muscles 2 posterior cervical muscles
Watson and Trott[194]	PTHAs had more tenderness findings than controls, particularly in upper cervical spine	Neck paraspinal muscles
Mercer, Marcus, and Nash[195]	HA subjects had higher values of tenderness than controls	Neck paraspinal muscles
Levoska, Keinanen-Kiukaanniemi, and Bloigu[196]	Test-retest correlation of manual palpation of scapular muscles was high; interrater reliability only fair	Scapular muscles
Levoska et al[197]	Neck pain sufferers had high number of tender points than controls	Neck paraspinal muscles
Hubka and Phelan[198]	Interrater reliability of segmental TTS scores were highly correlated (Kappa, 0.68)	Neck paraspinal muscles
Sandmark and Nisell[199]	Cervical tenderness was most sensitive (82%) and specific (79%) for neck pain patient discrimination	Neck paraspinal muscles
Nilsson[200]	TTS scores in neck pain patients high interrater reliability	Neck paraspinal muscles
Sandrini et al[201]	Mean TTS scores higher in ETTH and CTTH subjects than controls	Trapezius
Persson and Carlsson[202]	TTS scores higher in CH vs controls	Suboccipital, neck paraspinal, and scapular muscles
Stolk-Hornsveld et al[203]	Segmental tenderness on passive motion at C1-C4 higher in CH vs. other headache types; good interrater reliability	Suboccipital and neck paraspinal muscles

TTS, Total tenderness score; *TTH,* tension-type headache; *HA,* headache; *PTHA,* post-traumatic headache; *EMG,* electromyogram; *ETTH,* episodic tension-type headache; *CTTH,* chronic tension-type headache; *CH,* cervicogenic headache.

work[40,41] in particular enabled the standardization of this type of investigation. According to the clinician's protocol, side-to-side differences of 1 kg/cm² or absolute tender point values less than 2.5 kg/cm² in the cervical region indicate an active tender point. Table 24-5 lists studies

that used a pressure algometer to assess craniocervical tenderness in headache and neck pain subjects.

Motion palpation. One of the components of cervicogenic dysfunction most commonly cited

Table **24-5**   STUDIES OF PRESSURE ALGOMETRY IN NECK PAIN AND HEADACHE

Authors(s)	Findings	Location
Reeves, Jaeger, and Graff-Radford[204]	High correlation coefficients for intraexaminer and interexaminer reliability; average value for C0-C1, 3.0 kg/cm^2; for trapezius, 3.5 kg/cm^2	Occipital and suboccipital
Jensen et al[205]	Highly consistent values bilaterally and over 3-week interval in normals	Temporalis muscle
Drummond[206]	High intraexaminer reliability; HA subjects had lower algometer values than normals; no difference between TTH and migraine HA	Scalp and upper cervical muscles
List, Helkimo, and Falk[207]	High reliability coefficients; algometry scores highly correlated to manual palpation findings; TMJ pain subjects had lower values than normals	Temporalis and suboccipital
Langemark et al[208]	Temporalis algometry negatively correlated to headache intensity and to TTS on manual palpation; high correlation between temporal and occipital sites	Cranial muscles
Takala[209]	High intrarater and interrater reliability in normal subjects; women had lower algometry values than men; lower values in subgroup with minor neck pain and HA	Scapular muscles
Hogeweg et al[210]	Good reliability in normals; cervical points have lower algometry values than lumbar points	Spinal muscles
Bovim[211]	Lower algometry values in cervicogenic HA group vs. migraine, TTH, and controls; CH group had lower values in posterior cranial area and on the affected side	Cranial and suboccipital muscles
Chung, Un, and Kim[212]	Electronic pressure algometer showed good reliability and test-retest consistency in normals	TMJ and neck muscles
Jensen et al[213]	Algometry values lower in TTH vs controls	Cranial muscles

Continued

Table **24-5**   Studies of Pressure Algometry in Neck Pain and Headache—cont'd

Authors(s)	Findings	Location
Kosek, Ekholm, and Nordemar[214]	Algometry in normals showed good 1-week consistency; lower values in upper part of body	Whole body
Levoska, Keinanen-Kiukaanniemi, and Bloigu[196]; Levoska[197]	Reliability high in neck pain and normals; pain group had lower values	Scapular muscles
Mazzotta et al[215]	PPT values significantly lower in ETTH vs. controls	Temporalis
Sandrini et al[201]	PPT values significantly lower in ETTH and CTTH vs controls	Frontalis and trapezius
Stolk-Hornsveld et al[203]	High levels of interrater reliability; sensitivity and specificity for CH vs controls, 82% and 62%	Suboccipital and neck paraspinal muscles
Bendtsen et al[216]	Reported on an electronic finger pressure pad for palpating tenderness; high levels of interexaminer reliability	Cranial muscles

HA, Headache; *TTH,* tension-type headache; *TMJ,* temporomandibular joint; *TTS,* total tenderness score; *CH,* cervicogenic headache; *PPT,* pressure pain threshold; *ETTH,* episodic tension-type headache; *CTTH,* chronic tension-type headache.

by practitioners of manual therapy is disturbance of motion at individual spinal motion segments. This phenomenon has been variously termed *subluxation* or *fixation* by chiropractors, *joint* or *somatic dysfunction* by osteopaths, and *joint blockage* by manual medicine practitioners. The common feature of these terms is that they refer to *hypomobility* of the joints.

The procedures used to assess hypomobility are variations of manual palpation techniques of either the active, passive, or accessory motions of the individual spinal motions. These procedures have been devised and described by many experts in the manual therapy disciplines, from those in chiropractic,[159-163] to those in manual medicine.[4,164,165] The generic term for these procedures is *segmental motion palpation.* (For further detail on motion palpation, see Chapter 10.)

The interexaminer reliability of these procedures is unclear. Several authors have reported poor findings.[166,167] However, many methodologic flaws exist in these studies, including the use of asymptomatic students as subjects, the use of inexperienced students as examiners, and

the use of multiple replications of the procedures, such that the minor intervertebral derangements meant to be found were temporarily removed. In Watson and Trott's well-conducted study,[133] multiple outcomes of segmental dysfunction, including segmental motion palpation, were used to assess subjects with cervical headache. They reported on the reliability of posterior-to-anterior glide palpation in 12 of their subjects examined on two occasions by the same examiner. For these types of studies, the **Kappa Coefficient of Reliability** is typically calculated. This statistic indicates the degree above chance of the intraexaminer or interexaminer agreement. Their Kappa reliability values ranged from 0.67 to 1.00, depending on the segment.

More recently, Strender, Lundin, and Neil et al[168] reported poor interexaminer reliability for segmental motion assessment in 50 subjects, half of whom complained of neck or shoulder pain. On the other hand, Jull and colleagues[169] reported very high rates of agreement between several pairs of examiners in their ability to detect the presence or absence of any "treatable upper cervical dysfunction." Agreement levels as to the exact segment of dysfunction were somewhat lower but still acceptable (70% overall agreement). The C1-C2 segment showed the highest frequency of joint dysfunction.

With regard to the validity of the notion of spinal joint hypomobility in cervical headache patients, several studies have used both noncontrolled and controlled comparisons. Jull[170-172] compared motion palpation findings in headache and nonheadache subjects. Hypomobility was found at C0-C1, C1-C2, and C2-C3 in 60%, 40%, and 55% of headache subjects and 5%, 12%, and 22% of nonheadache subjects, respectively. These findings were later confirmed in a study comparing motion palpation findings (with tenderness) to anesthetic blockades to Z-joints in neck pain and headache subjects.[172] The sensitivity of motion palpation was reported as 100%. Jull and colleagues[169] also reported high levels of agreement between examiners' motion palpation findings that were obtained *without* pain cues from headache subjects and the subjects' subsequent report of pain during each procedure at each cervical segmental level. In other words, joint dysfunction can be validly determined without the subject providing pain-related feedback. Much greater levels of significant joint dysfunction were found in the upper cervical segments of cervical headache subjects versus controls in this study.

Jensen, Nielsen, and Vosmar's treatment study[173] of 19 posttraumatic headache patients reported on the findings of hypomobility before and after treatment with a short course of spinal manipulation. Fourteen of the subjects had at least one level of joint blockage in the upper cervical and upper thoracic region, whereas four had blockage only in the upper cervical region, for a total of 18 of 19 patients with upper cervical hypomobility. The most frequently blocked segment was C1-C2.

Vernon, Steiman, and Hagino[56] found that 54% of TTH sufferers had hypomobility at two upper cervical segments, whereas 30% had all three levels affected at least unilaterally. In the group of migraine headache sufferers, these figures were 42% and 42%, respectively. In both groups a total of 84% had at least two upper cervical segments demonstrating hypomobility.

In Watson and Trotts' study,[133] far more headache subjects than controls demonstrated painful segmental hypomobility, with the most frequent blockage at C0-C1.

Treleaven, Jull, and Atkinson[134] reported on 12 subjects with posttraumatic headache compared with an age- and gender-matched control group. Joint dysfunction (with tenderness) was rated as mild, moderate, or marked; 10 of 12 subjects with headache had at least one segment demonstrating marked hypomobility in the upper cervical spine. Much more significant joint dysfunction was noted between C0-C3 in the headache group as compared with the control group.

Stodolny and Chmielewski[144] reported that all 31 of their cervical migraine cases had significant joint dysfunction at C0-C1 on manual palpation. Over 80% of subjects had at least 2 cervical segments demonstrating joint dysfunction, which is remarkably similar to the findings of Vernon, Steiman, and Hagino[56] in TTH and migraine subjects.

SELF-RATED QUESTIONNAIRES

A variety of pencil-and-paper questionnaires provide patients with an opportunity to self-rate their experience of pain or disability related to headaches. Both practicing chiropractors and clinical researchers find these questionnaires very helpful for diagnosis and for monitoring the outcome of treatments.

Neck Disability Index

The first instrument designed for assessing self-rated disability as the result of neck pain in particular was the NDI.[174] Designed as a modification of the **Oswestry Low Back Pain Disability Index** (OLBPDI),[175] the NDI is a 10-item questionnaire with well-established **psychometric** properties such as high test-retest reliability, good internal consistency, and good sensitivity to change. Hains, Waalen, and Mior[176] recently established a single factor structure to the Index and reported that no response bias could be found among the items.

Riddle and Stratford[177] have recently added to the psychometric profile of the NDI by determining three important values for its use in clinical and research settings. These are "variation around a measured value," minimal detectable change (MDC), and minimal clinically important difference (MCID). The former of these values addresses the error margin inherent in any single use of the NDI, typically in a practice setting. This value was found to be 5 NDI points (at a 90% confidence interval). To paraphrase a recent review article by Binkley,[178] "If the error associated with a 50 point scale (such as the NDI) is 5 points, with a 0.09% confidence interval, the interpretation of this is that given a score of 20/50, a clinician can be 90% sure that the true score lies between 15 and 25."

According to Riddle and Stratford,[177] the MDC and the MCID values are both 5 NDI points. This means that the sampling error of the instrument limits the range of MDC in a patient's status to 5 NDI points. However, as a result of its use in a cohort of neck pain patients, the researchers determined that the MCID is also 5 NDI points. Several studies have reported mean change scores well beyond that level.[179,180]

In a recent study of 44 chronic WAD claimants,[154] Vernon reported on additional psychometric features of the NDI. First, the sample's responses were in almost identical rank order as the initial sample.[174] The items "headache," "lifting," "recreation," and "reading" were still among the five most highly rated items, confirming their importance in chronic WAD. Second, NDI scores were not well correlated with age and gender, as in the original work; however, in this new sample, duration of complaint was also not well correlated (r = 0.17, not significant [NS]). This was explained as follows: "Whiplash-injured patients who go on to experience chronic difficulties may reach a plateau of pain, impairment and self-rated disability, the complex of which (may remain) approximately static from that time onwards."[154] Third, two subsets of items (symptoms [four items] and activities [six items]) were compared with one another, with a moderate but significant level of correlation (r = 0.55, p = 0.05). The lack of strong correlation may mean that these two sub-

sets may offer unique information on the WAD sufferer's perception of the effect of their condition on their ADL. Finally, NDI scores in this sample were correlated with scores on a newer "generic" instrument for self-rating of disability, the Disability Rating Index.[181] The two questionnaires correlated very well (r = 0.89, p = 0.001). This finding further confirms the construct validity of the NDI as a measure of physical disability.

Neck Pain Questionnaire

In 1994, Leak and colleagues[182] reported on their development of the Northwick Park Neck Pain Questionnaire (NPQ). The authors reported that, as with Vernon and Mior,[174] they used the OLBPDQ as a basis for their instrument. No report of the methodology for adapting the OLBPDQ was given.

The NPQ contains nine items that are scored from 0 to 4 (for a total score out of 36). The nine items are (1) pain intensity, (2) sleeping, (3) numbness, (4) duration, (5) carrying, (6) reading and television, (7) work, (8) social life, and (9) driving. These items represent a mix of symptoms and activities thought to be important to neck pain patients. Of these "activity items," all but one (i.e., carrying versus lifting) had already been incorporated in the NDI, published 3 years earlier. Both instruments also retained the "pain intensity" item of the original OLBPDQ.

Forty-four subjects completed an NPQ at their original consultation, and 31 completed a second NPQ 3 to 5 days later. Thirty-five of these subjects also completed NPQs 4 and 12 weeks later. No formal treatment was offered in the study, but many subjects did receive some form of treatment.

Short-term repeatability was reported as high, with a Pearson's coefficient of r = 0.84 and Kappa = 0.62. Interitem agreements ranged from K = 0.53 to 0.76. Internal consistency was not formally tested but was graphically depicted as adequate.

Initial NPQ scores did not correlate well with age, gender, duration, or previous history of neck pain. Although NPQ scores did not change significantly over the 3-month study interval, they did correlate well with a separate question rating the subject's perception of improvement. This was cited as an indicator of "sensitivity to change." Subsets of subjects who either received physiotherapy or performed home exercises had what was described as "significant improvement" in their NPQ scores.

Given the similarities between the NDI and the NPQ, this author considers Leak and colleagues' report to be essentially a replication study of the NDI. The fact that the same set of psychometric properties was reported (namely, high levels of test-retest reliability, internal consistency, and sensitivity to change, as well as poor correlations with age, gender, and duration of complaint) is therefore not surprising and confirms the original report.[174] To this author's knowledge, no additional studies on the NPQ have been reported since 1994.

Copenhagen Neck Functional Disability Scale

Jordan and colleagues[183] devised the CNFDS as an attempt to improve the existing questionnaires (i.e., NDI, NPQ) for assessing disability caused by neck pain. The researchers asserted that because both previous instruments incorporated some items related to "symptoms" (pain, numbness, and duration in the NPQ; pain, headache, and concentration in the NDI), these questionnaires lacked some precision for measuring *solely* the disability caused by neck pain. This assertion was based on the theory that pain, disability, and impairment are separate but interrelated constructs.

The CNFDS contains 15 items with a three-point scale (yes = 0, occasionally = 1, no = 2) for a maximum of 30 points. Many of the item constructs are similar to those in the NDI (i.e., sleep, personal care, lifting, reading, headaches, concentration, recreation), whereas three additional items focus on psychosocial issues.

Jordan and colleagues reported very high test-retest reliability (r = 0.99), excellent internal consistency (Cronbach's alpha = 0.89), and no significant correlation between initial scores and age or gender. Additionally, initial CNFDS scores

were highly correlated with patients' global assessment of their conditions (r = 0.83) and moderately correlated with doctors' global assessments (r = 0.56). Initial scores also correlated highly with a separate 11-point pain ratings for neck and arm pain, which somewhat deflates the authors' original premise of a clinically important distinction between self-ratings of pain and disability.

Finally, the authors reported good sensitivity to change in a larger sample of subjects enrolled in a clinical trial for neck pain.[155] At 6, 24, and 52 weeks of this trial, changes in pain scores correlated with changes in CNFDS scores at r = 0.49, 0.48, and 0.54, respectively. Table 24-6 provides a comparison of the different items in each of these instruments.

Headache Disability Inventory

Jacobson and colleagues[184] developed this 25-item scale to assess the influence of recurrent headaches on daily function. The items are organized into two scales: (1) emotional and (2) functional. Good stability of scores has been reported over 1-week and 8-week intervals. Unfortunately, the authors[184] reported very poor sensitivity to change in a sample of treated patients. In addition, they reported that change in HDI was not well correlated with change in frequency of headaches. As such, the HDI is likely useful in the initial workup of a patient to assess self-perception of the daily burden imposed by the headache condition, but it may not be useful in monitoring the clinical outcome of a patient under treatment.

Activities of Daily Living

A series of validated questions to monitor the influence of headaches on ADL has been developed by von Korff, Stewart, and Lipton.[185] These ADL-related questions employ a relatively long interval of 6 months; however, for clinical use, the interval may be shortened. Some answers require the subject to rate a response using a zero to 10 scale, where zero represents "no interference" and 10 represents "unable to carry out any activities."

Table **24-6** Item Comparison of Neck Disability Scales

Items	NDI (pub. date, 1991)	NPQ (pub. date, 1994)	CNFDS (pub. date, 1998)
1	Pain†	Pain†	Sleeping‡
2	Personal care†	Sleeping‡	Daily activities*
3	Lifting†	Numbness*	Daily activities‡
4	Reading‡	Duration*	Dressing†
5	Headache†	Carrying*	Washing†
6	Concentration†	Reading and television‡	At home*
7	Work‡	Work‡	Lifting†
8	Driving†	Social†	Reading‡
9	Sleeping‡	Driving†	Headaches†
10	Recreation†		Concentration†
11			Recreation†
12			Resting*
13			Family*
14			Social†
15			"Future"*

*Item found in only one instrument.
†Item found in two instruments.
‡Item found in all three instruments.

The questions include the following:
- How many days in the last 6 months have headaches prohibited participation in usual activities (e.g., work, school, housework)?
- In the past 6 months, how much have headaches interfered with daily activities?
- In the past 6 months, how much have headaches interfered with the ability to take part in recreational, social, or family activities?
- In the past 6 months, how much have headaches interfered with the ability to work (including housework)?

Holroyd and colleagues[186] have recently reported that these questions loaded most highly on a separate factor labeled "headache disability" in the responses of their headache sample. Scores from the "disability" scale were not highly correlated to "pain intensity" scores, indicating that self-rated disability is a separate construct in the experience of headache sufferers

and should be assessed separately by clinicians and researchers.

Dizziness Handicap Inventory

This instrument was developed in 1990[187] as a 25-item scale used to assess the influence of dizziness and vestibular problems on daily life. The **Dizziness Handicap Inventory** (DHI) is composed of three subscales: (1) functional, (2) emotional, and (3) physical. The original paper reported good test-retest reliability and internal consistency. DHI scores were found to correlate well with increasing frequency of dizziness episodes and with scores from balance tests.[187]

Headache Diary

The primary instrument for monitoring headache activity is the **headache diary.** Numerous versions of such diaries exist, depending on the particular interest of the research involved.[188] For typical clinical use, the once-daily diary recording format is optimal. This type of diary permits calculations of the following parameters:

- Frequency of headache days per week and month
- Headache severity for any particular day or averaged over any interval
- Peak headache severity per any interval (i.e., worst headache in a month)
- Medication use

Some diaries record the duration of headaches; however, often the use of analgesic medications will shorten the duration, thereby providing false impressions of the true duration of ongoing headaches.

For clinical purposes, it is often sufficient to monitor the frequency and average severity of headaches. The desirable outcome of clinical management would be a reduction in both of these parameters. This is typically the kind of outcome that has been reported in clinical trials of prophylactic treatments for TTH or CH.

Review *Questions*

1. What are the three most common types of benign headaches? In what major ways do they differ from one another?
2. Which of the three types is the most prevalent? Which is generally the least painful?
3. What are some of the psychosocial factors influence headaches?
4. What percentage of TTH sufferers use OTC medications?
5. Paraspinal tenderness at what spinal level is a hallmark of CH?
6. What are the distinguishing characteristics of migraine headaches?
7. What are the primary pharmacologic and nonpharmacologic interventions used for migraines?
8. Discuss the examination procedures a chiropractor should use when evaluating a patient whose primary complaint is suboccipital headaches and neck pain.
9. Summarize the current scientific evidence on the effectiveness of spinal adjustment/manipulation for TTH, migraine, and CH.

10. How can self-rated questionnaires help the chiropractor when working with headache patients?

Concept *Questions*

1. If chiropractic spinal adjustment/manipulation and a certain prescription medication are both found to be effective in controlling a particular type of headache pain, on what basis would a patient decide that one method is preferable to the other?

    Consider all possible reasons for patient preference.
2. A migraineur arrives at the office in the midst of a full-blown episode. Aside from skillfully applying diagnostic and treatment procedures, what else might the clinician do to minimize the patient's suffering while the patient is in the office?

REFERENCES

1. Silberstein SD: Tension-type headaches, *Headache*, 34:82, 1994.
2. Leonardi M, Nusicoo M, Nappi G: Headache as a major public health problem: current status, *Cephalalgia* 18:66, 1998.
3. Waters WE: The Pontypridd headache survey, *Headache* 14:81, 1974.
4. Diamond S, Baltes BJ: Management of headache by the family physician, *Am Fam Phys* 5:68, 1972.
5. Ad Hoc Committee on Classification of Headache: Classification of headache, *Arch Neurol* 613:6, 1962.
6. International Headache Society: Classification and diagnostic criteria for headache disorders: cranial neuralgias and facial pain, *Cephalalgia* 8(suppl 7):1, 1988.
7. Pryse-Phillips W et al: A Canadian population survey on the clinical, epidemiologic and societal impact of migraine and tension-type headache, *Can J Neurol Sci* 19:333, 1992.
8. Schwartz BS et al: Epidemiology of tension-type headache, *J Am Med Assoc* 279:381, 1998.
9. Rasmussen BK: Epidemiology of headache, *Cephalalgia* 15:45, 1995.
10. Gobel H, Peterson-Braun M, Soyka D: The epidemiology of headache in Germany: a nationwide survey of a representative sample on the basis of the headache classification of the international headache society, *Cephalagia* 14:97, 1994.
11. Honskaalo M-L et al: A population-based survey of headache and migraine in 22,809 adults, *Headache* 33:403, 1993.

12. Edmeads J et al: Impact of migraine and tension-type headache on life-style, consulting behaviour, and medication use: a Canadian population survey, *Can J Neurol Sci* 20:131, 1993.

13. Wober-Bingol C et al: Tension-type headache in different age groups at two headache centers, *Pain* 67:53, 1996.

14. Graff-Radford SB, Reeves JL, Jaeger B: Management of chronic head and neck pain: effectiveness of altering factors perpetuating myofascial pain, *Headache* 27:186, 1987.

15. Waalen DP, White TP, Waalen JK: Demographic and clinical characteristics of chiropractic patients: a five year study of patients treated at the Canadian Memorial Chiropractic College, *J Can Chiropr Assoc* 38:75, 1994.

16. Kelner M, Wellman B: Who seeks alternative health care? A profile of the users of five modes of treatment, *J Altern Comp Med* 3:127, 1997.

17. Hurwitz et al: Use of chiropractic services from 1985 through 1991 in the United States and Canada, *Am J Public Health* 88:771, 1998.

18. Vernon HT: Spinal manipulation and headaches of cervical origin, *J Manipulative Physiol Ther* 12:455, 1989.

19. Vernon HT: Spinal manipulation and headaches of cervical origin: a review of literature and presentation of cases, *Man Med* 6:73, 1991.

20. Vernon HT: Spinal manipulation and headaches: an update, *Topics Clin Chiropr* 2:34, 1995.

21. Vernon HT: The effectiveness of chiropractic manipulation in the treatment of headache: an exploration in the literature, *J Manipulative Physiol Ther* 18:611, 1995.

22. Vernon HT: Cervicogenic headache. In Gatterman M, editor: *Foundations of chiropractic: subluxation,* Chicago, Ill, 1988, Mosby.

23. Sjaastad O et al: Cervicogenic headache: an hypothesis, *Cephalalgia* 3:249, 1983.

24. Sjaastad O, Fredrickson TA, Stolt-Neilsen A: Cervicogenic headache, C2 rhizopathy and occipital neuralgia: a connection, *Cephalalgia* 6:189, 1986.

25. Fredrickson TA, Hovdahl H, Sjaastad O: Cervicogenic headache: clinical manifestations, *Cephalalgia* 7:147, 1987.

26. Pollmann W, Keidel M, Pfaffenrath V: Headache and the cervical spine: a critical review, *Cephalalgia* 17:801, 1997.

27. Vincent M, Luna RA: Cervicogenic headache: Josey's cases revisited, *Arq Neuropsiquiatr* 55:841, 1997.

28. Bartschi-Rochaix W: *Migraine cervicale: das encephale syndrom nach halswirbeltrauma,* Bern, 1949, Huber.

29. Hunter CR, Mayfield FH: The role of the upper cervical roots in the production of pain in the head, *Am J Surg* 48:743, 1949.

30. Campbell AMG, Hoyd IK: Atypical facial pain, *Lancet* 2:1034, 1954.

31. Pfaffenrath V et al: Cervicogenic headache: results of computer-based measurements of cervical spine mobility in fifteen patients, *Cephalalgia* 10:295, 1990.

32. Leone M et al: Possible identification of cervicogenic headache among patients with migraine: an analysis of 374 headaches, *Headache* 35:461, 1995.

33. Bogduk N, Marsland A: On the concept of third occipital headache, *J Neurol Neurosurg Psychiatry* 49:775, 1986.

34. Bogduk N: Cervical causes of headache and dizziness. In Grieve GP, editor: *Modern manual therapy of the vertebral column,* Edinburgh, 1986, Churchill Livingstone.

35. Lord SM et al: Third occipital nerve headache: a prevalence study, *J Neurol Neurosurg Psychiatry* 57:1187, 1994.

36. International Association for the Study of Pain (IASP): Cervicogenic headache. In Merskey H, Bogduk N, editors: *Classification of chronic pain. Descriptions of chronic pain syndromes and definitions of pain terms,* ed 2, Seattle, 1994, IASP Press.

37. Persson LCG, Carlsson JY: Headache in patients with neck-shoulder-arm pain of cervical radicular origin, *Headache* 39:218, 1999.

38. Sjaastad O, Fredriksen TA, Pfaffenrath V: Cervicogenic headache: diagnostic criteria, *Headache* 30:725, 1990.

39. Leone M et al: Cervicogenic headache: a critical review of the current diagnostic criteria, *Pain* 78:1, 1998.

40. Pfaffenrath V, Kaube H: Diagnostics of cervicogenic headache, *Funct Neurol* 5:159, 1990.

41. Nilsson N: The prevalence of cervicogenic headache in a random sample of 20-59 year olds, *Spine* 20:1884, 1995.

42. Edmeads J: Headaches and head pains associates with diseases of the cervical spine, *Med Clin North Am* 62:533, 1978.

43. Vernon HT: Vertebrogenic headache. In Vernon HT, editor: *Upper cervical syndrome: chiropractic diagnosis and management,* Baltimore, 1998, Williams & Wilkins.

44. Kapandji IA: *The physiology of the joints: the trunk and vertebral column,* Edinburgh, 1974, Churchill Livingstone.

45. Bogduk N et al: Cervical headache, *Med J Aust* 143:202, 1985.

46. Gobel S: An EM analysis of the transsynaptic effects of peripheral nerve injury subsequent to tooth pulp extirpations on neurons in laminae I and II of the medullary dorsal horn, *J Neurosci* 4:2281, 1984.

47. Kerr FW: Structural relation of the trigeminal spinal tract to upper cervical roots and the solitary nucleus in the cat, *Exp Neurol* 4:134, 1961.

48. Travell JG, Simons DG: Myofascial pain and dysfunction. The trigger point manual. Baltimore, 1983, Williams & Wilkins.
49. Dreyfuss P, Michaelsen M, Fletcher D: Atlanto-occipital and lateral atlanto-axial joint pain patterns, *Spine* 19:1125, 1994.
50. Feinstein B et al: Experiments on pain referred from deep somatic tissues, *J Bone Joint Surg* 36A:981, 1954.
51. Bogduk N, Marsland A: The cervical zygapophyseal joints as a source of neck pain, *Spine* 13:610, 1988.
52. Dwyer A, April C, Bogduk N: Cervical zygapophyseal joint pain patterns. I. A study in normal volunteers, *Spine* 15:453, 1990.
53. Aprill C, Dwyer A, Bogduk N: Cervical zygapophyseal joint pain patterns. II. A clinical evaluation, *Spine* 15:458, 1990.
54. Barnsley L et al: The prevalence of chronic cervical joint pain after whiplash, *Spine* 20:20, 1995.
55. Lord SM, Barnsley L, Bogduk N: The utility of comparative local anesthetic blocks vs. placebo-controlled blocks for the diagnosis of cervical zygapophyseal joint pain, *Clin J Pain* 11:208, 1995.
56. Vernon HT, Steiman I, Hagino C: Cervicogenic dysfunction in muscle contraction and migraine headache: a descriptive study, *J Manipulative Physiol Ther* 15:418, 1992.
57. Bouquet J et al: Lateralization of headache: possible role of an upper cervical trigger point, *Cephalalgia* 9:15, 1989.
58. Jaeger B: Cervicogenic headache: a relationship to cervical spine dysfunction and myofascial trigger points, Cephalalgia 7 (suppl 7):398, 1987.
59. Langemark M et al: Pressure pain thresholds and thermal nociceptive thresholds in chronic tension-type headache, *Pain* 38:203, 1989.
60. Bovim G: Cervicogenic headache, migraine and tension-type headache: pressure-pain threshold measurements, *Pain* 51:169, 1992.
61. Bendtsen L et al: Pressure-controlled palpation: a new technique which increases the reliability of manual palpation, *Cephalalgia* 15:205, 1995.
62. McCarthy DJ, Gatter RA, Phelps P: Dolorimeter for quantification of articular tenderness, *Arth Rheum* 8:551, 1964.
63. Merskey H, Spear FG: Reliability of pressure algometry, *Br J Soc Clin Psychol* 3:130, 1964.
64. Fischer AA: Pressure threshold measurement for diagnosis of myofascial pain and evaluation of treatment results, *Clin J Pain* 2:207, 1987.
65. Fischer AA, Chang CH: Temperature and pressure thresholds over trigger points, *Thermology* 1:212, 1986.
66. Reeves JL, Jaeger B, Graff-Radford SB: Reliability of pressure algometer as a measure of myofascial trigger point sensitivity, *Pain* 24:313, 1986.
67. Jensen K et al: Pressure pain threshold in human temporal region: evaluation of a new pressure algometer, *Pain* 24:322, 1986.
68. Kosek E, Ekholm J, Nordemar R: A comparison of pressure pain thresholds in different tissues and body regions, *Scand J Rehabil Med* 25:117, 1993.
69. Wallace HL et al: The relationship of changes in cervical curvature to visual analogue scale, Neck Disability Index scores and pressure algometry in patients with neck pain, *J Chiro Res Clin Invest* 9:19, 1994.
70. Vernon HT et al: Pressure pain threshold evaluation of the effect of spinal manipulation in the treatment of chronic neck pain, *J Manipulative Physiol Ther* 13:13, 1990.
71. Bogduk N: The clinical anatomy of the cervical dorsal rami, *Spine* 13:26, 1982.
72. Terrett A: Neck-tongue syndrome and spinal manipulative therapy. In Vernon HT, editor: *Upper cervical syndrome: chiropractic diagnosis and treatment,* Baltimore, 1988, Williams & Wilkins.
73. Hack GD, Koritzer RT: Anatomic relation between the rectus capitis posticus minor muscle and the dura mater, *Spine* 20:2484, 1995.
74. Elvidge AR, Choh-Luh L: Central protrusion of cervical intervertebral disc involving the descending trigeminal tract, *Arch Neurol Psychiat* 63:455, 1950.
75. Sessle BJ, Hu JW, Yu X: Brainstem mechanisms of referred pain and hyperalgesia in the orofacial and temporomandibular region. In Vecchiet L et al, editors: *New trends in referred pain and hyperalgesia,* Amsterdam, 1993, Elsevier.
76. Olesen J: Clinical and pathophysiological observations in migraine and tension-type headache explained by integration of vascular, supraspinal and myofascial inputs, *Pain* 46:125, 1991.
77. Olesen J: *Headache classification and epidemiology,* New York, 1994, Raven Press.
78. Blau JN: A clinicotherapeutic approach to migraine. In Blau JN, editor: *Migraine: clinical and research aspects,* Baltimore, 1987, Johns Hopkins University Press.
79. Davidoff RA: *Migraine: manifestations, pathogenesis and management,* Philadelphia, 1995, FA Davis.
80. Wolff HG: *Headache and other head pains,* ed 2, New York, 1963, Oxford University Press.
81. Rasmussen BK: Migraine and tension-type headache in a general population: precipitating factors, female hormones, sleep pattern and relation to lifestyle, *Pain* 53:65, 1993.
82. Van den Bergh V, Amery WK, Waelkens J: Trigger factors in migraine: a study conducted by the Belgian Migraine Society, *Headache* 27:191, 1987.
83. Blau JN: Pathogenesis of migraine attack: initiation, *J R Coll Physicians Lond* 19:166, 1985.
84. Blau JN, Thavapalan M: Preventing migraine: a study of precipitating factors, *Headache* 28:481, 1988.
85. Rasmussen BK, Olesen J: Migraine with aura and migraine without aura: an epidemiologic study, *Cephalalgia* 12:221, 1992.

86. Lipton RB et al: Prevalence and burden of migraine in the United States: data from the American Migraine Study II, *Headache* 41:646, 2001.

87. Stewart WF et al: Prevalence of migraine headache in the United States: relation to age, income, race and other sociodemographic factors, *J Am Med Assoc* 267:64, 1992.

88. Dalsgaard-Nielsen T, Engberg-Pederson H, Holm HE: Clinical and statistical investigations of the epidemiology of migraine, *Dan Med Bull* 17:138, 1970.

89. Stewart WF et al: Age- and sex-specific incidence rates of migraine with and without visual aura, *Am J Epidemiol* 134:1111, 1991.

90. Stewart WF, Lipton RB: Migraine headache: epidemiology and health care utilization, *Cephalalgia* 13(suppl 12):41, 1993.

91. Ziegler DK: Epidemiology of migraine. In Rose CF, editor: *Handbook of clinical neurology,* vol 48, Amsterdam, 1986, Elsevier.

92. Leao AAP: Spreading depression of activity in cerebral cortex, *J Neurophysiol* 7:359, 1944.

93. Lauritzen M: Pathophysiology of the migraine aura: the spreading depression theory, *Brain* 117:199, 1994.

94. Lauritzen M: Cortical spreading depression in migraine, *Cephalalgia* 21:757, 2001.

95. Goadsby PJ, Duckworth JW: Low frequency stimulation of the locus ceruleus reduces regional cerebral blood flow in the spinalized cat, *Brain Res* 476:71, 1989.

96. Moskowitz MA et al: Pain mechanisms underlying vascular headaches, *Rev Neurol* 145:181, 1989.

97. Moskowitz MA: Neurogenic versus vascular mechanisms of sumatriptan and ergot alkaloids in migraine, *Trends Pharmacol Sci* 13:307, 1992.

98. Strassman A et al: Response of brainstem trigeminal neurons to electrical stimulation of the dura, *Brain Res* 379:242, 1986.

99. Goadsby PJ, Edvisson L, Ekman R: Vasoactive peptide release in the extracerebral circulation of humans during migraine headache, *Ann Neurol* 28:183, 1990.

100. Goadsby PJ, Edvisson L, Ekman R: Release of vasoactive peptides in the extracerebral circulation of humans and the cat during activation of the trigeminovascular system, *Ann Neurol* 23:193, 1988.

101. Edvinsson L: Sensory nerves in man and their role in primary headaches, *Cephalalgia* 21:761, 2001.

102. Edvinsson L, Goadsby PJ: Neuropeptides in headache, *Eur J Neurol* 5:329, 1998.

103. Goadsby PJ, Edvinsson L: The trigeminovascular system and migraine: studies characterizing cerebrovascular and neuropeptide changes seen in human and cats, *Ann Neurol* 33:48, 1993.

104. Russell MB: Genetics of migraine without aura, migraine with aura, migrainous disorder, head trauma migraine without aura and tension-type headache, *Cephalalgia* 21:778, 2001.

105. Ulrich V et al: Evidence of a genetic factor in migraine with aura: a population-base Danish twin study, *Ann Neurol* 46:606, 1999.

106. Edmeads J: Emergency management of headache, *Headache* 28:675, 1988.

107. Edmeads J: Management of the acute attack of migraine, *Headache* 13:91, 1973.

108. Peatfield RC, Fozard JR, Rose F: Drug treatment of migraine. In Rose CF, editor, *Handbook of clinical neurology*, vol 4, Amsterdam, 1986, Elsevier.

109. Diamond S, Freitag FG: Do non-steroidal antiinflammatory agents have a role in the treatment of migraine headaches? *Drugs* 37:755, 1989.

110. Elkind AH: Interval therapy of migraine: art and science, *Headache Quar Curr Treat Res* 1:280, 1990.

111. Klapper JA: The efficacy of migraine prophylaxis, *Headache Quar Curr Treat Res* 2:278, 1991.

112. Blanchard EB: Psychological treatments of benign headache disorders, *Behav Ther* 18:375, 1987.

113. Turk DC, Meichenbaum DH: A cognitive-behavioral approach to pain management. In Wall PD, Melzack R, editors: *Textbook of pain*, ed 2, Edinburgh, 1989, Churchill Livingstone.

114. Blanchard EB, Andrassik F: Biofeedback treatment of vascular headache. In Hatch JP, Fisher JG, Rugh JD, editors: *Biofeedback studies and clinical efficacy*, New York, 1987, Plenum Press.

115. Diamond S, Montrose D: The value of biofeedback in the treatment of chronic headache: a four-year retrospective study, *Headache* 24:5, 1984.

116. Friedman H, Traub HA: Brief psychological training procedures in migraine treatment, *Am J Clin Hypnosis* 26:187, 1984.

117. Smith WB: Biofeedback and relaxation training: the effect on headache and associated symptoms, *Headache* 27:511, 1987.

118. Chapman S: A review and clinical perspective on the use of EMG and thermal biofeedback for chronic headaches, *Pain* 27:1, 1986.

119. Pryse-Phillips WEM et al: Guidelines for the nonpharmacologic management of migraine in clinical practice, *Can Med Assoc J* 159:47, 1998.

120. Vernon H, McDermaid C: Chiropractic management of episodic tension-type headaches: a survey of clinical specialists, *J Can Chiropr Assoc* 42: 209, 1998.

121. Hoyt WH et al: Osteopathic manipulation in the treatment of muscle contraction headache, *J Am Osteopath Assoc* 78:322, 1979.

122. Jensen OK, Nielsen FF, Vosmar L: An open study comparing manual therapy with the use of cold packs in the treatment of post-traumatic headache, *Cephalalgia* 10:241, 1990.

123. Nilsson N: A randomized controlled trial of the effect of spinal manipulation in the treatment of cervicogenic headache, *J Manipulative Physiol Ther* 18:435, 1995.

124. Nilsson N, Christensen HW, Hartvigsen J: The effect of spinal manipulation in the treatment of cervico-

genic headache, *J Manipulative Physiol Ther* 20:326, 1997.

125. Boline PD et al: Spinal manipulation vs. amitriptyline for the treatment of chronic tension-type headache: a randomized clinical trial, *J Manipulative Physiol Ther* 18:148, 1995.
126. Bove G, Nilsson N: Spinal manipulation in the treatment of episodic tension-type headache: a randomized controlled trial, *N Engl J Med* 280:1576, 1998.
127. Parker GB, Tupling H, Pryor DS: A controlled trial of cervical manipulation for migraine, *Aust N Z J Med* 8:589, 1978.
128. Parker GB, Pryor DS, Tupling H: Why does migraine improve during a clinical trial? Further results from a trial of cervical manipulation for migraine, *Aust N Z J Med* 10:192, 1980.
129. Nelson CF et al: The efficacy of spinal manipulation, amitriptyline and the combination of both therapies for the prophylaxis of migraine headache, *J Manipulative Physiol Ther* 21:511, 1998.
130. Tuchin PJ, Pollard H, Bonello R: A randomized controlled trial of chiropractic spinal manipulative therapy for migraine, *J Manipulative Physiol Ther* 23:91, 2000.
131. Awalt P, Lavin NL, McKeough M: Radiographic measurements of intervertebral foramina of cervical vertebra in forward and normal head posture, *J Craniomandibular Practice* 7:275, 1989.
132. Darnell MW: A proposed chronology of events for forward head posture, *J Craniomandibular Practice* 1:50, 1983.
133. Watson DH, Trott PH: Cervical headache: an investigation of natural head posture and upper cervical flexor muscle performance, *Cephalalgia* 13:272, 1993.
134. Treleaven J, Jull G, Atkinson L: Cervical musculoskeletal dysfunction in post-concussional headache, *Cephalalgia* 14:273, 1994.
135. Grimmer K, Blizzard L, Dwyer T: Frequency of headaches associated with the cervical spine and relationships with anthropometric, muscle performance and recreational factors, *Arch Phys Med Rehabil* 80:512, 1999.
136. Placzek JD et al: The influence of the cervical spine on chronic headache in women: a pilot study, *J Manipulative Physiol Ther* 7:33, 1999.
137. Nagasawa A, Sakakibara T, Takahashi A: Roentgenographic findings of cervical spine in tension-type headache, *Headache* 33:90, 1993.
138. Zachman Z et al: Inter-examiner reliability and concurrent validity of two instruments for the measurement of cervical ranges of motion, *J Manipulative Physiol Ther* 12:205, 1989.
139. Cassidy JD, Lopes AA, Yong-Hing K: The immediate effect of manipulation versus mobilization on pain and range of motion in the cervical spine: a randomized controlled trial, *J Manipulative Physiol Ther* 15:570, 1992.

140. Tucci SM et al: Cervical motion assessment: a new, simple and accurate method, *Arch Phys Med Rehabil* 67:225, 1986.
141. Rheault W et al: Intertester reliability of the cervical range of motion device, *J Orthop Sports Phys Ther* 15:147, 1992.
142. Capuano-Pucci D et al: Intratester and intertester reliability of the cervical range of motion device, *Arch Phys Med Rehabil* 72:338, 1991.
143. Youdas JW, Carey JR, Garrett TR: Reliability of measurements of cervical range of motion: comparison of three methods, *Phys Ther* 71:98, 1991.
144. Stodolny J, Chmielewski H: Manual therapy in the treatment of patients with cervical migraine, *Man Med* 4:49, 1989.
145. Kidd RF, Nelson R: Musculoskeletal dysfunction of the neck in migraine and tension headache, *Headache* 33:566, 1993.
146. Sandmark H, Nisell R: Validity of five common manual neck pain provoking tests, *Scan J Rehab Med* 27:131, 1995.
147. Stolk-Hornsveld F et al: Impaired mobility of cervical spine as a tool in the diagnosis of cervicogenic headache, *Cephalalgia* 19:436, 1999 (abstract).
148. Dvorak J et al: Age and gender related normal motion of the cervical spine, *Spine* 17:S393, 1992.
149. Hildingsson C, Toolanen G: Outcome after soft-tissue injury of the cervical spine: a prospective study of 93 car accident victims, *Acta Orthop Scand* 61:356, 1990.
150. Hohl M: Soft tissue injuries of the neck in automobile accidents: factors influencing prognosis, *J Bone Joint Surg* 56A:1675, 1974.
151. Gargan MF, Bannister GC: The rate of recovery following whiplash injury, *Eur Spine J* 3:162, 1994.
152. Osterbauer PJ et al: Three dimensional head kinematics and clinical outcome of patients with neck injury treated with spinal manipulative therapy: a pilot study, *J Manipulative Physiol Ther* 15:501, 1992.
153. Hagstrom Y, Carlsson J: Prolonged functional impairments after whiplash injury, *Scand J Rehabil Med* 28:139, 1996.
154. Vernon HT: Correlations among ratings of pain, disability and impairment in chronic whiplash-associated disorder, *Pain Res Manag* 2:207, 1997.
155. Jordan A et al: Intensive training, physiotherapy or manipulation for patients with chronic neck pain: a prospective, single-blind, randomized clinical trial, *Spine* 23:311, 1998.
156. Vernon HT et al: Evaluation of neck muscle strength with a modified sphygmomanometer dynamometer: reliability and validity, *J Manipulative Physiol Ther* 15:343, 1992.
157. Lewit K: Ligament pain and anteflexion headache, *Eur Neurol* 5:365, 1971.
158. Sachse J, Erhardt E: Phenomenological investigation in migraine patients, *Man Med* 20:59, 1982.

159. Gillet H: *Belgian Chiropractic research notes*, ed 10, Huntington Beach, Calif, 1970, Motion Palpation Institute.

160. Gillet H, Liekens M: A further study of spinal fixations, *Ann Swiss Chiropr Assoc* 4:41, 1969.

161. Faye LJ: *Spine II. Motion palpation and clinical considerations for the cervical and thoracic spine*, Huntington Beach, Calif, 1986, Motion Palpation Institute.

162. Grice AS: A biomechanical approach to cervical and dorsal adjusting. In Haldeman S, editor: *Modern developments in the principles and practice of chiropractic*, New York, 1980, Appleton-Century-Crofts.

163. Fligg B: Motion palpation of the upper cervical spine. In Vernon HT, editor: *The upper cervical syndrome: chiropractic diagnosis and treatment*, Baltimore, 1988, Williams & Wilkins.

164. Lewit K: *Manipulative therapy in the rehabilitation of the locomotor system*, London, 1991, Butterworth.

165. Mennel JM: *Joint pain*, Boston, 1964, Little, Brown.

166. DeBoer KF et al: Reliability study of the detection of somatic dysfunctions in the cervical spine, *J Manipulative Physiol Ther* 8:9, 1985.

167. Mior SA et al: Intra- and inter-examiner reliability of motion palpation in the cervical spine, *J Can Chiropr Assoc* 29:195, 1985.

168. Strender L-E, Lundin M, Neil K: Interexaminer reliability in physical examination of the neck, *J Manipulative Physiol Ther* 20:516, 1997.

169. Jull G et al: Inter-examiner reliability to detect painful upper cervical joint dysfunction, *Aust J Physiother* 43:125, 1997.

170. Jull GA: Clinical observations of upper cervical mobility. In Grieve GP, editor: Modern manual therapy of the vertebral column, Edinburgh, 1986, Churchill-Livingstone.

171. Jull GA: Manual diagnosis of C2-C3 headache, *Cephalalgia* 5(suppl 5):308, 1985.

172. Jull GA, Bogduk N, Marsland A: The accuracy of manual diagnosis of cervical zygapophyseal joint pain syndrome, *Med J Aust* 148:233, 1988.

173. Jensen OK, Nielsen FF, Vosmar L: An open study comparing manual therapy with the use of cold packs in the treatment of post-traumatic headache, *Cephalalgia* 10:241, 1990.

174. Vernon H, Mior S: The Neck Disability Index: a study of reliability and validity, *J Manipulative Physiol Ther* 14:409, 1991.

175. Fairbank JCT et al: The Oswestry Low Back Pain Index, *Physiotherapy* 66:271, 1980.

176. Hains F, Waalen J, Mior S: Psychometric properties of the Neck Disability Index, *J Manipulative Physiol Ther* 21:75, 1998.

177. Riddle DL, Stratford PW: Use of generic versus region-specific status measures on patients with cervical spine disorders: a comparison study, *Phys Ther* 78:951, 1998.

178. Binkley J: Measurement of functional status, progress and outcome in orthopedic clinical practice, *Orthop Div Res* Fall:7, 1998.

179. Vernon HT et al: Chiropractic rehabilitation of spinal pain: principles, practice and outcomes data, *J Can Chiropr Assoc* 39:147, 1995.

180. Giles LGF, Muller R: Chronic spinal pain syndromes: a clinical pilot trial comparing acupuncture, a non-steroidal anti-inflammatory drug and spinal manipulation, *J Manipulative Physiol Ther* 22:376, 1999.

181. Salen BA et al: The Disability Rating Index: an instrument for the assessment of disability in clinical settings, *J Clin Epidemiol* 47:1423, 1994.

182. Leak AM et al: The Northwick Park Neck Pain Questionnaire: devised to measure neck pain and disability, *J Rheumatol* 33:469, 1994.

183. Jordan A et al: The Copenhagen Neck Functional Disability Index: a study of reliability and validity, *J Manipulative Physiol Ther* 21:520, 1998.

184. Jacobson GP et al: The Henry Ford Hospital Headache Disability Inventory (HDI), *Neurology* 44:837, 1994.

185. von Korff M, Stewart WF, Lipton RB: Assessing headache severity, *Neurology* 44:S40, 1994.

186. Holroyd KA et al: The three dimensions of headache impact: pain, disability and affective distress, *Pain* 83:571, 1999.

187. Jacobson GP, Newman CW: The development of the Dizziness Handicap Inventory, *Arch Otolaryngol Head Neck Surg* 116:424, 1990.

188. Blanchard EB, Andrassik F: *Management of chronic headaches: a psychological approach*, New York, 1985, Pergammon Press.

189. Lebbink J, Spierings EL, Messinger HB: A questionnaire survey of muscular symptoms in chronic headache: an age and sex-controlled study, *Clin J Pain* 7:95, 1991.

190. Jensen R et al: Cephalic muscle tenderness and pressure pain threshold in a general population, *Pain* 48:197, 1992.

191. Jensen R et al: Muscle tenderness and pressure pain threshold in headache: a population study, *Pain* 52:193, 1993.

192. Jensen OK, Nielsen FF, Vosmar L: An open study comparing manual therapy with the use of cold packs in the treatment of post-traumatic headache, *Cephalalgia* 10:241, 1990.

193. Hatch JP et al: The use of electromyography and muscle palpation in the diagnosis of tension-type headache with and without pericranial muscle involvement, *Pain* 49:175, 1992.

194. Watson DH, Trott PH: Cervical headache: an investigation of natural head posture and upper cervical

flexor muscle performance, *Cephalalgia* 13:272, 1993.

195. Mercer S, Marcus D, Nash J: Cervical musculoskeletal disorders in migraine and tension-type headache, *Phys Ther* 73:105, 1993 (abstract).

196. Levoska S, Keinanen-Kiukaanniemi S, Bloigu R: Repeatability of measurement of tenderness in the neck-shoulder region by dolorimeter and manual palpation, *Clin J Pain* 9:229, 1993.

197. Levoska S: Manual palpation and pain threshold in female office employees with and without neck-shoulder symptoms, *Clin J Pain* 9:236, 1993.

198. Hubka MJ, Phelan SP: Interexaminer reliability of palpation for cervical spine tenderness, *J Manipulative Physiol Ther* 17:591, 1994.

199. Sandmark H, Nisell R: Validity of five common manual neck pain provoking tests, *Scan J Rehab Med* 27:131, 1995.

200. Nilsson N: Measuring cervical muscle tenderness: a study of reliability, *J Manipulative Physiol Ther* 18:88, 1995.

201. Sandrini G et al: Comparative study with EMG, pressure algometry and manual palpation in tension-type headache and migraine, *Cephalalgia* 14:451, 1994.

202. Persson LCG, Carlsson JY: Headache in patients with neck-shoulder-arm pain of cervical radicular origin, *Headache* 39:218, 1999.

203. Stolk-Hornsveld F et al: Pain provocation tests for C0-C4 in the diagnosis of cervicogenic headache, *Cephalalgia* 19:436, 1999 (abstract).

204. Reeves JL, Jaeger B, Graff-Radford SB: Reliability of pressure algometer as a measure of myofascial trigger point sensitivity, *Pain* 24:313, 1986.

205. Jensen K et al: Pressure pain threshold in human temporal region: evaluation of a new pressure algometer, *Pain* 24:322, 1986.

206. Drummond P: Scalp tenderness and sensitivity to pain in migraine and tension headache, *Headache* 27:45, 1987.

207. List T, Helkimo M, Falk G: Reliability and validity of a pressure threshold meter in recording tenderness in the masseter muscle and the anterior temporalis muscle, *J Craniomandibular Pract* 7:223, 1989.

208. Langemark M et al: Pressure pain thresholds and thermal nociceptive thresholds in chronic tension-type headache, *Pain* 38:203, 1989.

209. Takala E: Pressure pain threshold on upper trapezius and levator scapulae muscles: repeatability and relation to subjective symptoms in a working population, *Scand J Rehabil Med* 22:62, 1990.

210. Hogeweg JA et al: Algometry: measuring pain threshold, method and characteristics in healthy subjects, *Scand J Rehabil Med* 24:99, 1992.

211. Bovim G: Cervicogenic headache, migraine and tension-type headache: pressure-pain threshold measurements, *Pain* 51:169, 1992.

212. Chung S, Un B, Kim H: Evaluation of pressure pain threshold in head and neck muscles by electronic algometer: intrarater and interrater reliability, *J Craniomandibular Pract* 10:28, 1998.

213. Jensen K et al: Pressure pain threshold in human temporal region: evaluation of a new pressure algometer, *Pain* 24:322, 1986.

214. Kosek E, Ekholm J, Nordemar R: A comparison of pressure pain thresholds in different tissues and body regions, *Scand J Rehabil Med* 25:117, 1993.

215. Mazzotta G et al: Study of pressure pain and cellular concentration of neurotransmitters related to nociception in episodic tension-type headache patients, *Headache* 37:565, 1997.

216. Bendtsen L et al: Pressure-controlled palpation: a new technique which increases the reliability of manual palpation, *Cephalalgia* 15:205, 1995.

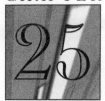

CHAPTER 25

Somatovisceral Research

Charles S. Masarsky, DC and Marion Todres-Masarsky, DC

Key Terms

ANGINA	ENCOPRESIS	RAND SF-36
AUTISM	ENDOSCOPIC	SKIN DRAG
CHIROPRACTIC ANALYSIS	ENURESIS	SNELLEN CHART
COLIC	FORCED EXPIRATORY	SOMATIC DYSFUNCTION
COMPUTERIZED	VOLUME	SOMATIC DYSPNEA
ELECTROENCEPHALOGRAPHY	FORCED VITAL CAPACITY	SOMATOVISCERAL
DESCRIPTIVE STUDIES	GRAND MAL SEIZURES	SPONTANEOUS REMISSION
DIPLOPIA	HORNER'S SYNDROME	STRABISMUS
DISEASE	HYPERTENSION	TACHYCARDIA
DYSFUNCTIONAL UTERINE	ISCHEMIC PENUMBRA	TINNITUS
BLEEDING	MERIC	TONE
DYSMENORRHEA	MYOPIA	ULCERS
DYSPNEA	NERVE TRACING	VASOMOTOR
DYSURIA	OUTCOME MEASURES	VERTEBROGENIC
EDGE LIGHT PUPIL CYCLE	PEAK EXPIRATORY FLOW	VITAL CAPACITY
TIME	PERIMETRY	
ELECTROCARDIOGRAPHIC	PROSTAGLANDIN	
ELECTROENCEPHALOGRAPHY	PUPILLARY RESPONSE	

Mainstream research organizations such as the Foundation for Chiropractic Education and Research (FCER) now actively support research on a wide range of **somatovisceral** disorders, and the definition of chiropractic provided by the Association for Chiropractic Colleges (ACC)[1,2] in 1996 (see Chapter 2 for the full ACC definition) appears to support the contention that somatovisceral considerations are part of mainstream chiropractic. However, a small sector of the profession still wishes to restrict chiropractic to the care of acute, uncomplicated musculoskeletal pain in adults.

Somatovisceral research findings are important, in part, because they represent the scientific study of chiropractic's role in maintaining wellness. Although wellness and general health can be studied in any patient, *whole-person benefits* are less obvious when attention is limited to

sprain and strain injuries. Research at the somatovisceral interface may provide a window into wellness.

Enhanced understanding of **somatic dysfunction** and the autonomic effects of the vertebral subluxation complex (VSC) can potentially improve chiropractic assessment methods. To the extent that measurement of autonomic **tone** becomes a routine step in evaluating VSC, every patient examination can serve as a lesson in the whole-person benefits of chiropractic care. This is no radical departure; the assessment of autonomic tone has a solid pedigree in chiropractic history (Fig. 25-1).

HISTORICAL PERSPECTIVES

An early method of **chiropractic analysis** was **nerve tracing**—the use of digital pressure to

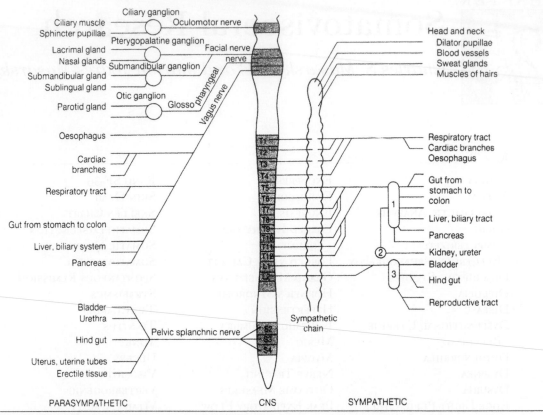

Fig. 25-1 The autonomic nervous system, showing at which levels and within which cranial and spinal nerves that autonomic fibers link with the central nervous system (CNS). *1,* Celiac ganglion; *2,* renal ganglion; *3,* pelvic ganglion. *(From Rogers AW:* Textbook of anatomy, Edinburgh, *1992, Churchill-Livingstone.)*

follow a line of hypersensitive tissue from an uncomfortable body part to the spine or vice versa. A nerve trace to a particular spinal segment was held to represent disturbed tone in the indicated spinal nerve. The chiropractor would suspect disturbed neurologic tone as a cause of dysfunction in all tissues (somatic or visceral) innervated by the indicated nerve.

D.D. Palmer's foundational concept of tone was understood to apply to any part of the body or the body as a whole[3]:

Life is the expression of tone. In that sentence is the basic principle of chiropractic. Tone is the normal degree of nerve tension. Tone is expressed in functions by normal elasticity, activity, strength, and excitability of the various organs, as observed in a state of health. Consequently, the cause of disease is any variation in tone.

In modern terms, *tone* would be defined as the rate or intensity of function of any tissue or organ, reflecting the neurologic integrity of that tissue or organ. Although the whole-body aspect of tone bears much resemblance to the contemporary concept of homeostasis, the segmental aspect of tone was the center of the nerve tracer's concern.

B.J. Palmer published photographs of many such nerve traces in a book written in 1911.[4] As the reproductions in Figs. 25-2 and 25-3 make clear, originating a nerve trace from an inguinal hernia or a deaf ear was held to be as legitimate as tracing from a sore shoulder or painful hip.

Nerve-tracing data, correlated with autonomic neuroanatomy, was systematized into the **meric** system of chiropractic analysis. This development was already under way when Mabel

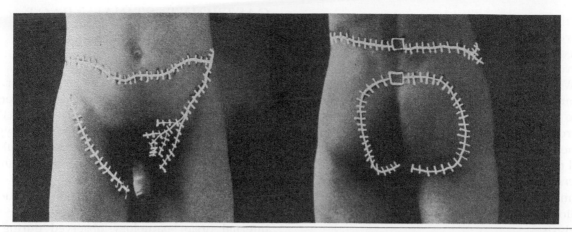

Fig. **25-2** Nerve trace of a patient with a history of inguinal hernia. The results of the nerve trace indicated an apparent relationship between the inguinal and scrotal areas and a lumbar and lumbosacral subluxation. (*Courtesy Palmer College of Chiropractic. From Palmer BJ: The philosophy, science and art of nerve tracing, Davenport, Iowa, 1911, Palmer School of Chiropractic.*)

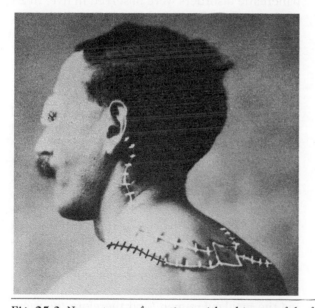
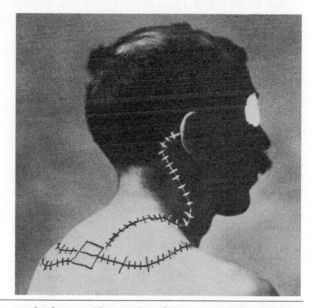

Fig. **25-3** Nerve trace of a patient with a history of deafness in both ears. The results of the nerve trace indicated an apparent relationship between the dysfunctional ears and a subluxation at T2-3. (*Courtesy Palmer College of Chiropractic. From Palmer BJ: The philosophy, science and art of nerve tracing, Davenport, Iowa, 1911, Palmer School of Chiropractic.*)

Palmer (the wife of B.J. Palmer) published *Chiropractic Anatomy* in 1918 and had reached maturity by the time R.W. Stephenson published his *Chiropractic Textbook* in 1927. In meric analysis, a clinical problem is considered in terms of the *zone* (the body section innervated by a particular pair of spinal nerves) in which it occurs. All tissue of a particular type within a zone is termed a *mere*. For example, a zone's muscle tissue is its *myomere*; its visceral tissue is its *viscemere*. This concept bears some resemblance to the contemporary concepts of the dermatome (i.e., the skin innervated by the sensory division of a particular spinal nerve) and the myotome (i.e., the muscles innervated by the motor division of a particular spinal nerve).

When a patient complained of stomach discomfort, the meric chiropractor would recognize the involved organ as part of the viscemere corresponding to the fifth through eighth thoracic vertebrae. The results of nerve tracing and the palpation of paraspinal *taut and tender fibers* would indicate the precise subluxated segment. If these results were ambiguous, a radiographic examination would clarify the analysis.[5]

By the early 1920s many chiropractors used the back of the hand to palpate for *hot boxes* (i.e., areas of increased temperature along the spine). Fascinated by this analytic method, Dossa D. Evins, a 1922 graduate of the Palmer School of Chiropractic, developed the neurocalometer, the first chiropractic heat-reading instrument. It consisted of two thermocouple probes and a galvanometer, which indicated left-to-right thermal asymmetry while the examiner glided the instrument up or down the spine. Persistent thermal asymmetry was taken to be a sign of disturbed **vasomotor** tone, consistent with the presence of VSC.[6]

To summarize, in chiropractic's early years, assessment of autonomic tone was an integral part of chiropractic analysis. This took the form of nerve tracing, meric analysis, and vasomotor analysis by instrument or by hand. The goal of this autonomic assessment was not to determine whether a patient could be cured of **hypertension,** asthma, constipation, or other visceral disorders. Rather, it was an essential part of characterizing a patient's state of disturbed tone (or *dis-ease*).

It was proposed that VSC could disturb the tone of any neurologically controlled function. Given this assumption, chiropractic analysis logically was not limited to muscular tone, but included vasomotor tone, bronchial tone, alimentary tone, and so forth. Contemporary somatovisceral research is best understood in the spirit of this traditional perspective. It is hoped that this research will encourage the modern evolution of D.D. Palmer's *science of tone.*

GASTROINTESTINAL TRACT

Clinical Research: Historical Perspectives

An early osteopathic research team, under the leadership of Louisa Burns, studied the effects of experimental spinal lesions on animals from 1907 to approximately 1948.[7] Hyperemia, hyperchlorhydria, petechial hemorrhages, and **ulcers** were found in the gastric mucosa of rabbits lesioned at T4-T7.

Medical researcher Henry K. Winsor[8] studied correlations between spinal curvatures and internal organ pathology observed during 50 autopsies at the University of Pennsylvania in 1922. Stomach pathology was identified in nine cadavers, liver **disease** was found in thirteen, gallbladder pathology was described in five, and pancreatic disorders were observed in five. In 28 of these 32 instances of alimentary pathology, curvature was noted in the T5-T9 area.

Chiropractic practitioner and educator Clarence Gonstead recorded a number of clinical insights relevant to the alimentary tract during his long career.[9] Gonstead found peptic ulcers and diarrhea to be most frequently related to upper cervical subluxation, and duodenal ulcers more frequently related to the T4-T10 region. Constipation was linked to multiple sites of subluxation, including T3-T5, T8-T12, L1-L4, and occasionally the upper cervical area.

Several osteopathic investigators have maintained that the upper cervical region and the area from T4-T10 were most often implicated in gastric, duodenal, and peptic ulcers.[10,11] Magoun,[12] an exponent of osteopathic cranial manipulation, has emphasized the importance of lesions affecting the jugular foramen (and therefore the vagus nerve) in the development of various kinds of ulcers and other gastrointestinal disease. An osteopathic study by Northup[13] and a study by Lindberg, Strachan, and Koehnlein[14] noted the association of the thoracolumbar area and colitis.

Controlled Experimental and Clinical Studies

Pikalov and Kharin[15] studied 11 adult patients with endoscopically demonstrated duodenal ulcer who received spinal manipulation supplemented with regional mobilization and manual soft tissue therapy. This group was compared with 24 ulcer patients receiving medication. Both groups were placed on a bland diet. Weekly physical and **endoscopic** examinations were the major **outcome measures.** Ulcer remission in the experimental group took place an average of 10 days earlier than in the control group. The most frequently manipulated segments were in the T9-T12 region.

The association of infantile **colic** and the VSC is controversial. To date, the published controlled clinical trials in this area have failed to settle the issue. A chiropractic team at the University of Odense in Denmark randomly assigned 50 colicky infants to chiropractic care or medication with the drug dimethicone.[16] Dimethicone, which decreases foam in the gastrointestinal tract, is prescribed for colic, although several controlled studies have shown it to be no better than placebo.[17,18] In the chiropractic group, adjustments were administered by light fingertip pressure at segments identified by motion palpation. Most of the adjustments were performed at the upper and middle thoracic regions. By day 12 of the study, the parents of the chiropractic group reported a 67% reduction in hours of crying; there was only a 38% reduction in the medication group. These results were statistically significant. The researchers concluded that, "either spinal manipulation is effective in the treatment of the visceral disorder infantile colic or infantile colic is, in fact, a musculoskeletal disorder."[16]

A contrasting view is provided by a study performed under the auspices of a University Pediatrics Department in Norway.[19] In this study, 86 infants were randomly assigned to chiropractic care or placebo (i.e., being held for 10 minutes by a nurse, rather than being given a 10-minute visit with the chiropractor). In the chiropractic group, adjustments were administered by light fingertip pressure. The methods used to identify involved segments were not described, and no mention was made of which regions were most frequently involved. Both groups experienced substantial decreases in crying—the primary outcome measure. Seventy

percent of the chiropractic group improved, compared with 60% of those held by nurses. However, no statistically significant differences were found between the two groups in terms of the number of hours of crying or as measured on a five-point improvement scale (from "getting worse" to "completely well"). The researchers concluded that, "chiropractic spinal manipulation is no more effective than placebo in the treatment of infantile colic."[19]

It is worth considering whether or not the descriptive literature, which is reviewed in the following section, indicates the existence of an important subset of colicky infants who do respond to chiropractic adjustments. It is suggested that the reader consider the implications of those cases in which the infant responded after a single adjustment, as well as cases in which previous medical intervention failed to resolve the colic. In addition, the reader should consider those cases in which well-described signs of VSC were reduced at the same time that symptoms of colic were reduced. In the absence of clear, effective medical protocols for infantile colic, and in view of the extreme distress that infants and their families can experience as a result of this disorder, the existence of a subset of VSC-related colic could justify a trial of chiropractic care for such infants.

Descriptive Research

A number of well-described cases and case series involving chiropractic care for colicky infants have been published. The most impressive case series to date was published by Klougart, Nilsson, and Jacobsen,[20] in which 38% of Denmark's chiropractors participated in a prospective study. According to parental reports, 90% of the infants improved within 2 weeks, with 23% improving after a single adjustment. The most commonly adjusted segments were occiput, C1 and C2.

A number of individual case reports are worthy of mention. Pluhar and Schobert[21] reported reduced crying, improved sleep, and increased formula consumption after a single adjustment of a 3-month-old girl with a 4-week history of colic. Previous medical intervention had not been successful. Hyman[22] reported alleviation of colicky crying, of back arching, and of flatulence after a single adjustment (at T9 and C1) of a 5-week-old boy with a 3-week history of colic.

In a case based on clinical records from the late 1940s and recently recovered from the files of the B.J. Palmer Research Clinic, Killinger and Azad[23] reported favorable results with a 5.5-month-old colicky infant after two modified Palmer upper cervical adjustments delivered over a period of 1 week.

Fallon and Lok[24] presented a case suggesting a possible cause for some cases of infantile colic. Their patient was a 3-week-old girl with a 2-day history of projectile vomiting, accompanied by colicky crying (up to 18 hours each day). Based on a previous medical diagnosis of pyloric stenosis, surgery had been recommended. The parents opted for a chiropractic consultation before surgery. Palpation of the right upper abdominal quadrant revealed a hard olive-shaped mass, consistent with hypertrophy of the pyloric muscles, thereby supporting the previous diagnosis of pyloric stenosis. A temperature asymmetry of 3° F was noted at the styloid fossae, and attempts to motion palpate the upper cervical spine produced a loud wail from the patient. Light-force upper cervical adjusting was the only intervention, with the exception of a T4 adjustment on one visit. The mother noted cessation of projectile vomiting and reduction in screaming at the fourth visit (eighth day of care); the temperature asymmetry was reduced to 2° F. By the tenth visit, screaming had ceased. The authors suggested that undiagnosed pyloric stenosis may be the cause of some cases of infantile colic.

A number of other **descriptive studies** in the gastrointestinal arena deserve mention. DeBoer, Schutz, and McKnight[25] demonstrated inhibition of stomach and duodenal smooth muscle in rabbits as a result of surgical misalignment of T6. Hewitt[26] described the case of a 7-month-old with chronic constipation. According to the patient's mother, the child had suffered from constipation since birth. At the initial examination, the mother reported that the child's bowel movements occurred between one time per day and one time every 3 days. Hours of straining and crying preceded each bowel movement, and

the consistency of the feces was described as similar to rabbit pellets. After chiropractic examination, gentle diversified adjusting was administered to L5-S1, L4-L5, T6-T7, to the atlantooccipital motion segments, and to the coronal suture. Four such adjustments were performed over a period of 8 weeks. During this time, the child had one to two soft, effortless stools per day, with the exception of 1 week of diarrhea secondary to chicken pox. At the time of publication, this improvement was stable at 1-year follow-up. In addition to the Hewitt study, cases involving constipation and other bowel disorders are described in the section on pelvic organic dysfunction.

Implications for Clinical Assessment

Much chiropractic clinical experience relevant to the gastrointestinal tract has been with pediatric patients. Nyiendo and Olsen[27] found that gastrointestinal problems were common primary complaints among pediatric patients attending a chiropractic teaching clinic. These investigators also found that pediatric patients were more likely than adult patients to have nonmusculoskeletal primary complaints. The widespread nerve supply to the gastrointestinal tract makes symptoms of distress in this system good general indicators of autonomic tone.

RESPIRATORY FUNCTION

Clinical Research: Historical Perspectives

Respiratory disorders attracted early and significant attention within the chiropractic and osteopathic research communities. As early as the 1920s, patients with asthma were routinely managed at the B.J. Palmer Clinic.

Of historic and scientific interest is a paper presented by Miller[28] at a 1975 Interdisciplinary Conference on Spinal Manipulation at the National Institutes of Health (NIH). In this study, 44 chronic obstructive pulmonary disease (COPD) patients underwent osteopathic examination. COPD is characterized by clinically significant, generalized obstruction of the airways associated with varying degrees of chronic bronchitis, loss of elastic fibers in the lung tissue, and rupture of the alveolar septa. The pathologic changes associated with COPD are generally considered to be irreversible.

Signs of somatic dysfunction noted in Miller's examination included asymmetry of paraspinal muscle tone, loss of intersegmental mobility, **skin drag** (i.e., palpatory assessment of asymmetry or local alteration in friction offered to the examiner's finger while it moves along the patient's paraspinal skin—a sign consistent with altered sweat gland activity caused by changes in autonomic tone), and *red reflex* (i.e., visual assessment of asymmetry or unusual intensity in reactive skin hyperemia after stroking with the examiner's fingertip or fingernail—a sign consistent with altered vasomotor activity caused by changes in autonomic tone). Based on this evaluation, the greatest number of abnormal findings was evident in the thoracic spine, particularly at T2-T5.

Miller's patients were randomly assigned to treatment and control groups. Both groups received standard medical interventions (including bronchodilators, postural drainage, and breathing exercises); the treatment group also received osteopathic manipulation, consisting of two visits per week (duration of care was not mentioned). Lung volumes were measured, and patients filled out a questionnaire on respiratory symptoms.

The lung volume results were inconclusive; both groups improved, with no significant difference between groups. However, more patients in the treatment group reported the ability to walk greater distances; they also reported fewer colds, less coughing, and less **dyspnea** than before treatment.

A case series by Hviid[29] failed to gather enough data to provide calculations of statistical significance. However, the preliminary data indicated that of 17 symptomatic asthma patients, more than 75% reported subjective improvement by the eighth chiropractic visit. More than 35% were symptom free by the eighth visit. Five of these patients demonstrated increased **vital capacity** (i.e., the amount of air expelled in a complete exhalation).

Controlled Experimental and Clinical Studies

Two controlled clinical studies have been published in this arena, both dealing with asthmatic patients. Nielsen and colleagues[30] reported a randomized controlled clinical trial of chiropractic care for adult asthma patients in which no statistically significant differences were found between sham adjustments and actual chiropractic intervention. The sham maneuver consisted of gentle, apparently specific manual pressure, with the patient positioned on a drop table. While this light pressure was applied with one hand, the drop mechanism was simultaneously released with the other hand. Because the whole patient sample experienced improvement by the end of the study, both in terms of asthma symptom severity and nonspecific bronchial hyperreactivity (i.e., a measure of resistance to histamine-induced bronchial obstruction), it is also possible that both the sham adjustments and the actual adjustments may have elicited healing effects.

An important and controversial study was published in 1998 by Balon and colleagues.[31] After a 3-week baseline evaluation period, 91 children who had continuing symptoms of asthma despite usual medical therapy were randomly assigned to receive either actual or sham chiropractic adjustments for 4 months. Morning **peak expiratory flow** (i.e., the maximum velocity of air during a forced exhalation) was the major outcome measure. Although both groups of children exhibited improved peak expiratory flow, no significant difference existed between groups. Both groups also demonstrated improvement in terms of secondary outcome measures such as quality of life, daytime symptoms, nighttime symptoms, and inhaler use. However no significant difference between groups was noted in terms of these secondary outcome measures.

The authors offer three possible explanations for the results of this study:

1. Patients in both groups may have responded favorably to frequent professional attention.
2. Patients in both groups may have been growing out of their symptoms at the time of the study.

3. Patients in both groups may have complied more with their medication schedules during the study than before the study.

Another possible explanation is that the sham treatment was not as biologically inert as a placebo should be. Simulated adjustive treatment included several distraction and low-amplitude, low-velocity impulse maneuvers to the cervical, thoracic, and lumbopelvic areas. As in the previously cited paper by Nielsen and colleagues,[30] Balon and colleagues[31] assumed that these simulated adjustments would not effect any correction of subluxation or elicit beneficial effects through other means. However, this assumption is questionable. The contemporary chiropractic perspective would anticipate that taking the spine through those movements could, in fact, affect the biomechanical integrity of spinal motion segments, influencing mechanoreceptor and nociceptor pathways. Such concerns are shared by Hondras, Linde, and Jones,[32] who noted in their Cochrane Collaboration review that sham-controlled trials may underestimate the actual benefit of manual therapy. Additional criticism of the sham procedure in the Balon study was offered by Jongeward[33] and Richards, Mein, and Nelson.[34]

Additional questions concerning the paper by Balon and colleagues was discussed by Rosner,[35] who noted that in a poster presentation at the May 1997 conference of the American Thoracic Society (17 months before publication in the *New England Journal of Medicine*), Balon and colleagues stated that the patients receiving real chiropractic adjustments improved in terms of nighttime symptoms to a significantly greater degree than those patients receiving the sham procedure. This important and encouraging result was not published in the *New England Journal of Medicine* paper authored by the same team. This discrepancy remains unexplained as of September, 2002.

Descriptive Research

The case of a COPD patient under chiropractic care was reported by Masarsky and Weber.[36] After a 2-week baseline period, diversified chiropractic adjustments were administered at various levels, usually including the upper cervical and upper thoracic regions. The frequency of visits was three times weekly for more than 14 months. Intersegmental traction, vitamin-C supplementation, cranial adjustments, and soft tissue procedures were also included in the chiropractic regimen. Outcome measures included **forced vital capacity** (FVC), a measure of the volume of air expelled in a single forceful exhalation; **forced expiratory volume** in 1 second (FEV_1), a measure of the volume of air expelled in the first second of a forceful exhalation; patient ratings on a 10-point severity scale (with *1* mildest and *10* most extreme) for coughing, dyspnea, and fatigue; and a daily count of laryngospasms. Up to three laryngospasms per week had been the norm for the subject for 17 years.

Mean scores during the last 7 months of this study were compared with the mean baseline scores. FVC increased by more than 1.0 L, and FEV_1 increased by more than 0.3 L. Coughing intensity, dyspnea, and fatigue all decreased sharply. The patient reported no laryngospasms during the final 5 months of the study. Improved lung volumes lagged behind the subjective improvements by several months. These functional improvements are very encouraging, given that the pathologic changes of COPD are generally considered irreversible.

Peet, Marko, and Piekarczyk[37] reported similarly encouraging results with a group of 8 pediatric patients with medically diagnosed asthma. After 10 adjustments according to Chiropractic Biophysics Technique (CBP) protocols, this patient group demonstrated an average increase in peak flow of 25%. The parents of seven of the eight children also reported a decrease in medication use.

Another instructive case involving pediatric asthma was presented by Bachman and Lantz.[38] After three Gonstead adjustments at T3, T12, and the sacrum, the 34-month-old patient experienced 8 weeks of freedom from symptoms. During the previous year, the patient had weekly asthma attacks, twenty of which were severe enough to require visits to the hospital emergency department. An exacerbation at 8 weeks followed a fall from a stepladder; this time the asthma symptoms were accompanied by nocturnal **enuresis.** Both sets of symptoms resolved after three more adjustments at the same levels. After a full year of freedom from symptoms, the boy fell from a horse and experienced a return of both asthma and enuresis. A single adjustment resolved this exacerbation. The researchers reported no recurrence after 2 years of follow-up evaluation. Peet[39] presented the case of an 8-year-old girl medically diagnosed with asthma 3 years before initiation of chiropractic care. Interestingly, this patient exhibited no evidence of respiratory disease until suffering a traumatic injury. This injury was severe enough to cause dislocation of the left elbow. Medication delivered by inhaler was used by this patient one to three times per day before the first chiropractic visit. After eight adjustments according to CBP protocols over a period of 2.5 weeks, the mother stated that the child had not used an inhaler for 2 days, was not wheezing, and could run without gasping. At the time of publication, the patient was reported to have been free of asthmatic attacks for 4 months without medication.

After a retrospective study of the files of 79 patients with medically diagnosed bronchial asthma, Nilsson and Christiansen[40] reported that patients likely to have a good response to chiropractic care tend to have less severe asthma symptoms at presentation and an earlier age of onset than do those patients with a poor response.

Masarsky and Weber[41] reported on six cases of dyspnea that resolved upon correction of VSC and related somatic dysfunctions. The term *somatic dyspnea* was coined to refer to such clinical situations. All six patients demonstrated midthoracic fixations on motion palpation, leading clinicians to suspect restriction of rib excursion, disturbance to the sympathetic nerve supply to the lungs and bronchi, or both of these problems. One patient reported a clear-cut association between a C2-C3 correction and relief from dyspnea, suggesting a connection to the phrenic nerve. The most common extravertebral dysfunction associated with somatic dyspnea was at the temporomandibular joint. Somatic dyspnea is a subjective symptom; it is not always accompanied by measurable depression of lung volumes. However, the improved subjective ease of breathing is often rapid and dramatic.

A small but important body of work has demonstrated improved lung volumes in patients without respiratory symptoms and with initial lung volumes within normal limits. Masarsky and Weber[42] presented a retrospective study in which FVC and FEV$_1$ improved in a sample of 50 chiropractic patients after one to three diversified adjustments. The majority of these patients had no respiratory complaints at initiation of care and demonstrated FVC and FEV$_1$ within normal limits at intake examination. An additional instance of spirometric improvement in a lung-normal patient appeared in a later case series published by the same authors (case 1).[43]

Kessinger reported FVC and FEV$_1$ improvement in a sample of 55 patients after they had received chiropractic care for the correction of upper cervical subluxation.[44] These improvements were significant in the 33 patients with depressed lung volumes at initiation of care and in the 22 patients with initially normal lung volumes.

Implications for Clinical Assessment

Although the lungs are visceral organs, skeletal muscles make inspiration and expiration possible. These include the diaphragm, external and internal intercostals, sternocleidomastoids, levator scapulae, serrati, scalenes, abdominals, trapezii, latissimus dorsi, pectoralis major, and pectoralis minor muscles. In other words, breathing is a musculoskeletal act. More than most bodily functions, breathing straddles the somatovisceral interface. Even if researchers never provided direct evidence that the chiropractic adjustment can improve the lung tissue of pulmonary patients, maintaining the tone of the respiratory muscles of such patients through the chiropractic adjustment would still be a worthy goal.

Although objective measures (e.g., lung volumes) and subjective measures (e.g., respiratory symptom severity) do not directly demonstrate the presence of VSC, such measures do help demonstrate the tone of skeletal and smooth respiratory muscles. As reflections of tone, respiratory observations and measurements can be useful to the chiropractor in assessing clinical outcome.

Taken together, the results on lung-normal patients reported in the two studies by Masarsky and Weber[42,43] and the Kessinger[44] study imply that even people with normal lung volumes may be functioning well below their potential, and that chiropractic care may improve this already normal physiology. The general health implications of improved pulmonary function cannot be overstated. Lung volumes have long been recognized as a biologic marker of aging. Improvement in these volumes may be seen as tantamount to enhancing vitality and reversing at least one effect of aging.

CARDIOVASCULAR FUNCTION

Clinical Research: Historical Perspectives

Chiropractic's concern with cardiovascular health goes back to the profession's earliest days. D.D. Palmer[45] described a case of "heart trouble" shortly after the Harvey Lillard case. A later contribution was made by chiropractic clinician, educator, and researcher Carl S. Cleveland Jr.[46] Using surgically implanted spinal splints, Cleveland produced segmental spinal misalignments in the spines of rabbits. Physiologic measures on live rabbits were correlated with postmortem findings. In this innovative first attempt by chiropractic investigators to use an animal model of subluxation, heart diseases, valvular leakages, arrhythmias, and vasomotor paralysis were noted, but the exact spinal levels were apparently not reported. (For further discussion of this study, see Chapter 7.)

Henry K. Winsor, the medical anatomist previously mentioned in the discussion of the gastrointestinal tract, reported autopsy results correlating regions of spinal curvature to 20 cases of heart and pericardium pathology.[8] Spinal curvature was found in the T1-5 region in 18 cases and at C7-T1 in two cases (see Chapter 8).

Osteopathic investigators conducted a great deal of the early research correlating spinal function to cardiovascular health. Louisa Burns' research team[47-49] found experimentally induced lesions from T2 to T4 to be most likely to be followed by cardiac pathology in rabbits. Clinical researchers Becker[50] and Koch[51] implicated dysfunction of the T1-T6 region in human heart disease.

In a small case series reported by Appleyard,[52] dysfunction in the upper cervical and upper thoracic regions was found to correlate with **angina** pectoris. **Electrocardiographic** (ECG) abnormalities noted before osteopathic manipulation were found to have normalized 30 minutes after treatment.

Northup[53] reviewed records of 100 hypertensive patients under osteopathic care and reported that dysfunction at T8-T9, the upper cervical area, and the occipitomastoid suture were most frequently found in those patient whose hypertension normalized under osteopathic manipulative therapy. Citing many years of clinical experience, Lewit,[54,55] a Czech medical physician and manual medicine practitioner, maintains that paroxysmal **tachycardia** with no organic heart lesion routinely responds to osteopathic spinal manipulation.

Controlled Experimental and Clinical Studies

The only recent chiropractic controlled clinical trial in the cardiovascular arena is the hypertension study by Yates and colleagues.[56] Although the number of subjects was small and the physiologic outcome was only measured for the short term (i.e., 1 to 10 minutes postadjustment), this carefully designed study provides a useful model for future work. Twenty-one patients with elevated blood pressure were randomly assigned to active-treatment (adjustments in the T1 to T5 region, based on Activator and protocols), placebo treatment (sham adjustments with the Activator instrument set on zero tension), and control (no intervention) groups. Noting that previous studies may have been confounded by elevated initial readings caused by anxiety (i.e., *white coat hypertension*), Yates and colleagues used a standard psychologic questionnaire before and after the intervention. They found a statistically significant decrease in both systolic and diastolic blood pressure in the active treatment group but not in the placebo or control groups. Because the active and control groups did not differ on anxiety reduction, this was ruled out as an explanation for the difference between groups. These findings support the hypothesis that short-term blood pressure reduction in hypertensives is a physiologic effect of the chiropractic adjustment.

Descriptive Research

A number of well-described cases involving patients with hypertension have been published in the recent chiropractic literature. Plaugher and Bachman[57] published an instructive case study involving a 38-year-old man with a 14-year history of hypertension. The patient also reported side effects caused by his two medications, including bloating sensations, depression, fatigue, and impotence. Low back pain was also reported as an incidental issue.

Examination according to Gonstead protocols revealed evidence of VSC at various levels, particularly in the midcervical, upper thoracic, and middle thoracic regions. Adjustments were administered once per week. After three visits, the patient's medical doctor was able to reduce the dose of one medication and stop administration of the other one. All medication was discontinued after seven visits. After this, the frequency of visits was reduced to twice per month. Follow-up at 18 months showed that blood pressure was stabilized within normal limits without medication. Bloating, depression, fatigue, and low back pain abated; normal sexual function returned.

Connelly and Rasmussen[58] reported favorable results with three hypertensive patients using the cranial procedures of DeJarnette's sacrooccipital technique (SOT). Particular attention was given to dysfunction of the occipitomastoid suture in these cases. DeJarnette theorized that opening the occipitomastoid suture decompresses the jugular foramen, resulting in a reduced interference to the vagus nerve and subsequent normal-

ization of blood pressure. SOT and osteopathic cranial theory are in apparent agreement in this regard; Northup[59] also emphasized the importance of the occipitomastoid suture.

A number of interesting studies involve ECG studies of subjects under chiropractic care. Lott and colleagues[60] reported ECG improvements in three of four patients after chiropractic adjustments in conjunction with diet and exercise advice. All four patients experienced improvement in blood pressure, heart rate, or both.

Implications for Clinical Assessment

From the perspective of chiropractic analysis, a history of cardiovascular disease does not isolate an area of subluxation with any certainty. However, increased suspicion is warranted regarding subluxation at the upper thoracic and upper cervical regions of the spine and the occipitomastoid suture of the cranium.

Plaugher and Bachman[57] note that the combined effects of antihypertensive medication and chiropractic adjustments can temporarily drive a patient's blood pressure below normal levels. A patient experiencing vertigo secondary to hypotension after a chiropractic adjustment may be concerned about the possibility of a stroke or some other form of damage. Explaining the possibility of transient hypotension to such a patient at the beginning of treatment is advisable.

PELVIC ORGANIC DYSFUNCTION

Clinical Research: Historical Perspectives

Current understanding of the influence of spinal dysfunction on the pelvic organs (i.e., urogenital tract, lower intestinal tract) owes much to early osteopathic and chiropractic investigators. Clarence Gonstead found that diarrhea was most frequently related to upper cervical subluxation.[9] Gonstead implicated multiple sites of subluxation in association with constipation, including T3-5, T8-12, L1-4, and occasionally the upper cervical area.

Osteopathic investigator Northup[13] emphasized the importance of lesions at the thoracolumbar junction in patients with mucous colitis. Lindberg, Strachan, and Koehnlein[14] demonstrated a correlation between spinal lesions from T6-L1 and colitis, based on analysis of 349 cases at the Chicago Osteopathic Hospital.

Controlled Experimental and Clinical Studies

To date, dysmenorrhea and pediatric nocturnal enuresis are the only pelvic organic dysfunctions subjected to controlled study in the chiropractic scientific community. In a 1979 study, Thomason and colleagues[61] looked at the responses of eleven women suffering from menstrual pain and dysfunction. Among women given lumbar side-posture adjustments, 88% demonstrated significant symptomatic improvement (as assessed by a menstrual symptom questionnaire), whereas none of the women in a control group or in a sham adjustment group reported significant improvement.

In another small trial, Kokjohn and colleagues[62] used both symptomatic measurements and serum **prostaglandin** levels as outcome measures. Citing previous biomedical research implicating elevated serum levels of prostaglandins as an important cause of symptoms of **dysmenorrhea**, Kokjohn's team theorized that chiropractic adjustments might reduce these levels. However, there was no statistically significant difference in serum prostaglandin levels between women receiving side-posture adjustments and women in the control or sham adjustment groups. Nevertheless, symptomatic improvement in the experimental group was approximately twice that of the control group, a statistically significant finding that confirmed Thomason's findings.

Hondras, Long, and Brennan's follow-up study[63] to the earlier study by Kokjohn and colleagues failed to find significant differences in pain (as measured by visual analog scales [VASs]), disability (as measured by questionnaire), or serum prostaglandin levels of dysmenorrhea sufferers receiving side-posture manipulation versus patients receiving a sham procedure. Patients in both the manipulation and sham groups demonstrated mild improvement.

It should be noted that the sham procedure in both the Kokjohn and Hondras studies may not have been as biologically inert as the investigators supposed. It involved a low-amplitude side-posture thrust with both of the patient's legs flexed, rather than one leg flexed. It was supposed that the flexion of both legs and the reduced amplitude of the thrust would constitute a maneuver that would not correct biomechanical dysfunction. The long history of minimal-force chiropractic adjusting techniques such as Logan basic and SOT pelvic blocking should serve as a caution against such an assumption. The absence of significant differences between the two procedures in the Kokjohn and Hondras studies could reflect that both procedures were corrective at least to the extent of affecting symptom severity, if not prostaglandin levels.

Leboeuf and colleagues[64] presented a study on nocturnal enuresis, in which the bedwetting children served as their own controls. Baselines were established by monitoring the children for 2 to 4 weeks before the administration of chiropractic adjustments. Based on parental records, no significant difference was found between the baseline and intervention periods. These investigators did not note which spinal levels were adjusted or the methods used to determine these levels.

A contrasting view is provided in a more recent study by Reed and colleagues,[65] in which after a 2-week baseline period the children were divided into two groups: (1) a group receiving sham adjustments administered with an Activator instrument set on zero tension and (2) a group receiving actual adjustments, generally in the upper cervical and pelvic areas. The group receiving actual adjustments experienced a statistically significant (17.9%) decrease in the frequency of wet nights, compared with a slight increase in wet night frequency among the group receiving sham adjustments.

Descriptive Research

Liebl and Butler[66] demonstrated substantial improvement in a patient suffering from dysmenorrhea, based on a daily symptom-intensity diary.

Hawk, Long, and Azad[67] presented a study of 19 women with pelvic pain of at least 6-months' duration, unrelated to the menstrual cycle. Concomitant complaints included constipation, diarrhea, painful intercourse, and urinary problems. After 6 weeks of flexion-distraction adjustments and manual trigger point work, statistically significant improvement was demonstrated in pain levels as measured by the Pain Disability Index and the VAS. Reduced emotional distress was also indicated by statistically significant improvement in the Beck Depression Inventory and the problems subscale of the RAND-36 Health Survey.

Perhaps the most compelling body of case studies and case series in this literature has been presented by Browning,[68-76] whose work demonstrates a relationship between pelvic pain and organic dysfunction and spinal nerve root irritation at the S2 to S4 levels. The dermatomes corresponding to these levels, which are most readily tested at the buttocks, are often overlooked in clinical examination. Straight-leg raising enhanced by suprapubic pressure will often provoke intrapelvic pain in these patients, as will digital pressure at the L5-S1 intervertebral space enhanced by lumbar lateral flexion. These sensory signs provide the practitioner with useful outcome measures for patients with VSC associated with lower sacral nerve root involvement.

Particularly interesting among Browning's cases was a woman who had undergone appendectomy, left oophorectomy and partial hysterectomy, three bowel surgeries, and four bladder surgeries over a period of 18 years.[68] These procedures failed to resolve many complaints related to pelvic organic dysfunction, and the patient presented to Browning with pelvic pain, rectal bleeding, diarrhea, bladder discomfort, pain on intercourse, and anorgasmy. Noting signs of S2-4 irritation, Browning began a course of lumbosacral flexion-distraction adjustments. Within 4 weeks the symptom complex was noticeably responding, and complete resolution was obtained by 30 weeks. A fascinating aspect of this patient's history was the conspicuous absence of one symptom in particular: low back pain.

Well-described cases of nocturnal enuresis have been presented by Gemmell and Jacobson[77] and more recently by Blomerth.[78] An interesting case involving daytime urinary incontinence in a 12-year-old girl was reported by Stude, Bergmann, and Finer.[79] This patient had to wear a sanitary pad every day for more than 1 year, because of unpredictable urinary leakage. Prior evaluation by a medical pediatrician and an urologist had failed to provide a definitive diagnosis. Three months of diversified adjusting focusing on the sacroiliac and L3-4 segments provided only slight relief from this problem. At 3 months, periarticular pain was noted during an examination of the sacrococcygeal joint. At this time the patient remembered a slip-and-fall injury to that area just before the urinary incontinence made its appearance. After coccygeal adjustments were added to the regimen, the incontinence resolved in four visits, with no recurrence of the urinary symptoms during 4 years of follow-up.

Eriksen[80] presented the case of a 5-year-old girl who reportedly experienced constipation since beginning to walk. This problem had become more severe during the course of the year before chiropractic care began; at the time of the first examination, the patient was experiencing only one bowel movement per week, despite medication. The patient's mother and grandmother indicated that the child was also becoming increasingly lethargic. Examination results indicated upper cervical VSC, which was addressed with Grostic upper cervical adjusting. The day after the first adjustment, the patient experienced a bowel movement without medication; over the next 2 weeks the child had four to six bowel movements per week. The family noted increased energy levels during this time. An exacerbation of the constipation and VSC signs occurred 10 weeks into care after a fall. These were quickly resolved, and at the time of publication the patient was experiencing daily bowel movements without medication.

Falk[81] reported a series of three adult male patients with low back pain and associated pelvic organic problems. Two of the men suffered work-related injuries to the low back with concomitant difficulty in voiding. In both cases the low back pain and **dysuria** were resolved after 2 weeks of diversified side-posture adjusting of the L5-S1 motion segment. The third man experienced low back pain and sciatica unrelated to any known trauma, with concomitant constipation. A brief course of side-posture L5-S1 adjusting resolved these symptoms. Since the original episode, the patient experienced several exacerbations; each instance of low back pain was accompanied by constipation, and each episode was rapidly resolved under chiropractic care. Citing years of clinical experience, Falk maintains that most patients with low back pain have associated pelvic organic problems; however, most clinicians focus on the musculoskeletal complaint and may miss these important and interesting visceral concomitants.

Dysfunctional uterine bleeding (DUB) is nonmenstrual bleeding of unknown cause. Medical management includes the use of progestin therapy, estrogen therapy, dilation and curettage, and hysterectomy. Stude[82] reported the case of a 40-year-old woman with primary complaints of low back pain and bilateral leg pain; the patient was also 6 days into an episode of DUB. Within 1 day of the first chiropractic adjustment, which focused on the lumbar spine, uterine bleeding diminished to mild spotting. All symptoms were resolved after the second adjustment. One year after the initial visit, the patient experienced a new DUB episode with no concomitant musculoskeletal symptoms. Two weeks of chiropractic care resolved the symptoms and VSC signs, and a medical examination resulted in a clean bill of health. Although this patient's episodic DUB may have been self-limiting, the rapidity of response suggests a possible physiologic effect of the chiropractic adjustment.

Wagner and colleagues[83] reported the case of a 25-year-old woman with a 5-year history of irritable bowel syndrome (IBS). The patient's major symptoms were sharp intestinal pain and diarrhea. Diversified adjustments focusing on the upper cervical and thoracolumbar regions resulted in cessation of symptoms immediately after the first adjustment. After 2 years the patient was being seen approximately once per month and had not experienced any recurrence of IBS symptoms.

Implications for Clinical Assessment

In the private clinical setting, the practitioner is not primarily concerned with populations or statistical norms but with the situation of one unique patient at a time. Although it would be irresponsible for doctors of chiropractic to promise the treatment or cure of pelvic organic disorders, such disorders clearly may be among the clinical expressions of a particular patient's VSC. Careful attention to any history of such disorders is especially warranted when pain in the upper neck or lower back are the primary initial complaints. As the case unfolds, the pelvic organic symptoms may rise and fall along with signs of VSC. When the clinician is aware of this possible linkage, the pelvic organic disorders can be monitored as part of assessing patients' progress and arriving at recommendations for frequency of visits, return to normal daily activities, and so forth. When patients are aware of this linkage, it can reinforce their understanding that spinal pain is not the only manifestation of VSC and therefore not the only rationale for a chiropractic evaluation.

Signs of lower sacral nerve root involvement, when present, can provide the clinician with an additional dimension of clinical assessment. Browning[76] has proposed a system of categorizing patients with pelvic pain and organic dysfunction into Type I (in which the pelvic organic complaints are relatively mild) and Type II (in which the pelvic organic complaints are more severe and widespread). Although a detailed discussion of this system is beyond the scope of this chapter, the reader is encouraged to explore its potential use in clinical decision making.

SPECIAL SENSES

Clinical Research: Historical Perspectives

D.D. Palmer's first patient suffered from hearing loss.[4] According to Palmer, the following occurred:

On Sept. 18, 1895, Harvey Lillard called upon me. He was so deaf for seventeen years that he could not hear the noises on the street. Mr. Lillard informed me that he was in a cramped position, and felt something give in his back. I replaced the displaced fourth dorsal vertebra by one move, which restored his hearing fully.

Detractors of the chiropractic profession have challenged this case description for more than a century. A frequently cited argument against the possibility of VSC affecting the special senses is that these senses are primarily mediated via cranial nerves, not spinal nerves. In the specific case of Harvey Lillard, it is often mentioned that the sense of hearing is served by cranial nerve VIII—rather far from the fourth thoracic vertebra.

Such arguments overlook the autonomic connection. All nerves, including cranial nerves, require a vascular supply. This vascular supply requires innervation by autonomic fibers, primarily from the sympathetic outflow (T1-L2) of the spine. Indeed, it may well be said that when the connection between a health problem and a subluxation is not apparent, the clinician should consider the nerve supply to the blood supply. Autonomic innervation also controls other structures essential to the special senses, such as the pupils of the eye. A small but growing area of chiropractic research is literature focusing on the special senses.

Controlled Experimental and Clinical Studies

The only controlled chiropractic study involving the visual system is the work on pupil diameter by Briggs and Boone.[84] During a 4-day baseline period, 15 subjects had their pupils photographed in a darkened room using infrared film. Chiropractic analysis was performed during this same period, primarily based on heat-reading instrumentation and the Derefield-Thompson leg check. Eight subjects were found to have signs of cervical subluxation, whereas seven did not. After adjustment of the subluxated subjects with toggle-recoil or diversified methods and light soft tissue massage of the unsubluxated subjects, a fifth pupil measurement was performed. Although the subjects receiving massage demonstrated no postintervention change in pupillary diameter, there was change in all of the adjusted subjects (dilation in some and constriction in others). Briggs and

Boone suggest that cervical subluxation creates imbalance in the tone of the sympathetic and parasympathetic innervation to the pupils. As such, pupillary diameter may provide a noninvasive method for studying autonomic balance.

Descriptive Research

Gilman and Bergstrand[85] reported the case of a 75-year-old man with a 6-month history of total blindness after a head trauma. After three upper cervical adjustments, the patient was able to tell the difference between light and darkness. After eleven adjustments administered over a 3-month period, the patient could distinguish colors and experienced a return of the normal pupillary response. After 5 months of care, the patient was able to read again.

Although spontaneous remission of posttraumatic blindness has been reported, it is rare after 6 months. Gilman and Bergstrand suggest that upper cervical VSC may cause retinal vasospasm if sufficient irritation to the superior cervical sympathetic ganglia exists.

A fascinating body of ophthalmologic clinical research features automated static **perimetry** as a major outcome measure.[86-92] In this technique, points of light of various intensities are projected at different spots on a hemispheric screen placed over a patient's head. The patient presses a button each time a point of light is seen. Computerized mapping of the patient's visual field based on these responses identifies perceptual defects not usually detected by less sensitive techniques. Gorman's work has proved controversial in the Australian medical community. For this reason the work appears primarily in chiropractic journals.

Gorman, an ophthalmologist, has repeatedly noted improved perimetry results after general (i.e., *panspinal*) manipulation, usually performed under anesthesia. Most of these results have been verified by an independent medical ophthalmologist. Patients have included adults and children, traumatic and nontraumatic cases, mildly depressed visual sensitivity, and overt bilateral tunnel vision. Concomitant problems, such as neck pain, headache, arm pain, dizziness, fatigue, and abdominal pain, often resolve with the visual problems. Gorman hypothesizes that microischemia of the retina, the optic nerve, or the visual cortex may be related to spinal dysfunction.

Alcantara and Parker[93] provided an instructive case study involving a 6-year-old boy with bilateral internal **strabismus.** The parents indicated that the patient's problem began to become noticeable at the age of 2 years. No other significant clinical history was noted, except for the child's umbilical cord being wrapped around his neck at birth. Analysis using Gonstead protocols revealed evidence of upper cervical, lower cervical, and sacral subluxations. Within 10 visits, based on optometric examination, the patient's internal strabismus was barely noticeable and vision was measurably improved.

Gibbons, Gosling, and Holmes[94] presented a promising pilot study using the **edge light pupil cycle time** (ELPCT). ELPCT is measured by focusing the beam of a slit lamp so that it overlaps the edge of the patient's pupil. The pupil then constricts until it is beyond the light beam. After a brief latency period it dilates again, until the edge of the pupil once again enters the beam of light. Simply by holding the beam in a steady position, the pupil is made to oscillate between constriction and dilation. The time that it takes the pupil to go through one cycle of such constriction and dilation is measured in milliseconds. Pupil constriction is controlled by parasympathetic fibers from the oculomotor nerve (cranial nerve III), whereas dilation is controlled by sympathetic fibers arising primarily from the cervical sympathetic ganglia. ELPCT therefore reflects pupillary control by both divisions of the autonomic nervous system. Normal values have been established for ELPCT, and cycle time is prolonged in whiplash, **Horner's syndrome**, diabetes mellitus, multiple sclerosis (MS), and other disorders.

In this study, 13 subjects received a single osteopathic manipulation at the C1-C2 level (the side to be manipulated was chosen at random). ELPCT after manipulation was reduced (i.e., improved) to a statistically significant degree when compared with premanipulation levels. This effect was more pronounced in the eye on the side to which the upper cervical manipulation was administered.

In a study making elegant use of ordinary examination procedures, Kessinger and Boneva[95] reported visual acuity of subjects as measured by standard **Snellen chart** testing before receiving and 6 weeks after receiving upper cervical chiropractic care. The 67 subjects in this study were between the ages of 9 and 79. The most interesting finding was that the percentage of distance visual acuity (%DVA) increased among all subjects, including those with normal distance vision at the initial examination.

Tinnitus, or ringing in the ears, is a disturbance of hearing that can be distressing, often leading to insomnia and occasionally even suicide. Blum[96] offered a case report of a shipping clerk who was exposed to a high-decibel noise at work. The patient was unable to hear anything for approximately 30 minutes. As the day progressed, the patient began to experience ringing, hissing, buzzing, and warbling sounds. Treatment by an ear, nose, and throat specialist was not promising. When first visiting Dr. Blum's office, the patient was sleeping no more than 2 hours per night and would experience crying spells for 6 hours per day.

Chiropractic adjustments using sacrooccipital technique protocols for category II were instituted. (Category II protocols focus on a type of sacroiliac subluxation and correlates it with temporomandibular joint, cervical and cranial dysfunction.) Relief was noted after the first visit. At the time the paper was written, the patient reported improved sleep and more than a 50% decrease in tinnitus intensity.

In an earlier paper on tinnitus, Terrett[97] extensively reviewed the literature. Based on this review, the author advised a trial of chiropractic care for tinnitus patients, with special emphasis on the cervical and upper thoracic regions of the spine. Of special interest was the review of a case by manual medicine practitioner John Bourdillon. A patient of Bourdillon's was being treated for Meniere's disease, with symptoms including vertigo, tinnitus, and unilateral deafness. Only transient relief was obtained by cervical manipulation. When the T4-T5 motion segment was addressed, the patient experienced "dramatic and lasting relief of all the symptoms, including deafness." The similarity of this case to D.D. Palmer's famous Harvey Lillard case is difficult to escape.

Implications for Clinical Assessment

Infrared pupillometry, automated static perimetry, and ELPCT are not commonly performed in chiropractic offices. However, research to date suggests that the special senses may be sensitive to VSC. Further study of the potential role of chiropractic care in improving special sensory function is warranted, perhaps in clinical collaboration with optometrists, ophthalmologists, and otolaryngologists.

IMMUNE SYSTEM

Clinical Research: Historical Perspectives

The competence of the immune system has been a concern of the chiropractic and osteopathic professions from their earliest days. Both professions maintained that the body's immunocompetence is a more important factor in disease than the pathogenicity of germs. Emphasizing the importance of normal nerve supply for the disease resistance of all body tissues, D.D. Palmer[3] directed the chiropractic clinician's attention to specific spinal levels for a variety of diseases. Elaborating on A.T. Still's concept that the goal of osteopathy is to see that circulation is unimpeded so that the body's inner "drug store" may be well run, Hazzard[98] discussed "the bactericidal power of the blood."

Controlled Experimental and Clinical Studies

In a 1991 study, Brennan and colleagues[99] injected a nontoxic sealant into the posterior facet joints of four dogs at various thoracic and lumbar levels, in an attempt to mimic VSC through surgical joint fixation. Four other dogs underwent sham surgery. White blood cell (WBC) functional activity was measured in both groups during postsurgical recovery. Although functional activity levels of lymphocytes and polymorphonuclear neutrophils were depressed in both groups, the dogs that underwent sham surgery recovered normal WBC function in a shorter time than did the dogs with spinal joint fixation.

Another study by Brennan and colleagues[100] used human volunteers; thoracic adjustment/ manipulation (diversified maneuvers at levels indicated by motion palpation), sham manipulation (light-force thrust with no audible or palpable joint release), and soft tissue manipulation (light massage at the gluteal area) groups were compared. Blood was drawn both before and after interventions. Both polymorphonuclear neutrophils and monocytes demonstrated increased functional activity after thoracic manipulation but not after sham or soft tissue manipulation. The difference between groups was statistically significant. A second component of this study explored the role of a particular neurotransmitter (substance P) in spine-to-WBC communication. The results were inconclusive.

Descriptive Research

Lewit,[54] studied 76 children with chronic tonsillitis under the care of an otolaryngologist and reported the following:

The most striking and constant clinical finding was movement restriction at the craniocervical junction, in the great majority between occiput and atlas (70 cases, or 92%). Twenty-eight cases underwent operation, without having been manipulated; 25 suffered from movement restriction, and in 19 of these cases blockage was unaffected by tonsillectomy and was treated later (i.e., 3 to 6 months after operation). Thirty seven children were given manipulative treatment and followed up for 5 years; in 18 cases tonsillitis never recurred after manipulation; however, in seven of them, movement restriction did recur and had to be treated.

Lewit noted that in addition to restriction at the atlantooccipital level (with spasm of the short neck extensors), increased tension in the muscles frequently existed below the mandible near the tonsils.

Alcorn[101] tracked the serum immunoglobulin (i.e., antibody) levels of four patients with musculoskeletal pain under chiropractic care. Among the three patients who experienced symptomatic relief, there were elevations in serum immunoglobulin levels; the one patient who made no symptomatic progress demonstrated a decrease in serum antibody levels. Alcorn suggested that **vertebrogenic** stress might have increased the serum levels of the adrenal hormone cortisol, which is known to suppress lymphocyte production of antibodies. Statistical analysis was not possible because of the small number of patients.

Among a group of eight patients with chronic musculoskeletal conditions under chiropractic care, Vora and Bates[102] reported changes in lymphocyte levels. Five patients exhibited an increase in levels of circulating B lymphocytes; levels of T lymphocytes increased in one patient. Again, the small number of patients precluded meaningful statistical analysis.

Thomas and Wilkinson[103] published a case study of an adult woman with frank spina bifida from T11 to L2. Among other problems, the patient suffered from long-standing recurrent bladder infections despite a daily regimen of antibiotics. With chiropractic care (a variety of techniques over 5 years), infections became less frequent; at the time of the report the patient had been infection free for more than 1 year without antibiotics.

Araghi[104] presented the case of a 2-year-old girl with myasthenia gravis (MG). After 5 months of steady deterioration despite medical attention, the patient began to respond after a single Gonstead adjustment at the upper cervical and sacroiliac levels. MG is now widely seen as an autoimmune condition, in which the acetylcholine receptors at the myoneuronal junction are attacked by the patient's own WBCs.

A second case of MG was presented by Alcantara and colleagues.[105] A 63-year-old man initiated chiropractic care (i.e., Gonstead protocols) with multiple MG-related complaints, including swelling of the tongue, dysphagia, nausea, digestive problems, weakness in the eye muscles, dyspnea, **myopia, diplopia,** and headaches. The patient also experienced difficulty in ambulation resulting from loss of balance and coordination. At the time of publication, the patient was reported to be living a normal life free of

medication, and the MG symptoms were no longer debilitating.

Implications for Clinical Assessment

The research cited previously indicates that aspects of the immune system may in some cases respond to chiropractic intervention. As such, certain types of blood analysis may provide useful outcome measures, especially in the research arena and in the chiropractic and medical comanagement of selected patients.

CENTRAL NERVOUS SYSTEM

Clinical Research: Historical Perspectives

In the first half of the twentieth century, it was not unusual for patients with central nervous system (CNS) dysfunction to seek help from chiropractors. Some of these patients made their way to the B.J. Palmer Research Clinic. Killinger and Azad[106] reported four cases of MS seen at this clinic between 1948 and 1953. In those years, diagnosis was based on history and physical examination signs.

The Kentuckiana Children's Center in Louisville, Kentucky, has been providing chiropractic care to children with learning disabilities, cerebral palsy, **autism,** seizure disorders, and other CNS manifestations in a nonprofit, multidisciplinary setting since 1957. Clinical researchers have recently made an effort to introduce some of the Kentuckiana cases into the indexed literature. (One of the results of this effort will be summarized in the following section on descriptive research.)

Controlled Experimental and Clinical Studies

Although not a controlled experiment in the classic sense, the study of hyperactive children by Giesen, Center, and Leach[107] is a type of controlled clinical study called a *time-series design*. In studies of this sort, the subjects serve as their own control group. During a placebo period, seven hyperactive children were given sham adjustments with an Activator instrument placed on zero tension. During this period, parents kept a diary of the children's activity levels. Electrodermal testing provided a measure of sympathetic arousal, and a motion recorder disguised as a wristwatch was used to measure activity during a simulated homework assignment.

After the placebo period, Gonstead, diversified, or upper cervical specific adjustments (depending on examination results and doctor and patient comfort) were administered at various levels once per week. Across all measures and across all seven subjects, improvement was noted from the placebo phase to the end of the treatment phase. This improvement was statistically significant, despite the small number of subjects.

Carrick[108] made use of visual function as a window into brain function in a recent paper. This study featured circumference measurement of maps of the left and right visual blind spots before and after chiropractic adjustment at C2. Although all people have a blind spot in each eye because of light insensitivity at the optic disk, enlargement of the blind spot is usually associated with problems in the visual cortex. Carrick discovered that when C2 adjustment was delivered to the side of the larger map, symmetry increased and, by implication, cortical function improved. When the adjustment was delivered to the side of the smaller map, symmetry decreased.

Descriptive Research

In addition to the time-series study by Giesen and colleagues, well-described cases of hyperactivity and other learning disabilities improving under chiropractic care have been presented by Phillips,[109] Thomas and Wood,[110] Arme,[111] Araghi,[112] Manuel and Fysh,[113] and Peet.[114] Moreover, the Kentuckiana Children's Center continues to provide chiropractic care for children with learning disabilities of all sorts.

A recent publication by Barnes[115] (reporting two cases of special needs children) is one of the few accounts in the indexed literature of Kentuckiana's work. One patient was a 9-year-

old girl with spastic cerebral palsy. At the beginning of chiropractic care, this patient was in a brace prescribed by a medical orthopedist to correct internal rotation of both hips. Adjustments were administered twice per week. At 7 months, the orthopedist reviewed follow-up radiographs of the patient and indicated that **spontaneous remission** permitted brace removal and release from further orthopedic treatment.

Barnes' second case was a 16-year-old boy with high-functioning autism and a 2-year history of failure of voluntary bowel control, with at least one **encopresis** incident per day. After 13 sessions of spinal and cranial adjusting over 22 weeks, the patient was able to resume after-school activities (because no encopresis episodes had occurred in 2 months). At 7 months of follow-up, no further encopresis episodes were reported.

Seizure disorders have been discussed in recent publications. Woo[116] and Duff[117] each presented cases of adult women with myoclonic seizures of 17-years and 18-months duration, respectively. Antiseizure medication was ineffective in both cases. Thoracolumbar adjustments in Woo's case[116] and upper cervical adjustments in Duff's case[117] brought about rapid resolution.

Goodman[118] described a 5-year-old girl with a 9-month history of **grand mal seizures.** Dramatic improvement followed upper cervical adjustments. Alcantara and colleagues[119] described a 21-year-old woman with a history of grand mal and petit mal seizures since childhood. At initiation of chiropractic care, the patient's seizure frequency was approximately one every 3 hours. During the intake examination, a grand mal seizure began. The seizure abruptly ended the moment a Gonstead adjustment was delivered at the C6 level. At publication the patient was reporting periods between seizures as great as 2 months.

Hospers[120] presented a series of five cases with complaints including seizures, hyperactivity, and inability to concentrate. The major outcome measure in the study was **computerized electroencephalography** (CEEG) or "brain mapping." In this procedure a computer software program analyzes brain activity measured from surface electrocardiographic (EEG) electrodes.

The display is in the form of a diagram of the brain, with the percentage of various types of brain waves written or color coded over the various lobes. Previous research had identified normal values for each type of brain wave (i.e., alpha, beta, delta, theta) from each cerebral lobe for various age groups. After Life upper cervical adjustments (four patients) or category II pelvic blocking according to SOT protocols (one patient), all five patients demonstrated improved CEEG results, with concomitant symptomatic relief.

Recently a number of papers have appeared on the subject of MS. Stude and Mick[121] described an MS patient who responded favorably to thoracolumbar adjustments. More recently, Kirby[122] provided a well-described case of an MS patient whose symptoms improved after upper cervical adjustments when steroid medication and a low-fat diet provided no relief. The results of these case reports must be approached with some caution. MS is characterized by frequent remissions and exacerbations. The cause of these cycles of improvement and worsening remains unexplained and is generally referred to as *spontaneous*. It is possible that a patient could experience such a spontaneous remission during the course of chiropractic care.

The only study in the indexed chiropractic literature involving Parkinson's disease was published by Elster.[123] A 60-year-old man with a 7-year history of Parkinson's disease initiated chiropractic care. Symptoms included rigidity and tremor in the left arm and leg, memory loss, poor balance, depression, slurred speech, fatigue, spinal pain, and insomnia. Substantial improvement in all of these manifestations was experienced after seven upper cervical adjustments over a period of 3 months, including such a dramatic improvement in balance that the patient was able to ride a bicycle for the first time in several years.

Woo[124] reported a case of myelopathy after a sports injury. Despite 3 months of steroid therapy, the patient continued to deteriorate. At initiation of chiropractic care, this young man had lost bladder and bowel control, was unable to stand, and suffered from iatrogenic Cushing's syndrome. After 2 months of adjustments at the C7-T1 level, the patient was able to walk with crutches. At 9 years of follow-up, the patient could run, needed no crutches, and had no bladder or bowel complaints.

Probably the most exceptional case involving a CNS disorder was described by Plaugher, Rowe, and Gohl.[125] A 21-year-old man had been comatose for more than 1 year after an auto accident. After three modified Gonstead upper cervical adjustments administered within 1 week, the patient woke up, with a concomitant return of pulse rate and blood pressure to normal levels. Adjustments were later performed at L5-S1 and various levels of the thoracic spine. At the time of publication, the patient was able to ambulate with the aid of crutches.

Implications for Clinical Assessment

Chiropractic clinicians are becoming increasingly familiar with the indications for magnetic resonance imaging (MRI), EEG, CEEG, evoked potential studies, and other technologies useful in assessing the CNS. In the research arena, these tools have the potential to elucidate the role of VSC in brain and spinal cord dysfunction. This type of research holds great promise. If VSC can disturb CNS function, all other functions are in jeopardy.

Terrett[126] broke new theoretic ground in this area. Reviewing an extensive body of evidence, the researcher suggests a possible mechanism for chiropractic resolutions of such complaints as visual problems, paresis, dizziness, depression, anxiety, and memory loss. Terrett cites previous research indicating that depressed oxygenation because of decreased circulation can cause electric silence in neurons without causing cellular death. This level of oxygenation is called the **ischemic penumbra.** When the oxygen supply is restored, normal function often returns to the involved neural structures. Based on this information, Terrett theorizes that cervical VSC can disrupt blood flow to the brain to a degree less than a stroke, plunging portions of the brain into the ischemic penumbra. Essentially a portion of the brain enters a state of functional hibernation. Terrett further theorizes that restoration of blood flow by VSC correction can reactivate these brain centers.

GLOBAL WELLNESS AND OPTIMAL FUNCTION

Clinical Research: Historical Perspectives

A corollary to the tenet that VSC can disturb physiologic tone is that correcting VSC can assist wellness in general. Historically this idea was taken so seriously that patients and the public would often be told that "chiropractic adds years to your life and life to your years." However, no studies indicate that chiropractic care extends the human life span.

Leo Spears, the founder of the Denver, Colorado, hospital that bore the clinician's name, undertook a study in 1954 to determine the characteristics of people beyond the age of 100 years from a chiropractic clinical point of view (Fig. 25-4).[127] The goal of the Spears Longevity Research Study was to further develop the clinician's chiropractic techniques, which Spears maintained had the capacity to "goad nature into creating greater energy and therefore longer life." Unfortunately, while the arrival of the first group of centenarians in Denver was a publicity triumph for Spears and his hospital, no actual research results were ever published. The study was quietly shelved some time in 1956.

Despite this lack of useful data from the profession's past, recent investigators have begun to address the issue of global wellness and optimal function.

Controlled Experimental and Clinical Studies

Athletes are a potentially valuable group of subjects for the study of global wellness and optimal function, because they are relatively healthy people who routinely stress their bodies to achieve maximal performance. Although cases involving athletic injuries are common in the chiropractic literature, the study of the well athlete under chiropractic care is in the preliminary stage.

Lauro and Mouch[128] studied 50 athletes involved in a variety of activities, including football, volleyball, track, cross-country running, weight lifting, body building, rugby, and aerobic dancing. A total of 11 tests were used to measure various aspects of athletic ability, including agility, balance, kinesthetic perception, power, and reaction time. After initial testing, the experimental group received a chiropractic analysis, which included Gonstead and Palmer upper cervical radiograph marking, thermoscope pattern analysis, Derefield leg check, static palpation, and motion palpation. Adjustment techniques included toggle-recoil, Gonstead, diversified, and Thompson. Technique and visit frequency were determined on an individual basis, and the control group was not adjusted.

After 6 weeks the control group exhibited statistically significant improvement in two of the 11 tests, whereas the experimental group exhibited statistically significant improvement in

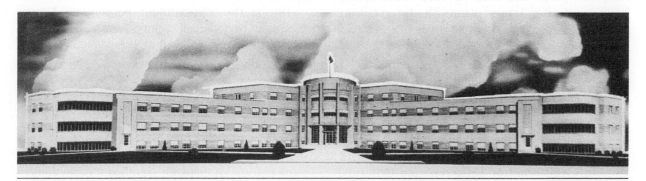

Fig. **25-4** The original building of Spears Hospital in 1943 was dedicated to chiropractic pioneer Willard Carver, DC. (*Courtesy William S. Rehm. From Masarsky C, Todres-Masarsky M:* Somatovisceral aspects of chiropractic: a evidence-based approach, *Philadelphia, 2001, Churchill-Livingstone.*)

eight tests. Of particular interest were the results of the Nelson hand reaction test—this is a measure of the speed of a manual reaction to a visual stimulus. After 6 weeks the control group exhibited less than 1% improvement in the test, whereas the experimental group exhibited more than 18% improvement.

A smaller but more focused study involving athletes under chiropractic care was conducted by a team under the direction of Schwartzbauer.[129] A total of 21 players on a men's college baseball team were randomly assigned to control (observation only) or experimental (upper cervical chiropractic care) groups. Statistically significant improvements were noted at 14 weeks in long jump distance and muscle strength in the experimental group; no statistically significant improvements were seen in the control group. The experimental group also exhibited statistically significant improvement in capillary counts, whereas the control group did not. Capillary counts were made by viewing the nail bed of the right and left middle fingers through a microscope at a 60x magnification. The number of capillaries visible in one microscopic field of view was recorded. An increase in capillary count represents improved microcirculation to the fingers.

Kelly, Murphy, and Backhouse[130] measured changes in reaction time after a single upper cervical adjustment delivered to asymptomatic chiropractic students. Thirty-six students found to have upper cervical subluxations during routine examination at their college's clinic were randomly assigned to treatment or control groups. All participants had their reaction times tested before and after intervention. The intervention for the treatment group was an upper cervical adjustment. The intervention for the control group was a brief rest.

The control group demonstrated an 8% improvement in reaction time postintervention. The treatment group demonstrated an improvement of more than 14%. The difference between groups was statistically significant. The results of this study are consistent with the improved reaction time reported by Lauro and Mouch[128] at 6 weeks of care and suggest that this improvement can begin with the first adjustment.

Descriptive Research

Previous sections of this chapter have included several studies in which the results of physiologic testing improved in subjects who were already within normal limits. These findings represent movement toward optimal function in the physiologic parameter in question. Masarsky and Weber[42] demonstrated improved lung volumes in lung-normal patients, as did Kessinger.[44] Improved visual acuity was demonstrated after chiropractic care of patients with initially normal vision by Kessinger and Boneva.[95] Brennan and colleagues[100] demonstrated improved function of lymphocytes and polymorphonuclear neutrophils in apparently healthy chiropractic students after thoracic manipulation.

Physiologic evidence of stress can often be found in patients with no apparent symptoms or active disease processes. However, this measurable physiologic stress has been identified as a risk factor for an entire constellation of health problems. Tuchin[131] presented a study of changes in salivary cortisol levels in a group of nine corporate employees. Cortisol is one of the glucocorticoids secreted by the adrenal cortex. Elevated serum levels of cortisol and other glucocorticoids have been found to correlate with disturbed concentration, tremors, elevated heart rate, and other signs consistent with high stress levels. Cortisol levels measured in the saliva closely reflect cortisol levels in the blood serum; as such, salivary cortisol levels are a practical noninvasive physiologic measure of stress.

During the pretreatment baseline and posttreatment periods, saliva samples were collected at noon each Wednesday and Sunday (these have been shown to be the most and least stressful times of the week, respectively, for these corporate employees). During the chiropractic spinal manipulative therapy period (four visits over 2 weeks), samples were collected before and after each session. Static and motion palpation were used for spinal analysis. Eight of the nine subjects demonstrated statistically significant reductions in salivary cortisol levels after chiropractic care.

In addition to physiologic testing, a number of pencil-and-paper instruments have been developed to measure general health and wellness. One such instrument is the **RAND SF-36** questionnaire, which includes 36 questions on such topics as vitality, mental health, and social functioning.[132] A simpler instrument, developed specifically for chiropractic use is the Global Well-Being Scale (GWBS).[133] The GWBS is essentially a modified visual analog scale (Fig. 25-5). A detailed discussion on the proper use of these instruments is beyond the scope of this chapter, but it is well-covered by Hawk.[134]

Implications for Clinical Assessment

Although the research implications in the arena of global wellness and optimal function are tantalizing, the working clinician can put many of these methods of measurement to work immediately. An ordinary Snellen chart or an inexpensive spirometer can provide the clinician with the capacity to measure physiologic improvement even in patients with no visual or respiratory complaints. The RAND SF-36 or the GWBS can be introduced into a clinician's intake protocols to provide a patient-centered measure that goes beyond mere pain. Such clinical procedures would not be appropriate for clinicians who limit their focus to the treatment of pain, but they are quite appropriate for those dedicated to assisting the body in the restoration of normal neurologic tone.

VERTEBROVISCERAL CORRELATIONS

To evaluate the apparent beneficial effects of adjustment or manipulation in the somatovisceral arena, it is important to consider all possible explanations. Lewit[54] proposes the following:

- The vertebral column (i.e., locomotor system) is causing symptoms that are mistaken for visceral disease.
- Visceral disturbance is causing symptoms simulating effects upon some part of the locomotor system.
- Visceral disease is causing a reflex (i.e., pseudoradicular) reaction in the segment, including blockage in the corresponding mobile segment of the vertebral column.
- Visceral disease that has caused segmental movement restriction has subsided, but blockage remains, causing symptoms of visceral disease.
- Disturbance of the locomotor segment is causing visceral disease (conjectural).

Although being careful not to reach beyond the available evidence, Lewit clearly has concluded from decades of work that chiropractic and osteopathic manual adjustment/manipulation is beneficial in many cases where (as in the tonsillitis study cited earlier) the presenting symptoms are primarily visceral.

Nansel and Szlazak[135] conclude, to the contrary, that all visceral benefits of the chiropractic

Pre

Number:_____ Date:____/____/____

Please think about how you are feeling right now, your general sense of health and well-being. On the line below, make a straight vertical (up-and-down) mark on the line to show how you feel right now.

| Worst you could possibly feel | | Best you could possibly feel |

Fig. **25-5** The Global Well-Being Scale (GWBS). *(From Hawk C et al: A study of the reliability, validity, and responsiveness of a self-administered instrument to measure global well-being,* Palmer J Res *2(1):15, 1995.)*

adjustment are apparent rather than real. Based on a literature review, they suggest that referred spinal pain mimics visceral disorders, and the relief of this referred pain creates the impression of a cure for a disorder that never existed. They assert that autonomic reflex disorders generated by VSC are highly localized and thus irrelevant to general health and wellness.

Taken as a whole, the literature reviewed in this chapter is difficult to reconcile with such a view.

FUTURE RESEARCH HORIZONS

Examples of cases and limited studies in the somatovisceral arena raise the possibility of chiropractic playing a role in the health care system beyond the care of musculoskeletal conditions. Pilot studies represent a foundation for further research into the chiropractor's role in systemic health and general wellness.

Chiropractic scientists and clinicians need more detail about subluxations and adjustments than has been provided in most previous studies. Authors of research papers on chiropractic need to address the following in all future studies:

- What signs were used to identify subluxations? "Chiropractic clinical criteria" is not an adequate description.
- What levels were found to be subluxated?
- What types of adjustments were administered? "High velocity, low amplitude" is not an adequate description.
- Did the subluxation signs and the disease-related signs and symptoms demonstrate any covariance? In other words, do measurements related to subluxation and measurements related to disease or symptoms increase and decrease together more frequently than one would expect from random fluctuation? This cannot be determined if subluxation signs were only recorded at the beginning and not the end of the study.
- Did the *sham* procedure inadvertently correct some of the subjects' subluxations? Again, this cannot be determined if subluxation data were gathered only at the beginning of the study.

These considerations must be attended to as fastidiously as the disease-related outcomes and randomization.

Taking the issue of optimal performance a step further, why stop with athletic performance? Why not find out whether VSC interferes with the voice quality of a singer, the accuracy of an accountant, or the creativity of a writer or painter?

The authors conclude with the hope that D.D. Palmer's science of tone will energize the chiropractic research community in coming years. If the traditional chiropractic tenets can be fully integrated with the field's scientific endeavors, the best days of chiropractic science lie ahead rather than behind.

Acknowledgments

The authors gratefully acknowledge the kind assistance of Mark T. Pfefer, DC, and research assistants Alexandra S. Cleveland, and Nathan Uhl, both of the Research Department of Cleveland Chiropractic College. Their preparation of an extensive literature search for this chapter was of inestimable value.

Review *Questions*

1. What methods of autonomic assessment were incorporated into chiropractic analysis during the profession's first 3 decades?
2. What methods has Browning proposed for assessing the lower sacral nerve roots?
3. Is somatic dyspnea always accompanied by reduced lung volumes?
4. What special measures should be taken in terms of clinical assessment and patient education when a patient is on antihypertensive medication?
5. What procedures are useful in monitoring CNS function? (Include physical examination, diagnostic imaging, and electrodiagnostic procedures.)
6. In what sense do WBCs resemble neurons?
7. What is the strongest evidence that can be cited from the scientific literature indicating that chiropractic adjustments may be beneficial for conditions other than musculoskeletal pain?

Concept *Questions*

1. How can the systemic benefits of chiropractic be explained to the general public, while avoiding unwarranted claims that the vertebral adjustment is a *cure-all?*
2. What are some possible implications of Terrett's theory of brain hibernation for society as a whole? (Address this question broadly. Consider traffic safety, learning disorders, domestic violence, creativity, and so forth.) What testable hypotheses are suggested by these implications?

REFERENCES

1. Association of Chiropractic Colleges: *Issues in chiropractic. Position paper #1. The ACC chiropractic paradigm.* Chicago, July, 1996, Association of Chiropractic Colleges.
2. Peterson DM: Chiropractic world meets in Paris: WFC adopts "ACC chiropractic paradigm," *Dyn Chiropr* 19(14):1, 2001.
3. Palmer DD: *The science, art and philosophy of chiropractic*, Portland, Ore, 1910, Portland Printing House.
4. Palmer BJ: *The philosophy, science and art of chiropractic nerve tracing*, Davenport, Iowa, 1911, Palmer School of Chiropractic.
5. Stephenson RW: *Chiropractic textbook*, Davenport, Iowa, 1948, Palmer School of Chiropractic.
6. Kyneur JS, Bolton SP: Chiropractic equipment. In Peterson D, Wiese G, editors: *Chiropractic: an illustrated history*, St Louis, 1995, Mosby.
7. Burns L, Candler L, Rice R: *Pathogenesis of visceral diseases following vertebral lesions*, Chicago, 1948, American Osteopathic Association.
8. Winsor HK: Sympathetic segmental disturbances, II. *Med Times* 49:267, 1922.
9. Plaugher G et al: Spinal management for the patient with a visceral concomitant. In Plaugher G, editor: *Textbook of clinical chiropractic: a specific biomechanical approach*, Baltimore, 1993, Williams & Wilkins.
10. Bondies OI, Stillman CJ: Notes on the diagnosis and treatment of ulcerative gastritis, *J Am Osteopath Assoc* 36:568, 1936.
11. Hay J: The importance of faulty structural relations in etiology and treatment of peptic ulcer, *J Am Osteopath Assoc* 39:162, 1939.
12. Magoun HI: Clinical application of the cranial concept, *J Am Osteopath Assoc* 47:413, 1948.
13. Northup TL: Manipulation in mucous colitis, *J Am Osteopath Assoc* 41:87, 1941.
14. Lindberg RF, Strachan WF, Koehnlein WO: The relation of structural disturbances to irritable colon ("colitis"), *J Am Osteopath Assoc* 41:253, 1941.
15. Pikalov AA, Kharin VV: Use of spinal manipulative therapy in the treatment of duodenal ulcer, *J Manipulative Physiol Ther* 17:310, 1994.
16. Wiberg JMM, Nordsteen J, Nilsson N: The short-term effect of spinal manipulation in the treatment of infantile colic: a randomized controlled clinical trial with a blinded observer, *J Manipulative Physiol Ther* 22:517, 1999.
17. Lucassen PL et al: Effectiveness of treatments for infantile colic: a systematic review, *BMJ* 316(7144): 1563, 1998.
18. Danielsson B, Hwang CP: Treatment of infantile colic with surface active substance (simethicone), *Acta Paediatr Scand* 74:446, 1985.
19. Olafsdottir E et al: Randomized controlled trial of infantile colic treated with chiropractic spinal manipulation, *Arch Dis Child* 84:138, 2001.
20. Klougart N, Nilsson N, Jacobsen J: Infantile colic treated by chiropractors: a prospective study of 316 cases, *J Manipulative Physiol Ther* 12:281, 1989.
21. Pluhar GR, Schobert PD: Vertebral subluxation and colic: a case study, *J Chiropr Res Clin Invest* 7:75, 1991.
22. Hyman CA: Chiropractic adjustments and infantile colic: a case study. In *Proceedings of the National Conference on Chiropractic Pediatrics*, Arlington, Va, 1994, International Chiropractors Association.
23. Killinger LZ, Azad A: Chiropractic care of infantile colic: a case study, *J Clin Chiropr Ped* 3:203, 1998.
24. Fallon JP, Lok BJ: Assessing the efficacy of chiropractic care in pediatric cases of pyloric stenosis. In *Proceedings of the National Conference on Chiropractic Pediatrics*, Arlington, Va, 1994, International Chiropractors Association.
25. DeBoer KF, Schutz M, McKnight ME: Acute effects of spinal manipulation on gastrointestinal myoelectric activity in conscious rabbits, *Man Med* 3:85, 1988.
26. Hewitt EG: Chiropractic treatment of a 7-month-old with chronic constipation: a case report, *Chiropr Tech* 5:101, 1993.
27. Nyiendo J, Olsen E: Visit characteristics of 217 children attending a chiropractic college teaching clinic, *J Manipulative Physiol Ther* 11:78, 1988.
28. Miller WD: Treatment of visceral disorders by manipulative therapy. In Goldstein M, editor: *The research status of spinal manipulative therapy*, Bethesda, Md, 1975, National Institute of Neurological and Communicative Disorders and Stroke.
29. Hviid C: A comparison of the effect of chiropractic treatment on respiratory function in patients with respiratory distress symptoms and patients without, *Bull Eur Chiropr Union* 26:17, 1978.
30. Nielsen NH et al: Chronic asthma and chiropractic spinal manipulation: a randomized clinical trial, *Clin Exp Allergy* 25:80, 1995.
31. Balon J et al: A comparison of active and simulated chiropractic manipulation as adjunctive treatment for childhood asthma, *N Engl J Med* 339:1013, 1998.

32. Hondras MA, Linde K, Jones AP: Manual therapy for asthma, *Cochrane Database Syst Rev* 2:1, 2001.

33. Jongeward BV: Chiropractic manipulation for childhood asthma (letter to editor), *N Engl J Med* 340:391, 1996.

34. Richards DG, Mein EA, Nelson CD: Chiropractic manipulation for childhood asthma (letter to editor), *N Engl J Med* 340:391, 1996.

35. Rosner AL: A walk on the wild side of allopathic medicine: going ballistic instead of holistic, *Dyn Chiropr* 17(9):10, 1999.

36. Masarsky CS, Weber M: Chiropractic management of chronic obstructive pulmonary disease, *J Manipulative Physiol Ther* 11:505, 1988.

37. Peet JB, Marko SK, Piekarczyk W: Chiropractic response in the pediatric patient with asthma: a pilot study, *Chiropr Pediat* 1:9, 1995.

38. Bachman TR, Lantz CA: Management of pediatric asthma and enuresis with probable traumatic etiology. In *Proceedings of the National Conference on Chiropractic Pediatrics*, Arlington, Va, 1991, International Chiropractors Association.

39. Peet JB: Case study: eight year old female with chronic asthma, *Chiro Pediatr* 3(2):9, 1997.

40. Nilsson N, Christiansen B: Prognostic factors in bronchial asthma in chiropractic practice, *Chiropr J Aust* 18:85, 1988.

41. Masarsky CS, Weber M: Somatic dyspnea and the orthopedics of respiration, *Chiropr Tech* 3:26, 1991.

42. Masarsky CS, Weber M: Chiropractic and lung volumes—a retrospective study, *J Am Chiropr Assoc* 20(9):65, 1986.

43. Masarsky CS, Weber M: Screening spirometry in the chiropractic examination, *J Am Chiropr Assoc* 23(2):67, 1989.

44. Kessinger R: Changes in pulmonary function associated with upper cervical specific chiropractic care, *J Vertebr Sublux Res* 1(3):43, 1997.

45. Palmer DD: *The science art and philosophy of chiropractic*, Portland, Ore, 1910, Portland Publishing House.

46. Cleveland CS Jr: Researching the subluxation of the domestic rabbit, *Sci Rev Chiropr* 1(4):5, 1965.

47. Burns L, Steudenberg G, Vollbrecht WJ: Family of rabbits with second thoracic and other lesions, *J Am Osteopath Assoc* 37:908, 1937.

48. Burns L: Preliminary report of cardiac changes following the correction of third thoracic lesions, *J Am Osteopath Assoc* 42:3, 1943.

49. Burns L: Tracings showing pulse changes following certain lesions, *J Am Osteopath Assoc* 44:4, 1945.

50. Becker AD: Manipulative osteopathy in cardiac therapy, *J Am Osteopath Assoc* 38:317, 1939.

51. Koch RS: A somatic component in heart disease, *J Am Osteopath Assoc* 60:735, 1961.

52. Appleyard EC: Angina pectoris with special reference to its mechanical causes, *J Am Osteopath Assoc* 37:245, 1938.

53. Northup TL: Manipulative management of hypertension, *J Am Osteopath Assoc* 60:735, 1961.

54. Lewit K: Vertebrovisceral correlations. In Lewit K: *Manipulative therapy in rehabilitation of the locomotor system*, Oxford, 1991, Butterworth-Heinemann.

55. Cleveland CSC III: Vertebrovisceral relations: a medical perspective, *California Chiropr Assoc J* 22(3):36, 1997.

56. Yates RG et al: Effects of chiropractic treatment on blood pressure and anxiety: a randomized, controlled trial, *J Manipulative Physiol Ther* 11:484, 1988.

57. Plaugher G, Bachman TR: Chiropractic management of a hypertensive patient: a case study, *J Manipulative Physiol Ther* 16:544, 1993.

58. Connelly DM, Rasmussen SA: The effect of cranial adjusting on hypertension: a case report, *Chiropr Tech* 10:75, 1998.

59. Northup TL: Manipulative management of hypertension, *J Am Osteopath Assoc* 60:735, 1961.

60. Lott GS et al: ECG improvements following the combination of chiropractic adjustments, diet, and exercise therapy, *J Chiropr Res Clin Invest* 5:37, 1990.

61. Thomason PR et al: Effectiveness of spinal manipulative therapy in treatment of primary dysmenorrhea: a pilot study, *J Manipulative Physiol Ther* 2:140, 1979.

62. Kokjohn K et al: The effect of spinal manipulation on pain and prostaglandin levels in women with primary dysmenorrhea, *J Manipulative Physiol Ther* 15:279, 1992.

63. Hondras MA, Long CR, Brennan PC: Spinal manipulative therapy versus a low force mimic maneuver for women with primary dysmenorrhea: a randomized, observer-blinded, clinical trial, *Pain* 81:105, 1999.

64. Leboeuf C et al: Chiropractic care of children with nocturnal enuresis: a prospective study, *J Manipulative Physiol Ther* 14:110, 1991.

65. Reed WR et al: Chiropractic management of primary nocturnal enuresis, *J Manipulative Physiol Ther* 17:156, 1994.

66. Liebl NA, Butler LM: A chiropractic approach to the treatment of dysmenorrhea, *J Manipulative Physiol Ther* 13:101, 1990.

67. Hawk C, Long C, Azad A: Chiropractic care for women with chronic pelvic pain: a prospective single-group intervention study, *J Manipulative Physiol Ther* 20:73, 1997.

68. Browning JE: Pelvic pain and organic dysfunction in a patient with low back pain, response to distractive manipulation: a case presentation, *J Manipulative Physiol Ther* 10:116, 1987.

69. Browning JE: Chiropractic distractive decompression in the treatment of pelvic pain and organic dysfunction with evidence of lower sacral nerve root compression, *J Manipulative Physiol Ther* 11:426, 1988.

70. Browning JE: The recognition of mechanically induced pelvic pain and organic dysfunction in the low back pain patient, *J Manipulative Physiol Ther* 12:369, 1989.

71. Browning JE: Chiropractic distractive decompression in treating pelvic pain and multiple system pelvic organic dysfunction, *J Manipulative Physiol Ther* 12:265, 1989.

72. Browning JE: Uncomplicated mechanically induced pelvic pain and organic dysfunction in low back pain patients, *J Can Chiropr Assoc* 35:149, 1991.

73. Browning JE: Distractive manipulation protocols in treating the mechanically induced pelvic pain and organic dysfunction patient, *Chiropr Tech* 7:1, 1995.

74. Browning JE: The mechanically induced pelvic pain and organic dysfunction syndrome: an often overlooked cause of bladder, bowel, gynecologic and sexual dysfunction, *J Neuromusculoskeletal Sys* 4:52, 1996.

75. Browning JE: Mechanically induced pelvic pain and organic dysfunction in a patient without low back pain, *J Manipulative Physiol Ther* 13:406, 1990.

76. Browning JE: Pelvic pain and organic dysfunction. In Masarsky CS, Todres-Masarsky M, editors: *Somatovisceral aspects of chiropractic: an evidence-based approach*, New York, 2001, Churchill Livingstone.

77. Gemmell HA, Jacobson BH: Chiropractic management of enuresis: time-series descriptive design, *J Manipulative Physiol Ther* 12:386, 1989.

78. Blomerth PR: Functional nocturnal enuresis, *J Manipulative Physiol Ther* 17:336, 1994.

79. Stude DE, Bergmann TF, Finer A: A conservative approach for a patient with traumatically induced urinary incontinence, *J Manipulative Physiol Ther* 21:363, 1998.

80. Eriksen K: Effects of upper cervical correction on chronic constipation, *Chiropr Res J* 3:19, 1994.

81. Falk JW: Bowel and bladder dysfunction secondary to lumbar dysfunctional syndrome, *Chiropr Tech* 2:45, 1990.

82. Stude DE: Dysfunctional uterine bleeding with concomitant low back and lower extremity pain, *J Manipulative Physiol Ther* 14:472, 1991.

83. Wagner T et al: Irritable bowel syndrome and spinal manipulation: a case report, *Chiropr Tech* 7:139, 1995.

84. Briggs L, Boone WR: Effects of a chiropractic adjustment on changes in pupillary diameter: a model for evaluating somatovisceral response, *J Manipulative Physiol Ther* 11:181, 1988.

85. Gilman G, Bertstrand J: Visual recovery following chiropractic intervention, *J Chiropr Res Clin Invest* 6:61, 1990.

86. Gorman RF: Automated static perimetry in chiropractic, *J Manipulative Physiol Ther* 16:481, 1993.

87. Gorman RF et al: Case report: spinal strain and visual perception deficit, *Chiropr J Aust* 24:131, 1994.

88. Gorman RF: The treatment of presumptive optic nerve ischemia by spinal manipulation, *J Manipulative Physiol Ther* 18:172, 1995.

89. Gorman RF: Monocular scotomata and spinal manipulation: the step phenomenon, *J Manipulative Physiol Ther* 19:344, 1996.

90. Stephens D, Gorman RF: The association between visual incompetence and spinal derangement: an instructive case history, *J Manipulative Physiol Ther* 20:343, 1997.

91. Stephens D, Gorman RF, Bilton D: The step phenomenon in the recovery of vision with spinal manipulation: a report on two 13-year-olds treated together, *J Manipulative Physiol Ther* 20:628, 1997.

92. Stephens D et al: Treatment of visual field loss by spinal manipulation: a report on 17 patients, *J Neuromusculoskel Sys* 6:53, 1998.

93. Alcantara J, Parker JA: Management of a patient with bilateral esothrophia and subluxations, *J Manipulative Physiol Ther* (in press).

94. Gibbons PF, Gosling CM, Holmes M: Short-term effects of cervical manipulation on edge light pupil cycle time: a pilot study, *J Manipulative Physiol Ther* 23:465, 2000.

95. Kessinger R, Boneva D: Changes in visual acuity in patients receiving upper cervical specific chiropractic care, *J Vertebr Sublux Res* 2(1):43, 1998.

96. Blum CL: Spinal/cranial manipulative therapy and tinnitus: a case history, *Chiropr Tech* 10:163, 1998.

97. Terrett AGJ: Tinnitus, the cervical spine, and spinal manipulative therapy, *Chiropr Tech* 1:41, 1989.

98. Hazzard C: The basis for immunity, natural or acquired, *J Am Osteopath Assoc* 37:327, 1938.

99. Brennan PC et al: Immunologic correlates of reduced spinal mobility: preliminary observations in a dog model. In Wolk S, editor: *Proceedings of the 1991 International Conference on Spinal Manipulation*, Arlington, Va, 1991, Foundation for Chiropractic Education and Research.

100. Brennan PC et al: Enhanced phagocytic cell respiratory burst induced by spinal manipulation: potential role of substance P, *J Manipulative Physiol Ther* 14:399, 1991.

101. Alcorn SM: Chiropractic treatment and antibody levels, *J Aust Chiropr Assn* 11(3):18, 1977.

102. Vora GS, Bates HA: The effects of spinal manipulation on the immune system: a preliminary report, *J Am Chiropr Assoc* 14:S103, 1980.

103. Thomas RJ, Wilkinson RR: Chiropractic care in adult spina bifida: a case report, *Chiropr Tech* 2:191, 1990.

104. Araghi HJ: Juvenile myasthenia gravis: a case study in chiropractic management. In *Proceedings of the International Conference on Pediatrics and Chiropractic*, Arlington, Va, 1993, International Chiropractors Association.

105. Alcantara J et al: Chiropractic management of a patient with myasthenia gravis and vertebral subluxations, *J Manipulative Physiol Ther* 22:333, 1999.

106. Killinger LZ, Azad A: Multiple sclerosis patients under chiropractic care: a retrospective study, *Palmer J Res* 2:96, 1997.

107. Giesen JM, Center DB, Leach RA: An evaluation of chiropractic manipulation as a treatment of hyperactivity in children, *J Manipulative Physiol Ther* 12:353, 1989.

108. Carrick FR: Changes in brain function after manipulation of the cervical spine, *J Manipulative Physiol Ther* 20:529, 1997.

109. Phillips CF: Case study: the effect of utilizing spinal manipulation and craniosacral therapy as the treatment approach for attention deficit hyperactivity disorder. In *Proceedings of the National Conference on Chiropractic and Pediatrics*, Arlington, Va, 1991, International Chiropractors Association.

110. Thomas MD, Wood J: Upper cervical adjustments may improve mental function, *J Man Med* 6:215, 1992.

111. Arme J: Effects of biomechanical insult correction on attention deficit disorder, *J Chiropr Case Rep* 1:6, 1993.

112. Araghi HJ: Oral apraxia: a case study in chiropractic management. In *Proceedings of the National Conference on Chiropractic and Pediatrics*, Arlington, Va, 1994, International Chiropractors Association.

113. Manuel JD, Fysh PN: Acquired verbal aphasia in a seven-year-old female: case report, *J Clin Chiropr Ped* 1:89, 1996.

114. Peet JB: Adjusting the hyperactive/ADD pediatric patient, *Chiro Pediatr* 2(4):12, 1997.

115. Barnes T: Chiropractic management of the special needs child, *Top Clin Chiropr* 4(4):9, 1997.

116. Woo CC: Traumatic spinal myoclonus, *J Manipulative Physiol Ther* 12:478, 1989.

117. Duff BA: Documented chiropractic results on a case diagnosed as myoclonic seizures, *J Chiropr Res Clin Invest* 8:56, 1992.

118. Goodman R: Cessation of seizure disorder: correction of the atlas subluxation complex. In *Proceedings of the National Conference on Chiropractic and Pediatrics*, Arlington, Va, 1991, International Chiropractors Association.

119. Alcantara J et al: Chiropractic management of a patient with subluxations, low back pain and epileptic seizures, *J Manipulative Physiol Ther* 21:110, 1998.

120. Hospers LA: EEG and CEEG studies before and after upper cervical or SOT category II adjustment in children after head trauma, in epilepsy, and in "hyperactivity." In *Proceedings of the National Conference on Chiropractic and Pediatrics*, Arlington, Va, 1992, International Chiropractors Association.

121. Stude DE, Mick T: Clinical presentation of a patient with multiple sclerosis and response to manual chiropractic adjustive therapies, *J Manipulative Physiol Ther* 16:595, 1993.

122. Kirby SL: A case study: the effects of chiropractic on multiple sclerosis, *Chiropr Res J* 3:7, 1994.

123. Elster EI: Upper cervical chiropractic management of a patient with Parkinson's disease: a case report, *J Manipulative Physiol Ther* 23:573, 2000.

124. Woo CC: Post-traumatic myelopathy following flopping high jump: a pilot case of spinal manipulation, *J Manipulative Physiol Ther* 16:336, 1993.

125. Plaugher G, Rowe DJ, Gohl RA: Chiropractic management of spinal fractures and dislocations with closed reduction methods: a report of nine cases. In Wolk S, editor: *Proceedings of the 1992 International Conference on Spinal Manipulation*, Arlington, Va, 1992, Foundation for Chiropractic Education and Research.

126. Terrett AGJ: Cerebral dysfunction: a theory to explain some of the effects of chiropractic manipulation, *Chiropr Tech* 5:168, 1993.

127. Rehm WS: Research: promise and hyperbole. In Rehm WS: *Prairie thunder: Dr. Leo L. Spears and his hospital*, Davenport, Iowa, 2001, Association for the History of Chiropractic.

128. Lauro A, Mouch B: Chiropractic effects on athletic ability, *J Chiropr Res Clin Invest* 6:84, 1991.

129. Schwartzbauer J et al: Athletic performance and physiological measures in baseball players following upper cervical chiropractic care: a pilot study, *J Vertebr Sublux Res* 1(4):33, 1997.

130. Kelly DD, Murphy BA, Backhouse DP: Use of a mental rotation reaction-time paradigm to measure the effects of upper cervical adjustments on cortical processing: a pilot study, *J Manipulative Physiol Ther* 23:246, 2000.

131. Tuchin PJ: The effect of chiropractic spinal manipulative therapy on salivary cortisol levels, *Austral J Chiropr Osteopath* 2:86, 1998.

132. RAND Health Sciences Program: *RAND 36-Item health survey 1.0*, Santa Monica, Calif, 1992, RAND.

133. Hawk C et al: A study of the reliability, validity and responsiveness of a self-administered instrument to measure global well-being, *Palmer J Res* 2(1):15, 1995.

134. Hawk C: Patient-based outcomes assessment: "pencil-and-paper" instruments. In Masarsky CS, Todres-Masarsky M, editors: *Somatovisceral aspects of chiropractic: an evidence-based approach*, New York, 2001, Churchill-Livingstone.

135. Nansel D, Szlazak M: Somatic dysfunction and the phenomenon of visceral disease simulation: a probable explanation for the apparent effectiveness of somatic therapy in patients presumed to be suffering from true visceral disease, *J Manipulative Physiol Ther* 18:379, 1995.

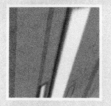

PART SIX

CONTEMPORARY ISSUES IN CHIROPRACTIC PRACTICE

Comparative Safety of Chiropractic

William J. Lauretti, DC

Key Terms

ABSOLUTE CONTRAINDICATIONS	HEMIPARESIS	OSTEOGENESIS IMPERFECTA (OI)
ATAXIA	HOMOCYSTINE	RANDOMIZED CONTROLLED TRIAL
CAUDA EQUINE SYNDROME	IATROGENIC DISORDER	
CEREBROVASCULAR ACCIDENT	ISCHEMIA	RED FLAG
	LOCKED-IN SYNDROME	RELATIVE CONTRAINDICATIONS
DOPPLER ULTRASONOGRAPHY	MARFAN'S SYNDROME	
EHLERS-DANLOS SYNDROME (EDS) TYPE IV	MEDLINE	VERTEBROBASILAR INSUFFICIENCY
	NONSTEROIDAL ANTIINFLAMMATORY DRUGS	
HEMIANESTHESIA	OSTEOARTHRITIS	WALLENBERG'S SYNDROME

Primum non nocere

I will follow that system of regimen which, according to my ability and judgment, I consider for the benefit of my patients, and abstain from whatever is deleterious and mischievous.

HIPPOCRATIC OATH[1]

The ancient Hippocratic appeal to physicians to "first, do no harm" has a powerful attraction among members of the health care professions and in the popular imagination. After all, if a physician's job is to heal, should not patients receive benefit from a physician's ministrations and not further injury? Unfortunately, the physician—as a professional, as a healer, and as a human being—must occasionally face the specter of inadvertently causing harm to a patient.

Chiropractic has come under increased scrutiny as a result of its widespread popularity and its recent entry into the health care mainstream. Considerable progress has been made in interprofessional relations between chiropractors and medical physicians in recent years, but the adversarial climate of the past has not entirely disappeared. In this context, the possibility of adverse reactions to chiropractic treatment is a politically and emotionally charged issue. In certain cases, the popular media and some biomedical journals have inflamed the issue by emphasizing the rare negative reactions to spinal adjustment/manipulation and evaluating its risks in isolation rather than comparing them with the risks of common medical treatments for similar problems.

Most chiropractors perform thousands of treatments annually without any serious complications, and they observe that many patients benefit greatly from adjustment/manipulation. Many of these therapeutic successes occur after more aggressive therapies, medications, and surgery have failed. Such personal experience with the safety and effectiveness of spinal adjustment/manipulation can lead individual chiropractors to devalue reports of adverse reactions. The incongruity between the positive personal experience of chiropractors using adjustment/manipulation and recurring negative stories about its alleged dangers sets the stage for a *chiropractic paradox*:

- According to certain medical authors, chiropractic spinal adjustment/manipulation has a very limited role to play in conventional health care, if any.[2] In some cases, particularly those involving the cervical spine, some medical authorities consider the procedure "too risky to perform."[3]

- Nonetheless, millions of people receive chiropractic spinal adjustment/manipulation each year, without apparent harm and with apparent benefit.

- Furthermore, the vast majority of doctors of chiropractic (DC) and non-DC practitioners of manual medicine have never personally experienced a serious complication during treatment. Most chiropractors view adjustment/manipulation as safe and noninvasive, and they frequently perform the procedure on family members and loved ones and receive it themselves with hardly a thought of potentially hazardous complications.

- In recent years, several reviews of the scientific literature from leading authorities have agreed that many chiropractic methods for treating neck-related conditions are safe, effective, and appropriate. For example, in a 1996 report published by the RAND Corporation,[4] a multidisciplinary expert panel found that adjustment/manipulation and mobilization of the cervical spine were appropriate treatments for patients with many common categories of neck pain and headache. In a 2001 systematic review of the scientific literature,[5] medical experts at the Duke University Evidence-Based Practice Center found cervical manipulation an appropriate treatment for both tension-type headaches and cervicogenic headaches (a specific category of headaches associated with neck symptoms). The Duke report also noted that "adverse effects are uncommon with manipulation and this may be one of its appeals over drug treatment."

It is crucial that the risks of chiropractic procedures not be evaluated in a clinical vacuum, with inappropriate emphasis on adjustment/manipulation's perceived risks and corresponding under-emphasis on the considerable scientific evidence favoring its safety and effectiveness. The solution to the *chiropractic paradox* lies in the answers to two key questions: how inherently risky is spinal adjustment/manipulation, and how do its risks and benefits compare with other conventional treatments for similar conditions?

CERVICAL ADJUSTMENTS: CONSERVATIVE CARE OR A RISKY GAMBLE?

The safety of cervical spine adjustment/manipulation has been questioned more frequently than any other commonly applied chiropractic procedure. Reports of serious complications from neck adjustment/manipulation have intermittently appeared in the medical literature since at least 1934.[6] The issue has been increasingly discussed in the popular media in the last decade. However, in early 2002, worries reached a crisis level in the Canadian press after a group of 60 Canadian neurologists issued press releases calling for a ban on neck manipulation.[7] Articles in newspapers published across Canada quoted the neurologists as asserting that the chiropractic procedure "causes strokes and crippling injury with alarming frequency."[8]

To most chiropractors, this article was deeply disturbing, not only for its overall alarmist tone, but also for its publication of blatantly inaccurate information. For example, it quoted one neurologist as saying that "the latest figures" estimating the risk of strokes from neck manipulation "have put it a little closer to one in 5,000 [manipulations]." However, one potentially positive effect of this story was that the need for chiropractors to fully inform themselves about the potential risks of neck adjustment/manipulation was highlighted. With accurate, up-to-date information, chiropractors can institute preventive measures to decrease risk to patients, as well as provide reasoned responses to journalists, patients, and medical colleagues who are concerned that chiropractic treatment is unacceptably hazardous.

Mechanisms of Stroke from Cervical Adjustment/Manipulation

The most likely mechanism of stroke from cervical adjustment/manipulation involves injury to the vertebral artery as it courses through the transverse foramina of the upper cervical vertebrae into the base of the skull. Between the first two cervical vertebrae, the vertebral artery makes a sharp bend upward and laterally to enter the transverse process of the atlas vertebra. The artery is relatively fixed to the transverse processes by fibrous tissue at this point and is less freely movable.

The vertebral artery emerges from the transverse process of atlas and winds posteriorly and laterally around the posterior arch of atlas. Then the artery ascends into the foramen magnum and joins with its counterpart to form the basilar artery. This vertebrobasilar (VB) system comprises the main blood supply of the brain stem.

Vigorous rotation of the neck may traumatize the vertebral artery along its course, most likely between atlas and axis or atlas and occiput (Fig. 26-1). This trauma may cause a dissection or tearing of the inner artery wall, or the trauma may lead to formation of a blood clot that can break free and lodge in one of the other ascending blood vessels. Either event can result in a **cerebrovascular accident** (CVA), or **ischemia** to the brainstem. Alternately, the force of rotation may cause vasospasm in one vertebral artery. If preexisting arteriosclerosis or a developmental anomaly has compromised flow in the contralateral artery, brainstem ischemia may also occur.

Cervical adjustment/manipulation is not the only mechanism to initiate this type of injury.

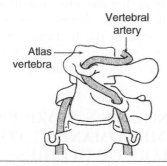

Fig. 26-1 The stretch applied to the vertebral artery with cervical rotation is a possible mechanism for vertebrobasilar stroke from adjustment/ manipulation. *(From Terrett AGJ: Current concepts in vertebrobasilar complications following spinal manipulation, West Des Moines, Iowa, 2001, NCMIC Group. Used by permission.)*

The literature contains numerous reports of similar vascular accidents resulting from common medical procedures, such as administering anesthesia during surgery[9,10] or during neck extension for radiography.[11] Cases of vertebrobasilar accidents (VBA) have been reported, which apparently occurred during normal activities such as swimming, yoga, stargazing, overhead work,[12] sexual intercourse,[13] and even during sleep.[14] "Beauty parlor stroke," caused by cervical hyperextension over a sink while washing the hair, is also well documented.[15] Cases of spontaneous VBAs, with no apparent precipitating event, have been reported as well.[16,17]

With the increasing availability of noninvasive imaging technologies, in particular magnetic resonance imaging (MRI), many patients who present with subtle manifestations of the condition are now being diagnosed as having a VB dissection. Although still considered an extremely rare form of stroke, the number of diagnosed cases of VBA has increased notably in recent years.

Based on the association between VBA and seemingly trivial stress to the artery, it is reasonable to conclude that this condition has a multifactorial etiologic aspect, likely involving both genetic and environmental factors. Several inheritable connective tissue disorders are associated with an increased risk of vertebral and carotid artery dissection.[18] These disorders include:

- **Ehlers-Danlos syndrome (EDS) type IV,** an inheritable disorder characterized by weakened linings of the walls of blood vessels and the intestine. Unlike more common types of EDS (sometimes referred to as the "rubberman" disease), type IV EDS is associated with minimal skin and joint hyperextensibility but is associated with a notable tendency toward easy bruising.
- **Marfan's syndrome,** a generalized disorder of connective tissue with skeletal, ocular, and cardiovascular manifestations. Characteristically, the affected person is tall and thin with long extremities, with an arm span greater than the height. These individuals often have long, thin, and hyperextensible fingers and commonly have a marked spinal kyphosis, deformities of the

sternum, or both, similar to pectus excavatum ("funnel chest") or pectus carinatum ("pigeon breast").

- **Osteogenesis imperfecta (OI),** a generalized inheritable disorder of the connective tissue associated with abnormal fragility of the skeleton, easy bruising, abnormal dentition, and blue sclerae. Milder cases of OI (type I) can also be associated with loose joints, low muscle tone, and a tendency toward spinal curvature.

Several recent studies have suggested a role for an infectious trigger in cervical artery dissections. One recent case-control study[19] established a recent respiratory tract infection as a possible risk factor of spontaneous carotid and vertebral artery dissections, a possibility supported by the seasonal variation in this condition, with a peak occurrence in the autumn.[20]

Other recent studies have suggested that mildly increased plasma levels of the amino acid **homocystine** (hyperhomocystinemia) might also be a risk factor for cervical artery dissections. One study[21] found that a series of 26 patients who had suffered a cervical artery dissection had higher plasma homocystinemia levels than controls, findings that were found to be statistically significant.

Mild to moderately increased levels of homocystine in the blood plasma (observed in 5% to 7% of the adult population) have been associated with an increased risk for a variety of cardiovascular diseases. This condition may be caused by congenital defects involving production of the enzyme 5,10-methylenetetrahydrofolate reductase (MTHFR). A chronic dietary deficiency of folate, vitamin B6, and vitamin B12 may also be an important cause.

Treatment of hyperhomocystinemia consists of vitamin supplementation and nutritional intervention, including direct supplementation with folic acid, vitamin B12, and pyridoxine. A diet rich in fruits, vegetables, and low-fat dairy products and reduced in saturated and total fat has been shown to lower serum homocystine.

Strokes of the posterior cerebral circulation (involving the posteriorly located VB arteries rather than the anteriorly located carotid arteries) usually present with signs of brainstem injury, such as severe nausea and vomiting, visual problems, or vertigo. Strokes of the posterior circulation also result in **Wallenberg's syndrome,** in which loss of pain and temperature of the face occurs on the ipsilateral (same) side of the lesion and of the body on the contralateral (opposite) side. Extreme cases can demonstrate the **locked-in syndrome,** during which the patient is conscious but completely paralyzed except for eye movements.

Although the outcome of VB strokes can be catastrophic, it is important to note that only a minority of these strokes are fatal or result in such severe disability. In 2001, Terrett[22] summarized the outcomes of the 255 cases of VBAs after spinal adjustment/manipulation reported in the worldwide medical literature from 1934 to 1999. Approximately 30% of the cases resolved completely or almost completely. Death occurred in 37 cases (15%), and 9 cases (4%) resulted in the locked-in syndrome with tetraplegia. In a retrospective analysis of hospital records, Saeed and colleagues[23] followed up on 26 patients who suffered VBA from a variety of causes. The authors found that 83% had a favorable outcome and the recurrence rate was low. A poor prognosis was usually associated with bilateral dissection and intracranial VB dissection accompanied by subarachnoid hemorrhage.

It has been proposed that the rate of strokes after adjustment/manipulation may be significantly underreported in the literature.[24] However, equally likely is that the cases resulting in death or major neurologic deficits are proportionally overreported in the literature. Serious and impressive cases appear more likely to warrant description in a published case report.

INCIDENCE OF STROKE FROM ADJUSTMENT/MANIPULATION: A SUMMARY OF STUDIES

Every reliable published study estimating the incidence of stroke from cervical adjustment/manipulation agrees that the risk is less than 1 to 3 incidents per 1,000,000 treatments and approximately 1 incident per 100,000 patients who are being treated with cervical adjustment/manipulation (Table 26-1). When discussing a numerical estimate of this risk, it is especially important to make a clear differentiation between the number of *chiropractic patients* and the number of *chiropractic visits*. Even some authorities on this subject have become confused because some studies have attempted to estimate the risks per visit, while other studies discuss the risk experienced by each chiropractic patient over an entire course of care, which may include a significant number of visits.

Several studies have documented large numbers of cervical adjustment/manipulations without any reports of stroke or major neurologic complication. One report[25] documents approximately 5 million cervical adjustment/manipulations performed at the National College of Chiropractic Clinic from 1965 to 1980 without a single case of vertebral artery stroke or serious injury. Henderson and Cassidy[26] reported a survey done at the Canadian Memorial Chiropractic College outpatient clinic in which more than

Table **26-1** STUDIES THAT HAVE ESTIMATED THE PROBABILITY OF STROKE (CVA) AFTER CERVICAL ADJUSTMENT/MANIPULATION

Source	Methods	Findings
Dvorak[28]	Survey of 203 members of the Swiss Society of Manual Medicine	One serious complication per 400,000 cervical adjustment/manipulations; no reported deaths
Jaskoviak[25]	Report based on clinical files of the National College of Chiropractic Clinic	No cases of vertebral artery injury or stroke in 5 million cervical adjustment/manipulations in a 15-year period
Patijn[29]	Review of computerized registration system in Holland	Overall rate of complication of 1 in 518,000 adjustment/manipulations
Haldeman[31]	Extensive literature review to formulate practice guidelines	1-2 incidences of stroke per million adjustment/manipulations
Carey[32]	Review of Canadian malpractice figures	1 CVA per 3,000,000 neck adjustment/manipulations
Klougart[34]	Survey of Danish Chiropractors' Association members, cross-referenced of CVA occurrences from published cases, official complaints and insurance data	1 CVA per 1,320,000 cervical spine treatment sessions and 1 CVA per 414,000 cervical spine sessions using rotation techniques in the upper cervical spine
Haldeman, Carey et al[33]	Updated review of Canadian malpractice figures	Risk of CVA 1 in 5.85 million cervical adjustment/manipulations, 1 in 1430 chiropractic practice years, and 1 in 48 chiropractic practice careers
Rothwell[35]	Case-control study, based on review of hospital records for VBA and insurance billing records for chiropractic visits	1 CVA per 3-4 million chiropractic cervical visits; "for every 100,000 persons aged <45 years receiving chiropractic, approximately 1.3 cases of VBA attributable to chiropractic would be observed within 1 week of their manipulation."

CVA, Cerebrovascular accident; *VBA*, vertebrobasilar accident.

500,000 treatments were given over a 9-year period, again without serious incident. Eder[27] offered a report of 168,000 cervical adjustment/manipulations over a 28-year period without a single significant complication.

A survey of 203 members of the Swiss Society for Manual Medicine[28] found a practitioner-reported rate of 1 serious complication per 400,000 cervical manipulations, without any reported deaths, among approximately 1.5 million cervical manipulations. Notably, these practitioners were nonchiropractors who received an average of approximately 38 days of training in manipulation. This survey represents the highest incidence rate of complications from cervical manipulation reported in the literature.

In another survey based on a computerized registration system in Holland, Patijn[29] found an overall rate of 1 complication in 518,886 manipulations. Other experts on adjustment/manipulation[30] have published opinions that the risk of stroke from cervical adjustment/manipulation is "two or three more-or-less serious incidents." per million treatments.

After performing an extensive literature review to formulate practice guidelines, the authors of a consensus document[31] concurred that, "the risk of serious neurological complications [from cervical adjustment/manipulation] is extremely low, and is approximately one or two per million cervical manipulations."

Carey,[32] the president of the Canadian Chiropractic Protective Association (CCPA), Canada's largest chiropractic malpractice insurance carrier, reviewed claims of CVA from chiropractic adjustment/manipulation in Canada between 1986 and 1991. Carey estimated that approximately 50,000,000 neck adjustment/manipulations were performed in Canada during that period, 13 of which resulted in significant CVA incidents, with no reported deaths. This article suggests that the incidence of CVA from neck adjustment/manipulation is approximately 1 incident per 3,000,000 neck adjustment/manipulations.

These figures were updated and republished in 2001[33] and found that 43 cases of neurologic symptoms after cervical adjustment/manipulation appeared in the malpractice database of the CCPA between 1988 and 1997. Based on a sur-vey questionnaire, estimates suggest that chiropractors covered by the CCPA performed approximately 134.5 million cervical adjustment/manipulations over that same time period. Based on these data, the authors concluded that the likelihood that a chiropractor will be made aware of an arterial dissection after cervical adjustment/manipulation is approximately 1 in 8.06 million office visits, 1 in 5.85 million cervical adjustment/manipulations, 1 in 1430 chiropractic practice years, and 1 in 48 chiropractic practice careers.

Klougart and Colleagues' 10-Year Danish Study

In one of the best-documented studies to date, Klougart and colleagues[34] sought to identify the total number of CVAs related to chiropractic adjustment/manipulation that occurred in Denmark over a 10-year period. All members of the Danish Chiropractors' Association were surveyed, and the members' reports of CVA occurrences were cross-referenced with published cases, official complaints, and insurance data. The authors then estimated the total number of neck adjustment/manipulations that chiropractors performed over the same time period from survey responses that were cross-referenced with insurance reimbursement data. Results indicated five cases of "irreversible CVA after chiropractic treatment." occurred in Denmark between 1978 and 1988 in the course of 6,600,000 cervical spine treatment sessions. Klougart estimated a risk of 1 CVA per 1,320,000 cervical spine treatment sessions and 1 CVA per 414,000 cervical spine sessions using rotation techniques in the upper cervical spine.

Rothwell and Colleagues' 5-Year Canadian Study with Statistical Control

A recent important population-based study published in the journal *Stroke*[35] has received much publicity, though its conclusions have been frequently misinterpreted. Rothwell and colleagues reviewed all hospital billing records in the province of Ontario between 1993 and 1998, and found a total of 582 VBA cases from all causes. Presumably, this search identified all cases of VBAs in this population because medical costs in Ontario are all recorded and paid by the provincial health plan; however, retrospective reviews of billing records are problematic because the diagnoses listed in billing records are often incomplete or inaccurate. Each VBA case identified was age and sex matched to four controls from the Ontario population who had no history of stroke. Public health insurance billing records were used to document use of chiropractic services for both the CVA patients and the four controls during the year before at the date of the VBA onset.

Based on the chiropractic billing history, the authors found that 27 of the 582 VBA cases were believed to have had a chiropractic cervical treatment in the year previous to the stroke. Of these, four individuals visited a chiropractor the day immediately preceding the VBA, five in the previous 2 to 7 days, three in the previous 8 to 30 days, and 15 in the previous 31 to 365 days. Compared with the controls, an increased incidence of VBA occurred among patients who saw a chiropractor within 8 days before the VBA event, but a decreased incidence of CVA occurred among patients who saw a chiropractor 8 to 30 days before the reference date.

This study found no correlation between recent chiropractic visits and VBAs in patients over age 45. However, patients under age 45 were five times more likely than the controls to have had a chiropractic neck treatment within the week before the VBA. Patients with VBA were also five times more likely to have had three or more chiropractic visits with a cervical diagnosis in the month preceding the VBA. Some media outlets and several chiropractic critics reported these findings with alarm.

It is important that the Rothwell group's findings be placed in proper perspective. Analysis of their raw data reveals that their findings relating cervical adjustment/manipulation to an increased incidence of VBA are based on fewer than five cases that occurred among the study's entire population over a 5-year time frame.

Stated another way, the data from the Rothwell and colleagues study show that the 11.5 million people of Ontario (approximately one third the population of Canada) had approximately 50 million chiropractic visits over the 5 years analyzed, some 15 to 20 million of which involved a cervical adjustment/manipulation. Among this population, approximately five incidences of VBA occurred that were statistically related to cervical adjustment/manipulation. Therefore this study actually found that the risk of a chiropractic-related VBA for the entire population was approximately *1 per 10 million chiropractic office visits* and on the order of *1 per 3 to 4 million chiropractic cervical visits.* "Despite the popularity of chiropractic therapy," the authors wrote in their conclusion,

[The] association with stroke is exceedingly difficult to study. Even in this population-based study the small number of events was problematic . . . . Our analysis indicates that, for every 100,000 persons aged <45 years receiving chiropractic, approximately 1.3 cases of VBA attributable to chiropractic would be observed within 1 week of their manipulation."

Even if one concedes that a statistically significant correlation exists between cervical adjustment/manipulation and VBA in the under-45 age group, correlation does not necessarily imply causation. Accumulating evidence suggests that sudden onset of headache pain, neck pain, or both may be an early indication that a VBA has occurred or is imminent. That many of these patients might present to a chiropractor for evaluation, treatment, or both of such symptoms appears likely. Given the established demographic patterns of chiropractic patients, also likely is that patients in the under-45 age group would be more likely than older patients to see a chiropractor for such symptoms. It would have been informative if the authors of this study had performed a similar study looking at how frequently patients of VBA saw *any* health care practitioner for a cervical-related diagnosis in the days or weeks preceding the stroke. Such a study might help clarify the early warning signs of this enigmatic condition and help all types of health care practitioners recognize a VB dissection before it becomes irreparable.

To their credit, Rothwell and colleagues recognized the limitations of this study and were duly cautious to not conclude that cervical adjustment/manipulation *causes* VBA. In contrast, an accompanying editorial[36] by a neurologist went much further, noting that, "For neurologists there is little doubt that chiropractic manipulation can cause vertebral artery dissection." As previously discussed, any such certainty—at least for the neurologists practicing in Ontario—would have been based on an average of a 1 case among some 100 annual cases of VB stroke. The same editorial goes on to state that this study demonstrated that the incidence of VBA dissection is "far more than the 1 case per million generally believed." However, this one-in-a-million figure is usually based on the risk of serious complications *per chiropractic visit*, or *per cervical adjustment/manipulation*. As previously noted, this study actually found that the risk of a chiropractic-related VBA for the entire population was on the order of *1 per 3 million chiropractic cervical visits*. Even in the apparently high-risk under-45 age group, the risk per cervical *visit* is still consistent with the widely quoted one-in-a-million figure.

Other data appearing in the Rothwell study found that only 2.1% of the 582 cases of VBA they identified had at least one cervical chiropractic visit in the month previous to the stroke versus 1.7% of controls that had a chiropractic cervical visit in the same time frame. In other words, VBA was correlated with a recent chiropractic neck treatment in only 0.4% of the 582 VBA cases they identified. These figures contrast sharply with the claim previously made by Norris and colleagues[37] that, "stroke resulting from neck adjustment/manipulation occurred in 28% of our cases [of VBA]." This data was collected from a survey of neurologists who treated patients of VBA. However, Norris' criteria for inferring this claimed relationship—much less their basis for presuming causality—have never been adequately described.

Relative Consistency of Data on Stroke

Taken together, the best quality studies form a remarkably consistent pattern regarding the frequency of stroke from cervical adjustment/ manipulation. In summary, a reasonable estimate of the risk of stroke from cervical adjustment/manipulation ranges between 1 in 400,000 to 1 in 5 million cervical adjustment/manipulations performed, and the risk of death from adjustment/manipulation-induced stroke is between 1 in 4 million to less than 1 in 10 million cervical adjustment/manipulations.

Research Challenges

Researching this issue more thoroughly presents many difficulties. Ideally, a **randomized controlled trial** (RCT) should be used to explore prospectively the relation between neck adjustment/manipulation and stroke. However, a reliable RCT requires the researcher to follow three times as many patients as the reciprocal of the expected reaction rate so as to be 95% confident that a single reaction will occur.[38] Thus, based on the best estimates currently available, an RCT would require observing 1.5 to 15 million neck adjustments to be valid. The time, money, and personnel required for such a prospective study would appear prohibitive.

Retrospective case studies may be the only feasible way to study this phenomenon. Unfortunately, many published case reports have serious drawbacks. Some reports are poorly documented and fraught with serious questions regarding the cause-and-effect relationship between the adjustment/manipulation and stroke. Other reports have misrepresented the profession of the practitioner, using the term *chiropractic* despite the fact that the involved practitioner was not a chiropractor.[39]

REDUCING THE RISKS

Although all the available evidence makes clear that stroke after adjustment/manipulation is quite rare, this is no reason for complacency on the part of chiropractors. Strokes from adjustment/ manipulation appear to fall into three patterns: manipulating the high-risk patient, inappropriate manipulative technique, and strokes occurring in patients who apparently who were unable to have been previously identified as being high risk.

Identifying the Patient at Risk

Certain patients have an identifiable preexisting abnormality that neck adjustment/manipulation can exacerbate into a completed stroke. In some cases, the problem can be identified by risk factors in the health history, by a **red flag** in the presenting complaint, or by a reaction to a provocative test that makes their preexisting condition apparent.

Occasionally, authors identify smoking and using birth control pills as risk factors for stroke from adjustment/manipulation.[40] These circumstances are established risk factors for most strokes; however, it is doubtful they are significant risk factors for strokes from adjustment/manipulation.[41] Characteristics such as advanced age, gender, and the presence of cervical **osteoarthritis** (OA) also do not appear to be significant risk factors for stroke from adjustment/manipulation.

Perhaps the most significant risk factors are found in the nature of the patient's presenting complaints. Case reports suggest that some patients may have shown signs and symptoms of VB insufficiency before the adjustment/manipulation that went unrecognized until it was too late. In these cases, the adjustment/manipulation probably exacerbated the preexisting condition. In other cases, the condition may have inevitably worsened as part of its natural course, though adjustment/manipulation was blamed for causing the stroke.

It is vital for chiropractors and other practitioners of manual therapies to recognize the signs and symptoms of VB ischemia, which Terrett[22] refers to as the **5Ds And 2Ns**:

1. Dizziness, vertigo, or light-headedness
2. Drop attacks (sudden fainting)
3. Diplopia (double vision) or other visual problems
4. Dysarthria (speech difficulty)
5. Dysphagia (difficulty in swallowing)
6. **Ataxia** (unsteadiness) of gait or **hemiparesis** (lack of voluntary movement on one side of the body)
7. Nausea or vomiting
8. Numbness or **hemianesthesia** (lack of sensation on one side of the body)

If a patient presents with any of these signs or symptoms, the practitioner should carefully consider the possibility of VB insufficiency. Another potential warning sign is the sudden onset of severe pain in the side of the neck, head, or both or in the occipital region, particularly if the pain is different than any pain the patient has had before. This case may represent referred pain from a trauma that has already occurred to the pain-sensitive wall of the vertebral artery and may herald the onset of a dissection. Significantly, patients may seek care at the chiropractor's office for treatment of this type of pain, and it may be misdiagnosed as musculoskeletal in origin.

A patient complaining of dizziness presents a particular diagnostic challenge. The dizziness or vertigo may have its origin in a musculoskeletal dysfunction of the cervical spine, in which case cervical adjustment/manipulation may be the treatment of choice.[42,43] However, the dizziness or vertigo might be an early sign of VB compromise, in which case a neck adjustment might precipitate a stroke. No simple and reliable method has been found to differentiate these entities. The practitioner should determine if neck rotation and extension aggravate the dizziness (which suggests a vascular cause), if any other of the **5Ds And 2Ns** are present, or whether cervical adjustment/manipulations have aggravated the symptoms in the past. The presence of any of these factors may suggest a vascular origin. *When in doubt, a prudent course is to treat the neck with other nonmanipulative conservative methods, such as soft tissue procedures, massage, physiologic therapeutics, or nonforce chiropractic techniques.* If the dizziness improves under this course of care, a musculoskeletal, nonvascular cause is likely.

Screening Tests

Various authorities recommend premanipulative screening maneuvers to identify high-risk patients.[44] These tests generally involve rotating and extending the cervical spine and holding it at the end-range of motion for a period while the practitioner watches for dizziness or other adverse effects suggesting VB insufficiency.

However, the literature offers little evidence supporting the validity of these tests.[45] Using these measures may only serve to give the practitioner a false sense of security. In Haldeman's[46] review, the practitioner described performing this screening test with negative results in 27 of the 64 cases of VBA that occurred after cervical adjustment/manipulation. In the past, this type of premanipulative maneuver was the de facto legal standard of care in many areas, but in light of recent findings, this test should rationally no longer be viewed as a standard. Preadjustment/manipulation screening tests are generally safe and may reveal patients with gross cerebrovascular pathologic conditions. However, the value of these tests in predicting the safety of a neck adjustment in any particular patient is doubtful.

Advanced Imaging Methods

In recent years, the possibility has been discussed that high technology imaging methods may offer a reliable means of screening out patients who are at risk of developing VB ischemia from adjustment/manipulation. Two of the most advanced imaging modalities considered in this regard are Doppler ultrasonography and duplex ultrasound scanning.

In theory, **Doppler ultrasonography,** particularly with duplex scanning, should allow blood flow in the vertebral arteries to be imaged and assessed in a noninvasive manner. One study[47] showed that duplex sonography could be used to record Doppler signals in the vertebral arteries in 89% of healthy volunteers. However, the clinical utility of these tools for screening high-risk patients before cervical adjustment/manipulation is far from established. For example, Thiel and colleagues[48] used duplex scanning to study the vertebral arteries in 42 subjects. Thirty of these subjects were controls with no signs or symptoms of VB insufficiency, and 12 subjects previously had a positive functional vertebral artery (VA) vascular test (i.e., clinical symptoms of arterial insufficiency on sustained neck rotation and extension). Duplex scanning detected no differences in VA diameter between the right and left sides in any of the subjects (whether experimental or control), and the

investigators found no difference in VA blood flow when any of the subjects held the various head positions that simulated the functional VA vascular tests. The results of this study may cast serious doubt on the utility of duplex scanning to correlate clinical findings from VA vascular tests with true VA insufficiency. However, problems with this study include the questionable validity of VA functional testing and the lack of a "gold standard" test for VA insufficiency.

If the value of duplex ultrasonography is uncertain for assessing reduced VA blood flow with neck rotation, its value is even more questionable in predicting whether cervical adjustment/manipulation will injure the artery by causing a dissection or vasospasm. At this time, Doppler and duplex ultrasonography have not been established as reliable or specific screening tools to determine in advance the safety of neck adjustment/manipulation in a particular patient.

Using Appropriate Manual Technique

In reviewing case reports of CVA after neck adjustment/manipulation, two points are apparent. First, when the reports describe the technique used, the vast majority apparently occurred with rotary cervical adjustments, particularly in the upper neck. Second, inexperienced, poorly trained, or untrained personnel appear to have performed the adjustment/manipulation in a disproportionate number of cases in which a serious injury occurred. Only properly trained, experienced, and qualified individuals should perform neck adjustment/manipulation.

Upper cervical adjustment/manipulations that use a strong rotary motion appear to be the most risky. One authority suggests discontinuing rotary upper cervical adjustments entirely.[49] Other authors have suggested that family physicians not refer to practitioners who perform rotary cervical adjustment/manipulation.[50] Given the good clinical results many practitioners report with this technique and the infrequent incidence of adverse effects, these suggestions appear extreme. However, the importance of good technique is underscored. If a rotary adjustment/manipulation is used, it is important to deemphasize excessive neck rotation and hyperextension and to emphasize lateral flexion to bring the joints to their physiologic end-range before thrusting.

Although no empirical evidence has been found that more forceful adjustment/manipulations are riskier, given what is known about the pathophysiology of VA dissections, the practitioner should apply only the amount of thrust necessary to bring the joint just beyond the elastic barrier and barely into the paraphysiologic range. This technique generally yields adjustments in which only a single audible "pop" is heard, rather than multiple cavitations. *Avoiding a follow-through in neck adjustments appears especially important*—the practitioner should release the force immediately after feeling the joint cavitate. Cervical rotation should not be continued to the anatomic end-range of the joint.

Another group of patients with strokes apparently resulting from improper care are those who experienced a mild or possibly uncompleted stroke from an initial adjustment/manipulation but whose condition was then greatly exacerbated by another adjustment/manipulation from a practitioner who ignored the early signs of a lesser stroke. If a patient exhibits any of the key warning signs or symptoms (the **5Ds And 2Ns**), experiences visual field disturbances (particularly seeing zigzag lines or flashing lights), or experiences other neurologic complications after a neck adjustment/manipulation, *the patient must not be remanipulated.* The literature contains reports in which a practitioner remanipulated a patient hoping to correct what appeared to be a mild "bad reaction."[51] In some cases, the second adjustment/manipulation appears to have changed what might have been a mild and temporary case of reversible ischemia into a completed and irreversible stroke.

If a patient shows any of the signs or symptoms as previously described after a neck adjustment, he or she should be allowed to rest quietly and should be observed closely. If the symptoms do not resolve or if they worsen, the patient needs to be hospitalized immediately. The emergency room physician should be told what happened so that the patient can receive proper care as soon as possible. The emergency treatment of choice for cervical artery dissection is immediate anticoagulant therapy.

Unpredictable Strokes

In some cases, a stroke occurs in the absence of identifiable risk factors despite a skillfully applied adjustment/manipulation. For practitioners, the existence of such cases is a humbling, even frightening, prospect because it means that even responsible and highly skilled doctors are capable of initiating strokes through adjustment/manipulation.

This sort of unpredictable adverse reaction is comparable to a severe idiosyncratic allergic reaction (e.g., anaphylactic shock) to an analgesic or an unpredictable severe complication from a routine surgery. The possibility of being injured by an unforeseen event is a fact of modern life, whether that event is an unavoidable auto accident, an unexpected adverse reaction to medication, or an unpredictable stroke from adjustment/manipulation.

OTHER ADJUSTMENT/MANIPULATION RISKS

Although the possibility of stroke from cervical adjustment/manipulation is the most publicized and serious complication from adjustment/manipulation, other cases of adverse effects from adjustment/manipulation have been reported.

Cauda Equina Syndrome

Cauda equina syndrome is usually described as the most serious accident that can result from lumbar spine adjustment/manipulation. This condition results from compression to the nerves running through the lower part of the spine—the cauda equina—as they pass through the lower part of the lumbar spinal canal. Cauda equina syndrome usually results from a large posteromedial disk herniation. The immediate effect can be a dramatic loss of bowel and bladder function. This condition appears to be an exceedingly rare complication from lumbar adjustment/manipulation.

In a detailed literature review of spinal adjustment/manipulation for low back pain, Shekelle and colleagues[52] estimated the occurrence of cauda equina syndrome from lumbar adjustment/manipulation to be less than 1 case per 100 million adjustment/manipulations. Terrett and Kleynhans[53] analyzed other disk-related complications from low back adjustment/manipulation and found only 65 cases reported in the worldwide literature in the 80 years from 1911 to 1991. The authors also noted that manipulative iatrogenesis is more common with adjustment/manipulation under anesthesia (usually performed by orthopedic surgeons), accounting for over 44% of the reported cases.

Additional Major Complications

Other major complications from adjustment/manipulation occur from missed diagnosis and inappropriate use of adjustment/manipulation. A variety of conditions are **relative** or **absolute contraindications** for adjustment/manipulation. These complications include metastatic tumors, unstable fractures, osteopenia, free disk fragments, and space-occupying lesions. Other authors have described these contraindications in detail.[54,55] All clinicians should also be familiar with the diagnostic red flags that indicate a patient with back or neck pain might have a potentially serious condition (Table 26-2). The presence of any of these red flags should alert the clinician to the possibility that the pain is nonmechanical in origin and suggests that further diagnostic procedures are warranted.

Less Serious Complications

Other less serious complications of adjustment/manipulation include sprains or strains, rib fractures, posttreatment soreness, and exacerbation of symptoms. Although these milder adverse reactions are far more common than the major complications of adjustment/manipulation, their self-limiting and relatively benign nature makes them a less pressing issue among chiropractors, patients, and chiropractic critics.

In a prospective clinic-based survey of 4712 treatments on 1058 new patients by 102 Norwegian chiropractors, Senstad[56] found that 55% of patients reported at least one unpleasant reaction during the course of a maximum of six visits. The most common complaints were local discomfort (53%), headache (12%), tiredness (11%), or radiating discomfort (10%) (Fig. 26-2). Reactions were mild or moderate in 85% of patients, and 74% of reactions had disappeared within 24 hours. No reports were found of serious complications in this study.

Good communication between doctor and patient can often help prevent a minor reaction from developing into a major issue. For example, advising a patient that he or she may experience some increased soreness or discomfort after an initial adjustment is prudent. If these reactions occur, they are usually mild and transitory, but they can be alarming to a new patient who is unaware that they may occur. New patients should be told to contact the doctor if a significant reaction occurs. This precaution allows the doctor to assess the situation and reassure the patient or advise some other course of action as needed.

RISKS OF CONVENTIONAL TREATMENT FOR NECK AND BACK DISORDERS

When considering the possible complications of chiropractic treatment, certain critics imply that nearly any degree of risk is unacceptable. The musculoskeletal conditions for which adjustment/manipulation is usually used are perceived to be self-limiting or unimportant. According to this logic, any complication encountered from treating such relatively benign conditions is unacceptable.

An example of this viewpoint is found in a 1993 *Neurosurgery* article,[3] which concluded the following:

[The] risk/benefit ratio for patients with midline neck pain is unacceptably high, and cervical SMT [spinal manipulative treatment] should be discouraged as treatment. Moreover, it is unlikely that a sufficiently high benefit for SMT in patients with benign disease processes will be achieved to justify the risk of severe complications, no matter how infrequent the occurrence.

The *Neurosurgery* article clearly implies that SMT is riskier than other options but provides no comparative analysis to justify this conclu-

Table **26-2** RED FLAGS FOR PATIENTS WITH BACK AND NECK PAIN

Musculoskeletal pain (such as back pain and neck pain) can sometimes be a sign of a serious underlying condition. Fortunately, the common pains that usually bring patients into a chiropractic office are rarely indicative of a serious disease. A number of signs should be considered reason for concern. A patient presenting with one or more of the symptoms listed in this table may require radiographs or further diagnostic studies to rule out potentially serious pathologic conditions. If these red flags are present, they are not necessarily contraindications to adjustment/manipulation; however, they do require further diagnostic investigation before even conservative care is initiated.

Sign or Symptom	Condition to be Ruled Out
History of a significant trauma, such as a fall or automobile accident	Possible traumatic fracture
History of osteoporosis, corticosteroid use, or endocrine disease; age over 50 years	Possible pathologic fracture
Recent unexplained weight loss or malaise; history of cancer or other serious disease	Possible pathologic fracture or metastatic disease
Nonmechanical pain pattern: constant, progressive pain unrelated to movement with no relief with rest; or severe pain during the night	Possible metastatic disease or referred pain from organ pathologic condition
Saddle anesthesia or sphincter disturbance, recent onset of bladder dysfunction (e.g., incontinence, increased frequency or urinary retention; bowel incontinence)	Possible cauda equina syndrome
Severe or progressive weakness or numbness in the legs or arms, particularly if it extends past the knee or elbow	Possible disk herniation with true radiculopathy
Neck pain that causes shooting pains into the arms or legs; or an extremely rigid neck when bending forward	Possible cervical disk herniation or meningitis
History of recent bacterial infection (e.g., urinary tract infection); intravenous drug use or immune suppression from steroid use, transplant or HIV infection; recent fever over 100° F	Possible spinal infection or meningitis
Constant headache or neck pain accompanied by numbness, weakness, dizziness, nausea, or vomiting	Possible CVA or CNS tumor
Headache or neck pain accompanied by confusion, visual disturbances, difficulties in speech or swallowing, or alteration in consciousness	Possible CVA or CNS tumor
Severe or constant and progressive headache or a sudden onset of "the worst headache ever"	Possible CVA or CNS tumor

HIV, Human immunodeficiency virus; *CVA,* cerebrovascular accident; *CNS,* central nervous system.

sion. To assess the risks of chiropractic treatment properly, the threat must be compared against the risks of other treatments for similar conditions. For example, even the most conservative conventional treatment for neck and back pain—prescription **nonsteroidal antiinflammatory drugs** (NSAIDs)—may carry significantly greater risk than adjustment/manipulation (see box, p. 575). Less conservative treatments such as neck surgery are also used for some condi-

tions similar to those chiropractors treat with spinal adjustment/manipulation. A 3% to 4% rate of complication exists for cervical spine surgery and 4000 to 10,000 deaths per million.[57] These risk rates are several orders of magnitude greater than the most extreme estimates of adjustment/manipulation risks.

Even bed rest, a mainstay of conservative treatment for back and neck pain in the past, carries substantial risks. These risks include

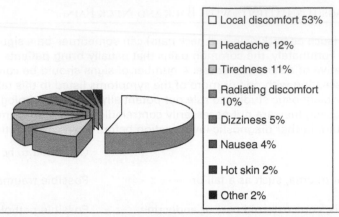

Fig. 26-2 Most commonly reported adverse reactions to spinal adjustment/manipulation, among the 55% of patients who reported at least one unpleasant reaction during a course of treatment. *(Based on Senstad O, Leboeuf-Yde C, Borchgrevink C: Frequency and characteristics of side effects of spinal manipulative therapy,* Spine *22:435 1997.)*

muscle atrophy (1.0% to 1.5% of muscle mass lost per day), cardiopulmonary deconditioning (15% loss in aerobic capacity in 10 days), bone mineral loss with hypercalcemia (increased blood calcium levels) and hypercalciuria (increased urine calcium levels), and the risk of thromboembolism.[58] The social and psychologic side effects of prolonged bed rest are also considerable. Current evidence suggests that more than 2 to 4 days of bed rest does more harm than good.

Moreover, doing nothing (i.e., not treating patients with neck and back pain) carries risks as well. These risks may include increased rates of disability, abuse of analgesics or illegal drugs for pain relief, and disruption of work and social activities.

DEALING WITH RISKS

Should chiropractors give routine informed consent warning patients of CVA from adjustment/manipulation? If the odds are truly one stroke in more than a million adjustment/manipulations, would a reasonable patient want to be informed of this risk? For comparison, are patients truly given informed consent before receiving treatments that are probably more risky, such as a prescription for an NSAID? In the experience of this author, standard practice does not include having patients sign informed

consent documents before receiving a prescription of Motrin. Is expecting chiropractors to provide a formal process of informed consent to every patient before performing a neck adjustment really reasonable?

Do most members of the public really have a concept of what a one-in-a-million chance means? As an illustration, the odds of winning the jackpot in most "Lotto" games is approximately 1 in 7,000,000; yet, millions of people spend large sums of money on a regular basis hoping to beat these astronomical odds. Indeed, many people treat the regular purchase of lottery tickets as a sound investment strategy. Is it reasonable to expect these same people to understand how rare a complication that can be expected to occur once in a million treatments is?

One in a million represents slim odds indeed. To illustrate this point, if a chiropractor performs 80 neck adjustments per week for 50 weeks per year, he or she would have to practice full time for 250 years before he or she might expect to cause one stroke. Statistically, for every 1.1 miles a person drives, a one-in-a-million chance exists that the driver will be involved in a disabling motor vehicle accident. If a patient comes to the doctor's office from the other side of town, is the care provider obliged to provide informed consent about the risk he or she takes driving to the office?

Currently in most communities in the United States, the standard of care for chiropractors does not require formal informed consent before performing routine cervical adjustment/manipulation. Canadian practice guidelines recommend using an informed consent form that specifically mentions the possibility of "stroke" and "serious neurologic injury" as a consequence of chiropractic treatment.[59] This issue continues to evolve throughout the world, and community standards of care are bound to change as more information becomes known about the frequency and mechanism of chiropractic complications.

Effectiveness of Chiropractic Adjustment/Manipulation versus Other Treatments

Numerous recent studies have found that spinal adjustment/manipulation provides superior clinical outcomes compared with other common treatments for neck and back complaints. These studies have been described in detail elsewhere in this text (see Chapter 23).

Ironically, despite their widespread use, the evidence supporting the effectiveness of NSAIDs for neck and back pain is limited. The Federal Agency for Health Policy and Research (AHCPR) Guideline for Treatment of Acute Low Back Pain[58] found that only 4 out of the 50 RCTs evaluating NSAIDs met their criteria for adequate evidence of efficacy, of which three found NSAIDs superior to placebo for short-term relief of low back pain. For comparison, the AHCPR found 12 RCTs for adjustment/manipulation that met the criteria for adequate evidence of efficacy. The evidence for NSAIDs in treatment of neck pain is even slimmer. A recent **MEDLINE** search (1966 to 1996) failed to identify even a single RCT examining the use of NSAIDs specifically for neck pain.[60]

Need for Consistent Standards

The history of pointed and often acrimonious criticism of spinal adjustment/manipulation in mainstream medical literature is long, although in the last decade, this criticism has been accompanied by increasing recognition of its value, as in the 1994 AHCPR Report, the 1996 RAND study, and the 2001 Duke University report.

The most common criticisms focus on the lack of definitive studies that clearly demonstrate the

NSAIDs: Is There Safety in Numbers?

The most common conventional first-line treatment for most musculoskeletal pain syndromes is NSAIDs.[61] These drugs are a broad class of prescription and over-the-counter drugs that include common aspirin, ibuprofen, Naprosyn, Voltaren, and similar drugs. NSAIDs are generally considered safe. These drugs are among the most prescribed drugs in the United States and represent approximately 5% of all prescriptions filled in the United States[62] or some 90 million prescriptions annually. NSAIDs also account for millions of dollars in annual sales of over-the-counter formulations.

In spite of their widespread use and perceived safety, NSAIDs have a significant risk of serious complications. The most common and most serious adverse effects associated with NSAIDs are gastrointestinal ulcers and hemorrhage. These complications of NSAIDs are likely an integral consequence of their pharmacologic components. NSAIDs probably provide their analgesic and antiinflammatory properties by inhibiting the synthesis of prostaglandins. However, prostaglandins are essential for promoting the health of the gastrointestinal mucus reducing gastric acid secretion and increasing the production of duodenal bicarbonate.[63] Unlike other common gastric ulcers, ulcers from NSAID use do not seem to be related to *Helicobacter pylori* infection and are not responsive to antibiotic therapy.

Although some people think of gastrointestinal ulcers as minor annoyances, they can often be very serious and can occasionally lead to fatal complications such as hemorrhage and perforation. At any given time, the chance of a patient on NSAID therapy having a gastric ulcer is 10% to 20%, a rate 5 to 10 times greater than nonusers.[64] One retrospective study[65] reported that nearly 80% of all ulcer-related deaths occurred in patients using an NSAID.

Continued

NSAIDs: Is There Safety in Numbers?—CONT'D

NSAIDs are often used for the long-term treatment of chronic conditions such as rheumatoid arthritis (RA). However, NSAIDs are also commonly used for symptomatic relief of musculoskeletal conditions. A diagnosis of OA accounts for over one half of NSAID prescriptions.[66] Many patients with symptoms of musculoskeletal pain, particularly chronic pain, receive a clinical diagnosis of OA or spondylosis. These individuals are exactly the type of patients chiropractors often treat effectively with adjustment/manipulation.

Fries[67] estimated 13 million regular users of NSAIDs in the United States. Eight million of these patients have OA or some other *miscellaneous condition*. The author used data from the Arthritis, Rheumatism and Aging Medical Information System (ARAMIS), a chronic disease database of 46,000 individuals in the United States and Canada. Fries found the rate of hospitalization from gastrointestinal (GI) bleeding was 0.4% per year higher than the expected rate among patients receiving NSAIDs for OA. Fries also estimated the death rate for NSAID-associated GI problems was 0.04% per year among patients with OA who are receiving NSAIDs or 3200 deaths in the United States per year.

A more recent study published in *The New England Journal of Medicine*[68] estimated that at least 103,000 patients are hospitalized each year in the United States for serious GI complications resulting from NSAID use. At an estimated cost of $15,000 to $20,000 per hospitalization, the annual direct costs of such complications exceed $2 billion. These authors also estimated that 16,500 NSAID-related deaths occur among patients with RA or OA every year in the United States. This figure is similar to the annual number of deaths from acquired immunodeficiency syndrome (AIDS) and considerably greater than the number of deaths from multiple myeloma, asthma, cervical cancer, or Hodgkin's disease. If deaths from GI toxic effects of NSAIDs were tabulated separately in the National Vital Statistics reports, these effects would constitute the fifteenth most common cause of death in the United States.

Complications from NSAID use apparently do not result only from chronic, long-term use. One meta-analysis[69] found short-term NSAID use was actually associated with a higher risk of GI complications than chronic use. The odds ratio for adverse GI events associated with NSAID use was 1.92 for more than 3 months of NSAID exposure but 8.00 for less than 1 month of NSAID exposure. (An odds ratio of 1.92 means that the odds that a person taking NSAIDs will develop an ulcer are 1.92 times the odds that a person not taking NSAIDs will develop an ulcer.) A double-blind trial found that 6 of 32 healthy volunteers developed a gastric ulcer that was visible on endoscopic examination after only 1 week's treatment with naproxen (at a commonly prescribed dose of 500 mg twice daily).[70] Although the risk of gastric complications varies widely among the different types of NSAIDs and is time and dose dependent, this study demonstrates that the risk can be significant even with short-term use of one of the most commonly prescribed NSAIDs at fairly low therapeutic doses.

Most studies of NSAID complications have dealt only with the prescription version of these medications. In recent years, an increasing number and variety of NSAIDs have become available in nonprescription strength. The widespread use of these over-the-counter NSAIDs may represent an increasing and underrecognized cause of peptic ulcer disease and ulcer-related hemorrhage.[71]

In the last decade, a new generation of NSAIDs, the cyclooxygenase (COX)-2 inhibitors, have been introduced amid claims of increased GI safety. These drugs are commonly marketed under the brand names Celebrex and Vioxx. Conventional NSAIDs reduce prostaglandin production by nonselectively inhibiting two forms of the COX enzyme: COX-1 and COX-2. Theories suggest that the inhibition of COX-1 is primarily responsible for inducing GI injury by impairing the production of the stomach's protective mucosal lining. COX-2 inhibitors selectively target the enzyme believed to be primarily responsible for pain and inflammation while sparing the COX-1 enzyme that allows for gut protection.

COX-2 inhibitors have still not been on the market long enough to determine if they have a significant safety advantage over conventional NSAIDs to justify their high cost (as much as 20 to 40 times the cost of a generic conventional NSAID). One recent review[72] article illustrated the way in which the initial enthusiasm for these drugs is gradually waning. "The promise (on theoretical grounds) of substantially improved safety" of the COX-2 inhibitors, they conclude, "has yet to be demonstrated convincingly in practice . . . . Most of the fully published evidence . . . points towards some reduction of

NSAIDs: Is There Safety in Numbers?—cont'd

risk but the advantage over conventional NSAIDs appears small," and the "spectrum of unwanted effects is similar to that of nonselective NSAIDs."

GI complications are not the only risks of NSAIDs. Uncommon side effects include hypersensitivity reactions, liver damage, and central nervous system damage.[73,74] Kidney disease is also an infrequent but potentially serious complication. One study[75] found NSAID use was associated with a fourfold increase in hospitalization for acute renal failure, a risk that was dose dependent and occurred especially in the first month of NSAID therapy.

Recent studies have raised serious questions regarding the appropriateness of using NSAIDs in cases of OA. Brandt[76] noted that no evidence was found that NSAIDs favorably influence the progression of joint breakdown in OA. The author also noted that several animal studies and human clinical studies have actually implicated NSAIDs in the *acceleration* of joint destruction.

Bogduk,[77] in reviewing the evidence supporting common treatments for neck pain, concluded that recommendations to use NSAIDs, exercise, and cervical collars were not valid. The author noted, "Of all the various therapies for neck pain, only early manual therapy for whiplash has been vindicated in the literature." Another review article[78] noted that, "although NSAIDs are good analgesics in many clinical settings, there are limited data supporting their use over pure analgesics or physical modalities in non-inflammatory musculoskeletal disorders." In a recent review of medications used for neck pain, the authors noted that the current standard of accepted practice "may rest on a quagmire of possibly valid, but unproven, treatments."[79]

To date, only one large-scale, randomized trial[80] has been conducted comparing manipulative therapy to general practitioner management (including NSAIDs) in treating back and neck pain. This trial found manipulative treatment significantly superior, with the advantages for the group treated with manipulation persisting at the 12-month follow-up (Table 26-3).

Table **26-3** Estimated Risks of Common Chiropractic Treatments and Common Medical Treatments and Accidents

Procedure or Activity	Estimated Risk	Source
Risk of developing cauda equina syndrome from lumbar adjustment/manipulation	1 in 100,000,000	(81)
Risk of death in fatal air crash, flying 425 miles (e.g., Boston to Washington, DC) on a scheduled commercial airline	1 in 4,000,000	(82)
Risk of death in motor vehicle accident, driving 14.5 miles	1 in 4,000,000	(82)
Risk of stroke or serious neurologic complication from cervical adjustment/manipulation	1 in 1,000,000- 5,000,000 treatments 1 in 100,000 patients	(34, 33)
Risk of being disabled in motor vehicle accident, driving 1.1 miles	1 in 1,000,000	(82)
Risk of death, per year, from GI bleeding due to NSAID use for osteoarthritis and related conditions	400 in 1,000,000	(69)
Overall mortality rate for spinal surgery	7 in 10,000	(58)
Death rate from cervical spine surgery	4-10 in 10,000	(57)
Rate of serious or life-threatening complications from spinal stenosis surgery	5 in 100	(58)

GI, Gastrointestinal; *NSAID*, nonsteroidal antiinflammatory drug.

effectiveness of adjustment/manipulation and on anecdotes illustrating the supposed dangers of the procedure. Much of the criticism appears to be sincere but misguided—motivated more by misunderstanding than by malice.

Of necessity, the healing arts have always been practiced-based both on pragmatism and on science. Even today, only a minority of mainstream medical methods has been exposed to careful scientific scrutiny.[83] On the level playing field of the contemporary health care system, each method must be fairly judged according to consistent standards. Spinal adjustment/manipulation should not be held to standards different than those required of other methods.

Review *Questions*

1. Which artery is most likely to be injured from cervical adjustment/manipulation? Other than cervical adjustment/manipulation, what are some other ways that this artery might be injured?
2. What is a reasonable estimate of the risks for a stroke following cervical manipulation?
3. What are the eight signs and symptoms of vertebrobasilar ischemia? Why is it important for chiropractors to be aware of and recognize the presence of these signs and symptoms?
4. Why does a patient with complaints of dizziness or vertigo present a dilemma to a practitioner of cervical adjustment/manipulation? What is a prudent course of action to take in treating these patients?
5. What specific type of neck adjustment seems to be most associated with an increased risk of vertebrobasilar stroke? How can technique be modified to decrease the risks?
6. What signs and symptoms might a patient experience following a neck adjustment that could indicate a potentially serious complication has occurred? What is a prudent course of action to follow if a patient presents with these signs and symptoms? What actions are imprudent?
7. Name five major contraindications for manipulation in general.
8. What are the red flags for possible fracture in a patient with back pain? What are the red flags for possible tumor or infection? What are the red flags for possible cauda equina syndrome?
9. What are some possible adverse effects from the use of NSAIDs for treatment of musculoskeletal pain? What is the most common and serious adverse effect?

Concept *Questions*

1. What factors should go into performing a risk/benefit analysis of a particular treatment? How do you determine if the risks are acceptable or not? Who should determine this?
2. For what types of conditions are the risks of spinal adjustment/manipulation acceptable and why? For what types of conditions are the risks unacceptable? Why? For these conditions, what are some alternative treatments a chiropractor could use with risks that are more acceptable?
3. How would you design a scientific study to better determine the risks of various chiropractic treatments? What strengths and weaknesses would your study have? How practical would it be to actually perform this study? How costly would it be to perform the study and where could you obtain funding?

REFERENCES

1. Thomas CL, editor: *Taber's cyclopedic medical dictionary,* Philadelphia, 1985, FA Davis.
2. Ernst E: Spinal manipulation: its safety is uncertain, *CMAJ* 166:40, 2002.
3. Powell FC, Hanigan WC, Olivero WC: A risk/benefit analysis of spinal manipulation therapy for relief of lumbar or cervical pain, *Neurosurgery* 33:73, 1993.
4. Coulter ID et al: The appropriateness of manipulation and mobilization of the cervical spine, Santa Monica, Calif, 1991, RAND Corporation Document No. MR-781-CR.
5. McCrory DC et al: *Evidence report: behavioral and physical treatments for tension-type and cervicogenic headache,* Des Moines, Iowa, 2001, Foundation for Chiropractic Education and Research.
6. Foster v. Thornton: Malpractice: death resulting from chiropractic treatment for headache, *JAMA* 103(16): 1260, 1934.
7. Anonymous: Neurologists issue public warning linking chiropractic and stroke, *eCMAJ* February 11, 2002, accessed 2/13/02. URL: www.cma.ca/cmaj_today/2002/02_11.htm.

8. Evenson B: MDs warn of chiropractic peril, *National Post* February 7, 2002.

9. Tettenborn B et al: Postoperative brainstem and cerebellar infarcts, *Neurology* 43:471, 1993.

10. Fisher M: Basilar artery embolism after surgery under general anesthesia: a case report, *Neurology* 43:1856, 1993.

11. Fogelholm R, Karli P: Iatrogenic brainstem infarction, *Eur Neurol* 13:6, 1975.

12. Okawara S, Nibblelink D: Vertebral artery occlusion following hyperextension and rotation of the head, *Stroke* 5:640, 1974.

13. Chang GY, Ahn PC: Postcoital vertebral artery dissection, *Am Fam Physician* 54:2195, 1996.

14. Hope EE, Bodensteiner JB, Barnes P: Cerebral infarction related to neck position in an adolescent, *Pediatrics* 72:335, 1983.

15. Weintraub MI: Beauty parlor stroke syndrome: report of five cases, *JAMA* 269(16):2085, 1993.

16. Swenson RS: Spontaneous vertebral artery dissection: a case report, *J Neuromusculoskeletal Syst* 1(1):10, 1993.

17. Mas J et al: Spontaneous dissection aneurysms of the internal carotid and vertebral arteries—two case reports, *Stroke* 16(1):125, 1985.

18. Schievink WI: The treatment of spontaneous carotid and vertebral artery dissections, *Curr Opin Cardiol* 15:316, 2000.

19. Grau AJ et al: Association of cervical artery dissection with recent infection, *Arch Neurol* 56:851, 1999.

20. Schievink WI, Wijdicks EFM, Kuiper JD: Seasonal pattern of spontaneous cervical artery dissection, *J Neurosurg* 89:101, 1998.

21. Gallai V et al: Mild hyperhomocystinemia: a possible risk factor for cervical artery dissection, *Stroke* 32:714, 2002.

22. Terrett AGJ: *Current concepts in vertebrobasilar complications following spinal manipulation,* West Des Moines, Iowa, 2001, NCMIC Group.

23. Saeed AB et al: Vertebral artery dissection: warning symptoms, clinical features and prognosis in 26 patients, *Can J Neurol Sci* 27:292, 2000.

24. Ernst E: Life-threatening complications of spinal manipulation, *Stroke* 32:809, 2001.

25. Jaskoviak P: Complications arising from manipulation of the cervical spine, *J Manipulative Physiol Ther* 3:213, 1980.

26. Henderson DJ, Cassidy JD: Vertebral artery syndrome. In Vernon H, editor: *Upper cervical syndrome: chiropractic diagnosis and treatment,* Baltimore, 1988, Williams & Wilkins.

27. Eder M, Tilscher H: *Chiropractic therapy: diagnosis and treatment (English translation),* Rockville, Md, 1990, Aspen Publishers.

28. Dvorak J, Orelli F: How dangerous is manipulation to the cervical spine? *Man Med* 2:1, 1985.

29. Patijn J: Complications in manual medicine: a review of the literature, *Man Med* 6:89, 1991.

30. Guttman G: Injuries to the vertebral artery caused by manual therapy (English abstract), *Man Med* 21:2, 1983.

31. Haldeman S, Chapman-Smith D, Petersen DM: *Guidelines for chiropractic quality assurance and practice parameters,* Gaithersburg, Md, 1993, Aspen Publishers.

32. Carey PF: A report on the occurrence of cerebral vascular accidents in chiropractic practice, *J Can Chiropr Assoc* 37:104, 1993.

33. Haldeman S et al: Arterial dissections following cervical manipulation: the chiropractic experience, *CMAJ* 165:905, 2001.

34. Klougart N, Leboeuf-Yde C, Rasmussen LR: Safety in chiropractic practice part I: the occurrence of cerebrovascular accidents after manipulation to the neck in Denmark from 1978-1988, *J Manipulative Physiol Ther* 19:371, 1996.

35. Rothwell DM, Bondy SJ, Williams JI: Chiropractic manipulation and stroke: a population-based case-control study, *Stroke* 32:1054, 2001.

36. Bousser MG: Editorial comment, *Stroke 32:1059, 2001.*

37. Norris JW, Beletsky V, Nadareishvili ZG: Sudden neck movement and cervical artery dissection (on behalf of the Canadian Stroke Consortium), *CMAJ* 163:38, 2000.

38. McGregor M, Haldeman S, Kohlbeck FJ: Vertebrobasilar compromise associated with cervical manipulation, *Top Clin Chiropr* 2:63, 1995.

39. Terrett AGJ: Misuse of the literature by medical authors in discussing spinal manipulative therapy injury, *J Manipulative Physiol Ther* 18:203, 1995.

40. Carver G, Willits J: Comparative study and risk factors of a CVA, *J Am Chiropr Assoc* 32:65, 1995.

41. Terrett AGJ: Vascular accidents from cervical spine manipulation: the mechanisms, *J Aust Chiropr Assoc* 17:131, 1987.

42. Chapman-Smith D: Vertigo, *Chiropr Rep* 5(5):1, 1991.

43. Fitz-Ritson D: Assessment of cervicogenic vertigo, *J Manipulative Physiol Ther* 14:193, 1991.

44. George PE et al: Identification of the high-risk pre-stroke patient, *J Am Chiropr Assoc* 15:S26, 1981.

45. Côté P et al: The validity of the extension-rotation test as a clinical screening procedure before neck manipulation: a secondary analysis, *J Manipulative Physiol Ther* 19:159, 1996.

46. Haldeman S, Kohlbeck FJ, McGregor M: Unpredictability of cerebrovascular ischemia associated with cervical spine manipulation therapy, *Spine* 27:49 2002.

47. Schoning M, Walter J: Evaluation of the vertebrobasilar-posterior system by transcranial color duplex sonography in adults, *Stroke* 23:1280, 1992.

48. Thiel H et al: Effect of various head and neck positions on vertebral artery blood flow, *Clin Biomech* 16:105, 1994.

49. Terrett AGJ: Vascular accidents from cervical spine manipulation: the mechanisms, *J Aust Chiropr Assoc* 17:131, 1987.

50. Assendelft WJJ, Bouter LM, Knipschild PG: Complications of spinal manipulation: a comprehensive review of the literature, *J Fam Pract* 42:475, 1996.

51. York v. Daniels: Medicolegal abstracts. Chiropractors: injury to spinal meninges during adjustments, *JAMA* 159:809; 1955.

52. Shekelle PG et al: Spinal manipulation for low-back pain, *Ann Int Med* 117(7):590, 1992.

53. Terrett AGJ, Kleynhans AM: Complications from manipulation of the low back, *Chiropr J Aust* 22;129 1992.

54. Dvorak J et al: Musculoskeletal complications. In Haldeman S, editor: *Principles and practice of chiropractic*, ed 2, Norwalk, Conn, 1992, Appleton & Lange.

55. Gatterman M: *Chiropractic management of spine related disorders,* Baltimore, 1990, Williams & Wilkins.

56. Senstad O, Leboeuf-Yde C, Borchgrevink C: Frequency and characteristics of side effects of spinal manipulative therapy, *Spine* 22:435 1997.

57. The cervical spine research society editorial committee: *The cervical spine*, ed 2, New York, 1989, JB Lippincott.

58. Bigos S et al: *Acute low back problems in adults.* Clinical Practice Guideline No 14, Rockville, Md, 1994, US Department of Health and Human Services, Public Health Service, Agency for Health Care Policy and Research, AHCPR Pub# 95-0642-3.

59. Henderson D et al: *Clinical guidelines for chiropractic practice in Canada,* 1993, Canadian Chiropractic Association.

60. Dabbs V, Lauretti WJ: A risk assessment of cervical manipulation vs. NSAIDs for the treatment of neck pain, *J Manipulative Physiol Ther* 18(8):530, 1995.

61. Dillin W, Uppal GS: Analysis of medications used in the treatment of cervical disc degeneration, *Orthop Clin North Am* 23:421, 1992.

62. Burke LB et al: *Drug utilization in the United States: 1989,* eleventh annual review, Rockville, Md, 1991, Department of Health and Human Services, Office of Epidemiology and Biostatistics, Center for Drug Evaluation and Research, Food and Drug Administration.

63. Bach GL: Introduction, *Scan J Rheumatol Suppl* 96:5, 1992.

64. Babb R: Gastrointestinal complications of nonsteroidal anti-inflammatory drugs. *West J Med* 157:444, 1992.

65. Armstrong CP, Blower AL: Nonsteroidal anti-inflammatory drugs and life threatening complications of peptic ulceration, *Gut* 28:527, 1987.

66. Savvas P, Brooks PM: Nonsteroidal anti-inflammatory drugs: risk factors versus benefits, *Aust Fam Phys* 20:1726, 1991.

67. Fries JF: Assessing and understanding patient risk, *Scan J Rheumatol* 92(suppl):21, 1992.

68. Wolfe MM, Lichtenstein DR, Singh G: Gastrointestinal toxicity of nonsteroidal anti-inflammatory drugs, *N Engl J Med* 340:1888, 1999.

69. Gabriel SE, Jaakkimainen L, Bombardier C: Risk for serious gastrointestinal complications related to use of nonsteroidal anti-inflammatory drugs. A meta-analysis, *Ann Int Med* 115:787, 1991.

70. Simon LS et al: Preliminary study of the safety and efficacy of SC-58635, a novel cyclooxygenase 2 inhibitor, *Arthritis Rheum* 41:1591, 1998.

71. Wilcox CM, Shalek KA, Cotsonis G: Striking prevalence of over-the-counter nonsteroidal anti-inflammatory drug use in patients with upper gastrointestinal hemorrhage, *Arch Int Med* 154:42, 1994.

72. Anonymous: Are rofecoxib and celecoxib safer NSAIDs? *Drug Therap Bull* 38:98, 2000.

73. Carson JL, Willett LR: Toxicity of nonsteroidal anti-inflammatory drugs; an overview of the epidemiological evidence, *Drugs* 46(suppl 1):243, 1993.

74. Saag KG, Cowdery JS: Nonsteroidal anti-inflammatory drugs: balancing benefits and risks, *Spine* 19:1530, 1994.

75. Gutthann SP et al: Nonsteroidal anti-inflammatory drugs and the risk of hospitalization for acute renal failure, *Arch Intern Med* 156:2433, 1996.

76. Brandt KD: Should osteoarthritis be treated with nonsteroidal anti-inflammatory drugs? *Rheum Dis Clin North Am* 19:697, 1993.

77. Bogduk N: Neck pain: how to treat, *Aust Dr Wkly* (August 21):i, 1992.

78. Saag KG, Cowdery JS: Nonsteroidal anti-inflammatory drugs: balancing benefits and risks, *Spine* 19:1530, 1994.

79. Dillin W, Uppal GS: Analysis of medications used in the treatment of cervical disc degeneration, *Orthop Clin North Am* 23:421, 1992.

80. Koes BW et al: Randomized clinical trial of manipulative therapy and physical therapy for persistent back and neck complaints, *BMJ* 304:601, 1992.

81. Shekelle PG et al: Spinal manipulation for low-back pain, *Ann Int Med* 117(7):590, 1992.

82. National Safety Council: *Accident facts,* 1995 ed, Itasca, Ill, 1995, National Safety Council.

83. Smith R: Where is the wisdom . . . the poverty of medical evidence (editorial), *BMJ* 303:798, 1991.

Chiropractic and the Law

Alan Dumoff, JD, MSW

Key Terms

I am not an advocate for frequent changes in laws and constitutions, but laws and institutions must go hand and hand with the process of the human mind. As that becomes more developed, more enlightened, as new discoveries are made, new truths discovered and manners and opinions change, with the change of circumstances, institutions must advance also to keep pace with the times. We might as well require a man to wear still the coat which fitted him when a boy as civilized society to remain under the regimen of their barbarous ancestors.

THOMAS JEFFERSON, IN A LETTER TO
SAMUEL KERCHEVAL, 1816

Several generations after these words were written, the art and science of chiropractic began its development. This development not only brought new ways of understanding and treating disease, but it also presented a challenge to state and private institutions developing to regulate, and in some cases, monopolize, the business of health care. Chiropractic has had many successes in crafting a role in the health care system and continues to face numerous challenges in an increasingly regulated and managed care system. Chiropractic has always reflected a somewhat idiosyncratic professional community, and many chiropractors are understandably uneasy with the unprecedented oversight and complexity in utilization reviews, quality assurance concerns, and the overarching control over all health care professions exercised by managed care and by governmental programs (see Chapter 29) for further detail on managed care and insurance issues).The intensity of the business development of health care has been counterbalanced to some extent by a resurgence of consumer interest in natural healing systems, creating additional opportunities and challenges for the chiropractic profession.

Although chiropractic is so well established that some ambiguity exists in referring to chiropractic as an "alternative" healing system, it clearly does offer an alternative to the dominant mode of allopathic* healing. As complementary and alternative medical (CAM) care takes an increasingly

---

*"Allopathic" medicine is now used as a synonym for "conventional" or "mainstream" medicine. Originally, the term was coined by homeopaths to describe medicines with allopathic, or oppositional, effects (i.e., antiinflammatory medicines used to combat inflammation) and to distinguish them from homeopathic medicines, which are asserted to work by the "law of similars."

stronger role in the health care system, chiropractic plays a unique role in this development. Chiropractic has the mixed blessing of being the best established and most widely used of all the alternative modalities, not only as a method of care for patients, but also as a target of old guard mainstream medical practitioners. Further development of chiropractic is advancing on many fronts. Legal actions against noncompetitive institutional practices and inappropriate denials by insurance companies, state laws banning discrimination against chiropractic in health care policies, reimbursement for a wider range of services by Medicare and worker's compensation programs, the continuing development of professional standards of care, and expanded interpretation of **scope of practice** are some of the most critical areas of continuing struggle as chiropractic seeks to make its legal purview expand to fit the range of competence it offers its patients.

HISTORICAL DEVELOPMENT

When D.D. Palmer began experimenting with spinal adjustments in the early 1890s, the professional landscape was composed of a lively competition between physicians and surgeons, osteopaths, homeopaths, eclectic herbalists, and a variety of other healers. At the turn of the century, what is now known as scientific medicine was at its very inception. Ether and antiseptics had been on the medical scene for only a generation, and the use of the "heroic" efforts of blistering, bleeding, and cathartics were in decline. Medical schools began to grow in earnest at this juncture, a growth that bloomed into a more professional education following the well-known Flexner report's recommendations in 1910.[1] By the time chiropractic was established in 1895, one half of the states had passed medical practice acts limiting the practice of medicine to those educated at allopathic medical schools.[2]

As medical schools became more professional in the early part of the century, many other professional and economic factors converged to accelerate the development of the medical profession. The development in the 1930s of third-party payers, including Blue Cross Blue Shield and **indemnity insurance** (fee-for-service) policies,

steered access to care sharply in the direction of medically trained providers. The development of medical hospitals and investment in the pharmaceutical industry also consolidated medical economic strength. These events established medical care as an industry and planted the seeds of the struggle between the professions of chiropractic and medicine.

Limited license statutes began shortly after the passage of the medical practice acts, as states recognized that practitioners such as dentists were required to focus on particular areas not within the training of medical physicians. Chiropractic was a principal part of this development. By the 1920s, chiropractic was flourishing with approximately 36,000 practitioners, a figure that has slowly grown to approximately 55,000 practitioners today.[3] Chiropractic at the beginning of the century was tolerated to the extent that many of the states without chiropractic licensing allowed large numbers of chiropractors to practice.[1] The Federation of Chiropractic Licensing Boards was established in 1933 to promote unified standards in licensing and to provide assistance to individual state licensing boards. By 1974, chiropractic was licensed in all 50 states and the District of Columbia.

Central to the development of any health occupation as a licensed profession is creating a standardized and accepted competency examination. The National Board of Chiropractic Examiners has been administering such examinations since 1965. All but a handful of states also require that chiropractors continue their training by imposing continuing education requirements before renewal of their licenses.

Current Efforts to Advance Chiropractic

The American Chiropractic Association (ACA), the International Chiropractors Association (ICA), and various state organizations have been actively working to further the legal framework under which patients have access to quality chiropractic care. The development of standardized practice guidelines, for example, has been a focus throughout the health care industry. The

Congress of Chiropractic State Associations has been developing such voluntary standards since 1992, referred to as the "Mercy Guidelines." The ACA was granted seats on two committees involved in periodically revising the **Current Procedural Terminology (CPT)** codes used to secure insurance reimbursement: the AMA/Specialty RVS [Relative Value Scale] Update Committee and the Health Care Professionals Advisory Committee (HCPAC). Another significant advancement in the acceptance of chiropractic was the creation of a "Chiropractic Health Care" section in 1995 in the American Public Health Association (APHA). The APHA had taken an antichiropractic posture until 1982, when it modified its stance resulting from efforts of the chiropractic community, including pressure from the historic lawsuit of *Wilk v. AMA*, highlighted later in this chapter.

Other recent developments are the successful campaign by the ACA, ICA, and the Association of Chiropractic Colleges (ACC) to secure inclusion of chiropractic care in the health services programs of the U.S. Department of Defense (2000) and Department of Veterans Affairs (2002); the addition of two doctors of chiropractic to the health services team serving members of Congress; and the appointment of Christine Goertz as the first chiropractor (she also holds a Ph.D.) to work in a full-time salaried position at the **National Institutes of Health,** as a program officer at the National Center for Complementary and Alternative Medicine (NCCAM).

Recent Growth in Alternative Practices

The last decade has seen phenomenal growth in the public and professional recognition of alternative and complementary health care approaches as a critical ingredient in health and wellness: the role of nutrition, exercise, and lifestyle; the contributions of alternative approaches, such as acupuncture, herbal approaches, and homeopathy; and the role of attitude and the responsibility of patients for their own health have all gained consumer and scientific acknowledgment. This growing interest is the result of the successes of alternative approaches and recognition of the limitations of conventional medicine as a complete

approach to health needs. Although still termed "alternative," these approaches are a significant aspect of our health care system; Americans make more visits to alternative practitioners than they do to primary care medical physicians (in 1997, 629 million visits to CAM providers versus 386 million visits to primary care physicians) and pay more out of pocket to see these providers than they do for all hospitalizations.[4,5]

The National Institutes of Health, through the NCCAM (formerly the Office of Alternative Medicine), is issuing grants as part of a new commitment to research the effectiveness of alternative treatments. Over 80 medical schools, including Harvard, are beginning to teach alternative medical practices, and a blue ribbon panel recently recommended that this practice be extended into all medical school curricula. These charges portend a growing integration of mainstream and alternative modalities, a shift that will create challenges and opportunities for chiropractors.

Criticisms of Medical Practice

Another influence affecting the public perception of chiropractic is increased attention to the iatrogenic hazards posed by medical science. In contrast to the drugless nature of chiropractic, the wisdom of pharmaceutical use has come under assault on a number of fronts, some debated more openly than others. A 1998 article in the *Journal of the American Medical Association*[6] noted that fatal reactions to properly prescribed, approved medications kill approximately 106,000 hospital patients per year, a staggering figure that makes this the fourth leading cause of death in the United States. This figure does not include outpatient deaths. The article also projected that 2.2 million patients are harmed in this fashion.

Other studies have raised serious issues about the objectivity of researchers whose funding depends on pharmaceutical companies, a source of income that creates an appearance, if not the reality of, a conflict of interest. This factor has also been quite public and has come from within segments of the medical profession itself, as has attention to the extent to which drug companies steer medical physicians and health organizations to use pharmaceutical therapeutics instead of other approaches.[7]

Although these stories do not by themselves suggest a sea change in public confidence in medical solutions, they are part and parcel of the consumer trend toward less technologic, invasive, and risky methods of healing.

SCOPE OF PRACTICE ISSUES

In the United States, regulating the practice of the healing arts is predominantly a state activity. Although the Federal government regulates some aspects of health care through food and drug law, administered by the **U.S. Food and Drug Administration (FDA),** and has a significant impact on what is deemed acceptable care through its regulation of third-party health insurance payment in the form of **Medicare, Medicaid,** and the Civilian Health and Medical Program of the Uniformed Services **(CHAMPUS),** as well as various health care fraud statutes, the vast majority of health care regulation is left to the states. This authority includes the licensing or certification of health care providers.

Each state decides which health care methods or types of provider it will authorize, the educational and other requirements for licensure, and the particular rules to which practitioners must conform their practice. Of particular importance, each state sets the nature and extent of practice allowable for each method. The amount of variation is significant among the 50 states in the scope of practice granted by the state, and chiropractors setting up practice must take special care to learn the nuances of these requirements in their own state. Some states have very narrow definitions restricting chiropractors to adjustment/manipulation of the spine, although most allow chiropractors a broader range of treatment modalities. Important to recognize is that just because a procedure is taught to chiropractors as a part of approved chiropractic curricula does not mean that the practice will be within the chiropractor's scope in a particular state.[8] Conversely, however, the lack of training in a procedure at a chiropractic college can be held to bar the practice.[9]

The grant given chiropractors to practice is considered a limited scope of practice. Every

health care provider other than medical and osteopathic physicians is given such a limited license. Most state statutes, for example, state that the grant of a scope of practice to one profession does not rule out its practice by another, that a licensed massage therapist, for example, has a right to perform massage does not prevent a physical therapist or a chiropractor from also performing massage. The grant of a right to perform spinal adjustment/manipulation to chiropractors does not, therefore, generally bar the unlimited rights of a physician. This issue provides an example of the convoluted relationship between state and federal laws. Although each state grants the right to practice, federal Medicare policy can have a direct impact on the practical realities of scope of practice. For example, The Center for Medicare and Medicaid Services (CMS), formerly the Health Care Financing Administration, will not allow a chiropractor to be supervised by a medical physician for the purposes of claim submission, because Medicare has correctly determined that chiropractic adjustment/manipulation is not within the training and scope of the medical physician. Therefore medical physicians generally may employ a chiropractor but cannot bill Medicare or most other third-party payer for the services of employee chiropractors, as they might, for example, a physician's assistant or nurse.

Although only medical and osteopathic physicians have a general license to diagnose and treat any disease or illness and under state laws can generally do so using virtually any treatment procedure, limited license practitioners (e.g., chiropractors, optometrists, podiatrists, dentists, acupuncturists, speech pathologists, audiologists) must make sure that they remain within the bounds of their licensed activities and do not infringe on the practice of medicine. Although courts may not always recognize the requirement, a disciplinary action against a chiropractor for exceeding the scope of chiropractic practice should arguably demonstrate that the statute did not authorize the practice in question and that the activity infringes on the practice of medicine.[10] Given the broad grant to medical physicians, demonstrating this infringement can often be accomplished.

Some chiropractors have attempted to avoid licensure by claiming that they are practicing naturopathy. This practice has been particularly true in states that allow the practice of naturopathy without regulation or based simply on registration, creating easier entry and less oversight. Because naturopaths may use manual manipulation as a part of their practice, these chiropractors have reasoned that they should be allowed to practice in this manner. The courts have disagreed, holding that the practice of adjustment or manipulation falls under the defined scope of chiropractic and thus requires such a license.[11] The trend in those few states that allow the practice of naturopathy is to require a license in any event. (Alaska, Arizona, Connecticut, Florida, Hawaii, Montana, New Hampshire, Oregon, Tennessee, and Washington license naturopathic physicians, and the District of Columbia requires registration rather than licensure.)

Scope of practice issues have also been the subject of heated disputes between groups of chiropractors with conflicting views of the role of chiropractic in health and the range of both illness and treatments that chiropractors should address. Disputes between "straights" versus "mixers," or "conservative" versus "broad scope" practitioners, have flared up in conflicts over which schools are accredited and how extensive a range of practices state licensing boards should accept. However, with Sherman College of Straight Chiropractic now holding full accreditation with the Council on Chiropractic Education (CCE), certain aspects of the decades-old accreditation controversy appear to have been resolved.

Debates on chiropractic scope of practice, however, continue to embroil the profession. In evaluating these disputes, understanding the broad ramifications is important. The acceptance of a particular school of thought at a regulatory level can affect whether a wide range of services can be delivered, such as adjunctive therapies (e.g., ultrasound, electronic muscle stimulation, hot and cold packs), nutritional counseling (including the recommendation of supplements), and extremity adjustment/manipulation, as well as procedures such as applied kinesiology, meridian therapy, and other services. Moreover, laws or regulations pertaining to certain diagnostic responsibilities and capabilities (e.g., diagnosing nonspinal conditions, performing **phlebotomies** for blood testing, ordering and interpreting magnetic resonance imaging films) may affect whether a chiropractor can act as a primary care physician and as a **gatekeeper** for the referral of covered services within a health plan. Because of the stakes involved, scope of practice limitations have been attacked in court, generally without success.[12] In the United States, chiropractic scope of practice issues are almost always resolved through state legislative action or interpretation of the law by chiropractic or other regulatory boards.

Legal Status of Chiropractors

Notwithstanding the limited scope of their license, chiropractors are considered **independent practitioners.** Independent practitioners are able to practice without a supervisory or collaborative relationship with a medical physician or other provider. In contrast, many health care occupations are dependent on some form of supervision or collaboration with a medical physician, such as nurses (except for advanced nurse practitioners) and physician assistants, among many others. Other practitioners, such as acupuncturists, physical therapists, and nutritionists, are treated as either an independent or dependent practice depending on the state.

The independent status of chiropractors allows them to play a role as a gatekeeper in various health care settings. Despite their independent status, some states bar chiropractors from using the term "chiropractic physician."[13]

As noted earlier, statutes also address chiropractors' ability to include a variety of particular modalities in their practice, such as acupuncture, acupressure, or meridian therapies; nutritional counseling; laboratory diagnostic procedures; ancillary or adjunctive procedures, such as electric muscle stimulators, hot and cold packs, diathermy, ultrasound, or massage; or even whether a chiropractor can perform either a physical or an x-ray examination that extends to parts of the body other than the spine.[14]

Chiropractors risk facing disciplinary proceedings by state regulatory authorities for practicing those activities that are not clearly within their scope of practice. Not surprisingly, these differences among state statutes reflect the political and legal struggle between the *straight* and *mixer* schools of thought within chiropractic,[15] as well as the concerns of medical physicians who have sought to limit the reach of chiropractic. Regarding conflicts between straights and mixers, an important aspect to note is that these categories do not reflect a sharp dichotomy in which all chiropractors are on one side or the other. The vast majority of chiropractors are in the middle ground between the extremes.

Acupuncture

In the United States and other Western nations, needle acupuncture has historically been considered to be a medical practice because it is offered for treating disease and also because it involves penetrating the skin. The practice of acupuncture by chiropractors has been addressed differently among the states. Some states allow chiropractors to practice as part of their standard scope of practice, others will allow practice after completing postgraduate training (commonly 100 to 200 hours), and approximately one half of the states do not allow such practice unless the chiropractor is separately licensed (Box 27-1). Some chiropractors practice a form of meridian

Box **27-1** STATES WHERE CHIROPRACTORS MAY PRACTICE NEEDLE ACUPUNCTURE

Alabama	Minnesota
Alaska	Missouri
Arizona	Montana
Arkansas	Nebraska
Colorado	New Mexico
Connecticut	North Carolina
Delaware	North Dakota
Florida	Oklahoma
Illinois	South Dakota
Indiana	Texas
Iowa	Vermont
Kansas	Virginia
Maine	West Virginia

therapy (via electric stimulation or digital acupressure) that does not involve the puncture of the skin. This technique is more likely to be acceptable given that it is not an invasive procedure, though results of disciplinary actions by state licensing boards have been mixed.[16]

Diagnostic Testing

Another issue of contention is the extent to which chiropractors may perform or order diagnostic testing. Some chiropractors perform complete physical examinations, including drawing blood for diagnostic testing or performing **Papanicolaou's smear.** Similar to most scope of practice questions, the answers at which chiropractic boards and state courts arrive have varied from state to state. The intent of the practitioner may govern the result; the procedure itself may be seen as within the competency of the practitioner, but in some states, an intent to diagnose human ailments *unrelated* to chiropractic practice can lead to **liability.**[17] However broad or restrictive the state law under which they practice, chiropractors (and all other health practitioners) are well advised never to exceed their scope of competence, even if a particular procedure beyond their competence is permitted by state law.

Nutritional Counseling

The right of a chiropractor to give nutritional advice has been the subject of much contention and confusion. Understanding allowable conduct under chiropractic practice acts is not always self-evident. Some courts have held, for example, that chiropractors cannot prescribe or otherwise suggest to their patients that they take a supplement available over-the-counter even when the state practice act allows for giving "dietary advice."[18] Nutritional advice has been problematic throughout the alternative health care community, though chiropractors have been a primary target for these actions despite the irony that many chiropractors are better trained in nutrition than most medical physicians. These disciplinary actions occur because of a concern that the chiropractor is *prescribing* for a particular ailment, which appears to the court to be counter to the established legal history of chiropractic as a "drugless art."[19] Courts are particularly concerned when specific remedies are suggested for particular ailments,[20] when the provider does not explain their educational background or limited scope of practice,[20] when blood work is used as a basis for nutritional guidance,[21] or when the provider has otherwise exceeded his or her scope of practice.[22]

The central basis for convictions is statements that can be interpreted as a prescription for a specific disease condition. However, many of these cases contain additional facts that may have added to the court's willingness to find the providers culpable of practicing medicine without a license. A chiropractor, for example, found guilty of medical practice act violations for giving nutritional advice was selling a line of nutritional products in his office. Although the language of the court suggests it may have upheld his conviction in any event, these sales may have undercut the argument that the statements were informational rather than prescriptive.[23] Of course, people holding themselves out as practicing chiropractic without a license are also subject to criminal prosecution.[24]

Although the scope of practice expressly arises only from the language of the state law, the standards of care established by the profession can influence a court in its interpretation of that scope when it is ambiguous. The ACA holds the position that "it is appropriate for doctors of chiropractic to recommend the use of vitamins, minerals, and food supplements for their patients, to the extent this is not in conflict with state statutes and regulations."[25] When weight loss is at issue, an assessment should be made, and the recommendations should not be for experimental products. The ACA also recommends that the chiropractor's suggestions be supported by independent laboratory data.[25] The ICA's policy on nutritional counseling and other ancillary procedures is as follows:

The Doctor of Chiropractic may elect to use appropriate ancillary and rehabilitative procedures appropriate to the area of the subluxation complex dysfunction in support of the chiropractic adjustment, nutritional advice for the overall enhancement of the health of the patient, and counsel for the restoration and maintenance of health.[26]

Providing information, as opposed to prescribing for a particular disease, may provide protection for chiropractors operating without a clear scope of practice allowing for nutritional consultation. Although this is a gray area of law, providing information and education rather than prescribing for a particular disease is on legally safer ground. Providing information is arguably protected by the First Amendment's guarantees of free speech. When one tells a patient, "If I had these symptoms, I would suspect a liver deficiency, and I would try to assist the liver using milk thistle herb," or "There is a significant body of evidence that daily use of feverfew can prevent migraines," this is providing information and is arguably protected speech. Although the protections of free speech are historically deeply honored and respected by our courts, the hoped-for protection in these statements might be rejected by a disciplinary body or the courts as merely an artifice meant to allow the practice of medicine, particularly when spoken within the context of a chiropractor-patient relationship.

A prerequisite to understanding this area of law is that the legal distinction that turns a substance into a drug is the purpose for which it is suggested. Any material intended for use to mitigate or cure a disease is a drug.[27] Most cases disciplining chiropractors for nutritional advice therefore involve the prescribing of a supplement for a particular disease condition.[28] When garlic is suggested because of its wonderful taste, it is a food; when garlic is suggested because it will mitigate arteriosclerosis by lowering cholesterol, it becomes a drug in the eyes of the law. Simply educating someone that evidence suggests that garlic lowers cholesterol, however, without mentioning arterial disease, references the nutritional impact on the structure and process of the body without going so far as to prescribe for disease. Such an approach may provide some protection, because it follows the approach taken by a compromise that Congress adopted in 1994 in its regulation of health claims on supplements and other natural products in the **Dietary Supplement Health Education Act** (DSHEA).[29]

This Act addressed the issue of health claims that may be made by supplement manufacturers, allowing claims regarding the impact on processes of the body but not with regard to disease or illness.[30] A supplement manufacturer may claim that calcium supplements improve the strength of bones, for example, but may not claim that calcium mitigates or cures osteoporosis. This distinction does not offer clear protection; important to recognize is that federal food and drug law holds that "articles (other than food) intended to affect the structure of any function of the body of man . . . " are a drug.[31] Nevertheless, discussing structure rather than disease in which the substance is at least arguably a food, as is the case for many supplements, serves to make the conversation more clearly educational and lessens, if not removes, the intent to prescribe a drug for a particular illness. Because state medical boards largely follow federal food and drug law in interpreting the scope of medical practice acts, framing advice in the same manner Congress allows manufacturers to label supplements under the DSHEA should have some weight in disciplinary matters.

ETHICAL ISSUES AND OTHER BASES FOR DISCIPLINE

Although ethical issues are not strictly legal in nature, violations of ethical principles can have legal consequences. State laws will generally make the violation of an ethical code a basis for discipline by the state chiropractic board. Ethical codes can also be considered standards of care, making their violation a basis for an action of **malpractice.** Substance abuse is a frequent basis for discipline. If a chiropractor has sexual contact with a patient, this ethical breach can be the basis for a malpractice action in addition to an action in **battery** (unlawful touching) and for a failure to obtain **informed consent** (a patient is often considered swayed by the authority of the health care provider and thus unable to grant informed consent for sexual

activity). Important to recognize is that risk is present even when the patient appears to be a willing participant. If the relationship turns sour, an action might ensue because the apparent consent might be held to have been manipulated under the influence of the doctor-patient relationship.

Some of the ethical issues somewhat unique to chiropractors involve various practice management procedures. Partly in response to difficulties in building a practice resulting from efforts by the allopathic community to marginalize chiropractic, many chiropractic colleges and practice management organizations teach a variety of techniques for building one's practice. Some of these suggestions raise concerns of professionalism or even of health and safety. Advertising free x-ray examinations, for example, may subject patients to unnecessary radiation without documented clinical need.[32] Efforts to incorporate mind-body or other holistic approaches into practice can in some instances also create exposure; informing patients that scoliosis is caused by emotional and psychologic problems, for example, has been a basis for discipline.[33]

MALPRACTICE AND DISCIPLINARY ISSUES

A health care provider becomes liable in malpractice when the provider (1) harms a patient (2) to which they owed a duty of due care (3) resulting from a negligent act (4) that violated the standards of care for the profession. The issue of harm and duty are usually clear in cases reaching the court. The issue on which litigation turns is generally whether the provider's negligence breached a **standard of care** and actually harmed the patient. Negligence can arise from commission, such as a forced adjustment that injures a patient, or omission, such as failing to diagnose a disease or contraindication or to make a referral to an medical physician or other professional when appropriate.

The rate of claims against chiropractors remained fairly steady throughout the 1990s; a chiropractor can expect to be sued at a rate of about 2.7 claims per 100 practitioners per year. Medical physicians are more than three times more likely to be subject to a malpractice claim, averaging about 9 claims per 100 practitioners during the same period. A malpractice carrier is more likely to reimburse a claim against a chiropractor. Slightly less than one half of claims against chiropractors are paid, with an average payment of approximately $60,000 per incident. Medical physicians claims are paid at a rate of approximately 30%, with a typical payment per incident of over $200,000.[34] The risk of malpractice claims is a fact of life for all health practitioners. Good rapport and communication with patients, including explanations of potential risks, is an important aspect of minimizing exposure.

Malpractice actions against chiropractors may be based on allegations that the patient was injured by an adjustment, such as one resulting in a stroke, that the chiropractor should have recognized that the treatment was contraindicated, or that the patient was misdiagnosed. One frequent basis for litigation is a claim that the chiropractor failed to take necessary x-ray examinations or other diagnostic tests.[35] Liability can also occur based on false representations of the reach of chiropractic care,[36] a claim in which the patient asserts that he or she was fraudulently induced into seeking a treatment for a medical condition not responsive to chiropractic and for which medical treatment would have been appropriate. Prescribing herbs for a serious infection or other medical condition is an area of definite malpractice risk.[37] Creating some pain during a procedure is by itself generally insufficient to create malpractice liability.[38]

Necessity for Referral

One critical area for chiropractors is the duty to refer to a medical or other provider for diagnosis or treatment if the chiropractor has reason to suspect a condition requiring such attention. Chiropractors are vulnerable to such suits given their limited scope of practice, particularly in some states whose statutes and judicial environment are not friendly to chiropractors. This obligation can even extend to a requirement that the chiropractor follow up with a patient to ensure that they follow up on the referral.[39]

Given the increasing interest in integrated

VARIATIONS IN INTERPRETATION

The law can be frustrating in the variable way it responds to issues of liability. In New York, a patient fell off an examining table, which was ruled to be ordinary negligence rather than professional malpractice, thus removing the matter from the hearing panel created for malpractice claims (*Rogers v. Schuyler,* 551 N.Y.S. 2d at 5 [A.D. 1st Dept., 1990]).

The exact opposite occurred in Louisiana. A patient fell off an x-ray table, which was held to be malpractice, resulting in the suit, brought as ordinary negligence, being dismissed for failure to bring the matter before the malpractice hearing panel (*Pitre v. Hospital Service District,* 532 So. 2d at 501 [La App. 1st Cir., 1988]).

Such distinctions, and their procedural results, can often drive the outcomes in malpractice litigation. (Source: *Chiropractic Legal Update,* June/July 1991.)

or multidisciplinary practices, chiropractors should be aware that collaborative practice has risks that, although manageable, are nonetheless real. A provider can be liable for the negligence of another because of association or because of joint work with the patient. An attorney can assist in limiting this liability by attention to the scope of practice governing the various providers, representations made to the patients, the legal structure of the practice, quality assurance efforts in choice of colleagues, and other such avenues.

Informed Consent

Similar to other health care professionals, chiropractors are also subject to liability for violating a patient's right to informed consent. This is an action in battery and is a modification of the long-established principle that people have a right to be touched only when they consent to that touch. Given the complexities of the professional health care relationship, the law has imputed a responsibility on the part of health care practitioners to educate their patients on the nature of procedures, including their risks and benefits, before touching patients in the clinical context. When such informed consent is not obtained, touching can be legally converted from a healing act into a battery.[40] A practice of adjusting patients who are unaware of the impending adjustment to minimize resistance makes the chiropractor vulnerable to such a suit, as does attempting to treat a presenting symptom from a part of the body distal to the spine without explanation or consent. A finding that the chiropractor misrepresented the treatment can lead to liability for failing to acquire informed consent.[41]

Informed consent forms can also provide some protection for alternative practices that fall outside the standard of care. Chiropractors who incorporate unusual approaches can inform their patients that the practice is not considered standard chiropractic care, as well as of the risks and benefits and alternatives to their techniques. A court might find, should an adverse reaction anticipated in the consent form occur, that the patient assumed the risk of the harm and thus find that the chiropractor is not liable. One medical case that accepted this argument involved the nonconventional cancer treatment of Emanuel Revici, M.D., whose finding of liability was overturned by an appeals court given this defense.[42]

Standard of Care

A primary concern for chiropractic has been to which standard of care the profession would be held in malpractice cases; early in the twentieth century, medical physicians would frequently testify against chiropractors despite their lack of education in and disdain for chiropractic care. Most courts now recognize that the standard of care to be applied for nonmedical health care practitioners is the standard of care for each particular nonmedical profession. The question is not what a medical physician should have done, but rather what a competent chiropractor (or acupuncturist, naturopath, or other relevant provider) would have done. Although the practices of chiropractic, for example, may seem *nonstandard* to a medical physician, the legal posture for chiropractic is that the chiropractic body of knowledge provides customary and stan-

dard practices for chiropractic.[43] Similarly, allegations that a chiropractor failed to diagnose an ailment accurately or recognize a contraindication would generally be tested not by whether a medical physician would have made the diagnosis, but rather whether a similarly trained provider would have done so. Testimony against a chiropractor therefore generally cannot come from a physician but must come from a person licensed in chiropractic.[44]

An important exception to this rule is when the chiropractor is found by the court to have exceeded his or her scope of practice and made what would be considered a medical determination. In that event, chiropractors will be held to a medical standard of care.[45] Chiropractors, similar to other limited-license practitioners, are limited in their legal ability to *diagnose and treat disease*, and face malpractice exposure when it can be shown that they exceeded their statutory scope of practice.

Malpractice insurance is an important aspect of protection against claims. Knowing one's policy and its exclusions is important. Intentional acts, such as sexual contact, will generally not be covered; this is also true of needle acupuncture or other modalities in states in which these techniques and modalities fall outside of the scope of chiropractic practice. Chiropractors should also be aware of their duties under their policy, such as reporting potential claims and advising of unusual practices.

Malpractice in Practice

An awkward dilemma that chiropractors face in some jurisdictions is that their liability in malpractice can arguably extend into areas for which it is difficult to protect themselves because of limitations in scope of practice. Chiropractors may be barred, for example, from performing a full physical examination, taking or ordering radiographs of the body other than of the spine, or ordering laboratory tests. Nonetheless, chiropractors may be liable in malpractice for failing to determine if a referral is necessary or if a procedure is indicated or contraindicated based on information that these tests would yield.[46]

One of the fronts along which the battle is fought for full recognition of chiropractic is inclusion as *primary care* physicians. The legal designation of primary care physician places principal responsibility for a patient's care on that physician and, in exchange, allows the physician greater participation in the health system. Depending on state law, designation as a primary care physician might, for example, create rights to contract with managed care organizations or health plans or to receive mandated coverage for a wider range of services. Such a determination has malpractice implications, as a primary care physician assumes broad responsibility for care, including missed diagnoses, and in some states, liability for referrals and other services the patient receives only indirectly to the physician's care. A threshold matter in this struggle is the extent to which the state law recognizes the chiropractor as a gatekeeper or physician with a broad scope of practice, a determination that allows the chiropractor to act as a first point of contact for assessment and care within managed care and insurance systems. When a chiropractor achieves some gatekeeper status (this is currently true in a small number of cases), the obligation to make proper referrals is increased when he or she finds signs or symptoms that may reflect a medical condition, particularly if that condition is outside the chiropractor's scope of treatment.

Even when the condition treated appears to be within the chiropractor's scope of practice, conservative practice still suggests that a referral be contemplated and discussed with the patient. Whatever the state law and regulations, the risk is that, should the symptoms turn out to signal a tumor or even a neurologic condition, a court may interpret a back or neck problem to be medical rather than chiropractic in nature, resulting in a malpractice finding against the chiropractor who failed to refer for a consultation.[47] The issue of referrals and missed medical diagnoses is less troublesome within current managed care networks because, in many cases, a medical physician will have referred the patient to the chiropractor. In this sense, the inclusion of chiropractors in managed care networks significantly lessens this primary area of exposure.

As chiropractors become gatekeepers in managed care settings, their liability will increase, and their scope of practice limitations may, in some cases, be inconsistent with full participation.

STRUGGLE BETWEEN CHIROPRACTIC AND MEDICINE: THE WILK CASE AND ITS PROGENY

The relationship between chiropractic and allopathic medicine has historically been uneasy at best. In a remarkable and significant decision, chiropractors Chester A. Wilk, James Bryden, Patricia Arthur, Steven Lumsden, and Michael Pedigo successfully sued the American Medical Association (AMA) for violations of federal antitrust laws[48] (Box 27-2). The **Wilk Case** suit alleged that the AMA "violated § 1 of the Sherman Antitrust Act[49] by conducting an illegal boycott in restraint of trade directed at chiropractors generally . . . . " The court found that the AMA had set out with clear intent to eliminate chiropractic and that the motive for this effort was focused not on protection of patients but based on the economic self-interest of its

BOX 27-2 DEFENDANTS IN THE WILK v. AMA ET AL ANTITRUST SUIT

American Medical Association
American Hospital Association
American College of Surgeons
American College of Physicians
Joint Commission on Accreditation of
  Hospitals
American College of Radiology
American Academy of Orthopedic Surgeons
American Osteopathic Association
American Academy of Physical Medicine
  and Rehabilitation
Illinois State Medical Society
Chicago Medical Society
Medical Society of Cook County
H. Doyl Taylor
Joseph Sabatier, MD
H. Thomas Ballantine, MD
James Sammons

membership. At the heart of this suit was the now infamous "Principle 3" of the AMA, which stated: "A physician should practice a method of healing founded on a scientific basis; and he should not voluntarily associate with anyone who violates these principles."

The evidence at trial clearly showed that the AMA branded chiropractic an "unscientific cult," and intended by Principle 3 to pressure medical physicians into boycotting chiropractors and anyone who associated with them. This boycott was managed by the AMA "Committee on Quackery," which moved to limit referral both to and from medical physicians, deny hospital privileges to chiropractors, and bar medical and chiropractic physicians from teaching in each other's schools.

In the middle of the trial, the plaintiffs dropped their money demand in an effort to focus on winning a declaration that the AMA had been conducting an illegal boycott. The plaintiffs had lost a jury verdict in a first trial but had that verdict vacated because improper jury instructions.[50] During the first trial, the AMA had presented the jury with a great number of practice management manuals in an effort to show that chiropractors are governed by greed rather than patient care. By removing the money demand,

this evidence was no longer relevant, and second trial focused on the issue of the AMA conduct.

The AMA argued at trial that their motive for the boycott was a genuine and reasonable concern for patient care. One of core successes of the Wilk legal team was that it presented enough evidence of the efficacy of chiropractic that the court found the "patient care defense" to be objectively unreasonable.[51] The court required the AMA to rescind its position with respect to chiropractic and to widely disseminate a new policy that did not discourage association with chiropractors by its members.

STATEMENT ON INTERPROFESSIONAL RELATIONS WITH DOCTORS OF CHIROPRACTIC

"The Illinois Medical Society, one of the *Wilk v. AMA et al* defendants, released the following statement as part of the case settlement.

The Illinois Medical Society declares that, except as provided by law (statute or final judicial opinion), there are and should be no ethical impediments to full professional association and cooperation between doctors of chiropractic and medical physicians. Individual choice by a medical physician voluntarily to associate professionally or otherwise cooperate with a doctor of chiropractic should be governed only by legal restriction, if any, and by the individual medical physician's personal judgment as to what is in the best interest of a patient or patients.

Professional association and cooperation to which the Illinois Medical Society's statement refers includes, but is not limited to, referrals, consultations, group practice in partnerships, health maintenance organization (HMOs), preferred providers organization (PPOs), and other alternative health care delivery systems; providing treatment privileges and diagnostic services, including radiologic and other laboratory facilities, in or through hospital facilities; working with and cooperating with doctors of chiropractic in hospital settings in which the hospital's governing board, acting in accordance with applicable law and that hospital's standards, elects to provide privileges or services to doctors of chiropractic; associating and cooperating in

PRE-WILK MEDICAL STANDARDS

One of the many practices of the AMA that came out at trial was the effort of AMA member physicians to subvert the customary handling of referrals that chiropractors made. The protocol for a referral between health professionals is ordinarily one in which the patient is sent to a specialist who sees the patient, suggests appropriate diagnosis and treatment, and then sends the patient back to the referring physician. AMA physicians were encouraged to give patients referred to them by chiropractors a "quack pack" that was used to discourage the patient from returning to the chiropractor. These clearly anticompetitive activities successfully denied patients both chiropractic services and the advantages of a team containing both medical and chiropractic physicians.

hospital training programs for students in chiropractic colleges under suitable guidelines at which the hospital and chiropractic college authorities arrive; participating in student exchange programs between chiropractic and medical colleges; cooperating in research programs and publishing research material in appropriate journals in accordance with established editorial policy of said journals; participating in health care seminars, health fairs, or continuing education programs; and any other association or cooperation designed to foster better health care for patients of medical physicians, doctors of chiropractic, or both."

Current Implications of the Wilk Decision

The court found that the conspiracy formally ended in 1980 but that the "lingering effects still threatened plaintiffs with current injury."[52] This finding is still as true today as it was when the opinion was written in 1990. Although an overt conspiracy may not be in evidence, these lingering effects are felt in the policies of third-party payers, the individual decisions of hospitals and other health care institutions, and efforts by some physicians and organizations still dedicated to eliminating chiropractic along with other forms of CAM health care.

One of the limitations of Wilk was that the court did not grant relief against the AMA's co-defendants. In addition to the AMA, the Wilk plaintiffs also pursued their action against the Joint Commission on the Accreditation of Hospitals (now the Joint Commission on Accreditation of Healthcare Organizations [JCAHO]) and the American College of Physicians (ACP), as well as several other medical societies. JCAHO and ACP were dismissed from the suit, and the plaintiffs settled with the American Hospital Association and other co-defendants.

As a result of the suit, however, JCAHO and AHA have taken the position that whether a hospital extends privileges is up to each individual hospital. The organizations no longer use the

threat of loss of accreditation or professional censure to force hospitals to exclude chiropractors. Whether position this brought an end to the conspiracy, or merely decentralized it to local communities, is open to debate and future litigation. Nothing in the Wilk opinion expressly prevents individual hospitals from choosing not to grant privileges to chiropractors. Suits since Wilk have been brought, often without success, because of immunity on the part of the hospitals or other defenses that have been upheld.[53] Progress in this regard has been definite but very slow; although some hospitals began extending privileges in the early 1980s when the Wilk case was first brought, to date only approximately 55 of the 6500 hospitals in the United States extend staff privileges to chiropractors, according to the ACA.

Staffing privileges allow chiropractors access to patients, their medical records, and some support services while patients are in the hospital. Some hospitals have taken the extra step of granting chiropractors "co-admitting" privileges under which they can admit a patient along with a medical physician. These privileges are generally granted either to individual chiropractors or to a group that contracts with the hospital to provide chiropractic services. A few hospitals have even set up a department of chiropractic within the hospital.

Current Litigation: Wilk Revisited in the Managed Care Setting

The dominant role managed care organizations (MCOs) play in the health care marketplace makes MCO policies toward chiropractic critical to the future of the profession. Some MCOs have been slow to accept the inclusion of chiropractic, and when services are covered, many MCOs do not accept the full range of chiropractic services. MCOs rarely afford chiropractors status as primary care providers with gatekeeping responsibility.

Whereas the battleground over unlawful boycotts by medical physicians against chiropractors in the 1980s included a significant emphasis on hospital privileges, the struggle has shifted to the more economically critical concern for full participation of chiropractors in managed care. A number of antitrust suits, including actions taken by the ACA and various state associations,[54] are being brought alleging a continuing conspiracy on the part of medical societies, hospitals, and MCOs to unlawfully boycott chiropractic services. The AMA, along with various MCOs, is once again being called to defend allegations of conspiring to restrain the delivery of health care services by chiropractors. At issue in these actions is the exclusion of chiropractors from participation in health plans as gatekeepers or providers, or when included, restrictions on the scope of benefits that effectively curtail the value that chiropractic offers. These limitations include restrictions on the conditions the plan will cover, limitations of treatment to only manual spinal manipulation, and denial of access to laboratories, x-ray facilities, and professional consultation and referral arrangements. Also at issue are the internal decision-making arrangements in which only medical physicians are enfranchised as decision makers, scientific studies demonstrating the superior efficacy of chiropractic for some conditions are arbitrarily dismissed, and excessive and improper utilization reviews target chiropractors. Some of these suits have been lost because of immunity or lack of evidence that HMO policy makers acted in concert or had a personal stake in the outcome of decisions that limited chiropractic care.[55]

A primary concern MCOs must address in choosing providers is the obligation to ensure professional quality. The profession of chiropractic, with its authorized scope of practice, well-established professional associations, credentialing bodies, **peer review** bodies, and established standards of care and ethical conduct, is clearly sufficiently developed to meet these quality assurance requirements. One difficulty health care institutions have faced in bringing chiropractors into their settings has been a perceived variability in chiropractic training. Some hospitals with experience working with chiropractors report considerable variation in the strength of the curriculum in the sciences and in the ability of chiropractors to provide effective relief for back injuries. Although the skills of medical physicians are also unquestionably vari-

able, a system based on medical **peer review** is understandably more comfortable dealing with such variation in their peers. Efforts are being made to incorporate chiropractors into the internal processes at health care institutions, which should eventually make these professional concerns more manageable.

REIMBURSEMENT ISSUES

Insurance Coverage

Coverage of chiropractic care has been increasingly incorporated into insurance contracts and currently represents approximately 60% of chiropractic income.[56,57] A December 1997 report from the federal Agency for Health Care Policy and Research (AHCPR) found that 80% of American workers in conventional insurance plans, PPOs, and point-of-service plans now have coverage that pays at least part of the cost of chiropractic care. Forty five states require insurers to reimburse for chiropractic services.[58] In forty five states Blue Cross Blue Shield Organizations are required to provide some chiropractic benefits.[58] A study by the Office of the Inspector General, Department of Health and Human Services, found that only 13 of 244 (5%) surveyed Medicare organizations do not use chiropractors to perform manual manipulations.[59] Coverage varies considerably by the type and extent of covered services and the diagnosis for which services will be covered. Even when a contract covers chiropractic services, chiropractors occasionally find that their claims are denied because the insurer claims that the treatments are not *reasonable and necessary*, or that payment amounts are capped or otherwise reduced contrary to the chiropractor's contract with the insurer or the patient's policy. These disagreements have been the subject of much litigation, based on varying theories[60] and with mixed success. One of the primary origins of this difficulty is the use of medical reviewers for chiropractic care, who may argue that no subluxations or musculoskeletal conditions exist or that conditions remediated by chiropractic would have resolved in any event. Chiropractors have sued a variety of decision makers, including peer review committees made up of other chiropractors, who oversee utilization decisions. Allegations have involved price fixing and limitations on the acceptable scope of practice. Whether peer review committees are immune from suit under federal law that protects the business of insurance is unclear, thus the results in such suits have been mixed.[61] Litigation generally arises either because of differences with medical review or because of differences of opinion within the chiropractic community. That effective practice management and proper billing procedures will help minimize such difficulties may be the case.

The opportunity to obtain improved reimbursement was enhanced with the report by the AHCPR, the federal agency charged with studying data on health outcomes. The agency's study on lower back pain, released in 1994, pointed to the success of spinal manipulation in both relieving pain and improving function. This recognition, in addition to numerous studies showing the positive impact of chiropractic,[62,63] may eventually result in increased payments and greater inclusion of chiropractors in the health care system. Unfortunately, the impact of this report will be somewhat diminished because the agency's role in setting standards has been reduced as a result of allopathic reaction to this report, especially by orthopedic surgeons. The AHCPR, now renamed the Agency for Health Research and Quality (AHRQ), no longer produces clinical guidelines.

Some state laws require that insurers grant parity or otherwise not discriminate against chiropractors in their payment of benefits. These laws are either specific to chiropractors or include **any willing provider law,** requiring that if a procedure is covered by the insurance policy, then a chiropractor or any provider who can perform that procedure within their scope of practice must be covered under the contract. However, even these laws have in some cases not achieved their purpose. A state may, for example, impose limitations on chiropractic care that indirectly affect insurance reimbursement. In Louisiana, chiropractors are barred from working in hospitals by statute. An insurance policy allowing 100% reimbursement for manipulations performed in a hospital (i.e., by osteopaths) but only 80% for outpatient work (i.e., chiropractors) was upheld as nondiscriminatory despite the disparate impact this had on reimbursement.[64] The court reasoned that the state can rationally limit chiropractors' access to hospitals and that procedures performed in hospitals can be billed differently than those done on an outpatient basis.

The state of Washington enacted a controversial requirement in 1995 that insurance policies allow "every category of health care provider to provide health services or care for conditions included in the Basic Health Plan."[65] This law requires that every health care plan sold in the state, including fee-for-service and managed care plans, must cover all services within the scope of practice of any licensed provider. As with an *any willing provider law,* if a "health plan covers rehabilitation therapy, that service must be covered whether treatment is rendered by an osteopathic physician, a chiropractor, a registered physical therapist, or a licensed massage therapist, so long as the practitioner is operating within his or her scope of practice."[66] What makes this law so unique is that it is based on covered conditions rather than on covered services. Any willing provider legislation generally requires that if a service (e.g., spinal manipulation) is covered, the policy cannot cover osteopaths and exclude chiropractors. The Washington law is much broader, requiring that if a person is covered for a condition (e.g., low back pain) that a licensed provider can treat within their scope of practice, the policy must cover the treatment.

A coalition of managed care and indemnity health insurance plans filed suit against the Washington State Insurance Commissioner, alleging that she misinterpreted that statute to require much broader mandatory coverage of alternative providers than the legislature intended.[67] The health insurance industry initially won a district court ruling that would have called into question the interpretation of Washington State's Insurance Commissioner requiring payments to a broad range of CAM practitioners. The appeals court reversed, allowing the insurance commissioner's ruling to stand.[68]

Many *any willing provider laws* have also been the subject of a great deal of litigation.[69] The legislative trend is expected to shift away from any willing provider laws, which some legislators believe were drafted too broadly. The legislative agenda may turn instead to **direct access laws,** which allow managed care plan members to access specialty care without having to access such care through a referral from a primary care gatekeeper. This legislation would allow patients to refer themselves to chiropractors and reduce the impacts of medical gatekeepers biased against chiropractic approaches.

Federal Programs: Medicare and Worker's Compensation

Insurance coverage for chiropractic has slowly and steadily grown. Although many third-party payers cover the range of services that are within the chiropractor's scope of practice, important limitations exist. Many contracts still specifically exclude chiropractors or limit payment to the diagnosis and adjustment/manipulation of spinal subluxations. These limitations are the result, in part, of the tendency of insurance policies to follow the lead of the federal government, a key player in the health care financing system, in determining compensable benefits.

Medicare limits payment to manual spinal manipulation for demonstrated subluxations of the spine. Medicare has also ruled that medical physicians can receive payment for manual spinal manipulation,[70] though some carriers that implement Medicare coverage have also determined that medical physicians cannot bill for the services of chiropractors who work under them, as they might for a physical therapist, for example, because manual manipulation is not within a medical physician's scope of practice. Once in practice, practitioners will learn that such seeming contradictions are not an unusual part of the regulatory environment.

Despite the fact that chiropractors handle many worker's compensation cases because of the success of the profession with work-related cervical and back injuries, federal worker's compensation similarly limits reimbursement. This requirement has, in some ways, limited chiro-

practic to a *one-procedure* profession, given that federal programs and some private insurance polices will reimburse only for CPT codes 98940, 98941, and 98942 (the codes for spinal manipulation/adjustment) despite the range of services chiropractic has to offer.

The federal limitations on payment for spinal adjustment/manipulation place undue hardship on chiropractors, not only because of the limitations on covered services, but also because of diagnostic requirements that must be met to obtain the payment that is available. From chiropractic's inclusion in Medicare in 1973 until January 1, 2000, Medicare would reimburse for chiropractic services only if an x-ray film demonstrated a subluxation and the chiropractor reasonably determined that the subluxation resulted in a neuromusculoskeletal condition for which adjustment/manipulation was appropriate. Nonetheless, Medicare still will not reimburse for the x-ray films used to support payment for the chiropractic care, nor will it yet cover other diagnostic efforts (such as a first-visit examination) in the patient's interest. The national associations continue to work to change this situation, seeking payment for a wider range of diagnostic categories and services and to add to the profession's success in gaining relief from the requirement that patients be exposed to x-ray regardless of clinical need. As a part of this effort, the ACA has been granted an unprecedented seat on the AMA committee in the process of developing recommendations to the Medicare system on reimbursement criteria and reasonable payment levels.

Many private insurers will pay for physical therapy codes, which are legally within a chiropractor's scope in nearly all states. Other codes present more complex difficulties and have even led to litigation. Texas, for example, ruled that manipulation under anesthesia and needle electromyography (EMG) were within the scope of chiropractic practice. An insurer brought suit because it would be obliged in worker's compensation cases to reimburse patients for a procedure it believed may not be legally performed by chiropractors. Practitioners must understand which codes their state board believes are within the proper scope of chiropractic and which codes will be paid by various programs and insurers.[71]

Although the courts allow the standard of care for chiropractic to be set by chiropractors in malpractice cases as previously noted, barriers to such professional self-direction still exist in the field of worker's compensation. Unlike malpractice, the issue of worker's compensation is statutory, and the language of some state statutes raises questions about whether a physician from one health care discipline (such as medicine) can offer an opinion that care being given by a practitioner of a different discipline pursuant to a worker's compensation claim is reasonable and necessary.[72]

A central issue in worker's compensation is whether chiropractors can serve as the primary physician in treating worker's compensation patients. Although chiropractors can generally serve in this capacity, certain mechanisms can work to exclude chiropractors. In some states, for example, employers are required to make a list of only a specified number of physicians available to a claimant, but there is nothing to require that the list include chiropractors.

Determinations in personal injury cases (primarily automobile accidents) are an important issue indirectly affecting reimbursement. These cases are an important source of income for many chiropractors, and the testimony of the chiropractor regarding the nature and extent of the injury is an important aspect of these recoveries. A primary issue here, once again, is the standard to be applied to testimony. The trend is to recognize that chiropractic issues are to be judged by chiropractic, not medical, standards.[73]

Reimbursement Mechanics

Utilization review (UR) committees are key centers of decision making in virtually all health care reimbursement systems. The function of UR is to review submitted claims to determine if the services provided are reasonable and necessary. Chiropractors often have particular difficulty with such review, in part because many UR committees still do not have chiropractors conducting the review of their work. Instead, this task is often assigned to nurses, medical physicians, or other nonchiropractors. Even when chiropractors sit on the UR committee, the pres-

sure to contain costs can result in determinations that do not follow the minimal standards of the profession. A chiropractic reviewer might, for example, deny payment for an x-ray examination with the conclusion that medical x-ray studies were available, even though the medical x-ray examinations were performed in a recumbent rather than weight-bearing position and thus were not acceptable for certain chiropractic purposes. These UR committee decisions to reject claims reflect the enormous pressure to contain costs. Unfortunately, UR committees and private companies performing UR functions enjoy limited immunity from civil action.[74]

Insurers and UR companies frequently refer patients for an **independent medical examination** (IME), which can include referral to a chiropractor for a second opinion. The IME raises numerous legal issues. When coverage for chiropractic is denied, one of the first places to seek information is the record by the examining physician. Unfortunately, this task can be difficult to accomplish because the records are not generally available to the claimant. Another issue is whether a chiropractor takes on malpractice liability by providing such an opinion. Courts generally conclude that no doctor-patient relationship is formed by such an examination, and thus no malpractice liability exists.[75] This same reasoning has also barred actions for simple negligence in performing the duties for an examining physician, the court reasoning that the only action in negligence that can be brought is one for professional negligence (i.e., malpractice), which requires a doctor-patient relationship.[76]

Careful record keeping is an important aspect of billing. One common pitfall is to record dates of services inaccurately. Such inaccuracy can lead to allegations of billing fraud. A surprising number of physicians alter charts in an effort to respond to litigation and are invariably caught.

Fraud and Abuse

Numerous federal statutes target kickbacks, overcharging, and other fraud and abuse issues. These laws are extremely complex, making it difficult for practitioners to follow the letter of the law. As a result, Congress passed the Health

Coverage Availability and Affordability Act of 1996 (HIPAA), under which the Secretary of Health and Human Services is required to provide advisory opinions answering questions on fraud and abuse issues.

A major area of enforcement activity are kickbacks and antireferral regulations in which an individual receives payment for referrals to an entity in which he or she has a financial interest or for merely making a referral. These referral fees generally include another provider, an attorney, or even a "runner" who receives payment, discounted office space, income guarantees, or other benefits for referrals. The issue is the intent of the parties and whether the scheme is intended to induce referrals. Marketing plans can be deemed legitimate or considered kickback schemes, depending on how they are structured. Kickbacks are also illegal when the provider refers to a laboratory or other venture in which the provider has a financial interest. The law provides "safe harbors" for many activities; any question about an activity should be addressed to legal counsel familiar with the area.

Overcharging is, of course, considered fraud, but it is important to recognize that this violation can occur in a variety of ways. **Miscoding, upcoding** to a CPT code with a higher fee, **unbundling** procedures normally billed together to bill the higher, separate amounts, and false reporting of time involved all can result in serious penalties. Many of these practices are of minimal concern to chiropractors given the few codes available to them, but as additional codes are developed for chiropractic use, chiropractors should familiarize themselves with these issues.

Some states regulate the waiver of **co-insurance** or a **co-payment,** * a few outlaw the practice outright, and others require that the insurer be notified of the practice. Failure to disclose waiver of

co-payment can be interpreted as evidence that the provider is not disclosing to Medicare or the insurer the true amount of the ordinary and customary charge and is inflating the fee to the payer.[77] If waivers are granted, they should be occasional, and the chart should reflect that the chiropractor did examine and base the waiver on the patient's circumstances rather than giving an across-the-board waiver. Medicare has taken the position that the routine waiver of co-payments is unlawful because it results in false claims by effectively overstating to Medicare the actual charge. This waiver is essentially considered a kickback to the patient, resulting in excessive utilization.[78]

Cash discounts for people who are not covered by insurance is also considered to be fraud. Just as with the waiver of co-payment, this conduct informs the insurer that they are being charged a premium rather than the provider's usual and customary rate. This issue not only arises under health insurance, but also in personal injury, worker's compensation,[79] and other third-party payment arrangements.

The question of whether certain services are unnecessary is a major area of controversy for chiropractors, given professional differences of opinion among chiropractors (for example, regarding scope of practice) and especially between chiropractors and the medical physicians who review many claims.

Other Practice Issues

Health care practice is a complex business, requiring attention to numerous details even beyond the central issues already described. One such issue arises when a practitioner provides inadequate services either because of a patient's limited resources or an insurer's restrictions on payment. Chiropractors should be cautious and not give an appearance of expressly withholding treatment they believe is indicated because of financial concerns once they accept a patient and become responsible for their treatment.[80]

Advertising is another area that requires some attention. An advertisement claiming, "Whatever the Cause, We Can Help," for example, can be

---

*Co-insurance is the percentage of the doctor's bill payable at each visit by the patient under the terms of some health insurance policies. *Co-payments,* or *co-pays,* which are required by some policies instead of co-insurance, are flat dollar amounts to be paid by the patient at each doctor visit.

interpreted as a guarantee, creating liability on the part of the practitioner for a poor result.[81] This type of advertising can also, of course, create disciplinary exposure for exceeding one's scope of practice.

HEALTH CARE FREEDOM

The current development of chiropractic in the health care system is occurring in the context of an overall renaissance in health care. The acceptance and potential for integration of complementary and alternative health care has been advancing rapidly over the last decade. Although this public development is positive, considerations of the legal rights one has to practice or to access the care of one's choice still have a direct impact on the development of chiropractic. The accelerating acceptance of alternative care, and the slow development of additional access to the range of alternative practice, have arisen from public demand rather than from recognition of such a right in the law. Courts generally hold that the U.S. Constitution does not provide a right to choose one's form of health care.

The **Ninth Amendment** and the "penumbra" of the Constitution have been held to create a right to privacy. The most famous opinion in this regard is *Roe v. Wade*,[82] which established a Constitutional right for women to have an abortion. This right of privacy has also been held to allow people the right to make end-of-life decisions.[83] Nonetheless, although courts recognize that the right to privacy and autonomy in one's decisions allows freedom at the beginning and end of life, they have been slow to extend such autonomy to choice of modality of treatment for the life lived in between. Courts do not extend this right to the practice of unorthodox medicine[84] or for patients to access the care of their choice. The issue has been raised in areas such as the right of a provider to practice an unconventional approach,[85] as well as nutritional and herbal treatments for cancer.[86]

The argument that the Ninth Amendment grants the right to seek the health care of one's choosing has been advanced without success.[87] The only rights courts have found within the meaning of the Amendment are those that sur-

vive scrutiny of the "'traditions and [collective] conscience of our people' to determine whether a principle is 'so rooted' [there] . . . as to be ranked as fundamental" (Griswold v. Connecticut, 381 U.S. 479, 493 [1965]) (J. Goldberg, concurring). Although individuals seeking alternatives to Western care would certainly rank such freedom as fundamental, the courts limit *retained* freedoms to such clearly, fundamentally, and universally held beliefs as the right to have a family, or, as in Griswold and its protection of birth control dissemination, to decide when to have a family.

The judicial opinions rejecting the Ninth Amendment as a Constitutional right to medical freedom are consistent with a vast and definitive array of case law that allows states the greatest possible latitude when regulating public health and safety. Potential rights under the Ninth Amendment must be balanced against the Tenth Amendment, which reserves all nonenumerated powers to the states. This power includes the so-called "police power," which allows the states virtually exclusive power to regulate matters of public health and safety. The state's police power almost always outweighs a call to what advocates of health care freedom might hope to see in the shadow of the Ninth Amendment.

One remarkable exception to this perspective is *Andrew v. Ballard*[88] in which the court in Texas found a statute restricting acupuncture to the hands of medical physicians irrational and unconstitutional. Whether chiropractors can practice acupuncture has been a frequent matter of dispute. In Andrew, the court found that the right to privacy includes the right to access the health care of one's choice, placing a limitation on the state's right to regulate health care practice and limit its practice to medical professionals. Unfortunately, courts have generally declined to follow Andrew.[89]

Instructive to note is that a careful reading of *Roe v. Wade* and its progeny suggest that the Court was not as impressed with the right of a woman to have an abortion as it was distressed at the idea that the state would have the right to limit the medical judgment of the physician. The courts have traditionally given great deference to medical physicians in virtually all areas of the law.

This deference, even in the face of demonstrated monopolistic practices, has been a significant source of the difficulty faced by chiropractors and other nonmedical providers. When the courts turn to the very profession whose professional bodies have opposed chiropractic, as well as other CAM approaches for guidance in how these matters should be addressed, it may be less surprising that a privacy right to choose one's treatment from a diverse array of modalities has not been widely adopted by the courts.

Review *Questions*

1. In what year did the final state in the United States pass a chiropractic licensure law?
2. Does the fact that a procedure is taught in chiropractic training institutions mean that the practice will be within the chiropractor's scope in a particular state?
3. Are there any circumstances in which sexual contact with a patient is legally acceptable?
4. What criteria determine malpractice?
5. Is the creation of pain during a procedure by itself sufficient to create malpractice liability?
6. Does the practice of adjusting patients unaware of the impending adjustment violate the principle of informed consent?
7. What was the AMA's primary defense in the Wilk case? How did the chiropractor plaintiffs overcome this defense?
8. What are some legal limitations of the Wilk decision?
9. How does Medicare define coverage for chiropractic services?
10. Name three fraudulent billing practices?

Concept *Questions*

1. Chiropractic scope of practice in the United States, unlike other nations, is governed by state laws that vary substantially from one to another. What do you believe is the proper scope of practice for the chiropractor?
2. What would be different now if the Wilk suit had never been filed?

REFERENCES

1. Starr P: *The social transformation of American medicine,* New York, 1982, Basic Books.
2. Thomas G. Moore: The purpose of licensing, *J Law Econ* 8(93):103, 1965.
3. American Chiropractic Association: *Frequently asked questions* [on-line] Internet, accessed June 6, 2003. URL: www.amerchiro.org/media/faqs.shtml
4. Eisenberg DM et al: Unconventional medicine in the United States, *N Engl J Med* 328:246, 1993.
5. Eisenberg DM et al: Trends in alternative medicine use in the United States, 1990-1997: results of a follow-up national survey, *JAMA* 280:1569, 1998.
6. Pomeranz BH: Adverse drug reactions may cause over 100,000 deaths among hospitalized patients each year, *JAMA* 279:1216, 1998.
7. Phillips P and Project Censored: Censored 2001: 25th anniversary edition: featuring 25 years of censored news and the top censored stories of the year, New York, 2001, Seven Stories Press.
8. See, e.g., *Van Wyk,* 320 N.W. 2d at 601.
9. See, e.g., *Jutkowitz v. Department of Health Services,* 596 A. 2d at 374, 384 (Conn, 1991).
10. See, e.g., *Beno,* 373 N.W. 2d at 548.
11. See, e.g., *Feingold v. State Board of Chiropractic,* 568 A. 2d at 1365 (Penn, 1990).
12. Sherman College of Straight Chiropractic v. American Chiropractic Association, Inc, 654 F, supp. 716; 1986-2 Trade Cas. (CCH) P67, 270 (N.D. Georgia, 1986).
13. In Maryland, e.g., see Op. Atty. Gen. 24:172, 1939.
14. See, e.g., *Attorney General on Behalf of People v. Beno,* 373 N.W. 2d at 544, 554 (Mich, 1985).
15. See, e.g., *State, Ex Rel. Iowa Department of Health v. Van Wyk,* 320 N.W. 2d at 599 (Iowa, 1982) (scope of practice would be not be expanded to include acupuncture, the drawing of blood for diagnostic procedures, or nutritional consultations despite suit by chiropractic board against the department of health); *Matter of Sherman College of Straight Chiropractic,* 397 A. 2d at 362 (NJ Sup. Ct., 1979) (chiropractors following "mixed" school of chiropractic sought to prevent accreditation of a school teaching "straight" chiropractic).
16. See, e.g., *State Board of Chiropractic Examiners v. Clark,* 713 S.W. 2d at 621 (Mo App., 1986) (laser stimulation of acupuncture points acceptable as a "reflex technique"); *Stockwell,* 622 P. 2d at 915 (meridian therapy allowed); cf., *State v. Wilson,* 528 P. 2d at 279, 282 (Wash, 1974) (galvanic stimulation "penetrates" skin and is therefore practice of medicine and barred to chiropractors).
17. See, e.g., *Spunt v. Fowinkle,* 572 S.W. 2d at 259, 264 (Tenn, 1978).
18. *Foster v. Board of Chiropractic Examiners,* 359 S.E. 2d at 877 (Georgia, 1987); *Stockwell,* 622 P. 2d at 914.

19. *Stockwell,* 622 P. 2d at 914. See also *Norville v. Miss. State Med Assn,* 364 So. 2d at 1084 (Miss, 1978); *State v. Wilson,* 528 P. 2d at 279 (Washington, DC App., 1974) (the American Chiropractic Association used the phrase "drugless profession" until 1974).

20. See, e.g., *State v. Hinze,* 441 N.W. 2d at 593, 594 (Neb, 1989).

21. See, e.g., *Foster,* 359 S.E. 2d at 878.

22. *Stockwell v. Washington State Chiropractic Disciplinary Board,* 622 P. 2d at 910, 914 (Washington, DC Ct. App., 1981) (chiropractor did meridian therapy as well as gave nutritional advice).

23. *Stockwell,* 622 P. 2d at 914.

24. See, e.g., *People of Michigan v. Rogers,* 2001 Mich. App. LEXIS 314 (Mich Ct. App., 2001).

25. American Chiropractic Association Policy ratified by the House of Delegates, June 1991.

26. International Chiropractors Association: *ICA policy statements,* [on-line] Internet, accessed June 5, 2003. URL: www.chiropractic.org/ica/policy.htm

27. See 21 U.S.C. § 321(g)(1)(B); *Foster,* 359 S.E. 2d at 880, 883.

28. See, e.g., *Norville,* 364 So. 2d at 1089.

29. Dietary Supplement Health and Education Act of 1994, codified at 21 U.S.C. §§ 321, 331, 342, 343, 343-2, 350, 350B; 42 U.S.C. §§ 281, 287C-11.

30. 21 U.S.C. § 343(r)(6)(B)(i).

31. 21 U.S.C. § 321(g)(1)(C).

32. See American Chiropractic Association Policy on X-Rays ratified by the House of Delegates, July 1993,

33. *Jutkowitz,* 596 A. 2d at 376.

34. Studdert DM et al: Medical malpractice implications of alternative medicine, *JAMA* 280(8):1610, 1998.

35. See, e.g., *Tilden v. Board of Chiropractic,* 898 P. 2d at 219, 221 (Ore App., 1995).

36. See, e.g., *Wengel v. Herfert,* 473 N.W. 2d at 741, 742 (Mich App., 1991).

37. See, e.g., Malpractice—no Virginia, herbs and oils will not clear up a virulent strep infection, *Chiropractic Legal Update* April-May 1, 1994.

38. *Boudreaux v. Panger,* 481 So. 2d at 1382, 1387 (La App. 5th Cir., 1986)

39. *Campbell v. F.H.P.,* No. 624061 (Orange County, Calif, 1994).

40. See, e.g., *Jones v. Malloy,* 412 N.W. 2d at 837 (Neb, 1987) (referral for possible myeloma not followed-up by chiropractor who continued to see patient for two years).

41. *Jones,* 412 N.W. 2d at 841.

42. *Boyle v. Revici,* 961 F. 2d at 1060 (2nd Cir., 1992).

43. See, e.g., *Clair v. Glades County Bd. of Comm,* 635 So. 2d at 84 (Fla App. 1st Dist., 1994); *Kerkman v. Hintz,* 406 N.W. 2d at 156, 161 (Wisc App., 1987).

44. *Kerkman,* 418 N.W. 2d at 800; *Wengel,* 473 N.W. 2d at 744; *Jones,* 412 N.W. 2d at 842.

45. See, e.g., *Kelly v. Carroll,* 219 P. 2d at 79 (Wash, 1950); *Boudreaux,* 481 So. 2d at 1488.

46. See, e.g., *Beno,* 373 N.W. 2d at 549; *Salazar v. Ehmann,* 505 P. 2d. at 387 (Colo App., 1972).

47. See, e.g., *Mostrom v. Pettibon,* 607 P. 2d. at 864, 867 (Washington, DC, 1980).

48. *Wilk v. American Medical Association,* 895 F. 2d at 352 (7th Cir., 1990).

49. 15 U.S.C. § 1.

50. *Wilk,* 895 F. 2d at 355.

51. 895 F. 2d at 356.

52. 895 F. 2d at 357.

53. See, e.g., *Cohn, D.C., v. Bond et al,* 953 F. 2d at 154; 1991-2 Trade Cas. (CCH) P69, 663 (4th Cir., 1991).

54. See, e.g., *American Chiropractic Association v. Trigon Healthcare, Inc,* 2001 US Dist. LEXIS 16057 (Case No. 1:00CV00113) (Va Dist. Ct., 2001) (antitrust matter still in progress).

55. See, e.g., *Solla et al v. Aetna Health Plans of New York, Inc et al,* 1999 US App. LEXIS 14628; 1999-2 Trade Cas. (CCH) P72, 570 (2nd Cir., 1999).

56. Goertz C: Summary of 1995 ACA annual statistical survey on chiropractic practice, *J Amer Chiropr Assoc* 33(6):35, 1996.

57. Hurwitz EL et al: Utilization of chiropractic services in the United States and Canada: 1985-1991, *Am J Publ Health* 88:771, 1998.

58. Anonymous: More states mandate new benefits, *Health Benefits Letter* 3(4):8, 1994.

59. Cited in *American Chiropractic Association, v. Donna E. Shalala,* Secretary of Health and Human Services, 131 F. Supp. 2d at 174 (DC, DC, 2001).

60. *Bumgarner v. Blue Cross & Blue Shield of Kansas,* 716 F. Supp. at 493 (Kans D., 1988) (alleged RICO violations, fraud, breach of contract, negligence, tortious interference with contractual rights, tortious interference with business relationships and defamation); *Waldroup, D.C. d/b/a Chiropractic Health Clinic and Healthbeat of Alaska v. Allstate,* 28 P. 3d at 293 (Alaska Sup. Ct., 2001) (insurer has a right to intervene on behalf of insured to argue that chiropractic care is not necessary).

61. See, e.g., *Bartholomew, DC v. Virginia Chiropractors Association, Inc* et al, 612 F. 2d at 812, 1980-1 Trade Cas. (CCH), P63, 075 (4th Cir., 1979) (peer review the business of insurance and therefore immune from suit under federal law); but see *Pireno v. New York State Chiropractic Association,* 650 F. 2d at 387, 1981-1 Trade Cas. (CCH) P64, 047 (2nd Cir., 1981) (peer review not directly involved with sharing of risk, so not immune).

62. Bigos S et al: Acute low back pain in adults, Clinical Practice Guideline No. 14, AHCPR Publication No. 95-0642, Rockville, Md, 1994, Agency for Health Care Policy and Research, Public Health Service, US Department of Health and Human Services.

63. Shekelle PG et al: Spinal manipulation for low-back pain, *Ann Int Med* 117:590, 1992.

64. *Guarantee Trust Life Ins. Co. v. Gavin,* 882 F. 2d at 178, 181 (5th Cir., 1989).

65. RCW § 48.43.045.

66. Bulletin issued by the Washington Insurance Commissioner (Dec. 19, 1995).

67. *Blue Cross of Washington and Alaska v. Senn, Washington, DC,* Sup. Ct., No. 96-2-00137-3 (filed 1/8/96).

68. *Washington Physicians Service Association et al v. Gregoire,* 147 F. 3d at 1039 (9th Cir., 1998).

69. See, e.g., *Prudential Insurance Co. of America v. Arkansas,* No. LR-C-95-514 (Ark E.D., 1995), arguing that the Patient Protection Act of 1995 is preempted by Federal law and is unconstitutional.

70. *American Chiropractic Association, Inc. v. Donna E. Shalala,* Secretary of Health and Human Services, 108 F. Supp. 2d at 1 (DC, DC, 2000).

71. *Continental Casualty Company v. Texas Board of Chiropractic Examiners,* 2001 Tex. App. LEXIS 2336 (Tex Ct. App., 2001).

72. See, e.g., *Clair v. Glades County Board of Commissioners,* 635 So. 2d at 84 (Fla App. 1st Dist., 1994).

73. See, e.g., *Dutcher v. Allstate,* 4th Dist. No. 94-0169 (May 24, 1995) (error to instruct the jury to find to a reasonable degree of "medical" possibility when one witness was a chiropractor).

74. See, e.g., *Corcoran v. United Health Care, Inc.,* 965 F. 2d at 1321, 1331 (5th Cir., 1992).

75. See, e.g., *Saari v. Litman,* 486 N.W. 2d at 813 (Minn App., 1992); *Rogers v. Coronet Insurance Co.,* 424 S.E. 2d at 338 (Georgia App., 1992).

76. *Rogers,* id.

77. See, e.g., *Kennedy v. Cigna,* 924 F. 2d at 698 (6th Cir., 1991); *Feiler v. New Jersey Dental Association,* 467 A. 2d at 276 (1983); *Reynolds v. California Dental Services,* 216 Calif, Rep. 331 (1988).

78. Office of Inspector General: *Special fraud alert, routine waiver of co-payments or deductibles under Medicare part B,* [on-line] Internet, accessed June 6, 2003. URL: http://oig.hhs.gov/fraud/docs/alertsand bulletins/121994.htm/

79. See, e.g., California Labor Code § 1871.7.

80. See, e.g., *Harris v. Friedman,* No. 75757 (Imperial County, Calif).

81. See Chiropractic Legal Update, April/May 1, 1990.

82. *Roe v. Wade,* 410 US 113 (1973).

83. See, e.g., *Matter of Quinlan,* 348 A. 2d at 801 (NJ Sup. Ct. Div., 1975), modified, 355 A. 2d at 647 (NJ, 1976); in *re Boyd,* 403 A. 2d at 744 (Washington, DC, 1979).

84. *Guess v. Bd. of Medical Examiners,* 967 F. 2d at 998 (4th Cir., 1992) ("there exists no protected privacy right to practice unorthodox medical treatment...").

85. See, e.g., *Majebe v. North Carolina Board of Medical Examiners,* 416 S.E. 2d at 404 (NC Ct. App., 1992) (finding that the right of privacy does not allow the unlicensed practice of acupuncture).

86. *Rutherford v. United States,* 442 U.S. at 544 (1979) (terminal cancer patients have no Constitutional right of privacy superior to the State's police power which allows them access to laetrile); *People v. Priviteria,* 591 P. 2d at 919 (Calif, 1979) (there is no right of privacy which requires the state allow access to laetrile).

87. *United States v. Vital Health Products,* 786 F. Supp. at 761, 777-78 (Wisc E.D., 1992), affirmed 985 F. 2d at 563 (1993).

88. *Andrew v. Ballard,* 498 F. Supp. at 1038 (Tex S.D., 1980).

89. See, e.g., *Potts v. Illinois Department of Regulation and Education,* 128 Ill. 2d at 322, 538 N.E. 2d at 1140 (1989) (there have been some other cases supporting such a right; see, e.g., *Rogers v. State Board of Medical Examiners,* 371 So. 2d at 1037 (Fla Dist. Ct. App., 1979).

CHAPTER 28

Appropriate Care, Ethics, and Practice Guidelines

J. F. McAndrews, DC

Key Terms

BOYCOTT
CHRONICITY
COMPENSATION
CULTISM

DURATION OF CARE
EMPIRICISM
JOINT DYSFUNCTION
LEVEL PLAYING FIELD

MERCY GUIDELINES
UTILIZATION REVIEW

A profession's maturity is defined by the knowledge and behavior of its members. True professionalism in health care requires that interest in economics be subordinated to the best interest of the patient, that guidelines based on objective information be developed and respected, that members of the profession be knowledgeable of the scientific literature relating to their practice, that research be encouraged so that the new knowledge it reveals can accrue to the benefit of present and future patients, and that those who aspire to professional stature interact with each other in a professional rather than political manner. By these measures, the chiropractic profession is now far more mature than it was a generation ago, but it still falls well short of its potential.

Chiropractic has made tremendous strides in the last quarter century with regard to educational standards and the development of a solid scientific research base. As a result, government agencies, private insurers, and the health care community as a whole have increasingly recognized chiropractic as a valid form of health care. Full integration into the mainstream health care system, however, still appears to be a generation or two away.

Why? After-effects of the decades-long antichiropractic **boycott** by organized medicine (for which the United States Supreme Court in 1990 affirmed liable the American Medical Association)

still cast a pall over chiropractors' relations with other health professions and the general public. However, blaming others is too easy. Chiropractors must also look within.

Substantial improvement is required in two critical areas: (1) respect for reasonable, objectively based practice guidelines and (2) development of a profession-wide ethic of financial fairness.

PRACTICE GUIDELINES: WHAT THEY ARE AND WHY THEY ARE NEEDED

Political Imperative

By the early 1990s, chiropractic leaders understood that a significantly more fact-based era had begun in which political muscle and agility could not be relied upon to take the place of objectively agreed-on measures of clinical efficacy. The profession faced an urgent need to design and develop its own practice guidelines. Failure to do so would have allowed the resultant vacuum to be filled by default, with guidelines prepared by medical directors, nurses, people with a master's degree in business administration, attorneys, managed care organizations, insurers, and third-party payers.

Guidelines for Chiropractic Quality Assurance and Practice Parameters,[1] which grew out of the

1992 Mercy Center Consensus Conference, placed the chiropractic profession at the cutting edge of the guidelines movement. In contrast to professions that attempted to delay the inevitable, or, similar to the orthopedic surgeons, to allow their guidelines to be prepared by a single individual, chiropractors convened a consensus conference representing an appropriate balance of opinions in the profession and then debated the issues until consensus was reached. Minority opinions were included in the published report, which is specifically intended to be a living document, open to ongoing revision as new information emerges.

Because chiropractic proactively moved forward with this project, the specter of chiropractic guidelines prepared by outsiders was averted. The consensus conference, by bringing together so diverse a profession, set a positive tone for chiropractic's future.

Need for Objectivity

Science seeks to counter the well-known inclination of the human mind to fool itself. That a particular patient, or group of patients, recovers from back pain or any other ailment after receiving chiropractic adjustments does not necessarily indicate a cause-and-effect relationship between the adjustments and the recovery. The placebo effect and the natural course of the illness must be factored into the equation.

To clarify these crucial issues, practice guidelines identify and organize available hard data in the peer-reviewed literature. When such data are lacking or inconclusive, a consensus process is used to determine which procedures are safe and appropriate. One of the great virtues of the guidelines development process is that identifying areas in which insufficient objective information exists encourages outcome studies and other research.

Most of chiropractic history has been marked by a freewheeling **empiricism** in which individual practitioners developed new techniques, applied them immediately in patient care, and then taught them to as many colleagues as possible. This process, in some ways, has served the

profession well—many current chiropractic techniques originated in this manner. However, anecdotal evidence, no matter how powerful, does not qualify as proof. All chiropractic methods, and those of other health care disciplines, must eventually be subjected to rigorous scientific investigation, facing what Thomas Huxley called "the great tragedy of science: the slaying of a beautiful hypothesis by an ugly fact."[2] Such scrutiny can cause intense uncertainty as the process unfolds. Possibly some widely used chiropractic methods may fail to pass muster. In the current era, however, no acceptable alternative to this system exists. If chiropractors wish to become full participants in the health care mainstream, they must abide by the emerging rules of the **level playing field**.

Because the Mercy conferees required that all claims either be documented in the scientific literature or acquire a measurable and significant level of consensus, the report they produced has stood up well when presented to agencies that require high standards of documentation, such as the Agency for Health Care Policy and Research (AHCPR) panel on acute low back problems in adults. Professions that appeared before the AHCPR panel lacking such documentation were markedly less successful than chiropractic. In the long run, such documentation spells the difference between integration and isolation. No responsible professional wishes to permanently relegate his or her profession to the fringe.

Key Areas in the Mercy Guidelines

The **Mercy Guidelines** address all key areas of chiropractic practice in a manner consistent with AHCPR procedures for guideline development. These guidelines cover a wide range of diagnostic and therapeutic procedures employed by contemporary chiropractors, determining in each case whether such procedures are supported by scientific data, evaluating and rating the quality of that data, and in the absence of conclusive data, seeking a consensus of clinical opinion.

Areas covered in Mercy Guidelines include the following:

1. History and physical examination
2. Diagnostic imaging
3. Instrumentation
4. Clinical laboratory
5. Record keeping and patient consents
6. Clinical impression
7. Modes of care
8. Frequency and duration of care
9. Reassessment
10. Outcome assessment
11. Collaborative care
12. Contraindications and complications
13. Preventive maintenance and public health
14. Professional development

Addressing all of these topics in detail is beyond the scope of this chapter. However, practicing chiropractors and chiropractic students have a responsibility to read the Guidelines and to consider the appropriateness of bringing their practices into accord with the consensus recommendations.

Critiques of the Mercy Guidelines

Probably the most common criticism of the Guidelines is that the document is difficult to read. Unfortunately, documents that committees prepare are seldom hailed for their high literary quality. Most other critiques of the Guidelines identify certain perceived failings, which on deeper analysis turn out to be failures of the profession, not the Guidelines. These failings include concerns about inadequate research, inadequate objective thinking, and inadequate organization of results and outcomes. All of these areas need improvement, but guidelines can only reflect the current state of professional development. Furthermore, although imperfections are certainly present, *Guidelines for Chiropractic Quality Assurance and Practice Parameters* compares quite favorably with guidelines prepared by other professions and specialties.

Other criticisms of the Mercy Guidelines relate to recommendations on duration of care, the appropriate number of visits for various conditions, and the suggestion that cases not demonstrating clear improvement within a 1-month period be referred out. In particular, strong concerns have been raised about insurance companies using the Guidelines as a basis for cutting off reimbursement for chiropractic care sooner than is warranted.

Instances undoubtedly exist in which the Guidelines have been misused, whether from malice or ignorance. The flaw, however, lies not in the Guidelines themselves, but in their misuse. The Mercy document specifically states that the purpose of such recommendations is "to assist the clinician in decision making based on the expectation of outcome for the uncomplicated case [emphasis in original]. They are NOT designed as a prescriptive or cookbook procedure for determining the absolute frequency and duration of treatment/care for any specific case."[1] Furthermore, guidelines should not be confused with standards. Guidelines are voluntary; standards are mandatory.

DURATION OF CARE

Duration of care is a major unresolved issue in chiropractic. Depending on which chiropractor a patient sees, the recommended course of care for the same condition may vary drastically, from several visits with one doctor to several dozen—sometimes hundreds—with another. Such variations appear in all regions, among graduates of all chiropractic colleges, and in urban, suburban, and rural settings.[3,4] Reducing these variations is crucial to the further advancement of the chiropractic profession.

Abuses of the System

The question of why a patient needs to return to a chiropractor for a series of visits is legitimate and controversial. Like it or not, chiropractors have a reputation for lengthy courses of care. In the absence of a rational, patient-centered explanation for this reputation, the unfortunate corollary assumption is that such extended care is primarily for the financial benefit of the chiropractor. Sadly, in some instances, this scenario is indeed the case. Such abuses of the system will be confronted first, and then how duration of care can be addressed within a patient-centered framework will be explored.

In the early 1990s, the author of this text participated in a retrospective review of a year's already-paid chiropractic claims, in which page after page of outrageous overtreatment by chiropractors was discovered. In one case, 278 visits for a diagnosis of mitral valve disorder occurred; in another, 155 visits for a uterine infection was recorded. *Such doctors are a danger to society.* In another case, a chiropractor had taken 70 x-ray films of a 12-year-old girl. The opinion of this author is that this person should be behind bars.

Honest chiropractors pay a high price for the fraudmerchants in the profession. One particularly disturbing example of overuse and its consequences involves the highly respected John Deere health maintenance organization (HMO), which initially included chiropractic benefits in its health plan. During the first year of Deere's HMO operation, two doctors of chiropractic who were involved in the highly dubious practice of "forgiving" deductibles and co-payments so that their patients had no out-of-pocket expenses, billed the HMO $1 million each! Almost immediately, chiropractic benefits were removed from the plan. The damage caused by unscrupulous practitioners such as these is incalculable. Many thousands of people with a genuine need for chiropractic care will not receive it as a result of these practitioners' unmitigated greed.

Unethical practices such as these have created a situation in which all chiropractors are tarred with the same brush. The title "doctor of chiropractic" is too often associated with "scam artist" or "trumped up" fraudulent insurance claims. In addition, when these cases of abuse are subjected to the glare of media attention, chiropractic care becomes associated with the 1½- to 3-minute office visits common in such assembly line operations. It is a sad state of affairs. Chiropractors cannot reform the entire health care system, but the profession can certainly clean up its own backyard. Unless honest chiropractors speak out against this behavior, the entire profession will continue to be judged guilty by association.

Guidelines for Duration of Care

What constitutes an appropriate course of care? How many visits are necessary? The North

American Spine Society (NASS), the RAND Consensus Panel, and the Mercy Consensus Conference have attempted to define a reasonable and customary number of visits relative to particular conditions, correctly distinguishing acute cases from chronic and complicated from uncomplicated.

NASS, for example, suggests two to five chiropractic treatments per week for the first 2 weeks in cases of acute low back pain, decreasing to one to two treatments per week, with an optimal treatment duration of 1 month and a maximal treatment of 2 to 4 months.[5]

The RAND Consensus Panel and the Mercy Guidelines recommend 2 weeks of initial care for the uncomplicated acute case. If no positive result is evident in this time frame and with this number of visits, 2 weeks of an alternative chiropractic method may be appropriately employed. However, if no demonstrable improvement is noted at the end of this second 2-week period, the patient should be referred. Profession-wide attention to this guideline would dramatically rein in overutilization.

Of course, if subjective and objective improvement is noted, treatment may continue, though with a decreasing frequency of visits. The following conclusions from a study by Haldeman and Nyiendo, cited in the Mercy Guidelines, are helpful in evaluating a reasonable course of care:

1. Patients with chronic disorders may require additional treatment or care to resolve symptomatic episodes.
2. Lordotic areas of the spine, on average, required twice the care compared with complaints involving the thoracic and transitional regions.
3. Most cases studied resolved well within 6 weeks of intervention consistent with the expectations from natural history.
4. Patients for whom care is necessary beyond 6 weeks may require up to 11 (mean = 3.8) additional sessions before reaching resolution.[1]

Why So Many Visits?

Determining a reasonable and customary number of visits for a particular condition is an important endeavor, but it does not confront the deeper issue of *why* such visits are necessary. What exactly does the doctor of chiropractic do, and why, during such time periods and visits?

Individuals and groups within the profession offer a wide variety of answers, the diversity of which adds to the confusion already felt by the public, as well as small and large purchasers of health care, particularly employers. Even **utilization review** companies often display uncertainty when this subject is examined. Though certain elements, including many medical physicians and some insurers, may not want to understand, others are diligently seeking a rational and objective explanation. Providing such an explanation is the responsibility of chiropractors.

The following is offered as a rational basis for chiropractors to explain to patients, insurers, and other health professionals what chiropractors do, and why multiple visits are often required for them to accomplish it.

FACT-BASED RATIONALE FOR CHIROPRACTIC CARE

Correcting malfunctioning musculoskeletal joints or articulations (subluxations) is a central goal of the chiropractor.[6] However, correcting joint function does not occur in a vacuum. Attending a dysfunctional joint may be:

1. A neurologic component
2. Muscular, ligamentous, disk, or other soft-tissue damage or derangements
3. Extensive and complex compensation to the original dysfunction, affecting the function of various other joints and tissues of the musculoskeletal system[7,8]

The neurologic component, which constitutes an important part of the chiropractic hypothesis, centers on the fact that nerve supply to the tissues surrounding the joint may exert either adverse or beneficial effects on the healing process. Time is required for healing to occur, even after **joint dysfunction** has been partly or completely corrected by the chiropractor.

Because soft tissue injury may result in adhesions, deformation of certain tissues, tearing, or rupture,[9] the chiropractor seeks to make joint function corrections, in many cases, over a period that allows maximal restoration of normal joint mobility, to avoid fixating the joint in either an abnormal position or within an abnormal range of motion. Because certain soft tissues have a minimal blood or nerve supply,[10] proper healing and normal repositioning or mobilization of the injured joint requires more time than, for example, a cut on the skin. Furthermore, the weight-bearing function of the musculoskeletal system also tends to interfere with this process of healing and normalization.[11]

During this healing process, periodic visits with the chiropractor are required to evaluate changes in structural balance and in the dynamic relationships among bones, disks, muscles, and ligaments. When necessary, the chiropractor shepherds the healing process by adjusting, manipulating, or otherwise intervening to aid these structures on their road to recovery.

Compensation

Compensation is a more complex phenomenon, but it follows a logical pattern. As an example, an office assistant is talking on the telephone, holding it by the force of neck muscles against the shoulder while taking notes. The sustained contraction of the neck musculature creates waste products in the muscles, which quickly become fatigued and will enter a phase of spasm. This condition may involve the large muscles of the neck or the small muscles that control, in part, relationships between the vertebrae.

When the office assistant puts the phone down and straightens the neck to its normal position, one or more of the muscles remains in a contracted state. The joint at this site cannot now move normally; it is dysfunctional. At this time, a state of pain and stiffness may or may not exist. All 24 movable segments of the spine function as a whole with each segment contributing its share of movement to the movement of the entire structure—somewhat similar to a shaft of wheat in the wind.[12] Thus one dysfunctional joint will alter, to some degree, the full and normal movement of the entire spine.[13] The normal part of the spine must compensate.

Certain segments will rotate in directions opposite to that of the *fixed* or dysfunctional neck joint. Other segments will rotate in the other direction. A mild compensatory S curve will develop.[14] To accomplish this movement, certain muscles throughout the spine must contract on one side while their counterparts on the opposite side relax. The spine is now in a state of substantial compensatory distortion, placing abnormal loading on many of the tissues and joints, downward to the lower back or even the ankle and upward to the skull. In time this compensation may create other symptoms, such as lower back pain and headaches. In some cases, symptoms will emerge in the arms and legs or in the rib cage.

If the original neck problem and its compensation are left untreated for a long period, other structures that articulate with the now abnormally curved spine (e.g., rib cage) may alter their configuration. This change might take the form of a bulge on one side of the back and on the opposite side in the front of the body. One shoulder may be carried higher than the other, or the pelvis may no longer move in symmetric motion when walking or running.

The longer this situation exists, the more established it becomes. Thus a fairly innocent, acute beginning—a small neck muscle spasm— has led to a chronic and extensive compensatory distortion that may, at any time and in many possible locations, result in pain or disability. If the condition began in the neck, it might ultimately result in lower back pain; if it began in an ankle, it might result in hip or knee pain; if it began in the lower back, the upper back or perhaps the upper neck might exhibit pain.

The entire musculoskeletal system may be affected. Balance between the right and left sides of the body may be substantially disrupted. If the office assistant in this example is a jogger, he or she may find that his or her otherwise very healthy attempt to exercise creates new problems arising from compensatory imbalances.

Chronicity

To carry further this example of the office assistant's neck muscle spasm, the assistant then vis-

its the doctor of chiropractic 5 years after the initial incident for pain in the back and shoulder. The chiropractor must rule out a range of potential causes with a broad screening diagnostic examination. He or she must ascertain that no contraindications are present to spinal corrective procedures (adjustments) and confirm that no parallel problems exist necessitating referral to a medical physician for additional evaluation.

Assuming that the problem originated as previously detailed, the chiropractor must evaluate the entire compensatory distortion, differentiating between the compensation and the original joint dysfunction in the neck. After locating the offending spinal segment, he or she works to restore it to its normal function and mobility. The chiropractor must then evaluate and treat the rest of the spine to reduce the compensatory distortions. Failure to do so may cause the original problem to return repeatedly. The spine, in effect, splints itself against further distortion but also against an unaided return to normal. The **chronicity** of the problem adds to the chiropractor's challenge.

Logically, a long-term distortion that alters the loading or foundational aspects of the human frame and spine may result in degenerative joint dysfunction, bulging disks, ligaments that have exceeded their coefficients of elasticity, and other changes that are not correctable.[15] These results must be included in the chiropractor's professional evaluation of the patient.

With this background, the answers to the original questions of why the chiropractor does not simply correct the neck problem in one or two visits and then dismiss the patient, as well as why the patient needs to return to the chiropractor for repeated visits, are answered. A well-reasoned explanation of compensation and chronicity is central to making the answers understandable not only to chiropractic patients, but also to employers, insurance companies, health consultants, and government officials. In the current political and economic environment of retrenchment in health care, the fact that a certain number of visits is usual and customary attains maximal viability when presented in a context of solid, patient-centered reasons that explain *why* it is usual and customary.

Chiropractors must evaluate each case on its own merits so that in the cases in which extended care is needed, a coherent, fact-based explanation can be provided. Practitioners who take advantage of patients' vulnerability by having them return to the office an unnecessary number of times or recommend the same large number of visits for virtually every patient have abandoned professionalism, and they bring disrepute on the entire profession. In addition to its inherent immorality, such unethical behavior makes it extremely difficult to collect meaningful data from the field to arrive at evidence-based mean values of visits required for a particular condition.

ETHICAL CHALLENGES

Confronting the Charge of "Unscientific Cultism"

As part of its former campaign to contain and eliminate chiropractic, the American Medical Association once charged that chiropractic was an "unscientific cult."[16,17] Directly confronting the questions raised by such charges as **cultism** is worthwhile. Appropriate responses include not only self-defense but also self-analysis and self-criticism.

The allegation that chiropractic is unscientific has been answered since the 1970s with an ongoing commitment to research and rigorous educational standards. As stated earlier, when the validity of chiropractic research has been subjected to rigorous scrutiny by independent bodies such as the AHCPR, it has stood up extremely well. Similarly, chiropractic educational institutions have demonstrated sufficient rigor to achieve and maintain accreditation by both the Council on Chiropractic Education and various nonchiropractic regional accrediting agencies.

Charges of cultism are less easily resolved. First, the qualities of cultism must be defined as follows:

- Unquestioning loyalty to the principles of a founder or leader
- Unwillingness to analyze information objectively that is in conflict with the received precepts of the founder or leader
- Unwillingness to change one's beliefs even when a preponderance of new evidence contradicts such beliefs
- The belief that one possesses the sole and singular truth
- Elevation of slogans to the status of ultimate truths

In this author's opinion, examples of jingoistic chiropractic slogans include "innate rules," "subluxation kills," and "above down, inside out." These precepts clarify nothing about chiropractic science and create an aura of strangeness that continues to hover over the profession.

Chiropractors are not unique in the healing arts in sometimes demonstrating cultist qualities. Nevertheless, the uncomfortable truth is that the persistence of such behaviors among a vocal minority of chiropractors is a continuing stain on the reputation of the profession. In this author's years as a chiropractic college president, as a representative of the chiropractic profession in Washington, D.C., with the International Chiropractors Association, and later with the American Chiropractic Association, the greatest obstacle to advancing the profession has been the persistence of stridently vocal chiropractors with irrational, cultlike opinions. These opinions are a minority, but they can and do cause the profession great harm.

Appropriate Terminology

In the first few decades of the twentieth century, development of a vocabulary unique to chiropractic was an astute survival tactic. Charged with and, in some cases, jailed for practicing medicine without a license, chiropractic leaders maneuvered brilliantly, denying the charges by asserting that:

1. Medicine is the diagnosis and treatment of disease.
2. Chiropractors do not diagnose or treat disease.
3. Therefore chiropractors are not guilty of practicing medicine.

This rationale required significant semantic contortions. Normal use of the English language includes as diagnosis all methods used by a doctor to determine the nature of the patient's condition and defines as treatment all measures that the doctor uses to influence that condition. Thus the average, intelligent English speaker would recognize analysis of spinal subluxations as diagnosis and application of chiropractic adjustments as treatment.

In the process of circumventing attempts to control chiropractic with medical practice laws, many chiropractors enshrined their tactic as something close to holy writ. At the more traditionalist schools, generations of chiropractic students were taught (and in a few cases are still taught) that chiropractors do not diagnose or treat disease. Instead of diagnosing, chiropractors *analyze*; instead of treating, they *adjust*.

In this author's opinion, such cultish language has become highly counterproductive. Chiropractic is now mature enough to converse with other health professions in a common lexicon. This growth does not mean that chiropractors must reject their natural healing roots and endorse allopathic principles, nor does it mean that all terminology developed by the chiropractic profession should be jettisoned. It does mean that members of all professions, and their patients, benefit from professionals speaking the same language.

Cooperation need not imply co-optation. Chiropractic terms such as *subluxation* and *adjustment* to a considerable degree have entered the common domain of scientific language. However, to vigorously assert, at the dawn of the twenty-first century, that the chiropractic adjustment is not a form of treatment borders on the absurd and is properly perceived as such by impartial listeners.

STEPS TOWARD INTEGRATION INTO MAINSTREAM HEALTH CARE

At a 1995 conference on alternative medicine sponsored by Harvard University's School of Graduate Education, it was noted that one of the most significant achievements for any group wishing to join the health care mainstream is the creation of an infrastructure.[18] Chiropractic stood out among the many groups represented because it already has a substantial portion of such an infrastructure in place: licensure laws, a national association, state associations, an accrediting agency, established and accredited colleges, and ongoing scientific research efforts. These elements constitute substantive movement toward full professional status.

What further steps are necessary to solidify mainstream status? At a minimum, the following are urgently required:

1. Assertive, ongoing efforts by chiropractors to foster collegial relations with medical professionals should be established.
2. A proper ethic of interprofessional referral should be established, in which medical physicians know which cases chiropractors should refer to them and which cases they should refer to chiropractors. In both cases, such referrals require that the patient be returned to the original referring doctor or physician, as is the case when medical physicians refer to other physicians. For many years, referrals from chiropractors to medical physicians constituted a transfer of the patient rather than a true referral, and remnants of this pattern still exist. Lack of an explicit ethic on referral between doctors of chiropractic and medical physicians remains a barrier to better interprofessional communication and thus to improved patient evaluation and care.
3. An organized effort by licensing boards should be established to acquire peer review authority immunized from antitrust laws, followed by the assertive use of this authority to change the behavior of practitioners who violate laws and ethical standards.
4. The "practice building" programs that celebrate and glorify practitioners on the basis of elevated income should be actively discouraged. One significant step in this direction would be for all chiropractic publications to refuse all advertising promising to increase the doctor's income.

These efforts will work best if pursued simultaneously. These steps include individual action (reaching out to medical physicians), group action (mutual agreement with the medical profession on interprofessional referral), legal action (securing immunized peer review and applying it in a rigorous effort to raise standards), and moral action (rejecting programs that identify income as the prime measure of success). Though the desired changes will not happen overnight, the actions required to secure their eventual accomplishment must be undertaken without delay. The future of chiropractic depends on such actions.

Review *Questions*

1. What are three characteristics of a mature profession?
2. Why did the chiropractic profession develop practice guidelines?
3. How did Mercy Consensus Conference deal with minority opinions?
4. What were some criticisms of the Mercy Guidelines?
5. According to the Mercy Guidelines, what is the longest period that a chiropractor should wait in most cases before referring a patient who is not showing clinical progress?
6. According to Haldeman and Nyiendo, which areas of the spine generally require longer periods of treatment?
7. What is musculoskeletal compensation?
8. Identify examples of unethical practices and describe why they are unethical.
9. What are the characteristics of cultism?
10. What are the key components of a health profession's infrastructure?

Concept *Questions*

1. Describe a fact-based rationale explaining why chiropractic care sometimes requires extended intervention over a period.
2. How should the chiropractic profession (or other professions) deal with practitioners who violate the profession's ethics?
3. How should the chiropractic profession distinguish between cooperation and co-optation in relations with the medical profession? What are some examples of each?

REFERENCES

1. Haldeman S, Chapman-Smith D, Peterson DM: *Guidelines for chiropractic quality assurance and practice parameters: proceedings of the Mercy Center Consensus Conference*, Gaithersburg, Md, 1993, Aspen Publishers.
2. Huxley T: *Lay sermons, addresses and reviews*, New York, 1871, Appleton and company, p 356.
3. Shekelle PG, Markovich M, Louie R: Comparing the costs between provider types of episodes of back care, *Spine* 20(2):221, 1995.
4. Hurwitz EL et al: Utilization of chiropractic services from 1985 through 1991 in the United States and Canada, *Am J Pub Health* 88(5):771, 1998.
5. North American Spine Society: Common diagnostic and therapeutic procedures of the lumbosacral spine, *Spine* 16(10):1161, 1991.
6. Gatterman MI: *Foundations of chiropractic: subluxation*, St Louis, 1995, Mosby.
7. Jirout J: Studies in the dynamics of the spine, *Acta Radiol* 46:55, 1965.
8. Lantz CA: The vertebral subluxation complex. In Gatterman MI, editor: *Foundations of chiropractic: subluxation*, St Louis, 1995, Mosby.
9. Frank W et al: Medial collateral ligament healing: a multidisciplinary assessment in rabbits, *Am J Sports Med* 11:379, 1983.
10. Hell JE: Vascular distensibility and functions of the arterial and venous systems. In Guyton A, editor: *Textbook of medical physiology*, ed 2, Philadelphia, 1996, WB Saunders.
11. Bullough, PG, Vigorita JJ: *Atlas of orthopedic pathology with clinical and radiological correlations*, New York, 1984, Gower Medical Publishers.
12. Blunt EL, Gatterman MI, Bereznick DE: Kinesiology: an essential approach toward understanding the chiropractic subluxation. In Gatterman MI, editor: *Foundations of chiropractic: subluxation*, St Louis, 1995, Mosby.
13. Goel et al: An in-vitro study of the kinematics of the normal, injured and stabilized cervical spine, *J Biomech* 17:363, 1984.
14. Hviid H: Functional radiography of the cervical spine, *Ann Swiss Chiropr Assoc* 3:37, 1965.
15. Lantz CA: Immobilization degeneration and the fixation hypothesis of chiropractic subluxation, *Chiropr Res J* 1:21, 1988.
16. Wardwell WI: *Chiropractic: history and evolution of a new profession*, St Louis, 1992, Mosby.
17. *Wilk v. AMA*, 895 F 2d at 352 Cert den, 112.2 Ed 2d at 524, 1990.
18. Mason M: Centering on alternatives, *Washington Post*, April 3, 1995.

Managed Care

Marino Passero, DC, and Daniel Redwood, DC

Key Terms

ALLOWED AMOUNT
ANNUAL CAP
ANY WILLING PROVIDER
  LAWS
BENEFIT PAYMENT SCHEDULE
BENEFITS
CLAIM
CLAIMS REVIEW
COMPLEMENTARY AND
  ALTERNATIVE MEDICINE
CO-INSURANCE
CO-PAYMENT
COVERED SERVICE (COVERED
  BENEFIT)
DEDUCTIBLE
DIRECT ACCESS

DISCOUNT PLANS
EXCLUSIONS
FEE-FOR-SERVICE PLANS
GATEKEEPER
HEALTH MAINTENANCE
  ORGANIZATION
INDEMNITY PLAN
INITIAL CONTACT
  PRACTITIONER
INSURER
MEDICAL NECESSITY
PARTICIPATING PROVIDER
POINT-OF-SERVICE PLAN
  (POS)
PORTAL-OF-ENTRY PROVIDER
PRECERTIFICATION

PREEXISTING CONDITION
  EXCLUSION
PREFERRED PROVIDERS
PREFERRED PROVIDER
  ORGANIZATIONS
PREMIUMS
PRIMARY CARE
PRIMARY CARE PHYSICIAN
PROVIDER
REFERRAL
REIMBURSEMENT
STAFF MODEL
SUBSCRIBERS
THIRD-PARTY PAYER
UTILIZATION REVIEW

Managed care includes a variety of methods that the health insurance industry uses in an effort to decrease the cost of health care and, secondarily, to increase its quality. In the United States during the early 1990s, managed care was touted as the cure for spiraling health insurance premiums, which were escalating by as much as 18%[1] (Fig. 29-1). Managed care has partially achieved its goals, providing some benefits to **providers,** patients, and shareholders and now appears to be a permanent part of the health care landscape in the United States. For the chiropractic profession, however, managed care has largely failed to reproduce the level of success it recorded in conventional allopathic health care. As of 2002, between 72% and 85% of American workers insured under managed care programs had coverage for chiropractic services[2] (Fig. 29-2). However, the extent and quality of that coverage varies widely. Chiropractors need to understand the managed care landscape to make well-informed decisions regarding participation in managed care plans.

HISTORICAL PERSPECTIVE

Managed care dates back to the turn of the twentieth century. The first managed care organizations (MCOs) were prepaid group practices, conceived and created by medical physicians. These organizations accounted for only a minuscule portion of medical care delivery and, in most cases, did not account for the majority of physicians' practices. Patients insured through

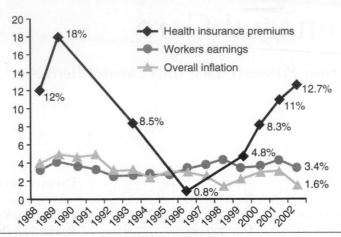

Fig. 29-1 The drop in the rate of increase for health insurance premiums, leading to its low in mid-1996, was a result of the spread of managed care. *(From* The New York Times, *September 6, 2001.)*

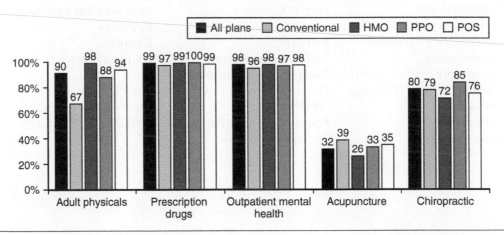

Fig. 29-2 Percentage of U.S. workers covered for selected benefits, by plan type, 2002. *(From NCMIC Managed Care Overview, November-December 2002, with permission.)*

MCOs paid a predetermined periodic fee in exchange for access to all necessary medical care.

As sociologist Paul Starr described in his landmark book, *The Social Transformation of American Medicine,*[3] members of labor unions and food cooperatives founded many early experiments in prepaid group practice programs. With the notable exception of the Group Health Cooperative of Puget Sound, most of these programs were financially too weak to survive. Crucial to the development of broad-based managed care was the program that industrialist Henry Kaiser initiated in the 1930s for the work-

ers at his west coast shipyards and steel mills. When World War II ended and the number of workers in the Kaiser plants declined, the Kaiser-Permanente health plans were opened to the public. These programs eventually grew to be far larger than their parent company.

Kaiser's goal, Starr writes, was to "reorganize medical care on a self-sufficient basis, independent of the government, to provide millions of Americans with prepaid and comprehensive services at prices they could afford." The Kaiser-Permanente program was a physician-operated **health maintenance organization** (HMO) that pioneered the **staff model** in which physicians are salaried employees of the HMO, and the economic incentives of private practice (in which increased services produce increased income) are eliminated. This model has the advantage of substantially decreasing overutilization of health services; conversely, it can have the disadvantage of encouraging underutilization whereby needed services may not always be provided.

After almost a century of direct involvement in the managed care process, allopathic medicine has secured a central role within managed health care. The same cannot be said for the chiropractic profession. Chiropractic, a relatively young profession today, was far less developed in the first half of the twentieth century. (One half of the chiropractors practicing today graduated within the last 10 years.) In the 1930s, when managed care was beginning, the profession was ill prepared to develop managed care strategies such as prepaid groups, much less grow them into huge corporate insurance entities such as Kaiser-Permanente; nor were any chiropractors invited to participate in medical managed care organizations, until many decades later.

As a result, managed care and the chiropractic profession had very little to do with each other until the late 1980s. Chiropractic grew rapidly through the 1970s and 1980s, enjoying significantly increased public recognition and improved interprofessional relationships. A decade or more of third-party reimbursement of chiropractic services (through **fee-for-service** insurance policies, automobile accident coverage, and worker's compensation plans) was beginning to foster a new sense of belonging and security in a profession that had long existed at the fringes of the health care industry. When chiropractors were first invited to participate in managed care on a large scale in the early 1990s, many practitioners eagerly joined. However, with rare exceptions, the profession was offered little meaningful input in developing managed care policy.

By the mid to late 1980s, managed care had evolved into a primarily corporate entity. About all that remained for full corporatization was purchasing and managing individual practitioners' practices, which for medical practices has proceeded at a rapid pace in recent years.

MANAGED CARE TERMINOLOGY

Allowed amount: Maximum charge permitted for a procedure under a health insurance policy.

Annual cap: Predetermined maximal amount payable by an insurance plan for a particular service within 1 calendar year. Many insurance policies have annual caps on spinal adjustment/manipulation or on chiropractic services.

Benefits: Services or goods covered under an insurance policy.

Benefit payment schedule: List of amounts an insurance plan will pay for covered health goods or services.

Complementary and alternative medicine (CAM): Health care interventions not taught widely in medical schools or generally available in hospitals. Under this definition, chiropractic is considered part of CAM.

Claim: Bill for services rendered that is submitted to a health benefit plan for payment.

Co-insurance: Percentage of the allowed amount of medically necessary services, which is paid by the patient to the provider after the annual deductible has been satisfied.

Co-payment: Flat dollar amount paid to the provider by the patient at each visit.

Covered service (covered benefit): Medically necessary procedures within the practitioner's scope of practice that are covered under the patient's health care insurance policy. Covered service is also called *covered benefit.*

Deductible: Flat out-of-pocket dollar amount that the patient must pay each year to providers before the insurer will pay for any covered benefits.

Direct access: Ability to consult a health care practitioner without a referral from a primary care physician.

Discount plan: Insurance arrangement under which the provider discounts the normal fee (usually by 20% to 30%). The patient pays the entire discounted fee, and the insurance company makes no payment to the provider. Discount plan is also known as *access plan* or *affinity plan.*

Exclusions: Services not covered under an insurance policy. See *Preexisting condition exclusion.*

Continued

MANAGED CARE TERMINOLOGY—CONT'D

Fee-for-service plan: Traditional health insurance policy that requires patients to pay an annual deductible after which the insurance plan pays a predetermined percentage of remaining costs for medically necessary care. Fee-for-service plan is also called **indemnity plan**.

Gatekeeper: Primary care physician designated as an HMO subscriber's **initial contact practitioner** and coordinator of care. Referrals from a gatekeeper are usually required before reimbursable services of specialists (including chiropractors) may be accessed. In HMOs the gatekeeper provides direct primary care services and also regulates and controls access to all other medical services.

Health maintenance organization (HMO): Organization that provides and manages the health services for plan members in exchange for payment of a fixed premium. In general, health care services are reimbursable by an HMO only when offered by providers who have contracted with the HMO.

Initial contact practitioner: See *Portal-of-entry provider*.

Insurer: Private or government insurance plan.

Medical necessity: Need for specific health care services based on clinical expectations that the health benefits will outweigh the health risks. Insurance policies require providers to certify that the services are medically necessary to qualify for reimbursement.

Participating provider: Provider who has entered into a contractual relationship with an insurer.

Point-of-service plan (POS): Arrangement under which HMO subscribers have the option to access out-of-network providers directly at an increased cost.

Portal-of-entry provider: Health care professional whose license permits him or her to see patients without referral from another practitioner. Such providers are expected to recognize clinical situations requiring referral. Chiropractors are portal-of-entry providers.

Precertification: Advance approval by a health insurance plan that allows the provider

MANAGED CARE TERMINOLOGY—CONT'D

to proceed with delivery of covered services. The precertification process may require some or all of the following: (1) written referral from a gatekeeper; (2) report of findings with diagnosis; and (3) goal-oriented treatment plan that includes the number of expected visits and anticipated date for completion of care.

Preexisting condition exclusion: Health condition not covered under an insurance policy because the condition existed before the date when the policyholder first subscribed to the plan. Under current law in the United States, preexisting conditions may only be excluded from reimbursement for patients who were uninsured immediately before enrolling in the plan. Preexisting condition exclusions generally have a time limit (commonly 12 months), after which the exclusion is removed.

Preferred provider: Health care practitioner who has entered into a contractual arrangement with a preferred provider organization.

Preferred provider organization (PPO): Insurance plan that offers subscribers incentives (e.g., lower deductibles and co-payments) to select in-network providers for accessing medical goods and services. PPO subscribers are also reimbursed for visits to non-network providers but at a lower rate. Preferred providers agree to charge no more than the plan's approved fees.

Primary care: No universally accepted definition of primary care exists. The Institute of Medicine defines **primary care** as "the provision of integrated, accessible health care services by clinicians who are accountable for addressing a large majority of personal health care needs, [for] developing a sustained partnership with patients, and [for] practicing in the context of family and community."[4] The American Chiropractic Association defines the role of chiropractic in primary care as "characterized by direct access, longitudinal, integrated, conservative ambulatory care of patients' health care needs . . . a first contact gatekeeper for neuromusculoskeletal conditions."[5] For a thorough discussion of issues relating to chiropractic and primary care, refer to the text provided by Gaumer and colleagues.[6]

MANAGED CARE TERMINOLOGY—CONT'D

Primary care physician (PCP): Medical physician who provides initial contact care and a broad range of conditions treated. The practice of the primary care physician includes overall health assessment, treatment of illness, management of illness, prevention of illness, and education.[4]

Premium: Amount paid by the subscriber (usually on a monthly or quarterly basis) to qualify for covered services under a health insurance policy.

Provider: Health care professional.

Referral: Recommendation by a health care practitioner that a patient consult another practitioner. Referral from a gatekeeper physician is required to access specialist services (including chiropractic services) under many managed care plans, particularly HMOs.

Reimbursement: Payment by an insurer under the terms of a health care insurance policy.

Staff model HMO: Health care maintenance organization that employs physicians and other providers to staff its facilities.

Subscriber: Individual covered by a health insurance policy. Many policies include coverage of the subscriber's spouse and children.

Third-party payer: Entity other than the subscriber or patient that is responsible for partial or complete payment of a claim. Virtually all third-party payers are private or government insurance plans.

Utilization review (UR): Procedures used by insurers to determine the appropriateness of care and to limit reimbursement for services deemed inappropriate or excessive. This review can involve a requirement for precertification before commencing care or periodic review by the insurer (or both) to determine whether continued care will be approved for reimbursement.

REIMBURSEMENT

Insurance **reimbursement** is regulated by statute and involves a contract between the reimbursing agent (insurance company) and the payer of **premiums** (generally either the consumer or the employer). Understanding the foundations of third-party reimbursement is essential to understanding managed care. The term *third party* refers to an entity other than the physician or patient (the first two parties) responsible for paying **claims** or otherwise involved in determining the circumstances under which care is delivered. For all practical purposes, the term *third-party payment* refers to payment by an insurance company.

Historically, methods of reimbursement have been based on one key underlying management concept: **medical necessity**. Although medical necessity, sometimes used interchangeably with *appropriateness*, might best be defined as "the need for specific health care services based on clinical expectations that the health benefits will outweigh the health risks."[4] In practice, the definition of medical necessity has remained vague and ambiguous, subject to interpretation by the individual **insurer**. Originally, medical necessity referred to any procedure or product that a duly licensed physician determined was needed by a patient. In this context, chiropractic services and goods that a duly licensed chiropractor delivered were considered to be medically necessary and were reimbursed, unless specifically excluded by the language of the individual policy. Over the years, the presence of such exclusionary language has been a continuing source of controversy between the chiropractic profession and the insurance industry.

Even under the broadest definitions of medical necessity, limits on necessary chiropractic services existed, and still do, in the form of an **annual cap** on the number of allowed chiropractic services or dates of service. Chiropractic services might be limited to a specific number of visits per year (averaging eight, occasionally as low as one or as high as 60) or an annual dollar limit per policyholder on the chiropractic services that would be reimbursed. These annual limits typically range from $200 to $2000 or more, depending on other policy issues, the most important of which is the subscriber's overall premium cost. In addition to caps on the number of visits and annual dollar caps, other management techniques include the use of deductibles, **co-insurance**, and **co-payments**, which are amounts of money the patient is required to pay "out of pocket" to the provider.

The **deductible** is usually a flat dollar amount per year (typically $100 to $400, but in some policies as high as $5000) that the patient must pay out of pocket to providers before the insurer pays its first dollar of reimbursement for health care services at a preset percentage (commonly 80% of the **allowed amount** but ranging between 50% and 100%). The patient then pays the remaining portion of the allowed amount (commonly 20%, but ranging between 0% and 50%) to the physician as a *co-insurance* payment. In place of co-insurance, some policies require *co-payments*, or *co-pays*, which are flat dollar amounts (typically $10 to $30 but sometimes lower or higher) to be paid by the patient at each doctor visit. All of the management techniques used in the early years of third-party reimbursement of chiropractic were financial tools such as these, employed to control the insurer's costs.

MANAGING DELIVERY OF CARE

Containing costs by shared expense (with payments to the physician by both the patient and the insurance company) and limitations on the yearly amount of reimbursable services played to the underlying strength of the insurance industry—financial analysis and management. However, attempts to manage care from a clinical perspective and to specifically define the concept of medical necessity brought the industry into areas where its qualifications were far weaker.

In the late 1980s and 1990s, a political movement spread across the United States, based on the dawning realization that tens of millions of Americans were uninsured or underinsured and that the cost of health care was excessive. In response, the insurance industry identified the provider of health care services, primarily the physician in the hospital, as a primary cause of this escalation of health care costs and of the system's inability to provide affordable health care for all Americans. Thus began a series of swift changes in health care reimbursement methods, culminating in the current version of managed care.

The key differences in the ways that care was managed before and after the great changes of the late 1980s and early 1990s can be summarized very simply: controlling the providers. The previous system of reimbursement included cost-control methods (deductibles, co-insurance, and annual caps) but made no sustained effort to control care from the perspective of medical necessity.

PROVIDER CONTRACTING

The system that emerged in the late 1980s and early 1990s focused on narrowing the definition of medical necessity and other techniques to control the delivery of services and therefore the provider of services. A prime mechanism for accomplishing these goals was the development of *provider contracting*, which brought pervasive and permanent changes to the American health care delivery system. Through provider contracting, the insurance industry sought to control delivery of care by establishing contractual relationships with providers (medical physicians, doctors of osteopathy, doctors of chiropractic, doctors of dental surgery, and so forth).

Provider contracting allows the insurer to limit the fees that contracting providers may charge to **subscribers.** For example, a chiropractic adjustment/manipulation, for which the chiropractor might normally charge $40, may be reimbursed at $35, $30, $25, or even less for patients subscribing to a particular insurance policy. Moreover, participating health care providers, in some cases, yield the right to be reimbursed for certain medically necessary services within their scope of practice. The providers may still make these services available but, under some contracts, agree to forego payment for these services not included under the contract.

For example, at a patient's first visit, the chiropractor might perform an initial examination, an adjustment/manipulation, and an ultrasound treatment. Some insurance policies that include chiropractic will cover the adjustment and the ultrasound but not the examination. Some policies will cover the examination and the adjustment but not the ultrasound. Some policies will cover all three. The possible variations of coverage for particular services are virtually infinite. Under some contracts, the provider may bill the patient for noncovered services (as long as the patient is notified in advance of the likelihood that the service is not covered), while other policies forbid billing the patient for certain noncovered services. The key point is that chiropractors who choose to enter into contractual relationships with managed care companies should familiarize themselves with the terms of their contracts and the specifics of reimbursement (which are not always included in the contract or attachments) *prior to signing any contract*. Consultation with an attorney may also be advisable.

One might ask why any provider would enter into such a limiting contract. In the early years of chiropractic participation in managed care, many providers accepted promises by managed care entities or insurance companies that contracting would streamline administrative processes, reduce paperwork, and enhance overall efficiency, thereby improving the provider's profit margin for each patient seen. In addition, many providers were fearful that by not entering into managed care contracts, they would lose access to the many patients in their communities who were insured under managed care policies. Further still was the implicit threat that unless they agreed to terms quickly, other chiropractors would be willing to take their place in the newly forming exclusive networks of **preferred providers.** In many cases, this concern was well founded.

Currently, few providers expect managed care to streamline administrative processes, reduce paperwork, enhance efficiency, or improve profit margins. Instead, concern about loss of access to potential patients and decreased market share is *the* driving force behind the willingness of providers to join managed care networks.

PREFERRED PROVIDER ORGANIZATIONS

Because chiropractors were never afforded the opportunity to join staff-model medical HMOs,

their earliest opportunities for managed care contracting were with **preferred provider organizations** (PPOs). PPOs provide incentives for patients to visit providers within their networks, through a reduction in fees. PPOs require payment of either a deductible (and co-insurance) or a per-visit co-pay. PPOs spread rapidly across the United States in the 1990s, with tens of thousands of chiropractors signing contracts that gave insurance companies great power to decrease levels of reimbursement and to limit services as they deemed necessary. Statistics from the year 2002 indicate that 85% of U.S. workers insured under PPO plans have chiropractic coverage, compared with 72% of those insured by HMOs and 79% insured by conventional, fee-for-service plans.[2]

Although HMO subscribers seeking to consult a specialist generally must have a **referral** from a **primary care physician** (PCP) who acts as a **gatekeeper,** PPO patients, in most cases, maintain **direct access** to all providers in the network and even to providers outside the network (though at a rate of reimbursement lower than for in-network providers). This relative freedom of choice comes at a price; PPO premiums are higher than those of HMOs.

UTILIZATION REVIEW

Chiropractors participating in either HMO or PPO plans find that their services are subject to **utilization review** (UR) by the insurer. This process can involve a requirement for **precertification** before commencing care, periodic reviews by the insurer to determine whether continued care would be approved for reimbursement, or both. In some insurance companies, URs are conducted by chiropractors; in others, they are conducted by medical personnel such as nurses. This aspect is another point of contention between chiropractors and insurance companies, because reviewers who are not doctors of chiropractic (DCs) may lack the qualifications to properly determine the indications for, and therefore the appropriateness of, chiropractic intervention.

Precertification refers to a requirement that the chiropractor receive advance approval from the insurer before undertaking the care of a specific patient. In policies in which referral from a PCP is required to see a specialist, the chiropractor must have a written referral from the PCP for such care to be reimbursable. Depending on the specifics of the policy, the chiropractor may then proceed with the initial examination and, in most cases, the initial treatment. Frequently, he or she will then be required to fill out a form summarizing the history, findings, diagnosis, and proposed treatment plan and to fax this information to the UR staff at the managed care organization. In some cases, a PCP gatekeeper will need to provide a signed approval of the chiropractor's proposed treatment plan before submitting it to the MCO. Then, the UR staff will respond within a prescribed period (usually 2 to 3 days). The response may take the following forms: approval of the treatment plan, approval of a modified version of the plan, rejection of the plan, or a request for further information. In the early years of chiropractic participation in managed care, many DCs were placed in the position of having to wait 3 days or more to receive permission to treat patients in acute pain. Such arrangements are now far more rare, as an increasing number of managed care companies allow an initial 3 to 5 visits before, or during, the process of determining whether longer courses of care will be approved for reimbursement.

DISCOUNT PROGRAMS

Some insurance policies offer a discount on the physician's services rather than a paid benefit, a marked departure from both the PPO and HMO models of managed care. Under PPO and HMO policies, the patient, physician, and insurance company all contribute financially to the arrangement. At each visit, the patient is responsible for a co-pay or co-insurance payment, the physician discounts his or her normal fee to a level set by the insurance company, and the insurance company pays the remainder as a **benefit**. In **discount plans** (sometimes called "affinity" or "access" programs), the physician discounts his or her normal fee (usually by 20% to 30%), the patient pays the entire discounted fee, and the insurance company pays nothing.

Discount plans, which identify chiropractic as part of **complementary and alternative medicine** (CAM), along with acupuncture and massage therapy, remain highly controversial in the chiropractic profession. Such plans have been criticized as an intentionally misleading marketing strategy, in which insurance companies advertise inclusion of chiropractic but in fact make no contribution toward the chiropractor's fee. Moreover, many chiropractors perceive discount plans as a means by which insurance companies seek to delay indefinitely the inclusion of chiropractic as a reimbursable benefit. Companies offering discount plans respond that subscribers benefit from paying lower fees and that providers participating in discount plans may attain a greater market share as a result of their participation. Another contention is that, in some cases, discount plans may be a first step toward a company's including chiropractic as a reimbursable benefit.

James Dillard, a chiropractor, medical physician, and acupuncturist who organized the complementary and alternative medicine (CAM) network for a large MCO in the Northeast United States, discussed discount programs in a 2000 article in *Topics in Clinical Chiropractic*. Acknowledging that managed care "represents more work at a lower rate of reimbursement for the practitioner," Dillard contends that the discount program "allows the practitioner to maintain somewhat of the old-style cash practice, albeit for a slight discount." This article is referring to the fact that unlike other managed care programs, discount programs require no medical referral, and no paperwork must be submitted to the insurer. The characterization of the discount as "slight," however, is not likely to find widespread agreement among practicing chiropractors.[5]

CONSIDERATIONS FOR CHIROPRACTIC STUDENTS AND PRACTITIONERS

In the United States, where the majority of the world's chiropractors practice, managed care is here to stay and has profoundly affected all major health care professions. Many of the difficulties that chiropractors face in managed care programs (e.g., decreased reimbursement, increased paperwork) are the same as those that medical practitioners encounter. Other challenges, especially the difficulty in securing chiropractic referrals from medical gatekeepers, are unique to chiropractors. DCs face important choices on whether to participate in managed care plans and, if so, which types of plans.

This choice is not an all-or-nothing decision. Most chiropractic practices in the United States are structured so that income relies on a blend of managed care, traditional fee-for-service insurance, automobile accident insurance, worker's compensation, and cash payments. Significantly, because chiropractic practice has as its centerpiece the adjustment/manipulation, a fundamentally low-tech, low-cost procedure, many chiropractic patients are willing and able to pay cash for their chiropractic services. Thus chiropractors enjoy a degree of choice unavailable to many medical practitioners (neurosurgeons and orthopedic surgeons, for example) whose high-tech, high-cost procedures rarely take place outside the context of insurance coverage.

For chiropractors and other health professionals, managed care participation entails a tradeoff as decreased revenue per patient and decreased control of one's practice is accepted in exchange for increased access to patients with managed care insurance. Plans that deliver what they promise—increased patient volume and streamlined reporting procedures—may be worth joining. Programs that fail to deliver should be avoided. Because the managed care marketplace continues to evolve, practitioners must stay abreast of policy changes, learning the basics and applying new information as it becomes available.

Review *Questions*

1. Who created the first managed care organizations?
2. What were the original goals of managed care?

3. How does managed care differ from traditional fee-for-service insurance plans?
4. Which difficulties with managed care are specific to chiropractic and which are common to all health professions involved in managed care?
5. What potential advantages does participation in a PPO or HMO bring to a chiropractor? What are the potential disadvantages?
6. In what ways do PPOs and HMOs differ from discount plans?
7. What is the primary driving force behind the willingness of providers to join managed care networks?
8. What is the role of the gatekeeper physician?
9. Aside from chiropractors, patients may need a referral from a gatekeeper physician to access the services of what other types of practitioners?
10. What does precertification of care usually involve?

Concept *Questions*

1. What are the similarities between American managed care and Canadian- or European-style national health care? What are the differences?
2. What has been the positive and negative impact of managed care on American society as a whole?

REFERENCES

1. *The New York Times*, September 6, 2001.
2. *NCMIC Managed Care Overview*, November-December 2002.
3. Starr P: *The social transformation of American medicine*, New York, 1982, Basic Books.
4. McAndrews JF: *Managed care: a guide for new practitioners*, Des Moines, 1996, National Chiropractic Mutual Insurance Company.
5. Dillard J: Chiropractic as a mainstream health benefit versus an alternative/complementary benefit, *Top Clin Chiropr* 7(1):57, 2000.
6. Gaumer G, Koren A, Gemmen E: Barriers to expanding primary care roles for chiropractors: the role of chiropractic as primary care gatekeeper, *J Manipulative Physiol Ther* 25(7) 427, 2002.

30 Pathways for an Evolving Profession

Daniel Redwood, DC

Key Terms

ACTIVE PREVENTION	NONPHYSICAL CAUSATION	PATIENT DEPENDENCY
HEALING PARTNERSHIP	PATIENT-CENTERED	SELF-CARE
GLOBALIZE	PRACTICE	

How can chiropractors and chiropractic students help the profession evolve so that it more fully reflects our noblest aspirations? For students immersed in mastering large quantities of technical information and field practitioners focused on day-to-day matters of patient care and practice management, such questions are usually crowded out by the press of immediate responsibilities. In the long run, however, the answers to these questions are crucial.

To survive for many generations, a healing art must be grounded in a system of enduring principles. Lacking that structure, the centrifugal force of new developments exerts too strong a destabilizing pull, eventually leading to loss of fundamental identity. To remain a distinct profession well into the future, chiropractors must hold fast to certain core principles. These principles include concepts shared with other natural healing arts along with unique chiropractic contributions to the overall body of healing arts principles and practice.

In addition to upholding the vital concepts of chiropractic and natural healing, individual chiropractors can influence the future path of the profession by doing the following:
- Distinguishing clearly among the proven, the probable, and the speculative
- Taking care to diagnose and prognose in ways that empower patients
- Minimizing patient dependency

- Serving people who cannot afford chiropractic services
- Making healthy lifestyle choices and thereby serving as a good example to others
- Modeling qualities of tolerance and openmindedness
- Learning about other healing traditions and interacting constructively with their practitioners

Although externally driven events will always exert an influence, the destiny of chiropractic is primarily in our own hands.

FOUNDATIONAL PRINCIPLES

Chiropractic could not have survived for a century without largely adhering to the tenets of natural healing enunciated by Daniel David Palmer and other chiropractic pioneers. These precepts include the following principles drawn from the common domain shared by all natural healing arts:

Natural Healing Principles[1]

1. Human beings possess an innate healing potential, an inner wisdom of the body.
2. Maximally accessing this healing system is the goal of the healing arts.
3. Addressing the cause of an illness should, in most cases, take precedence over suppressing its surface manifestations.

4. Pharmaceutical suppression of symptoms can, in some instances, compromise and diminish the body's ability to heal itself.

5. Natural, nonpharmaceutical measures, including chiropractic spinal adjustments, should, in most cases, be an approach of first resort, not last.

6. A balanced, natural diet is crucial to good health.

7. Regular exercise is essential to proper bodily function.

Endorsed and elucidated by chiropractors for more than a century, these precepts are recognizable today as the foundation of the emerging holistic health or wellness paradigm.

Core Chiropractic Principles[1]

The following constructs comprise the theoretical underpinning of chiropractic:

1. Structure and function exist in intimate relation with one another.

2. Structural distortions can cause functional abnormalities.

3. The vertebral subluxation is a significant form of structural distortion and dysfunction and leads to a variety of functional abnormalities.

4. The nervous system occupies a preeminent role in restoring and maintaining proper bodily function.

5. The subluxation influences bodily function primarily through neurologic means.

6. The chiropractic adjustment is a specific and definitive method for correcting the vertebral subluxation.

Although the precise definition of the subluxation has changed over the years (see Chapter 7), emphasis on the interplay among subluxation, the nervous system, and human health has been at the core of chiropractic concerns since the birth of the profession, and it remains so today.

TOUCHSTONES FOR FUTURE ADVANCEMENT

For individual chiropractors and the profession as a whole to rise to the challenges we face, we must draw upon the best of our history, looking inward with rigorous self-analysis and then acting based on a sense of higher purpose. To accomplish this task, the following points should be considered:

1. *Distinguish clearly among the proven, the probable, and the speculative.* Some of the most justifiable criticism of chiropractic has been in reaction to the tendency of some chiropractors to **globalize,**[2] making broad overarching claims on the basis of limited, though powerful, anecdotal evidence. Anecdotal information and case studies can be of genuine value in formulating the basis for further research; these elements should not be mistaken for scientific proof. Chiropractic's integrity and credibility, as well as its compliance with regulatory agencies, depend on its practitioners consistently making this distinction. To do so, we must stay well acquainted with current research. Keating (Internet communication, 1996) has noted that all health professions use unproven methods (the majority of conventional medicine's methods appear to be unproven)[3,4] but that it is *never* acceptable to make inaccurate claims about these methods and techniques.

2. *Recognize the power of your diagnoses and prognoses.* Doctors have the power to dramatically shape patients' views of their own health. Chiropractors have a responsibility to tell the truth, as well as a further responsibility to frame that truth in the manner most empowering to the patient. A patient once came to me with neck and shoulder pain, relating that she had been told by her previous chiropractor that on a scale of one to ten (ten being the ideal) the chiropractor rated her overall health at three. In my judgment, this was a healthy, vibrant young woman who happened to have some musculoskeletal pain. However, time and effort was needed to convince her that she was basically well. In our role as healing arts professionals, we need to be careful not to unthinkingly alter our

patients' self-perception for the worse. We can convey to them that they are fundamentally ill people or that they are healthy people who currently have certain symptoms or imbalances. There is a world of difference. Conveying confidence in patients' strength and healing potential is essential. Even with severely ill patients, tempering honest evaluation with hope is important.

3. *Minimize **patient dependency***. Most chiropractic cases require multiple visits. However, as J.F. McAndrews noted earlier in this text (Chapter 28), "depending on which chiropractor a patient sees, the recommended course of care for the same condition may vary drastically, from several visits with one doctor to several dozen—sometimes hundreds—with another. Such variations appear in all regions, among graduates of all chiropractic colleges, and in urban, suburban, and rural settings." Driven in some cases by perceived or real financial pressures and in other cases by a sincere belief that most or all patients require long-term, visit-intensive chiropractic care, chiropractors may discourage patient independence by scheduling more visits and performing more procedures than truly required for patients' well being.

Because some of these subliminal motivations reside in everyone, a conscious effort must be made to recommend only the treatment that is truly needed. Greater patient self-sufficiency can be encouraged through **active prevention,** teaching exercises and other **self-care** methods, and decreasing frequency of treatment as soon as appropriate. Kingsbury[5] notes that in the early days of the profession, doctors spoke with pride of how *few* visits were required to resolve a patient's condition and how long a patient was able to go without needing another adjustment. Such a mindset reflects a deep connection to the true purpose of chiropractic and is emblematic of a **patient centered practice.** This approach contrasts sharply with providers who include in their definition of

success maximizing the number of visits per case.

4. *Promote a healing partnership and patient-centered approach.* Doctor-patient relations are imbued with certain inherent inequalities. These differences include the physician's social status and specialized knowledge, as well as the patient's sense of insecurity resulting from his or her illness and disability.[6] Physicians should offer patients opportunities for empowerment so that the inequality created by their specialized knowledge is not generalized to all aspects of their relations with patients. Gordon argues persuasively for a **healing partnership**[7] in which the usual hierarchical model is transformed into a more egalitarian one whereby patients assume a significantly more active, responsible role. Gatterman makes a similar case in the context of chiropractic education and health care delivery.[8] Both Gordon and Gatterman call for a pattern of doctor-patient interaction that moves beyond the "men in white coats" hierarchical model that has currently become a cliché. These authors embrace a mutually respectful relationship that calls on patients to relinquish powerlessness and doctors to surrender some of their power.

5. *Do everything possible to create a positive public perception of the chiropractic profession.* Many people still retain negative stereotypes about chiropractors, and chiropractors must not act in ways that reinforce these ideas.

Patients and the profession can be better served by asking the following questions:

- Do I continue to treat patients who are showing no clinical progress after a reasonable (1 month in most cases) trial of care?
- Do I use x-rays only when clinically necessary?
- Do I perceive patients as spines to be adjusted, or do I also connect with them as people?
- Do my patients feel that I rush through their office visits?

- Do I encourage patients' questions and take time to answer them taken in sufficient depth?
- Is my primary focus the depth of the patient's healing or the size of my income?
- Are my billing practices honest?
- How informed am I about the latest research relating to chiropractic?
- How open to and knowledgeable about alternatives to chiropractic am I?

In recent years, the medical profession has faced a burgeoning grassroots movement seeking alternatives to conventional care; chiropractors are not immune to a comparable response to our own less-enlightened practices.

We can move proactively to avert this by clarifying our ideals through a process of serious self-examination and then changing those actions and attitudes that fail to measure up.

6. *Serve those who cannot afford your services.* In keeping with the spirit of healing and service that underlies the decision to pursue a career in chiropractic, chiropractors can serve people in the community by offering sliding-scale or no-fee services to patients whose financial status would otherwise prohibit them from seeking chiropractic care. This longstanding tradition in chiropractic dates back to D.D. Palmer and other guiding lights of the profession's early years. Less universal now than it was in the past, this practice is scorned in some chiropractic circles. When I was a new graduate, a colleague spoke of discouraging poor people from becoming patients, because "welfare refers welfare," a concept he had been taught at a practice management seminar. Aside from the fact that the basic premise is incorrect (poor people sometimes refer full-paying patients), this attitude is so insidious and uncompassionate that is deserves to be exposed to the cleansing light of day. Every spiritual tradition in the world speaks of the need to serve those less fortunate than ourselves. The admirable example of the profession's chiropractic forebears calls chiropractors to do no less.

7. *Model a healthy lifestyle.* Actions speak louder than words—we must walk our talk. Chiropractors whose lifestyles offer an example of health-affirming choices are in the best position to influence patients to do the same. This does not mean that we must be in perfect health before we can offer legitimate advice; it means that we need to make a sincere effort to choose a healthy lifestyle. This reflects on each chiropractor's integrity, as well as that of our profession.

Honest self-evaluation is required and should include questions such as the following:

- Is my diet consistent with what I know to be good nutrition?
- Do I smoke?
- Do I use alcohol or caffeine immoderately?
- Do I use other drugs?
- Do I exercise regularly?
- Do I get adequate rest?
- Do I use stress-reduction methods?

If there are areas in which our actions are inconsistent with our beliefs as chiropractors and natural health care practitioners, the relevant question is: why not make a change for the better today? Chiropractors should not expect patients to do for themselves what we are unwilling to do for ourselves.

8. *Cultivate tolerance and openmindedness.* In developing the clarity of awareness needed to attain mastery in healing arts practice, tolerance and openmindedness are among the most valuable tools. In health and healing, many questions have more than one correct answer. Back and neck pain, for example, can be remarkably responsive to chiropractic care but not in all cases. In certain instances, other methods, including acupuncture,[9,10] mind-body interventions,[11-13] or surgery,[14,15] bring improvement or resolution. In a time of worldwide interchange of health information,[16,17] we chiropractors should educate ourselves about other healing methods and traditions to deepen our understanding of alternative practices and paradigms, to know when to refer patients to practitioners of these healing arts, and

to incorporate into our own practices aspects of this knowledge that are compatible with our role as chiropractors. Calling on other qualified practitioners for assistance is sometimes precisely what the best interest of the patient requires. Informed people in all disciplines know that no method has all the answers and that those claiming to possess a panacea are unaware of their own blind spots.

9. *Acknowledge **nonphysical causation** of illness*. Contemporary chiropractic practice is largely geared to the assumption that physical symptoms have physical causes. This is not the whole truth. Emotional stress and belief patterns can strongly influence musculoskeletal pain and impairment.[18-21] Chiropractors can help in such cases by teaching patients to practice stress-management techniques and referring them to mental health professionals when appropriate.

10. *Recognize the hand of friendship when it is offered*. To develop cooperative relationships with other health professionals, a spirit of mutuality is essential. Chiropractors have made commendable efforts in recent years to build such bridges with both conventional and alternative practitioners. As we reach out to others, we must not allow fear to dominate our perception of those who reach out to us. An anecdote from former U.S. Surgeon General C. Everett Koop recounted by Marc Micozzi may be instructive here. According to Koop, in the 1950s, he and I.S. Ravdin, then the leading figure in surgery at the University of Pennsylvania, had concluded that drugs and surgery were proving inadequate for some patients with lower back pain. Koop and Ravdin believed that chiropractic might be helpful and approached chiropractors in Philadelphia about doing research on chiropractic, with the hope that this might lead to including chiropractic as part of standard care for lower back pain. The chiropractors refused to participate. Koop believes that they had

been persecuted for so long by organized medicine and local medical physicians that they had concluded that all medical physicians were their enemies. Fully appreciating the mindset of those 1950s-era chiropractors who had grown so accustomed to hostility from the medical profession that they were unable to recognize a sincere hand of friendship may not be easy for today's students and younger practitioners. Rather than judging them harshly, we should acknowledge that whatever challenges chiropractors now face pale in comparison with theirs. We can empathize with their situation and honor the legacy of their struggle for professional survival, from which we all have benefited greatly.

At the same time, however, we must remember that opportunity does not always knock twice on the same door. As we stride with backs unbent into this new century filled with potential, we must be willing to let go of old grievances against individuals and professions that have wronged chiropractic in the past. Openings will be presented in the coming years beyond what we can currently conceive. Let us evaluate these opportunities with clear minds, assume that people are sincere unless they prove otherwise, and then move forward together toward a future that fulfills D.D. Palmer's vision.

Review Questions

1. List seven common domain principles of natural healing shared by chiropractic and other natural healing arts.
2. List six core chiropractic principles.
3. How can a chiropractor's prognoses affect patients' self-perception of their own health?
4. What are the consequences of dependency?
5. How can chiropractors encourage greater self-sufficiency on the part of patients?
6. Why is it especially important for health practitioners to live in a healthy manner?
7. What reasons justify chiropractors seeing some patients on a sliding scale or no-fee basis?
8. What are three reasons chiropractors should learn about other healing traditions?

9. Name three methods other than spinal adjustments that can be helpful for some cases of lower back pain?

10. Do all physical symptoms have primarily physical causes?

Concept Questions

1. Why is it important to distinguish clearly among the proven, the probable, and the speculative? Have you seen cases where chiropractors failed to make this distinction? What are some possible negative consequences?

2. What are some stereotypes about chiropractors? What steps can the individual chiropractor take to overcome these stereotypes?

REFERENCES

1. Redwood D: Chiropractic. In Micozzi M, editor: *Fundamentals of complementary and alternative medicine,* New York, 1996, Churchill Livingstone.
2. Gellert G: Global explanations and the credibility problem of alternative medicine, *Adv Mind Body Med* 10(4):60, 1994.
3. Smith R: Where is the wisdom...? The poverty of medical evidence, *BMJ* 303:798, 1991.
4. Office of Technology Assessment: *Assessing the efficacy and safety of medical technologies,* Washington, DC, 1978, U.S. Government Printing Office.
5. Kingsbury GM: Does net worth equal self-worth? *J Am Chiropr Assoc* 33(8):23, 1996.
6. Brody H: *The healer's power,* New Haven, Conn, 1992, Yale University Press.
7. Gordon JS: *Manifesto for a new medicine: your guide to healing partnerships and the wise use of alternative therapies,* Reading, Mass, 1996, Addison-Wesley.
8. Gatterman MI: A patient centered paradigm: a model for chiropractic education and research, *J Altern Compl Med* 1(4):371, 1995.
9. Coan R et al: The acupuncture treatment of low back pain: a randomized controlled study, *Am J Chin Med* 8:181, 1980.
10. Coan R, Wong G, Coan PL: The acupuncture treatment of neck pain: a randomized controlled study, *Am J Chin Med* 9:326, 1982.
11. Caudill M et al: Decreased clinic utilization by chronic pain patients: response to behavioral medicine intervention, *Clin J Pain* 7:305, 1991.
12. Kabat-Zinn J, Lipworth L, Burney R: The clinical use of mindfulness meditation for the self-regulation of chronic pain, *J Behav Med* 8:163, 1985.
13. Kabat-Zinn J et al: Four year follow-up of a meditation-based program for the self-regulation of chronic pain: treatment outcomes and compliance, *Clin J Pain* 2:159, 1986.
14. Albert TJ et al: Health outcome assessment before and after lumbar laminectomy for radiculopathy, *Spine* 21(8):960, 1996.
15. van den Bent MJ et al: Anterior cervical discectomy with or without fusion with acrylate, *Spine* 21(7):834, 1996.
16. Bodeker G: Traditional health systems: policy, biodiversity, and global interdependence, *J Altern Compl Med* 1(3):231, 1995.
17. Bodeker G: Global health traditions. In Micozzi M, editor: *Fundamentals of complementary and alternative medicine,* New York, 1996, Churchill Livingstone.
18. Drottning M et al: Acute emotional response to common whiplash predicts subsequent pain complaints: a prospective of 107 subjects sustaining whiplash injury, *Nordic J Psychiatr* 49(4):293, 1995.
19. Klapow JC, Slater MA, Patterson TL: Psychosocial factors discriminate multidimensional clinical groups of chronic low back pain patients, *Pain* 62(3):349, 1995.
20. Lackner JM, Carosella AM, Feuerstein M: Pain expectancies, pain, and functional self-efficacy expectancies as determinants of disability in patients with chronic low back disorders, *J Consult Clin Psychol* 64(1):212, 1996.
21. Riley JF, Ahern DK, Follick MJ: Chronic pain and functional impairment: assessing beliefs about their relationship, *Arch Phys Med Rehab* 69:579, 1988.

Statistical Methods for Determining Reliability

John G. Scaringe, DC, DACBSP

Four commonly used methods to determine inter- and intra-examiner reliability are: (1) percentage agreement, (2) intraclass correlation co-efficient (ICC), (3) Pearson's product-moment correlation co-efficient (*r*), and (4) kappa statistic (*k*).

PERCENTAGE AGREEMENT

Percentage agreement is calculated by taking the number of agreements between two examiners divided by the total number of responses:

Agreements ÷ (Agreements + Disagreements)

Often, percentage agreement results represent elevated estimates of reliability because chance agreement between examiners is not corrected. A percentage agreement index is not a strong measure for inter- or intra-examiner reliability.

INTRACLASS CORRELATION CO-EFFICIENT (ICC)

ICC is often calculated when the consistencies of two or more examiners are studied. Unlike percentage agreement, ICCs correct for chance agreement between examiners and are computed with repeated measures of *analysis of variance* (ANOVA). Simply stated, ICCs reflect both the degree of consistency and agreement among ratings. Intraclass correlation co-efficients range from 0 to 1, with 1 representing high-reliability values. Huijbregts[1] reports the following recommendations for the interpretation of ICCs:

- <0.75   Poor-to-moderate agreement
- >0.75   Good agreement
- >0.90   Reasonable agreement for clinical measures

Pearson's Product-Moment Correlation Co-Efficient (*r*)

The *Pearson's r*, like other correlation co-efficients, describes the strength and direction of the relationship between two variables.[1] Pearson's *r* calculates the degree of association between two sets of data, not the extent of agreement. Correlation co-efficients range from −1.0, indicating a perfect negative correlation, to 1.0, representing a perfect positive correlation. Pearson's *r* is not recommended as a reliability measure. Interpretation of Pearson *r* values are as follows[1]:

- 0.00-0.25   Little-to-no relationship
- 0.25-5.50   Fair relationship
- 0.50-0.75   Moderate-to-good relationship
- >0.75   Good-to-excellent relationship

Kappa (*k*)

Kappa is appropriately used in situations with two examiners or two ratings (e.g., present or not present, yes or no, hypermobile or hypomobile). Although kappa can be reflected as a negative value (worse than chance), it usually varies between 0 and 1, with values closer to 1 representing higher reliability. Interpretation of kappa values includes[1]:

- <0.4   Poor-to-fair agreement
- 0.4-0.6   Moderate agreement
- 0.6-0.8   Substantial agreement
- >0.8   Excellent agreement
- 1.0   Perfect agreement

REFERENCES

1. Huijbregts PA: Spinal motion palpation: a review of reliability studies, *J Man Manipulative Ther* 10(1): 24, 2002.

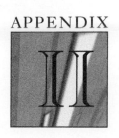

APPENDIX II

Relative Physical Invasiveness of Selected Techniques

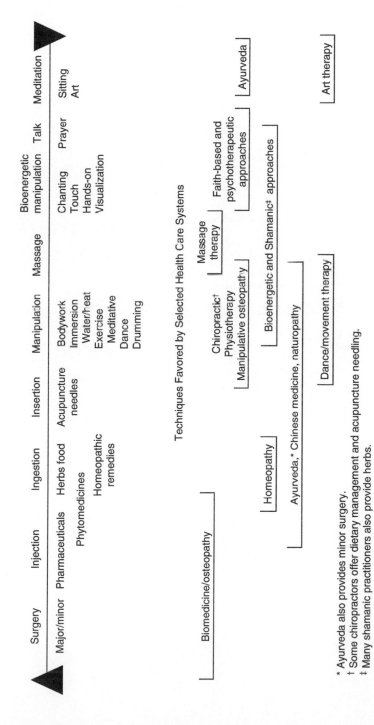

Surgery	Injection	Ingestion	Insertion	Manipulation	Massage	Bioenergetic manipulation	Talk	Meditation
Major/minor	Pharmaceuticals	Herbs food	Acupuncture needles	Bodywork		Chanting	Prayer	Sitting
	Phytomedicines			Immersion		Touch		Art
		Homeopathic remedies		Water/heat		Hands-on		
				Exercise		Visualization		
				Meditative				
				Dance				
				Drumming				

Techniques Favored by Selected Health Care Systems

Biomedicine/osteopathy

Homeopathy

Ayurveda,* Chinese medicine, naturopathy

Chiropractic†
Physiotherapy
Manipulative osteopathy

Massage therapy

Bioenergetic and Shamanic‡ approaches

Faith-based and psychotherapeutic approaches

Ayurveda

Dance/movement therapy

Art therapy

* Ayurveda also provides minor surgery.
† Some chiropractors offer dietary management and acupuncture needling.
‡ Many shamanic practitioners also provide herbs.

Adapted from Cassidy C. In Micozzi MS: *Fundamentals of complementary and alternative medicine*, ed 2, New York and London, 2000, Churchill Livingstone.

APPENDIX III

The ACC Chiropractic Paradigm

1.0 PREAMBLE

The Association of Chiropractic Colleges (ACC) is committed to affirming the profession by addressing issues facing chiropractic education. The ACC brings together a wide range of perspectives on chiropractic and is uniquely positioned to help define the chiropractic role within health care.

The ACC is committed to greater public service through reaching consensus on the following issues that are important to the chiropractic profession:

- Continuing enhancement of educational curricula
- Strengthening chiropractic research
- Participating and providing leadership in the development of health care policy
- Fostering relationships with other health care providers
- Affirming professional confidence and conduct
- Increasing public awareness regarding the benefits of chiropractic care

The member Colleges of the ACC represent a broad diversity of institutional missions. The presidents have drafted a consensus statement that includes the following:

- The ACC position on chiropractic
- A representation of the chiropractic paradigm
- Clarification regarding the definition and clinical management of the subluxation

Additional statements will be forthcoming as the ACC continues to provide meaning and substance regarding what is taught in chiropractic colleges and how this information influences the present and future of the profession.

2.0 ACC POSITION ON CHIROPRACTIC

Chiropractic is a health care discipline that emphasizes the inherent recuperative power of the body to heal itself without the use of drugs or surgery.

The practice of chiropractic focuses on the relationship between structure (primarily the spine) and function (as coordinated by the nervous system) and how that relationship affects the preservation and restoration of health. In addition, Doctors of Chiropractic recognize the value and responsibility of working in cooperation with other health care practitioners when in the best interest of the patient.

The Association of Chiropractic Colleges continues to foster a unique, distinct chiropractic profession that serves as a health care discipline for all. The ACC advocates a profession that generates, develops, and uses the highest level of evidence possible in the provision of effective, prudent, and cost-conscious patient evaluation and care.

3.0 THE CHIROPRACTIC PARADIGM (SEE FIG. A-1)

Purpose

The purpose of chiropractic is to optimize health.

Principle

The body's innate recuperative power is affected by and integrated through the nervous system.

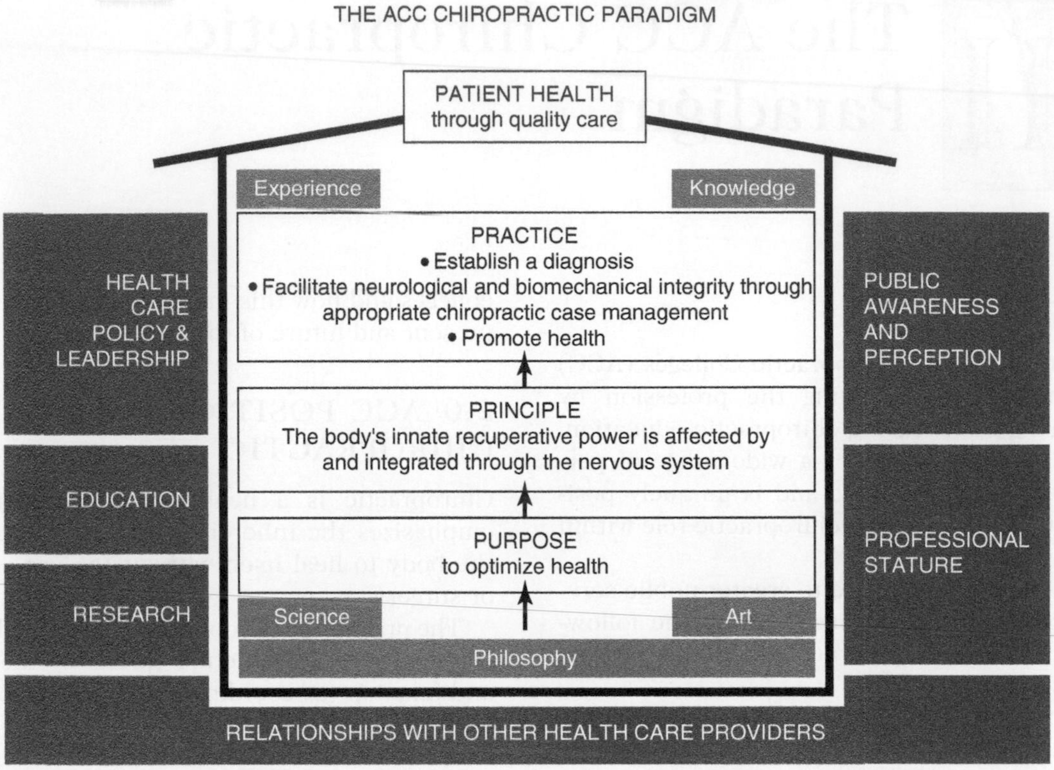

THE ACC CHIROPRACTIC PARADIGM

PATIENT HEALTH
through quality care

Experience   Knowledge

HEALTH
CARE
POLICY &
LEADERSHIP

PUBLIC
AWARENESS
AND
PERCEPTION

PRACTICE
• Establish a diagnosis
• Facilitate neurological and biomechanical integrity through
appropriate chiropractic case management
• Promote health

PRINCIPLE
The body's innate recuperative power is affected by
and integrated through the nervous system

EDUCATION

PROFESSIONAL
STATURE

PURPOSE
to optimize health

RESEARCH   Science   Art

Philosophy

RELATIONSHIPS WITH OTHER HEALTH CARE PROVIDERS

Fig. A-1   The ACC Chiropractic Paradigm. *(Association of Chiropractic Colleges, with permission.)*

Practice

The practice of chiropractic includes the following:

- Establishing a diagnosis
- Facilitating neurological and biomechanical integrity through appropriate chiropractic case management
- Promoting health

Foundation

The foundation of chiropractic includes philosophy, science, art, knowledge, and clinical experience.

Impacts

The chiropractic paradigm directly influences the following:

- Education
- Research
- Health care policy and leadership
- Relationships with other health care providers
- Professional stature
- Public awareness and perceptions
- Patient health through quality care

4.0 THE SUBLUXATION

Chiropractic is concerned with the preservation and restoration of health and focuses particular attention on the subluxation.

A subluxation is a complex of functional and/or structural and/or pathological articular changes that compromise neural integrity and may influence organ system function and general health.

A subluxation is evaluated, diagnosed, and managed through the use of chiropractic procedures based on the best available rational and empirical evidence.

THE ACC CHIROPRACTIC SCOPE AND PRACTICE

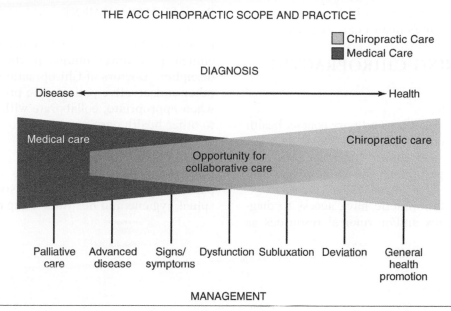

Fig. A-2 ACC Chiropractic Scope and Practice. *(Association of Chiropractic Colleges, with permission.)*

Chiropractic *Scope and Practice*

1.0 INTRODUCTION

The Association of Chiropractic Colleges (ACC) brings together a wide range of perspectives on chiropractic and is uniquely positioned to help define the chiropractic role within health care. In Position Paper #1 (July 1996), the ACC presidents described the practice of chiropractic within the chiropractic paradigm to include the following:

- Establishing a diagnosis
- Facilitating neurological and biomechanical integrity through appropriate chiropractic case management
- Promoting health

As part of its ongoing commitment to affirming the profession by addressing issues facing chiropractic education, the ACC presidents have drafted a consensus statement on chiropractic scope and practice.

ACC member colleges educate students for the competent practice of chiropractic. These academic institutions have a direct interest in the definition of the chiropractic scope and practice. Clarity on chiropractic scope and practice will do the following:

- Enhance the consistency and excellence of educational outcomes
- Contribute to a better understanding of chiropractic education and practice, both within the profession and by the public
- Provide direction to the profession for the advancement of chiropractic

This second position paper includes the following:

- Definition of the chiropractic scope
- A description of the practice of chiropractic with respect to diagnosis, case management, and health promotion

2.0 DEFINING CHIROPRACTIC SCOPE

Because human function is neurologically integrated, Doctors of Chiropractic evaluate and facilitate biomechanical and neurobiological function and integrity through the use of appropriate conservative, diagnostic and chiropractic care procedures.

Therefore direct access chiropractic care is integral to everyone's health care regimen.

3.0 DEFINING CHIROPRACTIC PRACTICE

A. DIAGNOSTIC

Doctors of Chiropractic, as primary contact health care providers, employ the education, knowledge, diagnostic skill, and clinical judgment necessary to determine appropriate chiropractic care and management.

Doctors of Chiropractic have access to diagnostic procedures and/or referral resources as required.

B. CASE MANAGEMENT

Doctors of Chiropractic establish a doctor/patient relationship and use adjustive and other clinical procedures unique to the chiropractic discipline. Doctors of Chiropractic may also use other conservative patient care procedures and, when appropriate, collaborate with and/or refer to other health care providers.

C. HEALTH PROMOTION

Doctors of Chiropractic advise and educate patients and communities in structural and spinal hygiene and healthful living practices.

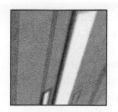

Glossary

Aberrant Deviating from the usual or normal.

Abdominal aortic aneurysm An aneurysm in the abdominal aorta, often the result of advanced atherosclerosis. Rupture of an abdominal aortic aneurysm is a life-threatening event. *See also* aneurysm.

Abnormality Condition that is not normal. Abnormality may be defined statistically or in terms of adverse health consequences.

Abortive therapy Treatment given to stop pain after it has begun. *See* Preventive.

Acceleration Change in velocity with respect to time.

Access plan *See* Discount plan.

Accessory joint movement Small specific joint movement that is independent of voluntary muscle action.

Accreditation Process through which educational institutions are evaluated. Accreditation has two fundamental purposes: (1) quality assurance and (2) institutional and program improvement. The Council on Chiropractic Education is the accrediting agency for chiropractic colleges in the United States.

Acetylcholine Neurotransmitter produced by nerve fibers in the somatic and parasympathetic portions of the nervous system.

Action potential Change in membrane potential that self-propagates along a neuronal axon or other excitable cell membrane.

Active analysis Worksite evaluation in which an occupational health physician observes, samples, measures, and records the presence of potential ergonomic hazards. *See* Passive analysis.

Active care Approach to case management that encourages patients to participate actively in the resolution of their conditions rather than relying solely on the intervention of a doctor. For musculoskeletal conditions, this approach emphasizes rehabilitation and exercise.

Active control Procedure that may have therapeutic effects and is performed on the control group in a clinical research trial.

Active coping Strategies in which patients make an effort to function in spite of pain.

Active prevention *See* Prevention, active.

Active range of motion Joint movements that are under the active muscular control of the patient.

Active-release technique Soft tissue technique in which the practitioner maintains pressure and tension while the patient moves the tissue from a shortened to a stretched position. This technique is used for the examination, diagnosis, and treatment of cumulative injury disorders.

Activities of daily living (ADLs) Personal care activities that are necessary for everyday living, such as eating, bathing, grooming, dressing, and toileting. Health care professionals often use ADLs as part of patient assessment in determining the need for care or type of care a person may require.

Activity intolerances Limitations (generally as a result of pain) in the activities a patient is able to perform.

Acupuncture Traditional Asian health practice in which fine needles are inserted into specific points on the body for a wide variety of therapeutic purposes, including the relief of pain. In approximately one half of the states in the United States, the chiropractor's scope of practice includes acupuncture. In almost all of these states, practitioners are required to demonstrate postgraduate training in acupuncture.

Adaptability Ability to change in response to stress.

Adhesions Abnormal adherence of biologic tissues as a result of scar development.

Adjunctive procedures Methods used by some chiropractors to complement manual adjustment/manipulation. Examples of commonly used adjunctive procedures include diet and nutritional supplementation and physical modalities such as massage, hot and cold applications, ultrasound, and electronic muscle stimulation. Also called *Pysiological Therapuetics*.

Adjustive lesion Complex clinical entity that serves as a basis for treatment by adjustive/manipulative procedures, as identified by observation, palpation, diagnostic imaging, and other procedures. This term may be applied to denote subluxation or vertebral subluxation.

Adjustive localization Preadjustive procedures that are designed to localize adjustive forces and joint distraction.

Adjustive thrust Application of a specific, controlled force that is applied with an impulse and accompanied with a specific vector (line of drive).

Adjustment 1. Maneuver that is specific in direction, point of contact, amplitude, and velocity. It is intended to correct a subluxation partly or wholly. 2. Manual procedure that is designed to effect improvement in the neurologic component of vertebral subluxation or joint dysfunction. Adjustment may or may not use a manipulative (i.e., thrusting) approach. 3. Any chiropractic manual procedure that uses controlled force, leverage, direction, amplitude, and velocity directed at specific joints or anatomic regions.

Admitting privileges Privileges extended to physicians by a hospital, permitting them to admit patients to the facility. Admitting privileges are generally based on whether the physician is permitted by credentials, law, and the Joint Commission on Accreditation of Hospital Organizations' policy to assume primary and full responsibility for the overall care of patients.

Adolescent idiopathic scoliosis Spinal curvature of unknown origin that develops around the age of puberty.

Adrenergic Pertaining to the secretion of the neurotransmitter adrenaline/epinephrine or noradrenaline/norepinephrine.

Aerobic fitness Fitness attained through aerobic exercise in which the heart rate reaches approximately 55% to 90% of maximum heart rate and 40% to 85% of maximum oxygen intake reserve. Aerobic exercise aids in maintaining cardiovascular fitness and weight control.

Affective Emotional.

Afferent Moving or carrying inward or toward a central part (e.g., blood vessels carrying blood toward the heart) or nerves carrying sensory impulses (i.e., information) toward the central nervous system.

Afferent fibers Nerve fibers that convey impulses to a ganglion or to a nerve center in the brain or spinal cord.

Afferent inhibition *See* Stimulus-induced analgesia.

Affinity plan *See* Discount plan.

A-fibers Large diameter, heavily myelinated axons that quickly convey impulses.

Agency for Health Care Policy and Research (AHCPR) An agency of the U.S. federal government that until the mid-1990s was given the responsibility of evaluating the effectiveness of various health care interventions. The AHCPR's 1994 guidelines on low back pain, which recognized spinal manipulation as one of only two professional interventions with substantial support in the scientific literature, marked a major breakthrough in the acceptance of chiropractic. The Agency for Health Research and Quality (AHRQ), the successor organization to the AHCPR, fulfills many of the functions of the AHCPR but does not have a mandate to prepare clinical guidelines.

Agonist A muscle that is the prime mover in eliciting a particular bodily movement.

Alar ligaments Ligaments extending upward and outward from the apex of the dens of the axis vertebra toward the occiput.

Alpha motor neurons Motor neurons that are responsible for innervating and activating skeletal muscle fibers through the myoneural junction. They are composed of large diameter, fast-conducting nerve fibers.

Algometry Measurement of pressure or painful stimuli.

Algorithm A step-by-step procedure for solving a problem.

Allodynia Pain as a result of a stimulus that does not normally induce pain. Allodynia describes an objective response to clinical stimuli, when the normal stimulus can be tested elsewhere in the body. Allodynia is a loss of specificity of any sensory modality, with the final perception being pain. A simple example of allodynia is the pain after light brushing of sunburned skin.

Allopath Practitioner of allopathic medicine. *See* Allopathy.

Allopathy 1. Practice of medicine based on using substances or procedures to counteract symptoms. 2. Conventional Western medicine.

Allostatic response Homeostatic, generalized adaptive response of the body to various stressors, resulting in increased circulating levels of substances including corticotropic-releasing hormone (CRH), adrenocorticotrophic hormone (ACTH), and cortisol.

Allowed amount Maximum charge permitted for a procedure under a health insurance policy.

Alternative therapy Treatment method not commonly taught in allopathic medical schools, not practiced in hospitals, nor reimbursed by third-party payers; an unconventional therapy.

American Chiropractic Association (ACA) 1. Largest national chiropractic organization in the United States, founded in 1963 as the successor to the National Chiropractic Association. 2. In the first half of the twentieth century, at least four organizations were also called the American Chiropractic Association.

American College of Chiropractic Radiology An organization representing board certified chiropractic radiologists, whose parent organization is the ACA Council on Diagnostic Imaging. Members of the ACCR are chiropractic radiologists who are members of the ACA and have successfully completed the examinations given by the American Chiropractic Board of Radiology.

Analgesic Medication that reduces or eliminates pain.

Anaphylaxis Immediate immune response, often allergic, characterized by vasoconstriction and capillary dilation, potentially leading to generalized tissue ischemia, cardiovascular failure, and death. Also called *anaphylactic shock*.

Anastomosis Connection of separate parts of a branching system, as occurs with blood vessels.

Anatomic barrier Limit of anatomic integrity or movement, as imposed by an anatomic structure. Forced movement beyond this barrier results in damage to the limiting tissues.

Anecdote Story about a clinical event or case.

Anesthetic blockade Anesthetic injection into a tissue for the purpose of blocking pain.

Aneurysm A pathologic sac formed by dilatation of the wall of a blood vessel. *See also* Abdominal aortic aneurysm.

Anisotropic Having mechanical properties that differ according to the direction of applied forces. Varying resistance to compression, torsion, or shear stresses demonstrates anisotropy of bone.

Ankylosis Union or linkage of adjacent bones or parts of bones to form a single unit.

Annual cap Predetermined maximum amount payable by an insurance plan for a particular service in 1 calendar year. Many insurance policies have annual caps on spinal adjustment/manipulation or on chiropractic services.

Annulus fibrosus Fibrous outer portion of the intervertebral disk.

Antagonist A muscle whose action directly opposes that of the muscle serving as the agonist or prime mover in a particular bodily movement.

Anterior longitudinal ligament (ALL) Broad, thick ligament extending from the occiput to the sacrum, attaching to the anterior surfaces of the vertebral bodies and intervertebral disks. The ALL limits anterior protrusion of the intervertebral disks and hyperextension of the spine.

Anterolisthesis Forward slippage of a vertebra in relation to the vertebra immediately inferior to it.

Anthropometric Pertaining to measurement of the size, weight, and proportions of the human body.

Antidromic Conducting nerve impulses in a direction opposite to the normal.

Antigenic Stimulating the production of antibodies.

Antioxidant Reducing agent. Dietary antioxidants counteract the negative effects of free radicals.

"Any willing provider" laws Statutes requiring that if a procedure is covered by an insurance policy, then providers licensed to perform that procedure within their scope of practice must be covered under the contract.

Apgar score Qualitative test developed by physician Virginia Apgar, which is used to determine the status of a newborn child at 1 minute and 5 minutes after birth. Scores between zero and two are assigned for heart rate, respiration, color, reflex irritability, and muscle tone. Ten is a perfect score. Children with scores between zero and three at 5 minutes tend to have higher rates of morbidity and mortality.

Apical ligament Ligament that extends from the tip of the dens of the axis and attaches to the occiput.

Apophyseal joints *See* Zygapophyseal joints.

Apposition Condition of being placed side by side.

Arachnoid mater Delicate, weblike, avascular membrane that constitutes the middle layer of the meninges.

Articular process Portion of a vertebra that projects superiorly or inferiorly from the lamina, forming part of the synovial joints with the vertebrae above and below.

Articulation Joint; the location where two bones meet.

Association of Chiropractic Colleges (ACC) Organization that represents chiropractic colleges and programs. Schools and programs that are accredited by Council on Chiropractic Education (CCE-USA) are eligible for membership, as are those accredited international schools and programs approved by agencies having reciprocity with CCE-USA.

Association neurons *See* Interneurons.

Ataxia Defective muscular coordination, especially exhibited when voluntary muscular movements are attempted.

Athletic trainer *See* Trainer, athletic.

Atlas First cervical vertebra.

Atonia Loss of normal muscular tone.

Atrophy Decrease in the size of a structure; wasting away.

Aura Sensation that precedes the onset of a migraine headache. Auras are often visual or auditory but may involve any of the senses.

Auscultation Act of listening to the sounds generated in the body.

Autonomic nervous system (ANS) Portion of the nervous system involved with involuntary functions. The ANS is subdivided into the sympathetic and parasympathetic systems.

Axis Second cervical vertebra.

Axon Neuronal cell process along which an action potential is propagated and transmitted away from the soma and dendrites.

Axon reflex Action potential propagation in an efferent direction on an afferent axon.

Axoplasmic flow Intracellular transport system that carries large molecules formed in the nerve cell body down the full length of the axon to the nerve fiber terminals.

Axoplasmic transport Intracellular transport system that carries large molecules formed in the nerve cell body the full length of the axon to the nerve fiber terminals and back again, at a rate faster than axoplasmic flow.

Ayurvedic medicine Traditional system of medicine in India. Also known as *Ayurveda*.

Babinski reflex Spreading of the toes and dorsiflexion of the great toe in response to stroking the sole of the foot. This reflex is normal up to 24 months of age. Beyond this age it indicates a neurologic deficit, as in lesions of the pyramidal tract.

Basic science laws Laws passed by some U.S. state legislatures beginning in the 1920s, which required that chiropractors seeking licensure demonstrate proficiency on basic science tests.

Basic science research Research that explores structures and mechanisms.

Battery Unlawful touching.

Benefits Services or goods covered under an insurance policy.

Benefit payment schedule List of amounts an insurance plan will pay for covered health services.

Bias Process that tends to produce results that systematically depart from true values.

Bifurcate To split into two parts.

Biomechanics Application of mechanical principles to living structures.

Biomedical Reflecting the values and/or practices of biomedicine. *See also* Biomedicine.

Biomedicine Currently dominant health care system in Western nations, in which biochemically based pharmaceutical intervention is the primary means of treatment. Synonyms are *conventional medicine, allopathic medicine,* and *Western medicine.*

Biopsychosocial Health care model that incorporates physical, mental, and emotional factors, as well as social and community relations.

Blepharoptosis Drooping of the upper eyelid.

Blinding Shielding the subject, the person administering the treatment, or the person assessing the outcome from knowledge that might compromise the integrity of a research study.

Blinded Study Clinical research trial performed so that the patients do not know (are blinded to) whether they are receiving the procedure

being tested or the control or placebo to ensure that the results of the study are not affected by a possible placebo effect (the power of suggestion).

Blockage, joint *See* Joint blockage.

Bone density Degree of bone mineralization.

Bone scan A procedure that begins with intravenous injection of a small amount of a radioactive marker, after which the patient is evaluated with a scanning device. Elevated concentrations of the radioactive marker are found in regions where the rate of bone turnover is high. Bone scans are highly sensitive tests for tumors, infections, or small fractures. In addition, they can be used to distinguish old from new compression fractures of a vertebral body.

Bonesetter Lay practitioner of joint manipulation, whose tradition is often passed down from generation to generation within families.

Bony landmark *See* Segmental contact point.

Botanic medicine System of healing that uses plants as medicines.

Boycott Organized refusal to do business with an individual or group. The Wilk v. American Medical Association (AMA) lawsuit reversed the medical profession's boycott of chiropractic.

Breech birth Birth where the presenting part is one or both feet or the buttocks.

Broad osteopath Historically, a practitioner of osteopathy who uses pharmaceuticals or surgery or both in preference to osteopathic manipulation.

Bruit Turbulence generated in an artery as a result of a loss of laminar flow.

Calor Localized increase in temperature; a cardinal sign of inflammation.

Calorie Quantity of heat required to raise the temperature of 1 gram of water by 1° C at 1 atmospheric pressure.

Canadian Chiropractic Association National association representing chiropractors in Canada.

Cardinal sign Definitive characteristic of an illness or condition.

Carpal tunnel syndrome (CTS) Complex of symptoms resulting from compression of the median nerve in the carpal tunnel of the wrist. Signs and symptoms of CTS can include numbness, tingling, burning sensations, pain, and weakness in hand, wrist, or entire affected upper extremity (or a combination of all three areas).

Case series Written report on the details of a series of related cases.

Case study Written report on the details of a single case.

Cauda equina Large group of nerve roots, extending from the end of the spinal cord in the lumbar region of the vertebral canal.

Cauda equina syndrome Injury to the nerve roots of the lumbosacral region as they pass through the lower spinal canal. This syndrome is usually caused by compression of the nerve roots from a large anteromedial disk protrusion or spinal stenosis.

Causalgia Burning pain, sometimes accompanied by trophic skin changes, caused by injury to a peripheral nerve.

Caveat Suggestion of caution.

Cavitation Formation of vapor and gas bubbles within fluid through local reduction of pressure. High-velocity, low-amplitude adjustments and manipulations are theorized to produce a cavity within a joint, eliciting a characteristic cracking sound.

Centralization Use of pain-centralizing or relieving positions and movement ranges for self-treatment with exercise. For example, if flexion peripheralizes symptoms and extension centralizes them, extension movements are indicated.

Central nervous system Brain plus spinal cord.

Cephalohematoma Unilateral or bilateral pooling of blood between the periosteum and underlying bone of the cranium. This pooling usually does not cross the suture line. The parietal bones are the most common site, but it can occur anywhere on the scalp.

Cerebrovascular accident (CVA) General term applied to conditions involving either ischemic or hemorrhagic lesions of the blood supply to the brain, usually resulting in injury or death of cerebral tissue. Also called *stroke*.

Cervicogenic headache *See* Headache, cervicogenic.

C-fibers Smaller diameter unmyelinated axons that convey impulses more slowly than A-fibers.

Civilian Health and Medical Program of the Uniformed Services (CHAMPUS) Health insurance plan for dependents of active members of the U.S. armed services.

Chemical mediators of inflammation Histamine, prostaglandin II, leukotrienes, kallidin, bradykinin, and serotonin.

Chemoreceptor Sensory receptor that generates an action potential in response to chemical stimulation.

Chiropractic Health care discipline founded by Daniel David Palmer in 1895, which emphasizes the inherent recuperative powers of the body to heal itself without the use of drugs or surgery. The practice of chiropractic focuses on the relationship between structure (primarily of the spine) and function (as coordinated by the nervous system) and how this relationship affects the preservation and restoration of health.

Chiropractic analysis Clinical assessment of a patient's state of biologic and neurologic integrity, primarily for the purpose of characterizing subluxation in general and vertebral subluxation complex in particular.

Chiropractic Health Bureau (CHB) Organization founded by B.J. Palmer in 1926. The CHB was renamed as the International Chiropractors Association in 1941.

Cholinergic. Pertaining to the secretion of the neurotransmitter acetylcholine.

Chondrocyte Cartilage cell.

Chronic cervical syndrome Condition marked by paroxysmal deep or superficial pain in parts of the head, face, ear, throat, or sinuses; sensory disturbances in the pharynx; vertigo; tinnitus, with diminished hearing; and vasomotor disturbances that include sweating, flushing, lacrimation, and salivation.

Chronic pain syndrome Ongoing pain, generally defined as lasting longer than 6 months. The etiology of chronic pain syndrome is unclear and no treatment or management method has consistently proven successful.

Chronicity Extended duration of a condition.

Cicatrisation Scar formation.

Cineradiography Fluoroscopic technique where the image is recorded on motion picture film.

Claim Bill for services rendered, submitted to a health benefit plan for payment.

Clinical epidemiology Application of epidemiologic principles to clinical case management. *See also* Epidemiology.

Clinical hypothesis Reasonable conjecture about the cause of a patient's problem.

Clinical research Research that addresses issues directly related to patient care.

Clinical trial Prospective longitudinal experiment that is designed to assess the comparative efficacy or effectiveness of a treatment. It is often labeled a randomized clinical trial (RCT) if the random assignment of subjects is made to each of the comparison treatment groups. *See also* Randomized clinical trial.

Clinical privileges Delineation of the roles of various members of hospital staffs. Categories of clinical privileges include fully qualified physicians, partially qualified physicians, nonphysicians, and staff affiliates.

Cluster headache Uncommon headache, mostly in men 35 to 60 years old, characterized by unilateral headache and facial pain of often excruciating intensity. Headaches come in clusters over periods of days and weeks.

Cochrane Collaboration International organization that prepares systematic reviews of the effects of health care interventions.

Cognitive-behavioral approach Structured, goal-oriented method emphasizing functional analysis and skills training.

Cognitive therapy Relatively short-term, focused psychotherapy for a wide range of psychologic problems including depression, anxiety, anger, marital conflict, loneliness,

panic, fears, eating disorders, substance abuse, and personality problems. The focus of therapy is on how an individual is currently thinking, behaving, and communicating rather than on early childhood experiences.

Cohort Defined group of people observed over a period of time.

Co-insurance Percentage of the allowed amount of medically necessary services that is paid by the patient to the provider after the annual deductible has been satisfied.

Co-morbid diseases Diseases existing simultaneously in the same body. Also called *comorbidities*.

Collateralize To branch.

Collimator Device that limits the area of the x-ray beam.

Colonoscopy Examination of the colon with an elongated endoscope.

Committee on Quackery Originally called the Committee on Chiropractic, this committee was a focal point of the efforts of the American Medical Association (AMA) to contain and eliminate chiropractic before the Wilk v. AMA lawsuit. *See also* Wilk v. AMA case.

Common domain Principles and practices shared by various healing arts.

Compensation Counterbalancing of a defect in structure or function.

Complementary and alternative medicine (CAM) Health care interventions not taught widely in medical schools or generally available in hospitals. Under this definition, chiropractic is considered part of CAM.

Compression Force applied to a body that decreases its volume and increases its density.

Computed radiography Radiographic method that uses a screen inside a conventional x-ray cassette to absorb the x-ray energy transmitted through a patient being x-rayed. This screen is then removed from the cassette and inserted into a laser reader. The stored energy is converted into electrical impulses that are interpreted by computer and converted into an electronic black and white image that can be viewed on a computer monitor or printed to film.

Computed tomography (CT) Procedure that produces cross-sectional images of the body by directing an x-ray beam through the structures of interest. Detectors surrounding the patient measure the x-ray attenuation. Axial images are produced using computer techniques. Data from the axial images may be reformatted to produce sagittal and coronal images.

Concomitant Occurring at the same time.

Concurrent Occurring at the same time.

Conduction velocity Speed at which action potentials are transmitted along a neuron.

Condyle Rounded prominence on a bone, generally a site for articulation with another bone.

Confounding bias Bias that results from the interaction of two or more factors in a cause-effect relationship such that the presence of one factor makes it difficult to evaluate the true effect of the other factors.

Congress of Chiropractic State Associations (COCSA) Not-for-profit organization consisting of state chiropractic associations. The mission of COCSA is to provide an apolitical forum for the promotion and advancement of the chiropractic profession through service-to-member state associations.

Consanguinity Genetic relationship; of the same bloodline.

Conservative methods Minimally invasive approaches to health care. *See also* Invasiveness.

Consolidation Increase in tissue substance that causes a structure to become more solid.

Consortial Center for Chiropractic Research (CCCR) Established in 1997 by the National Institutes of Health to build research capacity, bolster the chiropractic profession's research infrastructure, and initiate pilot studies. The CCCR has involved 13 chiropractic institutions and universities in basic and clinical science projects and other efforts. It also aims to develop an environment for training future scientists

and to encourage collaboration between basic and clinical scientists, and between the chiropractic and conventional medical communities.

Contact point *See* Segmental contact point.

Contraindication Any symptom or circumstance denoting the inappropriateness of a form of treatment or intervention that would otherwise be advisable.

Contraindication, absolute Set of circumstances where a particular treatment or intervention is always inappropriate.

Contraindication, relative Set of circumstances where a particular treatment or intervention may be appropriate, only if it is modified or applied in an unusual manner.

Contralateral On the opposite side.

Controlled movement Therapeutic movement of a body part within the limits imposed by wearing a brace.

Control group Comparison group in a clinical trial, whose members receive no treatment, a placebo treatment, or an alternative treatment. *See also* Placebo, active control.

Conus medullaris Tip of the spinal cord, located at the second lumbar level.

Conventional medicine Politically dominant form of health care in a particular country or culture. *See also* Biomedicine.

Convergence Termination at a single neuron of signals from multiple neuronal sources.

Co-payment Flat dollar amount paid by the patient at each visit to the provider.

Copenhagen Neck Functional Disability Scale Self-rating instrument for assessing disability caused by neck pain.

Correlation Consistent statistical relationship between two variables such that one variable tends to predict the other. Correlation may suggest but not prove a causal relationship.

Cortisol The major glucocorticoid synthesized by the adrenal cortex. It affects the metabolism of glucose, protein, and fats, regulates the immune system, and has many other functions.

Cost effectiveness Relative health value of an intervention compared with its financial cost.

Covered service Medically necessary procedures within the practitioner's scope of practice that are covered under the patient's health insurance policy. Also called *covered benefit.*

Cross sectional Measurements taken at one moment in time.

Council on Chiropractic Education (CCE) Accrediting agency for chiropractic colleges in the United States. Since 1974, the CCE has been recognized by the U.S. Department of Education to accredit chiropractic institutions and programs.

Counterstrain System of evaluation and treatment of joint pain in which treatment involves moving a muscle or joint to a position of comfort, holding it in that position for at least 90 seconds, and then slowly returning it to the neutral position.

Creep Increase in strain of a material that occurs during constant stress from loading. It is a deformation of a viscoelastic tissue to a constant, steadily applied load. In the body, the structure undergoing creep may or may not return to its original length or shape, depending on the load and whether the structure is damaged.

Crepitus Creaking or crackling sounds, as in a joint.

Cryokinetics Therapeutic application of ice, followed by or combined with motion of the affected body part.

Cryotherapy Therapeutic application of ice.

Cultism Membership in a group characterized by unquestioning loyalty to the principles of a founder or leader. Members are unwilling to analyze information objectively that conflicts with the received precepts of the founder or leader and are unwilling to change beliefs even when a preponderance of new evidence contradicts them.

Cumulative trauma disorder (CTD) Group of musculoskeletal disorders caused by repeated trauma to the body. Examples are carpal tunnel and thoracic outlet syndromes.

Current Procedural Terminology (CPT) System developed by the American Medical Association to code health care procedures for billing purposes.

DeQuervain's disease Painful tenosynovitis in the area of the thumb, caused by relative narrowness of the common tendon sheath of the abductor pollicis longus and the extensor pollicis brevis.

Decoaptation Increased separation or traction occurring at a local level by stretching the connected fasciae related to that area. (From *coapt*, to approximate or draw together.)

Deconditioning Diminishing ability to perform tasks involved in a person's ADLs.

Deductible In the context of the health insurance industry, a flat dollar amount that the patient must pay out of pocket each year to providers before the insurer will pay for any covered benefits.

Deep breathing Breathing that aerates all lung fields and has a relaxing effect.

Deformation Morphologic alteration of a normally developed structure during the fetal or postnatal period. *See also* Malformation and disruption.

Degeneration Breakdown, deterioration, falling from a higher to a lower level.

Degenerative joint disease Chronic disease involving the joints, which is characterized by joint pain, destruction of articular cartilage, and impaired function. Also called *osteoarthritis.*

Dendrite Branching process or extension from a neuron that carries electrical signals toward the nerve cell body, unlike an axon that carries electrical signals away from the cell body. Dendrites contain or are associated with receptors that are designed to sense specific stimuli or react to specific chemical transmitters. Neurons may have hundreds or even thousands of dendrites, depending on the size and complexity of their receptive fields.

Denervation Complete disruption of nerve supplies to a cell, tissue, or organ.

Dependency Doctor-patient relationship where the patient inaccurately believes that he or she requires ongoing intervention by the doctor or requires more frequent or intensive care than is actually necessary.

Depuytren's contracture Flexion deformity of one or more fingers due to shortening, thickening, and fibrosis of the palmar fascia, or a similar flexion deformity of one or more toes due to similar changes in the plantar fascia.

Dermatologist Medical physician specializing in diseases of the skin.

Dermatome Area or segment of skin innervated by the neurons within a single posterior spinal nerve root (sensory nerve).

Descriptive study Research report used to illustrate, initiate, disconfirm, or support a clinical hypothesis. Included in this category are nonexperimental research designs such as case studies and case series, as well as quasiexperimental approaches such as time-series designs.

Developmental milestone Specific point in a child's development, identified by the accomplishment of various psychomotor skills, such as sitting up, rolling over, crawling, creeping, and walking.

Diagnosis Identification and measurement of an abnormality in a particular patient that has clinical ramifications.

Dietary history Extensive history of a patient's dietary habits, including not only foods and beverages but also medications and vitamin, mineral, and herbal supplements.

Dietary Supplement Health Education Act (DSHEA) This 1995 U.S. law addresses the issue of health claims that may be made by supplement manufacturers. It allows claims regarding the impact on processes of the body but not with regard to disease or illness.

Diplomate of the American Chiropractic Board of Radiology (DACBR) Designation accorded to chiropractors specializing in radiology who have completed the required coursework and passed the diplomate examination of the American Chiropractic Board of Radiology.

Diplopia Double vision.

Direct access Ability to consult a health practitioner without previous referral from a primary care physician.

Direct access laws Statutes requiring managed care plans to permit their members to access specialty care without referral from a primary care gatekeeper.

Direct inquiry Method in which the examiner seeks particular information.

Disk bulge Bulging of discal material beyond the margins of the vertebral body, without herniation through the annulus fibrosus.

Disk extrusion Condition in which a portion of a displaced nucleus pulposus has penetrated the fibers of the surrounding annulus fibrosus and lies under the posterior longitudinal ligament.

Disk herniation Protrusion of the intervertebral disk from its normal anatomic position, usually in a posterolateral direction.

Disk, intervertebral Soft tissue component of the fibrous intervertebral joint. It is composed of a central, gelatinous nucleus pulposus and a peripheral, fibrocartilaginous annulus fibrosus. The intervertebral disk provides a cushioning support between adjacent vertebrae.

Disk sequestration Condition in which a displaced nucleus pulposus extends beyond the posterior longitudinal ligament into the epidural space or forms a free fragment.

Discount plan Insurance arrangement under which the contracted provider discounts the normal fee (usually by 20% to 30%), the patient pays the entire discounted fee, and the insurance company makes no payment to the provider or patient. Also known as *access plan* or *affinity plan.*

Disease Any morbid process altering the normal state of living tissue. It may be functional or physiologic and may affect the organism as a whole or any of its constituent parts.

Dis-ease Lack of physiologic efficiency that is due to disruption of coordination by the nervous system; aberrant tone.

Dislocation Displacement of a bone; a luxation.

Displacement 1. In biomechanics, a change in position of a body or body part. 2. In physics, the weight or volume of a fluid displaced by a floating body.

Disruption Morphologic defect resulting from the breakdown of a normally formed structure, during the fetal or postnatal period. The origin may involve altered growth patterns because of trauma, infection, tumors, or metabolic alterations.

Distraction Separation of joint surfaces without injury to the joint or its ligaments.

Distress Anxiety associated with pain or fear of pain.

Divergence Branching of axons, which allows a single neuron to communicate with and send signals to many other neurons.

Diversified technique A diverse collection of specific and nonspecific chiropractic adjusting methods that may be used with any manual technique analytic system.

Dizziness Handicap Inventory (DHI) Self-rating instrument used to assess the impact of dizziness and vestibular problems on daily life. The DHI is composed of three subscales: functional, emotional, and physical.

Dolor Localized pain; a cardinal sign of inflammation.

Doppler ultrasonography Diagnostic modality that transmits a high-frequency sound wave through tissue until it reaches an acoustic barrier, usually some other type of tissue. A portion of this pulsed sound wave is then reflected back toward the source where it is imaged or measured. Doppler ultrasonography can detect blood flow within arteries by measuring the frequency shifts of sound waves reflected off moving blood cells.

Dorsal root ganglion (DRG) Site of cell bodies of the sensory neurons of spinal nerves, located in the vicinity of the intervertebral foramen.

Double-blind study Experiment in which patients and either doctors or outcome assessors are blinded.

Duke Headache Evidence Report A systematic review of the scientific literature on physical and behavioral interventions for tension and cervicogenic headaches, performed at Duke University.

Duplex ultrasound scanning Diagnostic imaging modality that combines Doppler ultrasonography with a complementary modality called real-time B-mode ultrasonography. This scanning method allows an image to be created from the reflected sound wave, where the brightness of each picture element is dependent on the amplitude of the returning sound echo. The image is updated rapidly enough to allow the examiner to see real-time physiologic changes, such as the motion of blood vessel walls.

Dura mater Thick, tough connective tissue layer that constitutes the outer layer of the meninges and is continuous from the cranial cavity to the sacrum (S2).

Duration of care Length of professional treatment.

Dynamic palpation *See* Motion palpation.

Dynamic thrust High-velocity, low-amplitude procedures without recoil after the thrust. Also called *impulse thrust.*

Dysafferentation Abnormal afferent input as a result of joint restriction that involves a functional decrease in the activity of large diameter mechanoreceptor afferent fibers and a simultaneous functional increase in the activity of nociceptive afferent nerve fibers.

Dysautonomia Malfunction of the ANS.

Dyskinesia Distortions, difficulty with or impairment of voluntary movement.

Dysmenorrhea Painful menses.

Dysmetria Inability to judge distance during purposeful muscular movements.

Dysponesis Reversible physiopathologic state consisting of unnoticed, misdirected neurophysiologic reactions to various agents (e.g., environmental events, body sensation, emotions, thoughts) and the repercussions of these reactions throughout the organism.

Eccentric loading Lengthening of a muscle during its contraction.

Ectoderm Outer layer of the embryo after the establishment of the three primordial germ cell layers: ectoderm, mesoderm, and endoderm. The ectoderm is in contact with the mesoderm and amniotic cavity.

Efferent Moving outward or away from a central location (e.g., nerves carrying motor impulses [information] away from the CNS to the periphery or blood vessels carrying blood away from the heart).

Efferent fibers Nerve fibers that convey impulses to effector tissues, such as smooth, cardiac, or striated muscle or glands, in the periphery.

Effusion Escape of fluid (serous, purulent, or bloody) into a part or tissue.

Ehlers Danlos syndrome Congenital hereditary disorder marked by hyperextensible joints, hyperelastic and fragile skin, and fragile capillaries.

Eicosanoids Hormonally active products of free fatty-acid metabolism.

Elasticity Tendency of tissue under load to return to its original size and shape after removal of the load.

Electromyography (EMG) Recording and study of electrical muscular activity, most accurately performed with needle electrodes placed in the desired muscle.

Empiricism Reliance on direct experience.

Encopresis Fecal incontinence.

Endoderm Innermost layer of the embryo after the establishment of the three primordial germ cell layers, ectoderm, mesoderm, endoderm. The endoderm is in contact with the mesoderm and lines the primitive yolk sac.

Endogenous opiates Body's own internal pain relievers; neurotransmitters that shut off or decrease the perception of pain.

Endoneurium Connective tissue that surrounds individual nerve fibers. *See also* Epineurium.

Endorphin One of the body's endogenous opiates—a neuropeptide.

End organ Organ supplied or affected by a nerve.

End plate Superior and inferior cartilaginous borders of the vertebral body.

End play (end feel) Short-range movements or quality of resistance of a joint, determined by springing a joint at the limits of its passive range of motion.

End-play zone Area of joint movement past the physiologic barrier but before the anatomic barrier.

Enkephalinergic Mediated by enkephalins, part of the body's endogenous opiate system of pain modulation.

Entrepreneurship Art of developing and expanding a business in a private enterprise economy.

Enuresis Urinary incontinence; bedwetting.

Epineurium Connective tissue that surrounds an entire nerve and its major branches. *See also* Endoneurium.

Equilibrial triad Three bodily systems that control postural adaptation: (1) the proprioceptive system, found throughout the body in the Golgi tendon organs, the muscle spindles and the nerves that innervate these receptors; (2) the vestibular system, found in the inner ear, which signals the nervous system regarding the position of the head; and (3) the visual system. Each of these systems is coordinated and integrated (along with the cerebellum) within the CNS.

Ergogenic Tending to improve or enhance athletic performance.

Ergonomics Study of people in relation to their jobs.

Ergotamine Medication that induces vasoconstriction and is commonly used in treating migraine headaches.

Etiology 1. Cause of a problem. 2. Study of causation and origins.

Evidence-based health care Health care system in which, to the greatest extent possible, procedures used by health care providers have been subjected to rigorous standards of scientific observation, experimentation, and documentation.

Exclusions Services not covered under an insurance policy. *See also* Preexisting condition exclusion.

Experimental group Group in a clinical trial that receives the intervention that is being tested.

Expiration thrust Dynamic thrust manual adjustment performed at the end of expiration, when the patient's ribs are at their most flexed or "bent" position.

Extension 1. Act of straightening a joint. 2. In spinal motion, act of bending backward.

External validity Degree to which the results of a study can be expected to hold true in other settings.

Exteroceptors Sensory receptors that carry information originating outside or on the surface of the body. Because the force of gravity is considered to reside outside the body, and the proprioceptive and vestibular systems react to gravitational stimuli, these receptors (Golgi tendon organs, muscle spindles, hair cells) are considered exteroceptive mechanoreceptors.

Extrusion, disk *See* Disk extrusion.

Facet joints *See* Zygapophyseal joints.

Facet syndrome Sprain of the zygapophyseal joints, which elicits an inflammatory response and activation of nociceptors.

Facilitation 1. Increased or accelerated synaptic transmission by successive presynaptic impulses, usually the result of increased transmitter release. 2. Lowered threshold for firing of nerve cells (neurons) in a spinal cord segment, representing a hyperexcitable neurologic state with possible causes that include repeated use of a neural pathway or afferent nerve impulse bombardment associated with altered spinal biomechanics.

False positive 1. Test result that is positive, despite the absence of the disease or condition being tested. 2. Situation in which intervention A is no better than intervention B, but errors in the data or its interpretation lead to the reasonable conclusion that intervention A *is* actually better than intervention B. Also called *type I error.*

False negative 1. Test result that is negative, despite the presence of the disease or condition being tested. 2. Situation in which intervention A is actually superior to intervention B, but errors in the data or its interpretation lead to the reasonable conclusion that intervention A is *not* superior to intervention B. Also called *type II error.*

False pelvis Area between the ilia, above the pelvic brim.

Falx cerebelli Reflection of the meningeal dura from the inner surface of the cranial cavity, which, along with the falx cerebri, separates the cerebral and cerebellar hemispheres.

Falx cerebri Reflection of the meningeal dura from the inner surface of the cranial cavity, which, along with the falx cerebelli, separates the cerebral and cerebellar hemispheres.

Fascia Connective tissue that continuously runs through the body among muscles and other soft tissue structures.

Fasciculi Bundles of parallel anatomic fibers.

Faye model Five-component model of the vertebral subluxation complex proposed by Leonard John Faye. Components of this model include neuropathophysiology, kinesiopathology, myopathology, and histopathology, as well as a biochemical component.

Fear-avoidance behavior Pattern of response to a frightening situation in which the avoidance of fear becomes the dominant motivation.

Fee-for-service plan Traditional health insurance policy that requires patients to pay an annual deductible, after which the insurance plan pays a predetermined percentage of further medically necessary care. Also called *indemnity plan. See also* Deductible.

Fee splitting Paying or receiving any commission, bonus, kickback, or rebate, or engaging in any split-fee arrangement with the physician, organization, agency, or person, in any form whatsoever, either directly or indirectly, for patients referred to providers of health goods and services.

Femoral torsion Gait abnormality in toddlers; both the patellae and the toes point inward. This abnormality may result from pelvic rotation.

Fibromyalgia Painful musculoskeletal condition characterized by multiple trigger points.

Fibrosis Formation of fibrous tissue as part of the process of repair or replacement.

Filum terminale Long, slender connective tissue (pia mater) strand extending from the extremity of the medullary cone of the spinal cord to the internal aspect of the spinal dural sac (filum terminale internum) at the sacrum and coccyx. Broad strands of connective tissue that attach the spinal dural sac to the coccyx (filum terminale externum) are commonly called the coccygeal ligament.

Fixation Dysfunctional state of decreased or restricted joint motion.

Flexion 1. Act of bending. 2. In spinal motion, act of bending forward.

Flexion distraction technique A system of chiropractic analysis and adjustment/manipulation developed by James Cox that utilizes a specialized break-away flexion-distraction table that allows angled segmental traction in the lumbar region. Scoliosis and cervical spine protocols are also included in this system.

Flexner Report 1909 report on the status of medical education in the United States, which resulted in the closing of almost one half of medical schools and virtually all nonallopathic institutions.

Fluoroscopy An x-ray procedure that allows real-time visualization of physiologic motion within the human body.

Food and Drug Administration (FDA) The regulatory agency of the U.S. federal government that is responsible for ensuring the safety of foods and medications.

Food guide pyramid Visual depiction of U.S. Department of Agriculture recommendations on food choices, which takes into account factors of proportion, moderation, and variety.

Foramen, intervertebral Passage formed by the superior and inferior notches on the pedicles of adjacent vertebrae. Its anatomic contents include the spinal nerve, nerve roots, recurrent meningeal (sinuvertebral) nerves, blood vessels, lymphatics, and connective tissue.

Foramen magnum Large opening in the caudal portion of the occiput for passage of the spinal cord, meninges, cerebrospinal fluid, and vertebral arteries.

Foramen transversarium Space within the transverse processes of each cervical vertebra through which the vertebral artery travels.

Foramen, vertebral Space bounded by the posterior aspect of the vertebral body and the vertebral arch. It contains the spinal cord and nerves, the meninges and cerebrospinal fluid, and the vessels and nerves that supply these structures.

Force In biomechanics, force is a push or pull exerted on a body that tends to produce acceleration.

Frequency General or statistical expression of how often a condition or disease occurs. Statistical expressions of frequency take two forms, prevalence and incidence. *See also* Prevalence and Incidence.

Full-scope physician Medical or osteopathic physician licensed to practice medicine and perform surgical procedures.

Functio laesa Loss of normal function; a cardinal sign of inflammation.

Functional ailment Ailment with symptoms that are persistent, painful, and real, but where no underlying organic problem can be found.

Functional range Extent of a patient's capacities and limitations, based on evaluation of activity intolerances, mechanical sensitivities, and relevant pathologic function.

Functional spinal unit Two adjacent vertebrae and the joints and connective tissue structures that link them, as well as the skeletal muscles that move the joints and the nerves and vessels that supply these structures. Also called *intervertebral motor unit*.

Gait Manner or style of walking.

Gamma motor neurons Motor neurons responsible for the innervation of muscle spindles, which establish a set point for muscle tone. These neurons are somewhat smaller in diameter than alpha motor neurons and thus conduct impulses at a somewhat slower velocity.

Ganglion Collection of functionally related nerve cell bodies outside the CNS.

Gastroenterologist Medical physician specializing in diseases of the digestive tract.

Gate control theory A theory developed by Ronald Melzack and Patrick Wall proposing that mechanical intervention or noxious stimuli activate the large, fast-conducting tactile- or touch-responsive A-alpha fibers (mechanoreceptors), which in turn inhibit the synaptic transmission of the pain signals by blocking the synaptic "gates" normally used by the smaller C-fibers that convey pain signals, thereby suppressing the signals of pain. Also called *Gate theory* or *Pain gate theory*.

Gatekeeper Primary care physician designated as a health maintenance organization (HMO) subscriber's initial contact practitioner and coordinator of care. Many managed care plans require that patients have a referral from their gatekeeper physician to access specialty providers (including chiropractors) and laboratory or treatment services. In most HMOs, the gatekeeper physician provides direct primary care services and also regulates and controls access to all other services.

Gate-control theory Theory by Ronald Melzack and Patrick Wall proposing that mechanical intervention (e.g., rubbing a painful area) activates large, fast-conducting A-fibers (mechanoreceptors), which in turn inhibit the synaptic transmission of pain signals by blocking synaptic "gates" normally used by the smaller C-fibers that convey pain signals, therefore suppressing the signals of pain. Also called *gate theory* and *afferent inhibition*.

Genu valgus Abnormal postural variant in which the knees are unusually close together with the toes pointing outward.

Genu varus Abnormal postural variant in which the knees are separated with the toes pointing inward.

Geriatrics Health care related to older persons and the aging process.

Glia Nonneuronal supportive cellular elements of the central and peripheral nervous system. The three types of glial tissue are astrocytes, microglia, and oligodendrocytes. Unlike neurons, glial cells do not conduct electrical impulses.

Globalize To make broad overarching claims based on limited anecdotal evidence.

Global muscle hyperactivity *See* Synergist substitution.

Gold standard Measure of agreed-on accuracy and validity.

Golgi tendon organ (GTO) Proprioceptive sensory nerve that ends in the fibers of a tendon, frequently near the musculotendinous junction. GTOs are compressed and activated by increased tension in the tendon that results from active compression or passive stretch of the corresponding muscle.

Goniometer Instrument used for measuring joint motion in degrees.

Gonstead technique A system of chiropractic analysis and adjustment developed by Clarence Gonstead that utilizes specific x-ray analysis and dynamic thrust full-spine adjusting procedures performed on a flat bench, cervical chair, or knee-chest table, along with motion and static palpation, and instrumentation (Nervoscope) for level but not listing of subluxation.

Grade I sprain or strain Microscopic tear of a ligament, muscle, or tendon.

Grade II sprain or strain Macroscopic tear of a ligament, muscle, or tendon.

Grade III sprain or strain Complete tear of a ligament, muscle, or tendon.

Graded activity Exercise program that uses exercise to quota (a set amount) rather than being guided by pain (i.e., less on bad days and more on good days).

Grooving In rehabilitative exercise, reeducating and reprogramming appropriate movement patterns such as in agonist-antagonist co-activation or sensory-motor training.

Ground-reaction forces. Forces generated as a result of foot-ground interaction during locomotion.

Group III nociceptors Nociceptors with thinly myelinated axons (A-fibers) that subserve "fast" pain function.

Group IV nociceptors Nociceptors with unmyelinated axons (C-fibers) that subserve "slow" pain function.

Guarding Local response to internal inflammation brought on by injury or disease. This phenomenon occurs as a result of a viscero-somatic reflex, in which skeletal muscles of the body wall contract to protect internal structures from further damage. Guarding is usually found in the abdominal wall.

Habituation 1. Gradual adaptation. 2. Negative adaptation, in which a conditioned reflex is eliminated through excessive repetition of the stimulus.

Harrison model Postural model of subluxation developed by Donald Harrison, which emphasizes detailed radiographic evaluation of spinal curvatures. The Harrison model asserts that, over time, abnormal spinal postures result in degenerative changes in muscles, ligaments, and bony structures, as well as having a direct or indirect role in spinal pain syndromes.

Hawthorne effect Tendency of people in a research study to change their behavior, compromising the validity of the data.

Headache diary Self-rating instrument for monitoring headache activity. A typical version includes frequency of headache days per week and month, headache severity for any particular day or averaged over a specific interval, peak headache severity per any interval (i.e., worst headache in a month), and medication usage.

Headache, cervicogenic Headache whose site of origin is in the cervical spine.

Headache, migraine Headache characterized by unilateral location, pulsating quality, moderate or severe intensity, aggravated by routine physical activity, nausea or vomiting or both, and photophobia or phonophobia or both.

Headache, tension-type (TTH) Most prevalent form of benign, primary headache. TTH is typically bilateral, of mild-to-moderate intensity, experienced as an aching, tightening, or pressing quality of pain that lasts from 30 minutes to 7 days, with either photophobia or phonophobia (but not both), and not accompanied by nausea or vomiting.

Healing partnership Doctor-patient relationship based on mutual respect, which includes active effort by the patient and an openness to questions on the part of the doctor.

Health maintenance organization (HMO) Entity that provides and manages the health services for plan members in exchange for payment of a fixed premium. In general, health care services are reimbursable by an HMO only when offered by providers who have contracted with the HMO.

Health services research Research that studies the structure, process, and outcomes of the health delivery system and its role in society.

Heme iron Organic iron.

Hemianesthesia Complete loss of sensation on one side of the body.

Hemiparesis Unilateral muscular weakness.

Herniation Abnormal protrusion of a structure.

Heroic therapies Historically, extreme measures intended to elicit healing, including the use of leaches, bloodletting, purging, and excessive drugging.

High tech Tools and procedures that primarily rely on advanced machinery and the infrastructure that supports it.

High velocity, low amplitude (HVLA) adjustment/manipulation Dynamic thrust adjustment/manipulation.

Hippocrates Greek physician who lived in the fifth century BC and is considered the father of Western medicine.

Holistic 1. Viewing humankind in its totality within a wide ecologic spectrum, emphasizing the view that ill health or disease is brought about by an imbalance, or disequilibrium, of the individual in the total ecologic system and not only by the causative agent and pathologic evolution. 2. Whole person or systems approach to health care.

Homeopathy System of healing founded by the German physician Samuel Hahnemann in the late eighteenth century, which uses minute dilutions of substances for medicinal purposes.

Homocystine A disulfide homologous with the amino acid cystine. Elevated plasma homocystine levels have associated with an increased risk for a variety of cardiovascular diseases, and are a possible risk factor for cervical artery dissections.

Hooke's law Deformation of tissue increases in proportion to the load that is applied.

Howard, J.F. Alan Founder of the National School of Chiropractic, 1906.

Humors 1. Bodily moisture or fluids that include lymph, chyle, and vitreous and aqueous humors of the eye. 2. Four bodily fluids: blood, phlegm, yellow bile (choler), and black bile (melancholy). Proposed by ancient healing arts to determine temperament and health. 3. Energetic patterns used as diagnostic categories in some traditional systems of healing.

Hunchback Excessive thoracic kyphosis, usually associated with scoliosis.

Hydrotherapy Treatment of disease by the internal or external application of water; water cure.

Hygienic system System of natural healing developed in the 19th century, which amalgamated hydrotherapy and Nature Cure.

Hyperalgesia Increased response to a stimulus that is normally painful.

Hyperemia An increase in blood in an anatomical structure.

Hyperlipidemia Prolonged elevation of blood lipids.

Hypermobility Excessive joint motion.

Hypertonic Excessive tone or tension in skeletal muscles.

Hypochondriasis Deep anxiety about one's health, which may be expressed in a variety of symptoms not attributable to organic disease.

Hypomobility Restriction of joint movement; the fixation component of subluxation.

Hypermobility Excessive joint movement, often involving laxity of ligaments.

Hypertonus Excessive muscular contraction.

Hypothalamic-pituitary axis Central neurohormonal system that controls various other systems.

Hysterectomy Surgical removal of the uterus.

Hysteresis Effect of repeated loading and unloading of a tissue; the tissue does not return to its original shape after many repetitions over a long period of time. Although a tissue may resist one or many loads, the constant repetition of loading may cause the elastic limit to be exceeded. In the human body, hysteresis can be thought of as *overuse*.

Iatrogenic disorder Any adverse mental or physical condition induced in a patient by unwanted effects of a therapeutic intervention.

Imbibition The absorption of a liquid.

Ibuprofen Nonsteroidal antiinflammatory medication.

Iliolumbar ligaments Ligaments extending between the transverse processes of L4 and L5 and the iliac crest.

Iliotibial friction syndrome Common injury in runners; a tight tensor fascia lata causes the iliotibial band to snap over the lateral femoral epicondyle.

Image intensifier Tube used in videofluoroscopy to amplify the intensity of the image, reducing the amount of radiation necessary to perform the procedure.

Impulse 1. In biomechanics, the force of two colliding bodies that is exerted on one another. 2. In neurology, the transmission of a signal over a nerve. 3. Act of impelling forward with sudden force or thrust.

Impulse-based neural mechanisms Mechanisms of nerve transmission via nerve impulse or action potential. Progressive electro-chemical change occurs in the membrane of a nerve fiber following stimulation, transmitting sensation from a receptor or instructions to an effector. Conduction velocity of the impulse may range from as little as 0.25m/sec in small unmyelinated fibers to as high as 100 m/sec (the length of a football field in 1 second) in very large myelinated fibers. *See also* Non impulse-based neural mechanism, action potential.

Impulse thrust *See* Dynamic thrust.

Indemnity insurance Traditional prepaid health care insurance; health care expenses are reimbursed on a fee-for-service basis. Usually an annual deductible and a percentage of the fees are due from the patient as co-insurance.

Incidence Proportion of a clearly defined group (population) that is initially free of a condition but develops the condition over a given period.

Independent medical examination (IME) Examination in which a claimant for worker's compensation, personal injury protection benefits, or some other form of compensation for a health condition is assessed and an opinion provided for the payer of the claim as an independent evaluation of the merit and value of the claim.

Independent medical examiner Doctor who is paid by a third party (usually an insurance plan) to examine a patient and submit a report including history, examination findings, diagnosis, appropriateness of past care, and recommendations for possible future care.

Independent practitioner Health care provider legally permitted to practice without a supervisory or collaborative relationship with a medical physician or other provider.

Indifferent hand *See* Support hand.

Inertia Property of a body to remain at rest or in uniform motion in a straight line unless acted upon by an external force. This is *Newton's first law.*

Infarction Necrosis (tissue death) as a result of diminished blood supply, generally caused by an obstruction.

Inflammation Localized protective reaction of tissue characterized by five cardinal signs: (1) pain (dolor), (2) swelling (tumor), (3) redness (rubor), (4) heat (calor), and (5) loss of function (functio laesa). Inflammation can occur in response to injury or tissue destruction.

Informed consent Legal doctrine that requires health care providers to obtain consent for treatment based on the patient's informed and knowledgeable understanding of the risks, benefits, and alternatives to treatment.

Inion Midline external occipital protuberance.

Initial contact practitioner *See* Portal of entry provider.

Innate intelligence 1. Inborn healing wisdom of the body. 2. Intrinsic biologic ability of an organism to react physiologically to the changing conditions of the external and internal environments. *See also* Vis medicatrix naturae.

Insertion More distal or mobile attachment of a muscle.

Inspection Visual observation.

Instrument-assisted techniques Methods that utilize adjusting instruments to assist or replace manual adjustment/manipulation. Examples include the use of the Terminal Point Drop table, Cox Flexion Distraction table, Activator Adjusting Instrument, and SOT blocks and boards.

Insurance equality laws Laws that require health insurance plans to avoid discrimination against certain types of licensed practitioners. For example, some insurance equality laws require that if spinal adjustment/manipulation is a covered service when performed by a medical or osteopathic physician, it must also be covered when performed by a chiropractor.

Insurer Private or government insurance plan.

International Classification of Disease (ICD) codes Standardized numerical diagnostic codes utilized for insurance reimbursement.

Interneurons Neurons in the gray matter of the central nervous system, which connect sensory neurons to each other and to motor neurons. Also called *association neurons.*

Interoceptors Sensory receptors that convey information originating inside the body (e.g., sensory end organs in the walls of viscera such as the gastrointestinal and respiratory tracts).

Interpedicular zone Intervertebral foramen is viewed as a zone that represents an anatomic canal or tunnel between pedicles of adjacent vertebrae, not as a two-dimensional hole. Such a zone or canal provides for the passage of the spinal nerve and other related structures.

Interspinous ligaments Ligaments extending between spinous processes of adjacent vertebrae.

Intercristal line Line drawn between the two iliac crests, usually passing through the inferior end of the fourth lumbar vertebra.

Intertransverse ligaments Ligaments extending between transverse processes of adjacent vertebrae.

Intervention Health care procedure that is intended to prevent or alter the course of a condition, illness, or pathologic process.

Intervertebral foramen *See* Foramen, intervertebral.

Internal validity Degree to which the results of a study are correct for the methods and sample of patients included in the study. *See also* Validity, external validity.

International Chiropractors Association (ICA) Second largest national chiropractic association in the United States, founded in 1926 as the Chiropractic Health Bureau and renamed as the International Chiropractors Association in 1941.

Inter-observer reliability Consistency of measured results among different practitioners evaluating the same thing. *See also* Intra-observer reliability.

Interphalangeal Between the bones of a finger.

Intervention Procedure intended to prevent an illness or alter the course of an illness or pathologic process.

Intervertebral disk *See* Disk, intervertebral.

Intraclass correlation co-efficient (ICC) Method of statistical analysis that corrects for chance agreement between examiners. ICCs reflect both the degree of consistency and the agreement among ratings, ranging from 0 to 1, with 1 representing high-reliability values.

Intra-observer reliability Consistency with which one practitioner can consistently arrive at the same result. *See also* Inter-observer reliability.

Intravenous pyelogram (IVP) A radiographic study in which iodinated dye is injected into the bloodstream and the dye is then filtered by normally functioning kidneys. If calcification is shown to displace the dye as it collects in the renal pelvis, diagnosis of a renal stone is confirmed.

Intrinsic muscles Deep muscles that are responsible for joint stability on an involuntary or subcortical basis.

Invasiveness 1. Degree to which a health intervention intrudes on the physical body.

Invasiveness may be ranked on a scale ranging from the least invasive methods (e.g., meditation, art therapy) to the most invasive (e.g., pharmaceuticals, surgery). Using this definition, dynamic thrust chiropractic adjustments are near the middle of the scale. *See also* Appendix II. 2. Involving puncture or incision of the skin. Using this definition, dynamic thrust chiropractic adjustments are noninvasive.

Ipsilateral On the same side.

Ischemia Deficiency of the local blood supply that is a result of the obstruction of circulation to a part of the body.

Ischemic penumbra State of decreased blood flow not sufficiently low to cause neuronal death, but low enough to bring about electrical silence.

Isometric exercises Exercises in which a muscle is tightened, held in that position for a few seconds, and then relaxed without moving the joint.

Isotonic exercises Exercises that involve movement against resistance, often taking the form of repeated motions while holding light weights.

Joint blockage Hypomobility of a joint.

Joint Commission on Accreditation of Healthcare Organizations (JCAHO) Evaluates and accredits more than 15,000 health care organizations in the United States, including hospitals, health care networks, and health care organizations that provide home care, long-term care, behavioral health care, laboratory services, and ambulatory care services. An independent, not-for-profit organization, JCAHO is the United States' oldest and largest standards-setting and accrediting body in health care.

Joint dysfunction Joint mechanics that show functional disturbances with or without structural changes.

Joint fixation (restriction) Temporary immobilization of a joint in a position that it may normally occupy during any phase of normal movement.

Joint play Qualitative evaluation of the joint's resistance to movement when it is in a neutral position.

Kappa co-efficient of reliability Statistical test to determine whether dichotomous findings (present or absent) occur at a rate more likely than chance. Although kappa can be reflected as a negative value (worse than chance), it usually varies between 0 and 1, with values closer to 1 representing high reliability.

Kent model Developed by Christopher Kent, this three-component model of vertebral subluxation emphasizes the roles of dyskinesia, dysponesis, and dysautonomia.

Kickback Offering, paying, soliciting, or receiving of any form of direct remuneration intended to induce referrals.

Kilovolts Peak (KvP) A measurement of the quality and penetrating power of an x-ray beam. One kilovolt equals 1000 volts.

Kinematics Branch of mechanics that deals with motion of the body but not with the forces involved in that motion.

Kinesiology Study of muscles and the mechanics of motion.

Kinesiopathology In chiropractic, a major component of vertebral subluxation complex related to abnormal joint motion. It may include hypomobility, hypermobility, or altered joint play.

Kinesthesia Sense perception of movement, or muscular sense.

Kinesthetic 1. Relating to kinesthesia. *See also* Kinesthesia. 2. Characterized by reliance on the sense of touch.

Kinetic chain 1. Sequence of links between bones in which forces generated by muscles create movement. 2. Orderly function of all musculoskeletal structures required to perform an activity.

Kinetic chain, closed Kinetic chain in which the terminal joint of a moving limb is fixed to or supported by an immobile object.

Kinetic chain, open Kinetic chain in which the terminal joint of a moving limb is able to move freely. Throwing a ball is a classic example of an open kinetic chain activity.

Kinetics Study of motion.

Klippel-Feil syndrome Condition characterized by short neck, low posterior hairline, and limitation of cervical spine motion, due to congenital fusions of cervical vertebrae.

Kyphosis Spinal curvature with an anterior concavity. *See also* Lordosis.

Lacto-ovo-vegetarian Person whose diet includes eggs and dairy products but no meat.

Lamina Portion of a vertebra that projects posteromedially from the transverse process or pedicle to the base of the spinous process.

Laminar Layered.

Lantz model Nine-component model of the vertebral subluxation complex developed by Charles Lantz. It describes a hierarchy of organization and a pattern of interrelatedness among its components. Components of this model are connective tissue pathology, vascular abnormalities, inflammatory response, and pathophysiology, as well as the five components of the Faye model: (1) neuropathophysiology, (2) kinesiopathology, (3) myopathology, (4) histopathology, and (5) biochemical. *See also* Faye model.

Lateral flexion Act of bending to the side without flexion, extension, or rotation.

Layer palpation Method of assessing the mobility and condition of myofascial and other soft tissue structures. Palpation begins with the most superficial structures and proceeds to deeper tissues.

Legg-Calvé-Perthes disease Avascular necrosis of the femoral epiphysis.

Legume Vegetable group that includes peas and beans.

Lesion Pathologic change or discontinuity in an anatomic structure.

Lesion, adjustive *See* Adjustive lesion.

Lesion osteopath Historically, a practitioner of osteopathy who used osteopathic manipulation as a central part of practice.

Lesion, osteopathic *See* Osteopathic lesion and Somatic dysfunction.

Leukotrienes Lipid compounds (eicosanoids) related to prostaglandins that help mediate the inflammatory response.

Level playing field Political arrangement in which the claims of competing parties are evaluated according to a fair, mutually agreed upon set of rules.

Liability Legal exposure, either civil or criminal, to a patient or a payer of care for errors in diagnosis or treatment or for fraudulent billing or other financial violations such as kickbacks. *See also* Malpractice.

Lifestyle interventions Health care techniques seeking behavioral change.

Ligament Fibrous tissue structure consisting of dense regular connective tissue, principally collagenous, which connects one bone to another. This term is also used to describe soft tissue attachments in the viscera (e.g., gastrocolic ligament).

Ligamentum flavum Ligaments that extend from the articular process laterally to the spinous process medially and connect adjacent vertebral laminae. These ligaments are the most important of the posterior ligaments in limiting flexion of the spine.

Ligamentum nuchae Ligament that virtually surrounds the tips of the cervical spinous processes in the sagittal plane and functions as a major muscle attachment in the cervical region as a midline raphe. It extends from the seventh cervical vertebra to the occiput and is a specialization of the supraspinous ligament. Also called *nuchal ligament.*

Limited license practitioner Health professional whose license is limited by law to certain anatomic parts of the body or certain procedures (e.g., doctors of chiropractic, psychology, dentistry, optometry, podiatry, audiology).

Line of correction *See* Line of drive.

Line of drive Direction of dynamic thrust. Also called *line of correction.*

Listing Specific description of abnormal joint position or movement.

Locked-in syndrome Condition in which patients are awake and retain mental content but cannot express themselves because of paralysis of efferent motor pathways that prevent speech or limb movement. This syndrome usually involves a lesion of the motor pathways in the base of the pons or midbrain, whereas the dorsal gray matter is spared from injury.

Load External forces that may include compression, torsion, translation (shearing), and/or tensile loading.

Logan Basic technique A system of chiropractic analysis and adjustment developed by Hugh Logan that seeks to bring about spinal balance by correctly positioning the sacrum, which is considered the "keystone" of the spine. Logan Basic technique emphasizes the use of a light contact, nonthrusting thumb adjustment involving a sustained contact on the sacrotuberous ligament, while the opposite hand contacts the site of vertebral subluxation.

Longevity Long life, extended survival.

Longitudinal Involving serial measurements taken over time.

Long-lever adjustment/manipulation Procedure in which the doctor's manual contact point is located some distance from the targeted lesion or lesions. Once contact and stabilization are established, the doctor delivers a controlled dynamic thrust, initiating the adjustment. This method of manipulation tends to be considerably less specific than the short-lever technique and is generally better suited for targeting an area or region of the body rather than a specific joint.

Long-term depression Long-lasting decrease in synaptic efficacy, which can be established by both high- and low-frequency conditioning stimuli.

Long-term potentiation Long-lasting increase in synaptic efficiency after a high-frequency conditioning discharge by the primary afferent neuron.

Lordosis Spinal curvature with a posterior concavity. *See also* Kyphosis.

Low tech Tools and procedures that rely primarily on human effort rather than advanced machinery.

Lumbago Low back pain.

Lumbar facet syndrome *See* Facet syndrome.

Lumen Cavity or channel within a tube or tubular organ.

Lycopene The red carotenoid pigment in tomatoes, various berries, and fruits.

Lymphatics Vascular channels that transport lymph, a fluid that drains from the interstitial body space.

Magnetic healing Nineteenth century healing method, practiced by D.D. Palmer before his discovery of chiropractic, that included "laying on of hands" to transmit healing energy. It may also have included vigorous rubbing and manipulation.

Magnetic resonance imaging (MRI) Technique that produces images of the body through analysis of signals produced after the area of interest is placed in a magnetic field and exposed to radio frequency pulses. Images may be produced in axial, sagittal, coronal, or oblique planes. MRI does not use ionizing radiation.

Magnitude Size of an effect.

Maintenance care Health promotion and preventive care that involves periodic chiropractic adjustments/manipulations, along with other interventions that may include adjunctive therapies and education on exercise, nutrition, and relaxation.

Malformation 1. Anomaly. 2. Morphologic defect resulting from dysfunctional embryogenic development of an anatomic structure.

Malingering Intentional falsification or overstatement of illness or injury.

Malleability Quality of being easily deformed by external forces.

Malnutrition Faulty nutrition resulting from poor diet or poor assimilation.

Malpractice Liability for causing injury to a patient that arises as a result of a failure to meet the standards of care for the practitioner's profession.

Mammillary process In the lumbar spine, a ridge lateral to the superior articular process that serves as an attachment site for the multifidus muscle.

Mammography X-ray examination of the breast.

Managed care Form of insurance coverage that seeks to oversee and guide appropriate care. In exchange for cost savings, members agree to see contracted plan providers and to abide by cost-containment mechanisms, such as utilization review and precertification for certain procedures.

Manipulable subluxation Subluxation in which altered alignment, movement, or function can be improved by manual thrust procedures.

Manipulation Passive manual maneuver during which a joint is quickly brought beyond its restricted physiologic range of movement and beyond its elastic barrier without exceeding the boundaries of anatomic integrity.

Manipulation under anesthesia Manipulative procedure that is performed in a hospital or ambulatory surgical center, during which the patient is anesthetized.

Manual procedures Procedures by which the hands directly contact the body to treat the articulations or soft tissues. Also called *manual therapy.*

Manual therapy *See* Manual procedures.

Marfan's syndrome Congenital hereditary connective tissue disorder characterized by abnormal length of the arms and legs (especially fingers and toes), subluxation of the lens, cardiovascular abnormalities, and other deformities.

Massage Manual therapy (rubbing and kneading) applied to the muscles and other soft tissues of the musculoskeletal system, without cavitating joint manipulation or adjustment. Massage seeks to relax muscles and aid circulation.

Maximum medical improvement Point at which no further recovery from injury or illness can be reasonably expected.

Measurement bias Systematic error in data, resulting from poor methods of observation.

Mechanoreceptors Sensory receptors that generate an action potential in response to physical deformation or distortion, such as those responding to sound, touch, and muscular contractions.

Medicaid U.S. federal government health care plan for economically disadvantaged individuals and families. State governments administer Medicaid. Chiropractic care is covered in some states and excluded in others.

Medical necessity Need for specific health care services, based on clinical expectations that the health benefits will outweigh the health risks. Insurance policies require providers to certify that services are medically necessary to qualify for reimbursement.

Medicare U.S. federal government health plan for older and disabled individuals.

Mediterranean diet Dietary pattern of many Mediterranean nations, which includes fruits, vegetables, grains, fish, and olive oil. The Mediterranean diet is high in omega-3 fatty acids and fiber and is low in red meat.

MEDLINE Computerized health research data base maintained by the National Library of Medicine in Bethesda, Maryland, and partially supported by the U.S. federal government.

Meninges Connective tissues that cover and protect the spinal cord from excessive movement and damage. These tissues are arranged in three distinct layers: dura, arachnoid, and pia mater.

Meric analysis Chiropractic analytic system in which clinical manifestations or symptoms are considered in terms of the "zone" (body section innervated by a pair of spinal nerves) where it occurs. All tissue of one type within a zone is considered a *mere*.

Meric recoil (full spine specific) technique A specific, prone adjusting system that utilizes the toggle recoil dynamic thrust. Analysis is done through the use of full spine x-rays and the application of static and motion palpation.

Mercy Guidelines Guidelines for Chiropractic Quality Assurance and Practice Parameters, developed at the Mercy Center Consensus Conference.

Mesmer, Anton German physician (1734-1815) who lived in France and Switzerland and developed the theory of animal magnetism, which formed the basis for magnetic healing. *See also* Magnetic healing.

Mesoderm Intermediate layer of the embryo after the establishment of the three primordial germ cell layers (ectoderm,

mesoderm, and endoderm). It is in contact with the ectoderm and endoderm.

Meta-analysis Systematic review of the scientific literature on a specific topic that usually includes a ranking of the quality of each study plus statistical pooling of the data from all studies to determine the average effect of treatment. *See also* Systematic review.

Metaphysical healing Mind-body-spirit theories that influenced the early concepts of osteopathy and chiropractic, as well as some branches of modern alternative medicine.

Metastasis Transfer of cancer cells or other pathologic cells from one site in the body to another site.

Microbubbles Tiny bubbles of gas used as a vascular contrast agent during Doppler ultrasound to assess myocardial perfusion. The microbubbles of gas enhance ultrasound backscatter, so that flowing blood stands out from the surrounding soft tissues.

Microneurography Process in which fine-needle electrodes are placed into nerves, and the receptive fields of identified axons are characterized.

Migraine *See* Headache, migraine.

Migraineur Person who experiences migraine headaches.

Mineral Nonorganic substance from the earth's crust. Major minerals and trace minerals in the diet are required for normal physiologic function.

Miscoding Using a current procedural terminology (CPT) code incorrectly on an insurance claim, which becomes a legal concern when it is miscoded intentionally or negligently and results in overpayment.

Mixer chiropractor Term sometimes applied to chiropractors who depart from "hands only" or "straight" use of manual adjustments, including methods such as physiologic therapeutics and nutritional therapy. Also called *broad scope chiropractor. See also* Straight chiropractor.

Mobilization Movement applied singularly or repetitively within or at the physiologic range-of-joint motion without imparting a thrust or impulse and with the goal of restoring joint mobility.

Mobilization with movement Mobilization performed in symptom-free ranges of motion while the patient is moving either actively or passively or performing a resisted muscle contraction.

Morbidity Prevalence of a condition in a population.

Morphology 1. Structure or framework. 2. Study of form and structure.

Mortality Death rate within a defined population.

Motion Movement of a body part.

Motion palpation Manual palpation of bony structures and soft tissues that is performed with the patient in a variety of positions. In motion palpation of joints, the doctor applies pressure in the various directions of joint motion to ascertain areas of joint hypomobility or hypermobility.

Motion segment Functional unit made up of two adjacent articulating surfaces and the connecting tissues binding to them to each other. Also called *spinal motion segment.*

Motor 1. Producing motion. 2. Related to nerves that transmit electrical signals, causing muscle contraction (skeletal, cardiac, and smooth), epithelial secretion, or stimulation of lymphoid tissue.

Motor neurons, alpha *See* Alpha motor neuron.

Motor neurons, gamma *See* Gamma motor neuron.

Motor unit Spinal motion segment that is composed of two vertebrae and contiguous soft tissues. Also called *intervertebral motor unit.*

Mnemonic Memory aid.

Morphogenesis Formation and growth of organs and other body parts.

Muscle energy technique Soft tissue technique involving voluntary contraction of the patient's muscles in a precisely controlled direction, at varying levels of intensity, against a distinctly executed counterforce applied by the practitioner.

Muscle spindles Proprioceptive end organ that is located in skeletal muscle, which contains a subset of striated muscle fibers called

intrafusal fibers, innervated by gamma motor neurons, which maintain a set tension on the spindle. The sensory nerve endings of the spindle are called annulospiral or flower-spray endings and respond particularly to passive stretch of the muscle that they monitor.

Myelin Fatty material that covers certain nerve fibers.

Myelinated Covered with a myelin sheath.

Myofascial release Variety of soft tissue techniques for evaluating and treating the fascia.

Myopia Nearsightedness.

Myotome Muscle or group of muscles innervated by a spinal nerve.

Naproxen Nonsteroidal antiinflammatory medication.

National Board of Chiropractic Examiners (NBCE). Principal testing agency for the chiropractic profession. Established in 1963, the NBCE develops and administers standardized national examinations according to established guidelines.

National Center for Complementary and Alternative Medicine (NCCAM) One of 27 institutes and centers that make up the U.S. National Institutes of Health (NIH). NCCAM's mission is "to support rigorous research on complementary and alternative medicine (CAM), to train researchers in CAM, and to disseminate information to the public and professionals on which CAM modalities work, which do not, and why." NCCAM was founded in 1998, when the NIH Office of Alternative Medicine was upgraded to center status.

National Chiropractic Association (NCA) Chiropractic association founded in 1930 through the unification of the Universal Chiropractors Association and the third American Chiropractic Association. The current ACA is the successor organization to the NCA.

National Institute for Occupational Safety and Health (NIOSH) U.S. federal agency established by the Occupational Safety and Health Act of 1970. NIOSH is part of the Centers for Disease Control and Prevention (CDC) and is responsible for conducting research and making recommendations for the prevention of work-related illness and injuries.

National Institutes of Health (NIH) One of the world's foremost biomedical research centers, this branch of the U.S. Department of Health and Human Services has 27 separate institutes and centers at its campus in Bethesda, Maryland. The Consortial Center for Chiropractic Research was established and is funded by the NIH Center for Complementary and Alternative Medicine.

Natural healing 1. Ability of the body to heal itself. 2. Process through which health is restored through nonpharmaceutical, nonsurgical methods.

Natural history Usual progression of an illness in the absence of intervention.

Nature Cure Nineteenth century approach to natural healing that used a vegetarian diet along with light and air applied therapeutically.

Naturopathy Eclectic blend of natural healing modalities that include diet and nutrition, herbs, physical therapy, spinal manipulation, and acupuncture. Also known as *naturopathic medicine.*

Neck Disability Index Self-rating instrument for evaluating disability as a result of neck pain; designed as a modification of the *Oswestry Low Back Pain Disability Index.*

Nei Jing *The Yellow Emperor's Classic of Medicine,* a major Chinese medical text believed to have been compiled approximately 2000 years ago.

Neonate Newborn child.

Nephrolith Kidney stone.

Nephrologist A medical physician specializing in diseases of the kidney.

Neurogenic motor-evoked potentials A diagnostic method involving spinal cord stimulation, in which stimulating electrodes are placed percutaneously near vertebral bodies, and recording electrodes are placed near a peripheral nerve. This is proposed to elicit information on both the sensory and motor tracts of the spinal cord.

Nerve compression hypothesis Proposition that states that a nerve can become compressed through impingement from intersegmental spinal biomechanical derangements.

Nerve impulse Action potential.

Nerve interference 1. Compression of the spinal nerves in the environs of the intervertebral foramen. 2. Initiation of pain in the spinal joints that is capable of creating secondary aberrant reflex effects, such as increases in motor neuron or sympathetic neural activity.

Nerve sheath Structure consisting of an inner filamentous endoneurium, a thin but dense collagenous perineurium, and an areolar epineurium that protects the nerve and facilitates movement.

Nerve tracing Act of using digital pressure to follow a line of hyperpathia (tenderness or hyperesthesia) from a painful body part to the spine or vice versa. Nerve tracing is one of the earliest recorded methods of chiropractic analysis. Lines of hyperpathia may or may not correspond to named nerves.

Nervi nervorum Intrinsic innervation of nerves and their sheaths.

Neural Pertaining to nerves or to the nervous system.

Neural arch Posterior aspect of the vertebra, including the pedicles, transverse processes, laminae, and spinous process.

Neural crests While neural tube fusion is taking place in the embryo, a small number of cells at the apical region of the neural folds separate from the neural tube and come to lie just lateral to it. The cells migrate to various positions in the body and give rise to a wide variety of tissues.

Neuraxis Brain and spinal cord.

Neuritis Nerve inflammation.

Neurocalometer (NCM) Heat-sensing instrument consisting of two thermocouple probes and a galvanometer, which indicates left-to-right thermal asymmetry as the examiner glides the instrument up or down the spine.

Neurodesis Fibrosis around a nerve. *See* Traction neurodesis.

Neurodystrophic hypothesis Proposition that neural dysfunction is stressful to viscera and other body structures, which may modify immune responses and alter the trophic function of involved nerves.

Neurogenic inflammation Sterile inflammation that develops as a result of efferent nociceptor function.

Neuroma Tumorlike mass of regenerating axons that can result from nerve injury.

Neuron Impulse-conducting cell in the brain, spinal column, or nerves, consisting of a cell body with one or more dendrites and a single axon. Neurons are specialized to generate and transmit electrical impulses, carrying information from one part of the nervous system to another. Also spelled *neurone.* Also called *nerve cell.*

Neuropathic Relating to a nerve pathologic condition or a functional disturbance of a nerve or of some of the axons within a nerve.

Neurotransmitter Chemical substance that carries impulses from one nerve cell to another. It is found in the space (synapse) that separates the transmitting neuron's terminal (axon) from the receiving neuron's terminal (dendrite). Such chemicals elicit a change in the postsynaptic cell membrane potential and are either excitatory (depolarizing) or inhibitory (hyperpolarizing).

Neurotransmitter spillover Diffusion of specific neurotransmitters into adjacent tissue space, thereby exciting or inhibiting adjacent neurons.

Neurovascular bundle Spinal nerve and its associated artery, vein, and lymphatic vessels.

Newton (N) A unit of force that when applied in a vacuum to a body with a mass of 1 kilogram causes it to accelerate at a rate of one meter per second squared.

Newton's First Law of Motion Body remains at rest or in uniform motion until it is acted on by an external force. *See also* Inertia.

Newton's Second Law of Motion Force equals mass times acceleration.

Newton's Third Law of Motion For every action, there is an equal and opposite reaction.

Nimmo Receptor Tonus technique A method of chiropractic analysis and treatment developed by Raymond Nimmo that utilizes nonthrusting manual pressure to effect muscular trigger point release, thereby restoring muscular balance. Receptor Tonus technique is based on the hypothesis that irritated peripheral receptors overload and thereby cause disruption of the central nervous system.

Ninth Amendment Part of the U.S. Bill of Rights, the Ninth Amendment states: "The enumeration in the Constitution of certain rights shall not be construed to deny or disparage others retained by the people." This language has been interpreted to provide certain privacy rights, such as the right to an abortion, but it has not been interpreted to provide a constitutional right to the health care of one's choice.

Nociception Activity in a neural structure considered capable of leading or contributing to the sensation of pain.

Nociceptive Quality displayed by an active nociceptor. This term is often misused to modify the word "stimulus." A stimulus cannot be nociceptive, but it can be noxious.

Nociceptor Receptor preferentially sensitive to a noxious stimulus or to a stimulus that would become noxious if prolonged.

Nociceptor, group III Neural element innervating noncutaneous somatic tissues whose axons are small in diameter and lightly myelinated (A-fibers).

Nociceptor, group IV Neural element innervating noncutaneous somatic tissues whose axons are small in diameter and unmyelinated (C-fibers).

Nonimpulse-based neural mechanisms Mechanisms of neural transmission that are not based on the transmission of electrical impulses but instead rely on transport of macromolecular materials synthesized in the nerve cell body through the axon to the terminal endings for exchange at the synaptic terminals. These molecular materials exert a trophic influence on the target or postsynaptic cells. Contrasted to the conduction velocity of the nerve impulse (up to 100m/sec), the non impulse-based intra-axonal transport of macromolecular materials proceeds at a rate up to approximately 400mm/day. *See also* Impulse-based neural mechanisms and Axoplasmic transport.

Nonphysical causation Mental, emotional, social, or spiritual influences in the origin of illness.

Nonphysicians 1. Health professionals who have not received a doctoral degree. 2. The JCAHO classification for health care providers with a limited scope of practice (e.g., podiatrists, dentists, chiropractors), who are granted a limited degree of hospital clinical privileges. Nonphysicians are required to co-admit a patient with a medical or osteopathic physician who has full and active staff membership and admission privileges.

Nonspecific back pain Back pain not caused by nerve compression or "red flag" conditions, such as tumors or infections of bone. Based on this definition, 85% to 90% of back pain is nonspecific.

Nonsteroidal antiinflammatory drugs (NSAIDs) Broad class of drugs that reduce inflammation and decrease pain by reducing tissue concentrations of prostaglandins, which are hormones that produce inflammation and pain. NSAIDs are used for treatment of joint pain, inflammation, and stiffness. This class includes specific generic drugs such as ibuprofen, indomethacin, ketoprofen, naproxen, and sulindac.

Noxious stimulus Stimulus that damages normal tissue. Although most noxious stimuli are painful, some are not, including radiation injury and cutting the wall of the small intestine.

Nuchal ligament *See* Ligamentum nuchae.

Nuclear medicine Radiologic methods utilizing radioactive materials that are usually injected or sometimes inhaled into the body to demonstrate organ-specific pathology. This includes bone scanning to demonstrate bone tumors, osteomyelitis and other multicentric diseases, and positron emission tomography (PET) scanning that is useful for localizing brain and lung tumors.

Nucleus pulposus Gelatinous inner portion of the intervertebral disk.

Objective That which can be detected with the doctor's own senses or with diagnostic instruments. *See also* Subjective.

Observational study Study where the researcher observes events as they occur naturally or in the course of normal practice, without attempting to influence them.

Occupational Safety and Health Administration (OSHA) Established by the U.S. Congress in 1970, OSHA develops, implements, and enforces rules for workplace safety.

Oculomotion Movement of the eyes, controlled by the extraocular muscles.

Office of Alternative Medicine (OAM) Established as part of the National Institutes of Health by a 1992 congressional mandate, to "facilitate the evaluation of alternative medical treatment modalities" for the purposes of determining their effectiveness and to help integrate such treatments into mainstream medical practice. In 1998 the OAM was upgraded to center status within NIH as the National Center for Complementary and Alternative Medicine (NCCAM).

Oligodendrocytes Specialized supportive cells that are responsible for myelination in the central nervous system.

One cause–one cure Belief that all diseases have one cause (subluxation) and one cure (adjustment).

Ongoing activity Neural discharge in the absence of evident stimulus.

Open-ended inquiry Interview method that encourages patients to tell the story in their own words.

Operant conditioning Behavioral therapy that involves repeated exposures to activities inaccurately perceived to be harmful.

Ophthalmologist Medical physician specializing in the diseases of the eye.

Operational definition Description of the methods, tools, and procedures required to make an observation (i.e., a definition that is specific and allows objective measurement).

Opiates, endogenous *See* Endogenous opiates.

Origin More proximal or stable attachment of a muscle.

Orthogonal Relating to or composed of right angles in reference to the X, Y, and Z axes.

Orthopedic surgeon Medical physician specializing in the diagnosis and treatment (including surgery) of the musculoskeletal system. Also known as *Orthopedist.*

Orthopedic tests Simple motions that are designed to isolate particular tissues to determine whether those tissues are responsible for particular symptoms. In the case of pain, the test is considered positive if it reproduces the pain.

Osteoarthritis Chronic disease that involves the joints; characterized by joint pain, destruction of articular cartilage, and impaired function. Also called *degenerative joint disease.*

Osteogenesis imperfecta An inherited condition marked by brittle bones that fracture easily.

Osteomyelitis Inflammation of bone caused by infection.

Osteopath or osteopathic physician (DO) Full-scope physician with training in osteopathic manipulation who is a graduate of a school of osteopathic medicine.

Osteopath, broad See Broad osteopath.

Osteopath, lesion See Lesion osteopath.

Osteopathic lesion Disturbance of musculoskeletal structure or function that may include accompanying disturbances of other biologic mechanisms. This term has been replaced by *Somatic dysfunction. See also* Lesion osteopath.

Osteopathic medicine System of medicine that uses standard methods of medical diagnosis and treatment, which may include osteopathic joint manipulation to maintain structural balance and enhance overall health. Osteopathic medicine is based on the theory that the structure and function of the body are intimately related and that the body has substantial powers of healing when provided with proper nutrition and a supportive environment. Also called *osteopathy.*

Osteopathy, classical Practice of osteopathic medicine in which manual manipulation is accorded a central therapeutic role.

Osteophyte A bony outgrowth, or finger-like projection from the edge of a bone.

Osteophytosis Condition marked by the formation of osteophytes, or bony outgrowths. Osteophytosis is one of the hallmarks of moderate-to-advanced degenerative joint disease.

Osteoporosis Abnormal thinning of bone with reduced levels of mineralization; observed most frequently in older adults.

Oswestry Low Back Pain Disability Index Self-rating instrument for evaluating disability related to activities of daily living in patients with low back pain.

Otitis media Inflammation of the middle ear. The serous type is generally chronic, whereas the purulent type is generally acute.

Outcome measures Parameters that indicate a change in health status, used in studies of treatment effectiveness. These must be specifically defined at the beginning of a study.

Over-the-counter (OTC) medications Pharmaceutical medications available without a physician's prescription.

Overuse injuries Microtrauma that is the result of repetitive low-magnitude forces, causing microscopic disruption of the structure of the involved tissues.

Pain Unpleasant sensory and emotional experience associated with actual or potential tissue damage or described in terms of such damage.

Palmer, Bartlett Joshua (BJ) Named the "developer of chiropractic" and the son of founder D.D. Palmer, B.J. Palmer was a leading figure in chiropractic during the first half of the twentieth century.

Palmer, Daniel David (DD) Founder of the chiropractic profession who delivered the first chiropractic adjustment in Davenport, Iowa, in 1895 and founded the first chiropractic school in 1897.

Palpation Manual examination of a body part.

Palpation, dynamic *See* Motion palpation.

Palpation, layer *See* Layer palpation.

Palpation, motion *See* Motion palpation.

Palpation, pincer *See* Pincer palpation.

Palpation, static *See* Static palpation.

Papanicolaou's (Pap) smear A cytological staining procedure for the diagnosis of conditions of the female genital tract, including malignancies and premalignancies. Also called *Papinocolaou's stain test.*

Paradigm Explanatory model that helps clarify a complex process.

Paradigm shift Fundamental change in an explanatory model.

Parasympathetic Pertains to the craniosacral division of the autonomic nervous system.

Paravertebral sympathetic chain Group of sympathetic ganglia, connected in series, and extending from the upper cervical spine to the coccyx.

Parenchyma Tissue or structure of an organ.

Paresthesia An abnormal sensation, such as burning or prickling, that may occur with or without an external stimulus.

Participating provider Provider who has entered into a contract with an insurer.

PARTS An acronym used to describe five key diagnostic criteria (Pain/tenderness; Asymmetry; Range-of-motion abnormality; Tissue tone, texture, and temperature abnormality; and Special tests) for the identification of joint subluxation/dysfunction.

Passive analysis First step in ergonomic evaluation of workplace data, largely involving review and analysis of workplace documents. *See also* Active analysis.

Passive coping Personal self-care options that are dependent on following instructions rather than taking the initiative.

Passive modalities Treatment methods that rely completely or in large part on intervention by the doctor rather than active participation by the patient.

Passive range of motion Joint movements beyond the active range of motion that are carried through by the clinician without the conscious assistance or resistance of the patient.

Patellofemoral arthralgia Irritation of the patellofemoral joint, which is often the result of tight hamstrings, hyperpronation, or improper choice of running shoes. Also known as *runner's knee.*

Pathologic barrier *See* Anatomic barrier.

Pathophysiology Abnormal physiology; the stage before pathology or disease.

Patient-centered approach Mutually respectful doctor-patient relationship in which the doctor's emotional, social, or financial needs are not permitted to override the best interests of the patient.

Patient empowerment Active participation by patients in their own healing processes.

Pearson's r Pearson's r, or Pearson's product-moment correlation co-efficient, describes the strength and direction of the relationship between two variables. It calculates the degree of association between two sets of data, not the extent of agreement. Correlation co-efficients range from -1.0, indicating a perfect negative correlation, to 1.0, representing a perfect positive correlation. Pearson's r is not recommended as a reliability measure.

Pedicle Portion of the vertebra that attaches to the vertebral body posterolaterally and helps form the boundaries of the intervertebral foramina.

Peer review 1. Evaluation by members of one's own profession. 2. In insurance and reimbursement, a system of review used by hospitals, managed care, and insurance companies during which health care records are reviewed to determine whether services provided are medically necessary, meet the standards of care, and fulfill other cost containment criteria established by the payer of care. 3. In research, the evaluation of the scientific and technical merit of proposed research or research submitted for publication in a peer-reviewed journal. 4. In licensing and regulation, the process of evaluation and review in which members of one's own profession determine whether appropriate care has been rendered.

Pelvic girdle Articulation of the two coxal (pelvic) bones—the sacrum and coccyx.

Pennate Arrangement of muscle fibers at an angle to the direction of pull.

Percentage agreement Method of statistical analysis calculated by taking the number of agreements between two examiners, divided by the total number of responses (agreements 4 ÷ agreements + disagreements).

Percussion Inducing vibration into a part of the body.

Periaqueductal gray Column of gray matter in the brainstem whose neurons secrete endogenous opiates, which inhibit painful signals within the central nervous system.

Periarticular Surrounding a joint.

Perineurium Connective tissue that surrounds small bundles of nerve fibers.

Peripheral nervous system Portion of the nervous system that includes the spinal nerve roots, spinal nerves, and peripheral nerves.

Phasic Intermittent, occuring in alternating phases.

Phasic contraction Brief, forceful muscle activity. *See also* Tonic contraction.

Phasic receptor Rapidly adapting sensory receptor, which typically responds to alternating stimuli; rate or movement receptors (e.g., Pacinian corpuscles, Golgi tendon organs).

Phlebotomy Venipuncture for the purpose of drawing blood.

Phoria Weakness of the extraocular muscles.

Phonophobia Fear of or aversion to loud sounds.

Photophobia Fear of or aversion to bright light.

Physiatrist Medical physician specializing in physical medicine and rehabilitation.

Physical rehabilitation *See* Rehabilitation.

Physical therapy (PT) 1. For chiropractic context. *See also* Physiological therapeutics. 2. Health care profession specializing in the evaluation and rehabilitation of patients physically disabled by injury or illness. Sometimes called *physiotherapy.*

Physiologic barrier End point of a joint's active range of motion.

Physiologic hypermobility Joint flexibility as a result of the relative laxity of ligaments normally present in the pediatric spine.

Physiological therapeutics (PT) Therapies used by some chiropractors to complement manual adjustment/manipulation. Examples of commonly employed PT methods are massage, hot and cold applications, ultrasound, electronic muscle stimulation, and massage. Sometimes called *physiotherapy* or *physical therapy.*

Physiotherapy *See* Physiological therapeutics, physical therapy.

Pial arterial plexus Set of small arteries that course on the surface of the spinal cord, sending penetrating branches into the deeper layers.

Pia mater Innermost layer of the meninges, the pia mater is a connective tissue layer that adheres directly to the surface of the neural tissue, including the individual cranial and spinal nerve rootlets.

Piezoelectricity Electrical current generated by mechanical stress.

Pincer palpation Manual evaluation that is performed by grasping the muscle belly between the thumb and fingers while gently squeezing the tissues with a back and forth motion to locate taut bands.

Placebo Intervention designed to mimic a genuine treatment, performed on a control group in a clinical trial. Its purpose is to control for the nonspecific therapeutic effects of care, enabling the specific effects of an actual treatment to be measured.

Plasma extravasation Passive and active transmission of plasma elements through a blood vessel wall into the surrounding tissues.

Plasticity 1. In biomechanics, the property of a material that instantly deforms when a load is applied and does not return to its original shape when the load is removed. 2. In neurology, the ability of synapses to change as circumstances require, and the ability of the cell body to change its genetic expression to modulate its overall excitability and potential to excite other cells.

Pleural effusion Presence of fluid in the pleural space.

Pleximeter Finger that is struck in the act of percussion.

Plexor Striking finger in the act of percussion.

Pneumothorax Presence of air or gas in the pleural space.

Pocket mask Protective barrier with a one-way valve that allows a health practitioner to apply respiratory resuscitation without risk of disease exposure.

Point-of-service plan (POS) Arrangement under which health maintenance organization (HMO) subscribers have the option to directly access out-of-network providers at an increased cost.

Point-pressure techniques Soft tissue procedures that involve the application of digital pressure to specific target tissue areas. The applied pressure may be of a steady, sustained nature, or it may be increased progressively.

Polyunsaturated fats Fats with multiple double bonds (e.g., arachidonic acid).

Popular health movement Grassroots movement that emerged in the mid-nineteenth century, embracing many unconventional forms of healing and which emphasized a partnership role between practitioners and patients.

Population Group meeting a specific set of criteria.

Portal of entry provider Health care professionals whose licenses permit them to accept patients without referral from another practitioner. Such providers are expected to recognize clinical situations requiring referral. Chiropractors are portal of entry providers.

Positron emission tomography (PET) A form of nuclear medicine which uses radioactive substances such as 18F-fluorodeoxyglucose (FDG), a glucose analog that is radioactive and emits positrons (beta particles). Anywhere there is increased glucose metabolism within the body, such as tumor cells, there will be an increased concentration of the FDG, allowing differentiation of most malignant from benign tumors. PET scans are also used to measure the degree of plaque in arterial walls.

Posterior longitudinal ligament (PLL) Ligament extending from the occiput to the sacrum, attaching to the posterior surfaces of the vertebral bodies and intervertebral disks. The PLL limits posterior protrusion of the intervertebral disk and spinal hyperflexion.

Postfacilitation stretch Proprioceptive neuro-muscular technique that is primarily used to stretch chronically shortened muscles.

Postganglionic neuron Unmyelinated, C-fiber neuron whose cell body is located in an autonomic ganglion. Also called *postsynaptic neuron*.

Posturalist Chiropractor who asserts that subluxation consists of patterns of postural distortion rather than segmental joint dysfunctions and uses listings that describe the linear and angular relationship of entire regions of the axial skeleton. Also called *structuralist*.

Postisometric relaxation Manual soft tissue technique in which the doctor lengthens the muscle and after which the muscle is isometrically contracted and then relaxed by the patient.

Postsynaptic neuron *See* Postganglionic neuron.

Precertification Advance approval by a health insurance plan that allows the provider to proceed with delivery of covered services. The precertification process may require some or all of the following: (1) written referral from a gatekeeper physician, (2) report of findings with diagnosis, (3) and goal-oriented treatment plan including the number of expected visits and anticipated date for completion of care.

Preexisting condition exclusion Health condition not covered under an insurance policy because it existed before the date when the policyholder first subscribed to the plan. Under current law in the United States, preexisting conditions may only be excluded from reimbursement for patients who were uninsured immediately before enrolling in their current insurance plan. Preexisting condition exclusions generally have a time limit (commonly 12 months), after which the exclusion is removed.

Preferred provider Health practitioner who has entered into a contract with a Preferred Provider Organization (PPO).

Preferred provider organization (PPO) Insurance plan that offers subscribers incentives (e.g., lower deductibles and co-payments) to use in-network providers. PPO subscribers are also reimbursed for visits to nonnetwork providers, but at a lower rate. Preferred providers agree to charge no more than the plan's approved fees.

Preganglionic neuron First neuron involved in communicating a signal within the autonomic nervous system. The cell bodies of these neurons are located in the intermediate gray matter of the spinal cord in all segments between the first thoracic and the second or third lumbar. Also called *presynaptic neuron.*

Premium Amount paid by the subscriber (usually on a monthly or quarterly basis) to qualify for covered services under a health insurance policy.

Premonitory Providing a warning of the impending onset of more severe symptoms.

Presynaptic neuron *See* Preganglionic neuron.

Pretest-Posttest design Study design in which baseline (pretreatment) and outcome (posttreatment) measurements are performed.

Prevalence Proportion of a population that has a particular condition or outcome at a given time.

Prevention Process of anticipating an adverse outcome and taking steps to stop it from happening.

Prevention, active Preventive measures that rely primarily on the active commitment and participation of the individual, such as dietary changes, exercise, and stress management practices.

Prevention, primary Efforts to prevent a disorder before it has begun.

Prevention, secondary Efforts to prevent a subacute disorder from becoming chronic.

Primary care *There is no universally accepted definition of primary care.* The Institute of Medicine defines primary care as "the provision of integrated, accessible health care services by clinicians who are accountable for addressing a large majority of personal health care needs, developing a sustained partnership with patients and practicing in the context of family and community." The American Chiropractic Association defines the role of chiropractic in primary care as "characterized by direct access, longitudinal, integrated, conservative ambulatory care of patients' health care needs . . . a first contact gatekeeper for neuromusculoskeletal conditions."

Primary care physician (PCP) Physician whose role is characterized by initial contact care and a broad range of conditions treated and whose practice includes overall health assessment, treatment of illness, management of illness, prevention of illness, and education.

Primary contact practitioner *See* Portal of entry provider.

Primary prevention *See* Prevention, primary.

Primum non nocere "First, do no harm."

Prognosis Predicted course of an illness.

Prophylaxis Prevention.

Proprioception Sensory nerve information pertaining to movement, position, or tension of muscle, tendon, ligament, bone, or joint tissues. Proprioception is essential to self-regulation of posture and muscular movement.

Proprioceptive training Exercise that is used to build the coordination of proprioceptors and muscles to promote proper biomechanic function.

Proprioceptors Sensory receptors in muscles, tendons, and joint capsules that provide information on body position and movement. Examples are the *Golgi tendon organs* and *muscle spindles.*

Prospective study Study that generates new data based on events that occur after the study begins. *See also* Retrospective.

Prostaglandin Hormonelike substance derived from amino acids that mediates physiologic functions including nerve transmission, smooth muscle activity, and metabolism.

Proteolytic enzymes Enzymes that split proteins by hydrolysis of peptide bonds. Clinically, proteolytic enzyme supplements have an antiinflammatory effect.

Provider Health care professional.

Prudent diet A balanced diet characterized by high intake of vegetables, fruits, legumes, whole grains, fish, and poultry. This contrasts with the common Western dietary pattern, which is characterized by high intakes of red meat, processed meat, refined grains, sweets and desserts, fried foods, and high-fat dairy products.

Pseudosubluxation Spinal joint misalignment or dysfunction in a child that is due to the relative laxity of ligaments normally present in the pediatric spine. *See also* Physiologic hypermobility.

Psychiatrist Medical physician specializing in mental illness and dysfunction.

Psychogenic Arising from the mind rather than the body.

Psychometric Pertaining to the properties of an instrument related to its ability to measure accurately and reliably.

Psychosocial Incorporating emotional, interpersonal, and community-related factors.

P-values Statistical statement, generally representing the probability of a *false-positive* conclusion, or *Type I error*. P-values are used to account for the possibility of random error and to measure the statistical significance of a finding.

Pulmonary consolidation A process in which the lung becomes firm as air spaces are filled with exudates.

Quota In rehabilitation, a preestablished program of exercises.

Radiating pain Pain that is perceived to radiate away from the pathologic site or from the presumed pathologic site. Radiating pain can follow the pathologic condition of any component of the nervous system.

Radiculopathy Radiating pain caused by a pathologic damage of one or more dorsal roots.

Radiograph X-ray photograph.

Radiography Process of producing x-ray photographs.

Radiology The branch of the health sciences dealing with radioactive substances and radiant energy in the diagnosis and treatment of disease.

Radiolucent Easily penetrated by x-rays. Radiolucent structures appear dark on radiographs.

Rami communicantes Collections of presynaptic and postsynaptic sympathetic neurons, as well as visceral afferent axons, which form communicating branches between the spinal nerves and sympathetic chain.

Ramus Branch of a nerve or blood vessel.

RAND A nonprofit research and development company which first gained prominence with research for the U.S. military during World War II. In addition to defense, RAND's research fields include the health sciences, education, applied economics, sociology, and civil justice.

Random error Influence of chance variation.

Randomized controlled trial (RCT) Prospective, longitudinal study in which patients are divided into two groups, experimental and control, on a randomized basis. The experimental group receives the procedure being evaluated, whereas the control group does not. *See also* Clinical trial.

Rare earth screen Radiographic method in which intensifying screens utilize rare earth screen phosphors, which are doubly efficient at converting x-ray photon energy into light energy as compared to non-rare earth compounds like calcium tungstate. A significant reduction in patient exposure dose is realized through this innovation in x-ray image production.

Rarefaction Loss of tissue substance in which the structure becomes less dense.

Radiopaque Not easily penetrated by x-ray beams. Radiopaque structures appear white on radiographs.

Receptive field Area from which a receptor can be activated by a given stimulus.

Recoil thrust High-velocity, low-amplitude, ballistic thrust immediately followed by a passive recoil of the doctor's arms.

Recommended daily allowance (RDA) Level of a nutrient necessary to meet the needs of nearly all healthy persons.

Reconceptualizing Taking a different perspective.

Reconditioning Restoration of the ability to perform tasks involved in a person's usual activities of daily living.

Red flag Finding in a patient's history or physical examination that should raise the suggestion that a serious underlying condition is present. Red flags indicate the need for additional diagnostic tests or patient referral or both. Red flags contraindicating spinal adjustment/manipulation include tumors, infections, and fractures of bone.

Referral Recommendation by a health practitioner that a patient consult another practitioner. Referral from a gatekeeper physician is required to access specialist services (including chiropractic services) under many managed care plans, particularly health maintenance organizations (HMOs).

Referred pain Perception of pain in locations other than the site of generation and not localized to the distribution of a damaged nerve. Referred pain is rarely sharp, although it can be both intense and very unpleasant.

Refined sugars Products resulting from the refining of carbohydrates (e.g., sucrose).

Reflex Unconscious neuronal loop in which a stimulus and response occur as the result of a direct sensorimotor hookup.

Reflex arc Pattern of nerve transmission consisting of a stimulus-activated receptor, transmission over an afferent pathway to an integration center, transmission over an efferent pathway to the effector, and induction of a reflex response.

Rehabilitation Treatment intended to achieve restoration of optimal strength, stability, and integrity through a planned functional program. Rehabilitation can include aerobics, flexibility, and strength training.

Rehabilitation, vocational *See* Vocational rehabilitation.

Reimbursement Payment by an insurer under the terms of a health insurance policy.

Relaxation response A state in which the stress arousal threshold is raised, characterized by decreases in heart rate, blood pressure, respiratory rate, and muscle tension. Meditation has been shown to induce the relaxation response.

Relaxation training Physical approaches such as exercises to release muscular tension.

Reliability Consistency of a measurement when repeated.

Remak bundle Bundle of unmyelinated axons after they have invaginated a Schwann cell. *See* Schwann cell.

Repetitive stress disorders Conditions characterized by soft tissue damage that results from performing repetitive physical movements or holding a sustained posture over a long period of time. Among these disorders are carpal tunnel syndrome, De Quervain's Tenosynovitis, and lateral epicondylitis.

Report of findings Verbal or written report in which doctors describe to patients their diagnostic findings and recommendations for care.

Reticular formation Column of neural tissue, embedded in the central core of the central nervous system, which extends from the spinal cord to the rostral end of the diencephalon (hypothalamus). Several diffuse neural pathways are contained within it, which play roles in controlling autonomic nervous system and endocrine activity, behavior (e.g., responses to stress), as well as musculoskeletal reflex activity in controlling posture.

Retrospective study Study that reviews events that have already occurred. *See also* Prospective.

Rhoncus Deep rattling in the proximal airway as a result of obstruction or constriction.

Risk Likelihood of an adverse event or outcome. Risk is determined by measuring the relationship between the presence of possible risk factors and the subsequent incidence of particular conditions.

Roentgen, Wilhelm Discoverer of x-rays and recipient of the first Nobel Prize in physics.

Rotator cuff Muscles of the shoulder that include the subscapularis, infraspinatus, supraspinatus, and teres minor.

Rubor Localized redness; a cardinal sign of inflammation.

Runner's knee *See* Patellofemoral arthralgia.

Sacrospinous ligament Ligament extending from the sacrum to the spine of the ischium, just anterior to the sacrotuberous ligament.

Sacro-occipital technique A system of chiropractic analysis and adjustment developed by Major Bertrand DeJarnette that utilizes padded pelvic blocks and boards for adjustment of the pelvis and lower back and includes emphasis on analysis and adjustment of cranial bones.

Sacrotuberous ligament Ligament extending from the inferolateral aspect of the sacrum to the ischial tuberosity.

Sagittal plane Plane of the body running from front to back, parallel to the median plane.

Sample Subset of a population.

Schwann cell A large nucleated cell whose membrane spirally enwraps the axons of myelinated peripheral neurons, thus forming myelin. Some cells do not wrap, but rather evaginate to surround "unmyelinated" axons, forming Remak bundles. *See* Remak bundle.

Sclerotome Derivative of the embryonic somite, it ultimately forms the vertebrae and annuli fibrosi of the intervertebral disks.

Scoliosis Appreciable lateral deviation in the normally straight vertical line of the spine.

Scoliosis, adolescent idiopathic *See* Adolescent idiopathic scoliosis.

Scope of practice Range of diagnostic and treatment procedures that a given licensed professional is allowed to use. This scope is provided by the definition of the healing art in state statutes.

Secondary prevention *See* Prevention, secondary.

Segmentalist Chiropractor who asserts that subluxations occur at specific motor units consisting of two bones, rather than entire spinal regions.

Segmental contact point Anatomic structures, commonly referred as bony landmarks, located on the patient.

Segmental spinal stabilization exercises Training maneuvers designed to enhance coordination and endurance of the local, deep muscles responsible for segmental control of the spine.

Selection bias Bias that occurs when the group that has been selected for study differs in significant ways from the true population.

Self-care Methods used to restore or maintain one's own health.

Self-care contract Written agreement in which an individual commits to pursuing a personal wellness program.

Self-referral Arrangement in which the referring doctor has an ownership interest in an ancillary facility to which he or she makes referrals. Self-referral is illegal under the U.S. Medicare law.

Sensitivity Proportion of times that a diagnostic procedure yields a correct result in patients without a specific diagnosis. *See also* Specificity.

Sensitization 1. Process of becoming overly reactive to a stimulus after overexposure to the stimulus. 2. Phenomenon induced by stimulation of nociceptors and characterized by increased sensitivity to mechanical and chemical stimuli and by the development of ongoing activity.

Sensory 1. Related to the senses or sensation. 2. Afferent transmission of nerve impulses from the periphery to the central nervous system.

Sensory field Distribution of the sensory component of a neuron via peripheral collateralization (i.e., receptor distribution) or the distribution of cellular dendrites.

Septic arthritis Infectious arthritis, with inflammation of synovial membranes and purulent effusion into a joint.

Sequestration, disk *See* Disk sequestration.

Serotonin An endogenous chemical with found in the brain, blood serum, and gastric mucosa. Its functions as a neurotransmitter inhibits gastric secretion and stimulates smooth muscle.

Seven-day food diary Contemporaneously compiled list that records all foods and beverages consumed in a week.

Sham adjustment Manual intervention used for research purposes that must be convincing enough for research subjects to believe it is "real" adjustment/manipulation while having none of the specific physiologic or therapeutic effects of real adjustment/manipulation. Also called *placebo adjustment* or *placebo manipulation*.

Sham manipulation *See* Sham adjustment.

Shear (shearing) Forces that result when one body undergoes translation with respect to another body adjacent to it. *See also* Translation.

Sherrington's Law of Reciprocal Innervation Contraction of muscles is accompanied by the simultaneous inhibition of their antagonists. Also known as *reciprocal inhibition*.

Short-lever adjustment/manipulation Manual procedure in which the doctor applies a manual contact directly on or over some part of the soft tissue and osseous structures directly associated with the adjustive/manipulative lesion. Stabilization of the patient can be achieved with contacts in the immediate vicinity or at some distance away from the lesion. Once contact and stabilization are established, the clinician tensions the joint to the end of its normal physiologic range ("locks" the joint) and delivers a controlled thrust, taking the joint into its paraphysiologic range.

Shoulder impingement syndrome Condition in which the greater tuberosity of the humerus impinges on the supraspinatus tendon and subacromial bursa, resulting in pain and tendon degeneration. Also known as *swimmer's shoulder*.

Shoulder instability Pathologic condition in which the humeral head tends to slip out of the glenoid socket. Dislocation is the most severe presentation of shoulder instability.

Single-blind study Study in which the patients are blinded as to whether they are in the experimental group or control group, but researchers and outcome assessors are not blinded.

Sinuvertebral nerves Recurrent branches of the primary dorsal rami of the spinal nerves that supply the innervation to the vertebrae, joints, dura, and intervertebral disks.

Skin temperature differentials Differences of cutaneous temperature measured at like points on the left and right sides of the body.

Soft tissue Tissues including muscles, tendons, bursae, ligaments, and fascia, but not bone.

Soma 1. Cell body in which the cell nucleus resides along with other cellular organelles. 2. Body, in contrast to the mind.

Somatic dysfunction Impaired or altered function of the skeletal, arthrodial, myofascial, vascular, lymphatic, or neuronal components of one or more motion segments. This term was introduced in 1970 to replace "osteopathic lesion."

Somatic dyspnea Air hunger or shortness of breath that can be alleviated or eliminated by the correction of vertebral subluxation complex or other somatic dysfunction.

Somatoautonomic reflex *See* Somatovisceral reflex hypothesis.

Somatosensory-evoked potentials (SSEP) Waves recorded from the spinal cord or cerebral hemisphere after electrical stimulation or physiologic activation of peripheral sensory fibers. SSEP is used to determine the presence and nature of lesions of the peripheral or sensory conduction pathways.

Somatosomatic reflex 1. Reflex in which a stimulus to nerves or receptors related to somatic structures produces reflexive responses in other somatic structures.

Somatovisceral reflex Reflex in which a stimulus to nerves or receptors related to somatic structures produces reflexive responses in visceral organs, such as those of the digestive, cardiovascular, or respiratory systems.

Somatosympathetic reflex *See* Somatovisceral reflex.

Somites Segmented series of tissue blocks that extend from the occipital region of the head to the tail of the embryo and differentiate into a sclerotome and a dermomyotome, which in turn splits into a superficial dermatome and a deeper myotome.

Sonography Method of producing images of internal structures by exposing the area of interest to ultrasonic impulses and reconstructing the resulting echoes into an image.

Specificity Proportion of times a diagnostic procedure is correct in patients without a specific diagnosis. *See also* Sensitivity.

Spillover, neurotransmitter *See* Neurotransmitter spillover.

Spinal motion segment Two adjacent vertebrae and the connecting tissues binding them to each other. Also called *intervertebral motor unit.*

Spinograph Radiographic film that depicts the spine.

Spinography Technique for evaluating spinal biomechanics, which uses geometric analysis of radiographs.

Spinous process Portion of a vertebra that extends posteriorly from the midline junction of the laminae.

Spiritualism Belief that consciousness survives beyond death and that it is possible to contact the spirits of those who have died.

Spirituality Beliefs related to a nonmaterial dimension, religion, or soul.

Splinting Local response to tissue injury. Typically associated with the extremities, splinting occurs as a result of local edema, combined with hypertonicity of surrounding musculature. Splinting reduces joint mobility, in effect creating a natural splint.

Spondylolisthesis Forward displacement of a vertebra in relation to the vertebra immediately below it, usually due to a developmental defect of the pars interarticularis.

Spondylolysis Dissolution or breakdown of a vertebra, with separation of the pars interarticularis.

Spondylosis Degeneration of the spinal column.

Spontaneous remission Unexpected, complete recovery from a serious illness without an objectively verifiable reason for the recovery. This term is most commonly applied to cases of recovery from cancer.

Sports medicine team Interdisciplinary group of health professionals serving the health needs of an athletic team.

Sprain Joint injury that involves partial tearing of supporting ligaments.

Spray-and-stretch A method developed by medical physician Janet Travell, in which muscles with trigger points are sprayed with a vapocoolant substance before being stretched.

Springy end feel Quality of elasticity that may be present at the end of a joint's passive range of motion.

Staff model health maintenance organization (HMO) HMO that employs physicians and other providers to staff its facilities. *See also* Health maintenance organization.

Standard of care Consensus within a professional community regarding the appropriate methods of diagnosis and treatment that can be reasonably applied to the management of a patient's presenting difficulties. Standards of care set the legal obligation to which providers are held in malpractice actions.

Static palpation Manual palpation of bony structures and soft tissues, usually performed with the patient in a stationary position.

Statistical significance Statement, based on inferential statistics, that a good probability exists that a conclusion is not wrong as a result of random error. The magnitude of a therapeutic effect and the size of the sample are two key factors that influence statistical significance.

Stenosis Abnormal narrowing, as in *spinal stenosis* or *aortic stenosis*. Spinal stenosis (of the vertebral canal, nerve root canal, or intervertebral foramina) may be either congenital or due to degeneration.

Still, Andrew Taylor Founder of osteopathy.

Stimulus-induced analgesia Adaptive behavior used to distract the nervous system from the perception of pain. Examples include rubbing an elbow that has just been bumped, scratching an itch, or "shaking off" a traumatized joint. *See also* Gate control theory and Afferent inhibition.

Straight chiropractor Chiropractors whose case management includes spinal adjustments without the use of adjunctive therapies to correct subluxations.

Strain 1. Injury to a muscle as a result of excessive stretch. 2. In biomechanics, deformation of a body that is due to stress. *See also* Stress.

Stress 1. Response to adverse external physical, mental, and emotional influences. 2. In biomechanics, force per unit area, involving internal forces within a body that arise as a result of external loads applied to the body.

Stress fracture Microdisruption (fatigue fracture) of bone, often resulting from repeated low-force loading, that does not effect the overall integrity of the bone but may be symptomatic. Stress fractures can be visualized on both bone scans and radiographs, whereas *stress reactions* are visible on bone scans but not on radiographs.

Stress reaction An early stage of stress fracture, visible on bone scans but not radiographs.

Stroke *See* Cerebrovascular accident.

Structuralist *See* Posturalist.

Subjective Discernible by the patient but not directly discernible by the doctor. *See also* Objective.

Subluxation, chiropractic 1. Alteration of alignment, movement, integrity, or physiologic function (or any combination thereof) of a motion segment, while the joint surfaces remain in contact. Neurophysiologic disturbance may be local or widespread. 2. Aberrant relationship between two adjacent structures that may have functional or pathologic sequelae.

Subluxation, orthopedic Partial or incomplete dislocation.

Subluxation complex *See* Vertebral subluxation complex.

Subluxation syndrome Aggregate of signs and symptoms that relate to pathophysiology or dysfunction of spinal and pelvic motion segment or to peripheral joints.

Subscriber Individual covered by a health insurance policy. Many policies include coverage of the subscriber's spouse and children.

Substance P Peptide neurotransmitter in the peripheral nervous system that is excitatory for pain-transmitting neurons. It also acts peripherally as an inducer of the immune response.

Superior cervical ganglion Most superior of the sympathetic chain ganglia, it represents the termination of the sympathetic chain, located adjacent to the upper cervical vertebrae and carotid arteries.

Support hand Hand that is used to stabilize the patient, support adjacent joint structures, or reinforce the contact hand during an adjustive/manipulative procedure. Also called *indifferent hand*.

Supraspinous ligament Long, thick ligament extending between and over the tips of the spinous processes, from the axis to the sacrum. This ligament is specialized in the cervical region as the nuchal ligament (ligamentum nuchae), which extends to the occiput.

Sustainability Ability of a system to maintain healthy function over an extended period.

Swayback Excessive lumbar lordosis.

Swimmer's shoulder *See* Shoulder impingement syndrome.

Sympathetic Pertains to the sympathetic division of the autonomic nervous system. Also called *adrenergic*.

Sympathetic ganglion Collections of postsynaptic sympathetic neuronal cell bodies that are located either in the sympathetic chain (of ganglia) or on the anterior surface of the abdominal aorta (preaortic ganglia).

Synapse Microscopic gap between the ends of nerve fibers across which nerve impulses pass from one neuron to another. At the synapse, an impulse causes the release of a neurotransmitter, which diffuses across the gap and triggers an electrical impulse in the next neuron.

Synergist Muscle that works together with another muscle in performing a particular action.

Synergist substitution Muscular imbalance that occurs when superficial muscles compensate for inhibited deep, segmental (local) muscles. Also known as *global muscle hyperactivity*.

Synovial joint Joint that contains a connective tissue capsule, a specialized epithelial lining (synovial membrane), and a lubricating fluid (synovial fluid).

Systematic error Error reflecting bias. *See also* Bias.

Systematic review Summary of scientific knowledge in an area accomplished by a review of published research in which explicit objective methods are used to evaluate the methodologic quality and results. *See also* Meta-analysis.

Tactile Pertaining to the sense of touch.

Tenderness Excessive sensitivity to pressure or touch.

Tendinitis (tendonitis) Inflammation of a tendon. Most cases formerly termed *tendinitis* are now understood to be tendinosis because they are noninflammatory. *See also* Tendinosis.

Tendinosis Painful condition of a tendon caused by degeneration. Formerly called *tendinitis*. *See also* Tendonitis.

Tendon Fibrous tissue structure consisting of dense connective tissue, principally collagenous, that connects a muscle to a bone or to a ligament.

Tensegrity Concept originated by artist Kenneth Snelson and architect-inventor Buckminster Fuller, who posit a dynamic balance of compressional and tensional forces through a body that exists in a gravitational field.

Tensile loading Loading through elongation in the vertical axis.

Tension-type headache *See* Headache, tension type.

Therapy Treatment of disease, injury, or disability.

Thermoreceptor Sensory receptor that generates an action potential in response to changes in temperature.

Thompson technique A system of chiropractic analysis and adjustment developed by J. Clay Thompson that utilizes a mechanical drop-section table for the delivery of dynamic thrust adjustments. Analysis is primarily through the use of the Derifield Leg Check test (Romer Derifield).

Tinel's sign A tingling sensation in the distal portions of a limb when percussion is applied over the site of a divided nerve. Application of such percussion to the dorsum of the wrist is one of the tests for carpal tunnel syndrome.

Third-party payer Entity other than the subscriber or patient that is responsible for partial or complete payment of a claim. Virtually all third party payers are private or government insurance plans.

Thomsonianism System of healing founded by the early American herbalist Samuel Thomson, in which overexposure to cold was considered a central cause of disease.

Thoracic outlet syndrome (TOS) Compression of the brachial plexus nerve trunks. Signs and symptoms of TOS may include neck pain, occipital headaches, intermittent arm pain, numbness, paresthesia, fatigue, and weakness.

Traction neurodesis Fibrosis around a nerve resulting in the nerve being stretched rather than performing its normal gliding function.

Thrill Palpable vibration of turbulence that is due to loss of laminar flow in a vessel.

Thrombocyte Blood platelet.

Thrombosis Condition in which a stationary blood clot, or thrombus, has formed along the wall of a blood vessel. This may causes blockage of the vessel.

Tibial torsion With the patellae positioned normally, the toes turn inward (medially) as a result of primary rotation of the tibia. Tibial torsion is normal until age 6 to 18 months.

Tissue pull Part of the adjustive procedure in which a finger on the doctor's indifferent hand tractions the soft tissue overlying the segmental contact point in the direction of the adjustive thrust (line of drive). While maintaining the traction, the finger of the indifferent hand is withdrawn and simultaneously replaced by the doctor's contact point of the thrusting hand, allowing a secure and specific contact between doctor and patient.

Tone 1. In muscle, the normal degree of tension or resistance to stretch. 2. A healthy state of a bodily structure. 3. According to D.D. Palmer, tone was defined as the rate or intensity of function of any tissue or organ that reflected the integrity of transmission of neurologic information to and from tissue or organ.

Tonic 1. Of a continuous or sustained nature, as in *tonic contraction* of a muscle. 2. An herb or herbal formula believed to have strengthening effects.

Tonic contraction Sustained, low-level muscle activity. *See also* Phasic contraction.

Tonic receptor Slowly adapting sensory receptor, which typically responds to continuous stimuli (e.g., nociceptors, muscle spindles). *See also* Phasic receptor.

Torque Twisting movement or rotary force. *See also* Torsion.

Torsion Twisting movement or rotary force. *See also* Torque.

Traction-distraction Manual procedures designed to produce a pulling or distractive force at the target tissues and joints. Some traction-distraction procedures incorporate highly sophisticated mechanical tables, specifically designed to assist in precisely administering the appropriate force at a specific target joint or area.

Traditional medicine *This term has two very different meanings.* 1. Centuries-old healing art passed down through the generations in a particular culture, such as Chinese medicine or Ayurvedic medicine. 2. In Western industrial nations, the term is sometimes used as a synonym for *conventional Western medicine* or *allopathic medicine.*

Trainer, athletic Skilled paraprofessional who serves as a key member of a sports medicine team. *See also* Sports medicine team.

Training volume In athletic training, the duration of exercise multiplied by its intensity.

Transcutaneous electrical stimulation (TENS) A method of electrically mediated analgesia utilized for a variety of pain conditions. A TENS unit consists of one or more electric signal generators, a battery, and a set of electrodes. TENS is believed to reduce pain through nociceptive inhibition at the presynaptic level in the dorsal horn of the spinal cord.

Transforaminal ligaments Ligamentous bands that cross the intervertebral foramen.

Translation Motion in a body during which all particles in that body move in parallel at a given time.

Transverse friction massage Soft tissue technique usually administered to a ligament or muscle. Light friction may be used with caution on a recent partial tear or ligamentous sprain, whereas stronger friction is generally appropriate in the chronic stage.

Transverse process Lateral bony extensions of a vertebra.

Treatment Health intervention delivered in an attempt to aid recovery from disease or injury. Also called *therapy.*

Trendelenburg sign The patient, standing with his or her back to the examiner, lifts one leg with bent knee and then the other leg in like manner. A positive Trendelenburg sign is present when, with the weight supported by the problematic limb, the pelvis on the unaffected side rises rather than falling. This is related to dysfunction of the gluteus medius muscle.

Triage 1. Sorting and classifying injured individuals based on their need for or likely benefit from intervention by a health professional. 2. Process of prioritizing health needs.

Trigeminovascular reflex Sensory reflex that functions antidromically. Trigeminal neurons are activated; then pain-activating neurotransmitters are released at their peripheral terminals on cerebral vasculature, thus initiating a neurogenic inflammation, the mechanism thought to trigger migraine headaches.

Trigger points Tender, neurologically hyperactive loci in muscle that can produce referred pain.

Triple-blind study Study in which patients, doctors, and outcome assessors are blinded.

Triptans Class of medications that block the trigeminovascular reflex-generated release of serotonin in the cerebral vasculature.

Triptans are used as an effective abortive medication for migraine attacks.

Trophic 1. Related to nutrition and growth. 2. In the context of the neuronal function, trophic substances produced by nerves have been found to be essential for the development, growth, and maintenance of proper tissue structure and function. Trophic nerve influence affects those interactions between nerves and other cells that initiate or control molecular modification in the other cells.

Tropism In the vertebral column, asymmetry of the plane of the facet joints of a functional spinal unit.

True pelvis Area between the pelvic bones that is inferior to the pelvic brim. The true pelvis is supported from below by the muscular pelvic diaphragm and is superior to the perineum.

Tumor 1. Localized swelling; a cardinal sign of inflammation. 2. Benign or malignant neoplasm that results from uncontrolled growth of cells.

24-Hour recall diary Written list that is compiled by a patient recording everything he or she ate or drank the previous day, noting the time, place, type of food, and amount consumed.

Ultrasonography *See* Sonography.

Unbundling Taking current procedural terminology (CPT) codes that are intended to reference multiple procedures with a single code and instead billing each procedure using a separate code. Unbundling results in higher payment and is illegal.

Universal Chiropractors Association (UCA) Chiropractic organization founded by B.J. Palmer in 1906, which played a leading role in defending early chiropractors against charges of practicing medicine without a license. The UCA merged with the third American Chiropractic Association in 1930 to form the National Chiropractic Association.

Upcoding Using a more involved current procedural terminology (CPT) code than the appropriate code for the service actually provided. Billing for a complex office visit when the patient was seen only for a brief office visit is an example of upcoding. It results in higher payment and is illegal.

Utilization Review (UR) Procedures used by insurers to determine the appropriateness of care and to limit reimbursement for services deemed inappropriate or excessive. UR can involve a requirement for precertification before commencing care, or periodic reviews by the insurer to determine whether continued care will be approved for reimbursement or both.

Validity Degree to which an observation or measurement provides an indication of the true state of the phenomenon being measured. Also called *accuracy*.

Valsalva maneuver Forcible exhalation against a closed glottis. If the maneuver elicits pain, it may indicate increased intrathecal pressure, possibly due to the presence of a space-occupying lesion, such as a spinal disk herniation, osteophyte, or tumor. Also utilized in cardiovascular diagnosis.

Vasa nervorum Small arteries that provide a blood supply to nerves.

Vasoconstriction Temporary decrease in the diameter of a blood vessel.

Vasodilation Temporary increase in the diameter of a blood vessel.

Vegan Person whose diet includes no products of animal origin.

Vegetarian Person whose diet includes no meat. *See also* Lacto-ovo-vegetarian.

Velocity Change in position with respect to time. Velocity has both magnitude and direction, whereas speed has only magnitude.

Venous Plexus Network of veins.

Vertebral subluxation complex Model of motion segment dysfunction that incorporates the complex interaction of pathologic changes in nerve, muscle, ligamentous, vascular, and connective tissue.

Vertebrobasilar insufficiency Lack of normal blood supply to the brainstem, which is caused by a narrowing or blockage of one or both vertebral arteries or the basilar artery or all three. Vertebrobasilar insufficiency can result in symptoms such as dizziness, fainting, or double vision.

Vestibular system Sensory system with peripheral and central nervous system components are primarily responsible for coordinating eye and head movement.

Videofluoroscopy Technique for producing x-ray motion pictures that are recorded on videotape.

Vis medicatrix naturae Healing power of nature. *See also* Innate intelligence.

Visceral Related to the internal organs of the body.

Visceral disease simulation Proposition that somatic dysfunction or vertebral subluxation can often simulate, or mimic, the symptoms of visceral disease. Synonyms include *pseudovisceral disease, organ disease mimicry, somatic visceral disease mimicry syndromes,* and *somatic simulation syndromes.*

Viscerosomatic reflex Reflex in which a stimulus to nerves or receptors related to visceral structures produces reflexive responses that influence function in the musculoskeletal system.

Viscerovisceral reflex Reflex in which a stimulus to nerves or receptors in the visceral organs produces reflexive responses that influence function of other visceral organs (e.g., voiding reflex).

Viscoelasticity Property of a material to deform slowly and nonlinearly when a load is applied and to return to its original size and shape slowly and nonlinearly when the load is removed. Articular cartilage and intervertebral disks exhibit a combination of viscosity and elasticity.

Viscosity Property of a material that does not deform instantly when a load is applied. Stress develops, but strain is delayed; therefore deformation is time related. Failure to return to the original shape when the load is removed is a property of pure viscosity.

Vitalism Explanatory model that suggests the body requires a "vital energy," something

greater than physical and chemical processes to function. In its more extreme forms, "something greater" is given theologic significance.

Vitamin Organic substance found in food and required for normal physiologic function.

Vitamins, fat soluble Include vitamins A, D, E, and K. These vitamins tend to be stored in the body, are readily absorbable with dietary fats, and are unlikely to be excreted in the urine.

Vitamins, water soluble Include the B vitamins (B1, B2, B6, B12), niacin, pantothenic acid, biotin, folic acid, inositol, and choline, and vitamin C. These vitamins are not stored in the body and are readily excreted in the urine.

Video display terminal (VDT) worker Employee whose job includes work on a VDT such as a computer.

Vocational rehabilitation Programs designed to aid injured workers who are unable to perform their usual and customary preinjury work. Vocational rehabilitation often involves retraining in a less physically demanding job.

Wallenberg's syndrome Loss of pain and temperature sensation of the face on the ipsilateral side of the lesion and of the body on the contralateral side, usually resulting from a lesion to the brainstem within the distribution of the posterior cerebral circulation.

Weight-bearing exercise Activities involving muscular stress on the skeleton (e.g., walking, running).

Wellness A state of optimum physical, mental, and emotional health.

Whiplash Cervical acceleration-deceleration injury that is often the result of a motor vehicle collision.

Whole grains Unrefined carbohydrates such as brown rice, whole wheat, oats, barley, and millet.

Wilk v. American Medical Association (AMA) case Filed in 1976 by Illinois chiropractor Chester Wilk and four other doctors of chiropractic, this restraint of trade case represents a landmark antitrust suit. Chiropractor plaintiffs, with George

McAndrews as chief counsel, prevailed over the AMA and fourteen other medical organizations, ending a decades-long officially sanctioned medical boycott of chiropractic. In 1987, Judge Susan Getzendanner entered an injunction, national in scope, and still in force today. It prohibits the AMA and all who act in concert with the AMA from acting in any private manner to interfere with interprofessional relations between medical physicians and doctors of chiropractic and their institutions.

Windlass mechanism Tensing of the plantar fascia during the late stance phase of gait, which aids resupination of the foot and thus helps promote a smooth early propulsive phase of the gait cycle.

Windup Phenomenon of increasing response of a spinal cord cell to repeated stimuli.

Withdrawal reflex Reflex in which the body responds to pain by flexion of the extremities.

Wolff's law Bone is shaped by the forces or lack of forces exerted upon it. When stress is placed on a bone, it undergoes a tissue reaction during which its structure may change to fit its function.

Work In biomechanics, work is force acting over a distance or force times displacement.

Work hardening Structured rehabilitation program focused on training to restore skills needed for a return to employment.

Worker's compensation System of benefits designed to protect and assist workers who are suffering adverse health affects as a result of their employment.

World Chiropractic Alliance (WCA) Organization of subluxation-based chiropractors.

World Federation of Chiropractic (WFC) International chiropractic organization that represents all major national chiropractic organizations.

World Health Organization (WHO) United Nations health agency with headquarters in Geneva, Switzerland.

X-rays A form of electromagnetic radiation with sufficient energy to penetrate the body, produced in an evacuated glass tube when rapidly accelerated electrons collide with a dense target. The impact deceleration or «braking» of the electrons results in the production of x-ray photons.

Zygapophyseal joints Joints between the superior and articular processes of adjacent vertebrae. A zygapophyseal joint is a synovial, gliding type of joint, with a thin, loose, and somewhat elastic fibrous capsule. Also called *apophyseal joints, facet joints,* or *z-joints.*

Zygapophysis Articular process of a vertebra.

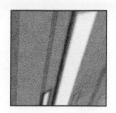

Index

A

A fibers, 93, 95
Abdominal aortic aneurysm, 244, 246, 247f
Abnormality, concept of, 450, 453
Abortive therapy, 499, 507
ACA. *See* American Chiropractic Association (ACA)
ACC. *See* Association of Chiropractic Colleges (ACC)
Acceleration, 125
ACCR. *See* American Chiropractic College of Radiology (ACCR)
Acetylcholine, 97, 101
Achilles tendonitis, 395
Action potential, 92-93
Activator instrument, 281f, 282f
Active motion, 219
Active release technique (ART), 297-298
Activities of daily living (ADL) questionnaire for headache, 521-522
Acupuncture, 586
Aδ fibers, 190, 195
Adhesions, 141
Adjustive localization, 260-263
Adjustive thrust, 260, 263-265
Adjustment, chiropractic. *See* Manipulation/adjustment, spinal
Adolescent idiopathic scoliosis (AIS), 351-352, 352f
Adrenal medulla, 105
Adrenalin (epinephrine), 101
Aerobic fitness, 427-428, 428
Aesculapius, 5
Afferent inhibition, 112, 164
Afferentation, 167-168
Agency for Health Care Policy and Research (AHCPR), 466
Aging
  chiropractic and, 444
  exercise and, 374
  intervertebral disks and, 53, 72
  joints and, 372-374
  lung volume and, 540
  statistics on, 366-374
  vision and, 375

Page numbers followed by *f* indicate figures; *t,* tables; *b,* boxes.

Aging patients
  avoiding adverse outcomes for, 381-382
  exercise for, 374, 376
  manipulation/adjustment in, 382-384
  resources for, 376-377
AHCPR. *See* Agency for Health Care Policy and Research (AHCPR)
AIS. *See* Adolescent idiopathic scoliosis (AIS)
Alar ligaments, 65
Alcoholic beverages, 425-426
Algometry, pressure, 212, 517-518t
Algorithm, 481
Allergies, 355, 358
Allodynia, 114, 188, 195
Allopathic medicine
  for back pain, 312
  cost of, compared to chiropractic, 489
  definition of, 581
  side effects of, 472
Allostatic response, 113-114
Alpha motor neurons, 97
AMA. *See* American Medical Association (AMA)
American Chiropractic Association (ACA)
  on nutritional counseling, 587
  origins of, 31
  on subluxation, 136
American Chiropractic College of Radiology (ACCR), 253
American Medical Association (AMA)
  objections of, to chiropractic, 35-36, 466, 603, 609
  Wilk v. AMA et al antitrust suit, 37-38, 591-594
Amputation, 200
Analgesics
  compounds for, 197-198
  for headache, 499-500, 508
  placebo effect of, 199
Anaphylaxis, 114
Anastomoses, 55, 97
Anatomic barrier, 220
Anecdotal evidence, 450, 456, 624
Anesthetic blockade, 500, 503
Angina pectoris, 540
Animal magnetism, 17
Anisotropy, 121, 123f
Annulus fibrosus, 51-53, 93-95
Antalgic gait and posture, 112, 213

Cervical vertebrae *(Continued)*
  strain and counterstrain on, 301
  surgery on, 573
  techniques for manipulation of, 271-273, 285-287,
    570-571
  tests for functional abnormalities in, 326-327
Cervicogenic headache
  definition and epidemiology of, 500-501
  diagnosis of, 214
  mechanisms of, 501-504, 502-503b
C-fibers, 190, 193, 195
CGRP. *See* Calcitonin generated peptide (CGRP)
CHAMPUS. *See* Civilian Health and Medical Program
    of the Uniformed Services (CHAMPUS)
Children. *See* Pediatric patients
Chinese medicine, 3-4
Chiropractic
  for aging patients, 374-376, 382t
  boycott of, 591-594, 603
  colleges of, 33, 36
  communication with/education of patient, 382,
    437-445
  in the community, 374-376
  comparative safety of, 572-574, 577t
  compared to medical approach, 417, 610-611
  complementary procedures and, 443-444
  controversy surrounding, 441, 458-459, 465, 466,
    545, 561-562, 603, 605-606, 609
  cost-effectiveness of, 399-400, 489
  definition of, 15-16, 22-23, 440
  diagnosis in, 23-24, 531-534
  diet/nutrition and, 586-588
  duration of care in, 605-608, 625
  future direction of, 623-627
  history of, 3-13, 31-33, 147, 149
  hospitals and, 12, 39, 593, 595
  insurance coverage for, 37, 40
  interprofessional relations and, 21, 142, 149
  language of, 3, 7-8
  legal issues and, 31, 34, 36
  managed care and, 613-615, 617-621
  military service and, 39
  osteopathy and, 11-12
  paradigm for, 17-18, 21-26, 439, 607-608,
    633-636
  for pediatric patients, 349-352, 443-444
  practice guidelines in, 603-606, 624
  radiology and, 237, 240, 249
  research essentials for, 449-461
  research in. *See* Research, chiropractic
  scope of practice in, 584-585, 635-636
  self-care at home, 445, 452
  sports chiropractic, 409-419
  statutes regarding, 133-135, 582-600
  techniques used in, 280b
  terminology for, 130-131, 137, 267, 609-610
  Worker's Compensation (WC) and, 398-399
  in the workplace, 389-404

Chiropractic technique, 384-387. *See also specific*
    techniques.
Chiropractors
  communication with/education of patient,
    437-445, 625
  in the community, 374-376, 390
  fraudulent practices of, 605-606
  in hospitals, 12, 39, 593, 595
  jailing of, 32, 34
  licensure of, 34, 582, 584
  managed care programs and, 620-621
  "mixer" vs. "straight", 33-34
  opportunities for, 39-40
  position of, during manipulation/adjustment,
    261-262
  as primary care providers, 366, 591
  scope of practice, 19, 24-25, 24f
  in sports chiropractic, 409-410, 412
Chondrocytes, 125
Chronic obstructive pulmonary Disease (COPD),
    536-537, 538
Chronic pain, 202-203
Chronic pain syndrome, 402
Chronicity (of dysfunction), 607-608
Cineradiography, 267
Circulatory system and osteopathy, 15-16
Civilian Health and Medical Program of the
    Uniformed Services (CHAMPUS), 584
Cleveland, Carl S. Jr., 147
Clinical Practice Guideline 14, 466
CNFDS. *See* Copenhagen Neck Functional Disability
    Scale (CNFDS)
Coaptation, 306-307
Coccyx, 47, 74
Cochrane Collaboration, 314, 316
Codes, current procedural terminology (CPT), 583,
    598
Cognitive therapy, 316, 423
Coiling reflex, 189
Colic, infantile, 165, 362, 535-536
Committee on Quackery, 35-36
Communication
  with adult patients, 437-445
  with aging patients, 375, 382
  palpation as, 211
  with pediatric patients, 354
  reassurance as form of, 328
  in the workplace, 392
Compartment syndrome, 302-303
Compensation (muscular), 607-608
Complementary and alternative medicine (CAM)
  definition of, 615, 620
  for headache, 500, 508
  natural healing principles of, 623-624
  for pediatric patients, 349
  prevalence of, 583
Compression, 119, 178-179
Computed radiography, 248-249

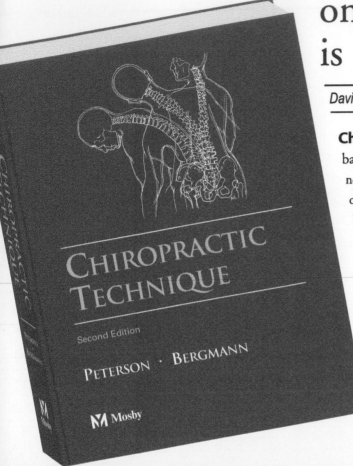

Printed and bound by CPI Group (UK) Ltd, Croydon, CR0 4YY

03/10/2024

01040364-0008